Obstetric Anesthesia

Obstetric Anesthesia

Sivam Ramanathan, M.D.

Professor, Department of Anesthesiology
New York University Medical Center
New York, New York

 LEA & FEBIGER

Philadelphia   1988

Lea & Febiger
600 Washington Square
Philadephia, PA   19106-4198
U.S.A.
(215) 922-1330

Library of Congress Cataloging-in-Publication Data

Ramanathan, Sivam.
    Obstetric anesthesia.

    Includes bibiliographies and index.
    1. Anesthesia in obstetrics. I. Title.
[DNLM: 1. Anesthesia, Obstetric.   WO 450 R165o]
RG732.R34   1988   617'.9682   87-17293
ISBN 0-8121-1118-4

PRINTED IN THE UNITED STATES OF AMERICA

Print No. 4   3   2   1

THIS BOOK IS DEDICATED
TO GERTIE F. MARX, M.D.
　　WHO TAUGHT ME HOW TO THINK CRITICALLY,
TO MY WIFE SITA
　　WHO PUTS UP WITH MY CRITICAL THINKING, AND
TO HERMAN TURNDORF, M.D.
　　WHOSE COMMITMENT TO OBSTETRIC ANESTHESIA MADE THIS WORK POSSIBLE

PREFACE

In the last two decades there has been significant progress in the field of obstetric anesthesia. The anesthesia departments of many schools and hospitals now offer advanced training in obstetric anesthesia. The practice of obstetric anesthesia has become increasingly difficult during this time because many more women with serious medical conditions now become pregnant.

Obstetric anesthesiologists are often assigned the unenviable task of simultaneously caring for two patients, the mother and her baby, both before and after birth. Because of their special skills, obstetric anesthesiologists are frequently called upon to manage many medical emergencies in the labor ward. In addition, the obstetric anesthesiologist is often required to make crucial medical decisions on which the welfare of the mother and the newborn may depend.

The practice of obstetric anesthesia requires not only technical skills but also a sound knowledge of the applied aspects of anatomy, physiology, pharacomology, internal medicine, obstetrics, and neonatology. This book provides a solid foundation of basic knowledge upon which is built a practical and sensible approach to the anesthetic management of patients with normal and complicated pregnancy. The third section, which discusses neonatal care, also includes problems faced by the premature neonate. This section will be particularly helpful to those interested in neonatal intensive care.

Throughout this book I have tried to steer clear of controversy and have in all my recommendations strictly adhered to the dictum "primum non nocere" (First of all, do no harm). In recommending anesthetic agents and techniques, my main consideration was their safety record rather than any minor theoretic advantages that they may offer. While discussing many key topics, I have avoided presenting just a summary of all the recent publications on these topics. Instead I have critically evaluated each publication and formulated an approach based on the combined experiences of myself and other investigators. This book includes many figures and tables that enable the reader to quickly grasp the situation and to also obtain an overall view of the problem.

I sincerely hope that this work will be a valuable aid to those whose primary concern is the care of the pregnant patient and her baby.

I am greatly indebted to Frank Parker, B.S., and James Arismendy, B.S. for preparing the illustrations for this book and for assisting me in the preparation of the manuscript.

New York, NY   Sivam Ramanathan, M.D.

CONTENTS

Section I. Normal Pregnancy

Section II. High-Risk Pregnancy

Section III. The Neonate

NORMAL PREGNANCY

1

INTRODUCTION

Perhaps no other specialty in anesthesiology provides as much personal gratification to the anesthesiologist as does obstetric anesthesia. The anesthesiologist not only becomes a part of the birth process but he also helps create a more pleasurable environment for future generations. The benevolent nature of this specialty is especially apparent to anyone who has experienced the great appreciation of a mother who has received lumbar epidural analgesia for labor. The practice of obstetric anesthesia is also gratifying because it is not concerned with terminal or degenerative conditions but rather with new life.

HISTORY

Obstetric anesthesia has taken almost two hundred years to evolve into its present form.[1–3] For centuries attempts have been made to relieve the pain of labor. Persian literature depicts how wine was given to a mother to facilitate the delivery of a mythical hero. Early Chinese writing includes description of the use of opiates and soporifics for the relief of labor pain. It was customary in some European communities to provide the mother with alcoholic beverages to ease the pain of childbirth. Also in use were plant extracts from hemp, hemlock, and hyoscyamus, which were ingested, externally applied, or inhaled. In some parts of Europe proponents of using analgesia for labor pain were considered witches and were persecuted for trying to alleviate the pain of labor. Obstetrics was mainly

practiced by midwives until the end of the 17th century. In the early 18th century, physicians began to take over the duties of the midwives. The first academic chair for midwifery was established in 1726, in Edinburgh.

The first ether anesthetic was administered by Crawford Williamson Long in 1842. He did not publish his results, however, until years later, thus William Morton is credited with having administered the first ether anesthesia. Morton had been a partner of a man named Horace Wells who had been successfully administering nitrous oxide for some time; however, Wells' demonstration of nitrous oxide's anesthetic property failed at the Massachusetts General Hospital, and he never recovered from this humiliation. Morton administered the first successful ether anesthetic soon after this event, on October 16, 1846. The operation and the use of the anesthetic were both successful.

James Simpson used ether in his practice of midwifery in January, 1847; because of the increased incidence of nausea and vomiting, however, he did not particularly favor the use of the agent in obstetrics. Simpson soon learned about chloroform, which had been in use for some time in London. He slowly dripped chloroform into a folded handkerchief or a hollow sponge, which was held over the patient's face. Simpsons' attempts to alleviate the pain of labor were heavily criticized by the clergy, who held that it was required of a woman to suffer pain during childbirth.

In April 1847, ether was used for the first time

in American obstetrics. This event was reported in the *Boston Medical and Surgical Journal*. Walter Channing published the classic *Treatise on Etherization in Childbirth–Illustrated by Five-Hundred and Eighty One Cases* in which Channing said that ether was administered to render the process of childbirth both pain-free and enjoyable.

John Snow was the first anesthesia specialist in the United Kingdom and was particulary fond of chloroform. Snow was invited to administer chloroform to Queen Victoria for the birth of Prince Leopold on April 7, 1853. He used an analgesic concentration of chloroform, which was dripped onto a handkerchief, a method that came to be known as "chloroform 'a la reine". On April 14, 1857, Queen Victoria received chloroform again for the birth of Princess Beatrice.

The next milestone in the history of obstetric analgesia was the isolation of morphine in the early 1800's. Use of the drug, however, was restricted until the discovery of the hypodermic syringe fifty years later. Before the syringe was discovered the drug was introduced into the circulation of the parturient either by scarifying the skin or by injection with a special syringe-like devise into a previously-made skin incision. A German physician, E. Kormann, recommended hypodermic administration of morphine along with scopolamine for the control of pain of parturition. This method of analgesia, called the twilight sleep, was popular until World War II. Soon, a multitude of sedatives and narcotics were being synthesized. Meperidine, which is still popular in obstetrics today, was first synthesized in Germany in 1939 by Eisleb and Schaumann.

The most important event in the history of obstetric anesthesia was the introduction of regional anesthesia. Carl Koller introduced cocaine into ophthalmic surgery in 1884. William Halstead performed the first nerve block. In 1898, August Bier performed the first clinical spinal anesthesia. In 1901, Sicard and Cathlein described the caudal approach to epidural anesthesia. In 1921, Fidel Pagés described the lumbar epidural approach; and that same year, spinal analgesia for vaginal delivery was first described by Kreiss in Germany. In Europe, von Stökel used caudal anesthesia in a parturient in 1909. George Pitkin popularized spinal anesthesia for obstetrics in this country. The lumbar epidural method was introduced to obstetrics in 1935 by Charles B. Odom. Continuous techniques came into existence in the 1940's. Procaine was synthesized by Alfred Einhorn in 1905, and lidocaine was developed by Löfgren of Sweden in 1943. Other important events that made obstetric anesthesia safer were the recognition of aortocaval compression and the introduction of prophylactic intravenous hydration as a method of preventing hypotension caused by regional anesthesia.[4]

VITAL STATISTICS

The aim of good health care is to reduce morbidity and mortality. It is vital to know how many maternal and neonatal deaths occur in this country and to identify factors contributing to these deaths. To help the numerous agencies report data accurately, the following standardized definitions of terms relating to obstetric events have been introduced:[5]

The term *birth* signifies the complete expulsion or extraction from the mother of a fetus, regardless of whether the umbilical cord has been cut or the placenta is still attached. In many states, fetuses weighing less than 500 g are considered abortuses, not births. When weight is not available, a crown to heal length of 25 cm is considered to be the equivalent of 500 g.

The *birth rate* is the number of births per 1000 people of a given population (also called crude birth rate).

A *live birth* occurs when the infant after birth breathes spontaneously, has a spontaneous heart beat, or moves voluntary muscles spontaneously.

A *stillbirth* (fetal death) occurs when none of the signs describing a live birth are present.

Neonatal death can be of two types. Early neonatal death of a live born infant occurs within 7 days of birth. Late neonatal death occurs 7 to 29 days after birth.

The *neonatal mortality rate* is the number of neonatal deaths per 1000 live births.

The *perinatal mortality rate* is the number of deaths per 1000 fetuses weighing 500 g or more (before or during birth) plus the number of deaths per 1000 live-born infants occurring within the first 28 days of life.

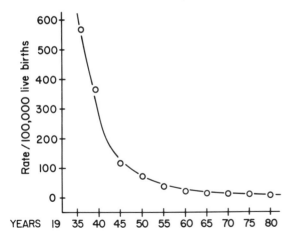

FIG. 1–1. Declining maternal mortality in the United States. (Adapted from Pritchard JA, McDonald PC, and Gant NF: Williams Obstetrics. 17th Edition. Norwalk, Appleton-Century-Crofts, 1985.)

MATERNAL MORTALITY

In the United States, maternal mortality rate (MMR) records have been kept since 1915. In the United Kingdom, triennial *Reports on Confidential Inquiries into Maternal Deaths in England and Wales* (CEMD) have been published since 1952. These reports are used as the standard for international comparison. Each triennial report covers 2 to 3 million births and 10 such reports are presently available. In the United States, the maternal mortality rate's (MMR) dramatic decline in the last 50 years is probably the result of the general improvement in medical care; availability of blood, blood products, and antibiotics; and an increase in the number of training facilities (Fig. 1–1).[5] The common

The *maternal mortality rate* represents the number of maternal deaths per 100,000 live births. Direct maternal death refers to deaths relating to obstetric factors such as complications of pregnancy, labor and puerperium, or deaths resulting from incorrect obstetric management. Indirect maternal death refers to death caused by preexisting disease or disease that developed during pregnancy, labor, or puerperium. Anesthetic deaths were listed as indirect deaths. In 1980, the International Classification of Diseases–9th Division–Clinical Modification (ICD–9–CM) listed anesthetic deaths under a special category.

causes of maternal mortality are abortion, pulmonary embolism, hemorrhage (antepartum and postpartum hemorrhage, ruptured uterus, ectopic pregnancy), hypertensive disorders of pregnancy, and anesthesia related causes (Fig. 1–2).[6] In most countries where reliable statistical information is available, the absolute number of deaths attributable to anesthesia have decreased; however, the ratio between the number of anesthesia deaths and the total deaths has not shown much decrease (Fig. 1–2). In the 1976–78 CEMD report, 18 maternal deaths occurred during anesthesia for emergency cesarean section compared to only 3 deaths during elective cesarean section.

CAUSES OF MATERNAL MORTALITY

General anesthesia is the single most important factor contributing to maternal death. Out of 61 maternal deaths reported in the triennial reports of 1973–1975 and 1976–1978, more than 47 deaths may have been caused by general anesthesia-related complications. Inhalation of gastic contents during induction of anesthesia, aspiration occurring during difficult intubation, hypoxia associated with unrecognized esophageal intubation, and apparatus mishap, were the most common causes. In the United States, similar factors contribute to deaths during general anesthesia. Another worrisome contributing factor to maternal death is the complication associated with intravascular injection of local anesthetic during an attempted regional block. In the state of Indiana, the cardiorespiratory problem associated with local anesthetic toxicity has replaced pulmonary aspiration as the major cause of maternal mortality.[7] Severe hypotension associated with spinal anesthesia, which used to contribute heavily to maternal death, has been practically eliminated by the practice of prophylactic fluid administration and avoiding aortocaval compression.

The overall perinatal mortality rate has been steadily declining. It is not known whether this decline is the result of an increase in the cesarean section rate or of the availability of improved facilities for neonatal care. Chapters 9 and 26 will provide more information on perinatal and neonatal mortality rates.

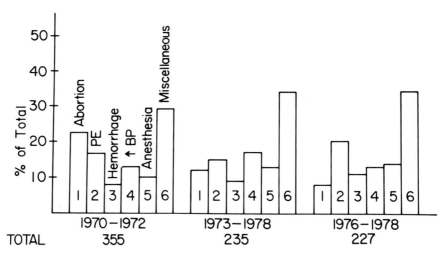

FIG. 1–2. Causes of maternal mortality in England and Wales. Note that the percentage of anesthesia related deaths fails to decrease appreciably. (Reports on Confidential Enquiries into Maternal Deaths in England and Wales, Triennial Reports: 1970–1972; 1973–1975; 1976–1978.)

REDUCTION OF MATERNAL MORTALITY

Adequate training of all anesthesia personnel in the art of administering obstetric anesthesia is the most important measure towards minimizing anesthesia-related mortality in obstetrics. The use of rapid sequence induction followed by endotracheal intubation must be done in all obstetric anesthetics. Although administration of antacids has been recommended to diminish the likelihood of acid-aspiration pneumonitis, it is not currently known whether this practice will have major impact on maternal mortality rates. Every institution must develop a failed-intubation drill, which must be put into practice immediately when endotracheal intubation is difficult (see Chapter 9). Avoiding general anesthesia will also help significantly reduce mortality. This measure requires that personnel be educated on the proper technique of administering regional anesthesia. Since intravascular administration of local anesthetic carries grave dangers, the drug should be administered in divided doses whenever possible.

Ideally, an anesthesiologist should be available to administer obstetrical analgesia or anesthesia on a 24-hour basis. The survey done by the Committee on Obstetric Anesthesia of the American Society of Obstetrical Anesthesiologists and the Liaison Committee for Obstetrics and Gynecology of the American College of Obstetricians and Gynecologists show that condi-

tions currently prevalant in United States hospitals are far from ideal.[8] Anesthesiologists are available on a full-time basis in only 21% of all hospitals and at nights and weekends in only 15% of hospitals. In many hospitals, obstetrical analgesia and anesthesia was being provided by nurse anesthetists (without the supervision of the anesthesiologist), obstetricians, and obstetric house staff. Regional anesthesia was being used for cesarean section in only 50% of patients. Obstetric units with less than 500 deliveries per annum are less likely to receive expert anesthesia care than are larger units. This might be explained by a possible lack of interest on the part of anesthesiologists to provide better organized obstetric anesthesia care because of the relatively inadequate remuneration provided for obstetric analgesia and the unpredictable work hours. Another critical factor may be the poor cost effectiveness of the field, especially in smaller units, where the income generated may not justify the number of man hours invested.

Anyone interested in reducing anesthesia-related mortality and morbidity must address the economic and materialistic conflicts affecting obstetrical anesthesia.

REFERENCES

1. Atkinson RS, Rushman GB, and Lee JA: A Synopsis of Anaesthesia. Baltimore, John Wright and Sons, 1982.

2. Churchill-Davidson HC: A Practice of Anaesthesia. Chicago, Year Book Medical Publishers, 1984.

3. Schaer HM: History of pain relief in obstetrics. *In* Obstetric Analgesia and Anaesthesia. (Edited by Marx GF and Bassell GM) New York, Elsevier, 1980.

4. Wollman SB and Marx GF: Acute hydration of prevention of hypotension of spinal anesthesia in parturients. Anesthesiology 29:374, 1968.

5. Pritchard JA, McDonald PC, and Gant NF: Williams Obstetrics. 17th Edition. Norwalk, Appleton-Century-Crofts, 1985.

6. Reports on Confidential Enquires into Maternal Deaths in England and Wales, Triennial Reports: 1970–1972; 1973–1975; 1976–1978.

7. Ravindran RS and Ragan WD: Anesthetic causes of maternal mortality in the state of Indiana from 1960–1980. *In* Abstracts of Scientific Papers, 15th Annual Meeting, Society for Obstetric Anesthesia and Perinatology, 1983.

8. Gibbs CP, et al: Obstetric Anesthesia: A National Survey. Anesthesiology 65:298, 1986.

MATERNAL ADAPTATION TO PREGNANCY

The requirements of the growing conceptus cause the maternal physiology to undergo enormous changes, which affect every organ function in the body. The maternal metabolism is altered to provide an abundant supply of fuel and oxygen to the fetus. If similar hormonal and physiologic changes occurred in a nonpregnant subject, she would be suspected of suffering from an incurable endocrine disorder. Some of these changes may dictate a different course of action in the evaluation and anesthetic care of pregnant patients. A working knowledge of the changes in normal pregnancy is essential in order to appreciate the interaction between pregnancy and many associated systemic diseases.

CARDIOVASCULAR SYSTEM

The changes in the cardiovascular system are important to the anesthesiologists.[1,2] The heart is pushed upward and shifted to the left and anteriorly. The cardiac size may be increased because of both hypertrophy and dilation. EKG may show apparently benign atrial and ventricular premature beats, left axis deviation, and nonspecific ST-T segment changes. Echocardiogram may show increased left ventricular end-diastolic volume (LVEDV). Both heart rate and stroke volume start increasing early in the first trimester and reach peaks at 28 to 32 weeks (Fig. 2–1). Cardiac preload is increased because of the expanded blood volume and increased EDV. Afterload is reduced as a result of decreased peripheral resistance and blood viscosity.

In auscultation, the first heart sound is accentuated, and it may also be split. By the 20th week, 84% of women with normal pregnancies have a third heart sound. Two types of functional murmurs may be heard: a pulmonary midsystolic murmur and a supraclavicular systolic murmur that is produced by blood flow in the brachiocephalic trunks. The hyperdynamic state may predispose to functional cardiac murmurs. In the early puerperium, the cardiac output is at least 50% above predelivery values. Thus pregnancy imposes a severe demand on the myocardium. Patients with cardiac diseases may poorly tolerate the increased myocardial oxygen consumption. Uterine blood flow and renal blood flow increase, but cerebral and hepatic blood flows remain unaltered in uncomplicated pregnancy.

BLOOD VOLUME CHANGES

The plasma volume and the red and white cell volumes begin to increase from the middle of the first trimester, peaking during the early third trimester.[3] The increase in plasma volume is greater than the increase in RBC mass, which leads to reduced hemoglobin concentration (Fig. 2–2). The specific gravities of whole blood and plasma are reduced and blood viscosity de-

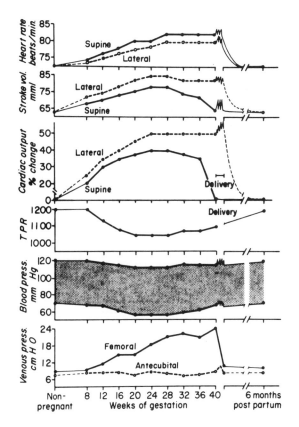

FIG. 2–1. Heart rate, stroke volume, cardiac output, total peripheral resistance (TPR), blood pressure, and venous pressure change during pregnancy. Note that in the lateral position the cardiac output is lower and the heart rate is higher than in the supine position because of compression of the inferior vena cava. Labor pains cause further fluctuations in hemodynamic parameters. (From Bonica JJ: Obstetric Analgesia and Anesthesia. 2nd Ed. Amsterdam, World Federation of Societies of Anesthesiologists, 1980).

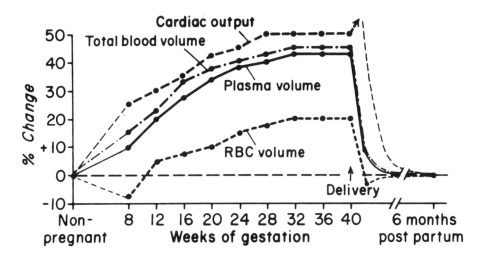

FIG. 2–2. Cardiac output, plasma volume and RBC volume increases in pregnancy. Note that in early pregnancy, the RBC volume tends to decrease before it starts increasing and that the increase in plasma volume is greater than the increase in RBC. (From Bonica JJ: Obstetric Analgesia and Anesthesia, 2nd Ed. Amsterdam, World Federation Society of Anesthesiologists, 1980).

clines approximately 12%. Despite the increase in blood volume, there is no evidence of circulatory overload. Central venous pressure (CVP) remains unaltered. In a healthy gravida, the CVP will rise from 8 to 10 cm H_2O, after a rapid infusion of one liter of crystalloid solution in 20 minutes. The increased blood volume during pregnancy not only facilitates transplacental gas exchange but also enables the parturient to tolerate the substantial blood loss that she is likely to incur during delivery.

There is a net gain of sodium, potassium, calcium, and water in pregnancy. Both intra and extracellular water compartments (ICF and ECF) increase in size, the increase being greater in the ICF compartment than in the ECF compartment[4] (see Fig. 10–4).[4] The increase in plasma volume accounts for only a 20 to 25% increase in ECF and the remaining increase is caused by the expanded interstitial fluid compartment. In normal gravidas, the greatest increase in the interstitial fluid compartment occurs in the third trimester, regardless of the presence or absence of edema. In contrast, the greatest increase in plasma volume occurs in the first two trimesters. The increase in interstitial fluid is caused by both the reduced plasma oncotic pressure and the augmented ability of the tissue ground substance to absorb more water.[5] Total gain in water and electrolytes, especially Na^+, in different body compartments are shown in Table 1.[6]

AORTOCAVAL COMPRESSION

Starting from 20 to 24 weeks of gestation, the gravid uterus may compress both inferior vena cava and the aorta (Figs. 2–3, 2–4, and 2–5).[1,7,8] Compression of the inferior vena cava, which

occurs in over 90% of term pregnant patients reduces the cardiac venous return, thus decreasing the maternal cardiac output.[7] The lower aorta and its branches may be compressed and shifted to the left,[8] which decreases the utereoplacental blood flow (Fig. 2–5). Vertebral venous plexus, which drains into the azygos vein, provides collateral circulation when the inferior vena cava is obstructed.[1]

The supine position causes profound changes in maternal hemodynamics (Fig. 2–6). Cardiac output, systemic blood pressure, and pulmonary blood volume decrease in the supine position.[9] The patient usually compensates for this decrease by increasing the peripheral vascular resistance (vasoconstriction) and/or her heart rate. The compensatory mechanism may maintain systemic pressure in 70% of patients. However, in the rest, the systemic pressure decreases and the patient faints, especially when collaterals are not well-developed. When the sympathetic tone is reduced by a regional block, the supine position causes a more profound and precipitous reduction in cardiac output because of the reduced compensatory vasconstriction.

The supine position should be avoided in late pregnancy. In order to minimize aortocaval compression patients should be prophylactically hydrated with crystalloid solutions before they are given a regional or general anesthetic, a non-compressible sandbag should be wedged under the patient's right hip to displace the uterus 15° to the left during anesthesia, and the femoral arterial pressure may be used as a guideline to assess the degree of aortic compression. Bienarz, et al.[10] showed that while brachial and femoral artery pressures are equal to each other in the supine normotensive patient, the femoral systolic pressure falls 20 mm Hg below the brachial

Table 2–1. Fluid and Electrolyte Gain in Pregnancy

Tissue/fluids	g	Water (L)	Na+ (mmol)	K+ (mmol)
Fetus	3400	2.0	290	155
Placenta	650	0.3	60	40
Uterus	800	1.2	100	5
Breasts	405	0.4	30	40
Plasma volume	1250	1.25	150	60
Interstitial fluid	1680	1.68	240	10
Maternal fat	3345	—	—	—
Totals	12500	7.53	950	360

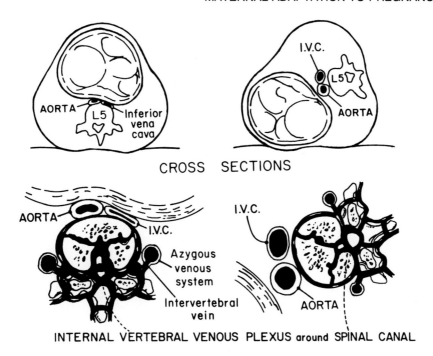

CROSS SECTIONS

INTERNAL VERTEBRAL VENOUS PLEXUS around SPINAL CANAL

FIG. 2–3. Compression of the aorta and the interior vena cava (IVC) by the gravid uterus. Note that both blood vessels are compressed against the 5th lumbar vertebra (L5): that the vertebral venous plexus are distended in the supine position because they provide the collateral circulation; and that the plexus are less distended in the lateral position because the IVC compression is relieved. (From Bonica, JJ: Obstetric Analgesia and Anesthesia. 2nd Ed. Amsterdam, World Federation Society of Anesthesiologists, 1980).

pressure when they are hypotensive. This occurs because the aorta is more easily compressible when the intraluminal pressure is reduced. Even in asymptomatic patients, the aorta may be significantly compressed in the supine position with significant reduction in lower limb blood pressures.[11] If systemic hypotension develops despite these measures, ephedrine should be injected in 5 mg increments until the systolic pressure reaches 100 mm Hg or above.

Although a decision is readily made to treat a systolic hypotension <90 mm Hg with a vasopressor, there may be a dilemma in deciding whether to treat borderline reduction in systolic pressure (e.g., a systolic pressure of 95 to 100 mm Hg). In this case, the patient's heart rate can be used as a guideline to help one decide the need for therapy. A 25% increase in heart rate over the preanesthesia value in this situation suggests inferior vena cava compression and compensatory tachycardia (concealed supine hypotension).

RESPIRATORY SYSTEM

The nasopharynx, the larynx, the trachea, and the bronchi may appear reddened and swollen because of capillary engorgement. The glottic opening may be narrower than in nonpregnant subjects. The vertical diameter of the chest decreases because of cephalad displacement of the diaphragm (4 cm) and the anteroposterior and transverse diameters increase as a result of rib flaring.[12] Because of an increase in pulmonary blood volume, lung markings are increased, simulating mild congestive heart failure. Tidal volume, respiratory rate, minute ventilation, and alveolar ventilation start increasing from early in pregnancy (Fig. 2–7, Table 2–2). Dead space does not change. Residual volume (RV), expiratory reserve volume (ERV), and functional residual capacity (FRC) consistently decrease. Closing capacity (CC) and closing volume (CV) remain unaltered.[13] However, the difference between FRC and CC is reduced, especially in the supine position, which may predispose to ventilation-perfusion anomalies.[13] At a fractional inspired oxygen concentration (FIO_2) of 1, the mean arterial oxygen tension (PaO_2) of a term pregnant patient is 60 to 70 mm Hg lower than that of a nonpregnant female.[14] The lung compliance (CL) and the forced expiratory volume at 1 second (FEV_1) do not change. The ratio of

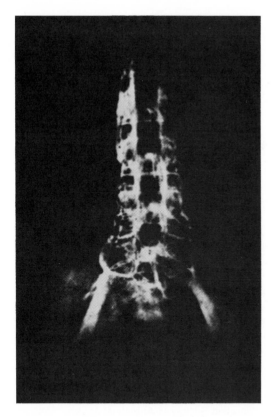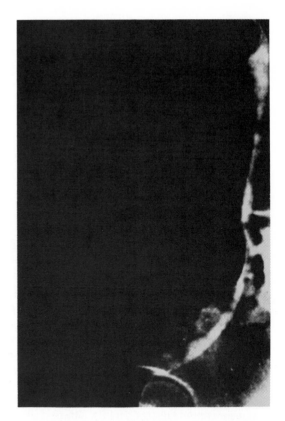

FIG. 2–4. Anterior and lateral views of the venogram of the inferior vena cava (IVC) in late pregnancy. Note the failure of the IVC to opacify and the ascent of the dye along the vertebral venous plexus. (From Kerr MG, Scott DB, and Samuel E: Studies of the inferior vena cava in late pregnancy. Br Med J, *1*:532, 1964).

FEV_1 to forced vital capacity (FEV_1/FVC) and the ratio of dead space volume to tidal volume (V_D/V_T) also do not change.[12,15] Similarly, the flow-volume loop parameters are not altered compared to nonpregnant subjects.[16]

The increased alveolar ventilation causes the arterial carbon dioxide tension (Pa_{CO_2}) to fall to 33 to 35 mm Hg by the third month and to remain unaltered through the rest of the pregnancy (Fig. 2–8).[1] Arterial blood pH increases slightly. The Pa_{O_2} is consistently greater than 100 mm Hg from the 12th week of pregnancy (hyperventilation).[15] Plasma $H_{CO_3}^-$ and base excess both decrease because of increased renal excretion of $H_{CO_3}^-$ to compensate for the respiratory alkalosis. The diminished FRC is of interest to anesthesiologists. Because of diminished oxygen stores in the lungs and increased total body oxygen consumption ($\dot{V}_{O_2}$), the rate and magnitude of decrease in Pa_{O_2} in an apneic pregnant patient is greater than in a

nonpregnant patient.[17] Pregnant patients should therefore inhale 100% oxygen for at least 5 minutes (whenever possible) to denitrogenate the lungs before induction of general anesthesia. This will minimize the risk of hypoxia that might otherwise develop during routine endotracheal intubation.

Because of the diminished FRC, the anesthetic uptake rate is faster in pregnant patients. Although the increased cardiac output of pregnancy is expected to decrease the uptake rate, the decrease in FRC, combined with increased alveolar ventilation, overrides any diminishing effect that the increased cardiac output may have on the uptake rate.

GASTROINTESTINAL SYSTEM IN PREGNANCY

The stomach and intestines are progressively displaced cephalad by the enlarging uterus. In

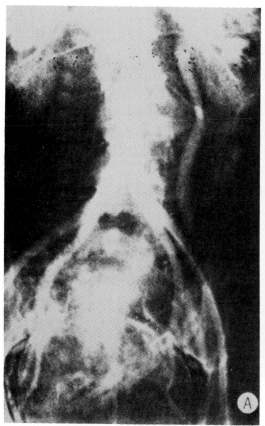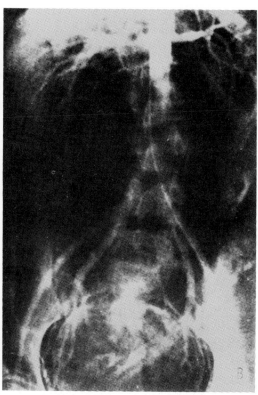

FIG. 2–5.   Aortogram in late pregnancy showing obstruction by the gravid uterus causing reduced placental perfusion (B). Note improved filling of the aorta and better placental perfusion in the lateral position (A). (Reprinted by permission from the *New York State Journal of Medicine,* copyrighted by the Medical Society of the State of New York, from Abitbol MM: Aortic compression by pregnant uterus. NY State Med Soc J, *76*:1470, 1976.)

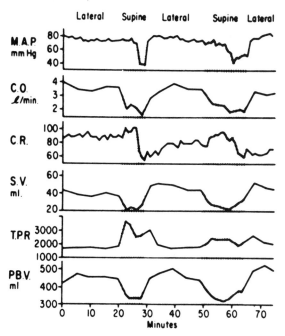

FIG. 2–6.   Hemodynamic effects of supine position in late pregnancy. Note the reduction in mean arterial pressure (MAP), cardiac output (CO), stroke volume (SV) and pulmonary blood volume (PBV) in supine position. The compensatory increase in cardiac rate (CR) and total peripheral resistance (TPR) maintains MAP for a short period of time, following which the patient develops a marked hypotension. (From Scott DB: Inferior vena cava occlusion in late pregnancy and its importance in anesthesia. *40*:120, 1968).

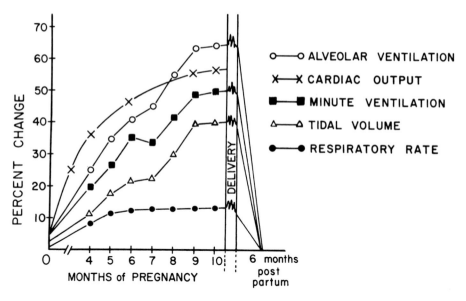

FIG. 2–7. Pregnancy induced changes in respiratory parameters. Note that changes begin to occur very early in pregnancy and that the increase in minute ventilation is mainly caused by increased tidal volume. (From Romero R: The management of acquired hemostatic failure in pregnancy. *In* Critical Care of the Obstetric Patient. (Edited by Berkowitz RL) New York, Churchill-Livingstone, 1983).

addition, the stomach may be divided into antral and fundal pouches by the gravid uterus, preventing proper admixture of antacids within the stomach.[18] Rotating the patient 360° may facilitate the admixture of antacids with the gastric fluid. Intragastric pressure rises during pregnancy and increases further in lithotomy and Trendelenburg position. Conflicting results have been reported on the pressure gradient between the stomach and the lower esophagus. However, there is little doubt that in those who complain of heartburn, the pressure gradient is reduced because of a feeble gastroesophageal sphincter (Fig. 2–9).[19] The prolonged gastroin-

testinal transit time is attributed to increased circulating progesterone concentrations.[20] Patients with decreased gastric motility may also complain of heartburn.[21] Although the total quantity of both basal and histamine-stimulated acid output decreases in midpregnancy, it increases above nonpregnant controls towards term (Fig. 2–10).[22]

During labor, there is further prolongation of gastric emptying time caused both by pain and anxiety and by use of sedatives and analgesics. Thus, the risk of pulmonary aspiration is greatly increased in a pregnant patient. A rapid sequence induction followed by endotracheal in-

Table 2–2. Lung Function in Pregnancy

Measurement	Change	% change over nonpregnant
Minute ventilation	increased	50
Dead space	no change	0
Alveolar ventilation	increased	70
Respiratory rate	increased	40
Tidal volume	increased	40
Airway resistance	decreased	36
Lung compliance	no change	0
Chest-wall compliance	decreased	45
Expiratory reserve volume	decreased	20
Residual volume	decreased	20
Functional residual	decreased	20
Closing volume	no change	0

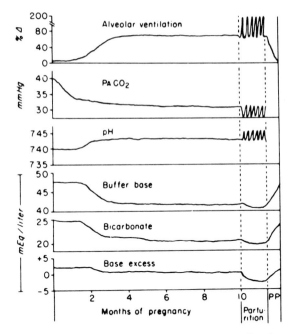

FIG. 2–8. Pregnancy induced changes in alveolar ventilation and blood acid-base indices (%Δ = percent change). Note that during labor alveolar ventilation, Pa_{CO_2} and pH fluctuate with uterine contractions. (From Bonica JJ: Obstetric Analgesia Anesthesia. 2nd Ed. Amsterdam, World Federation Society of Anesthesiologists, 1980).

tubation must be performed while cricoid pressure is being applied to occlude the esophagus. From the 18th week of pregnancy, inhalational anesthesia administered through a face mask without endotracheal intubation definitely risks aspiration of gastric contents. Generally, a gastric fluid pH of 2.5 or less, and a gastric fluid volume of 25 ml or more, increases the risk of acid aspiration syndrome in hospitalized patients. Judged by these criteria, several studies have shown that 60 to 90% of all surgical patients will be at risk. Regardless of the type of anesthesia, all pregnant patients must receive some antacid therapy prior to surgical intervention. Antacid therapy or other prophylactic measures are discussed in the chapter on cesarean section.

BLOOD COAGULATION

Blood is hypercoagulable during pregnancy. The serum fibrinogen concentration increases from 300 mg/dl to over 480 mg/dl.[23,24] A progressive rise in serum fibrin degradation prod-

ucts is also seen in the third trimester. The platelet count remains unchanged but concentration of factor VII (proconvertin), factor VIII (antihemophilic globulin), factor IX (Christmas factor), and factor X (Stuart-Prower factor) are increased. The levels of factors XI and XIII, however, decrease, probably because of consumption at the placental site. The consumption is partly the result of fibrin deposition occurring at the placenta.[23] Prothrombin time, partial thromboplastin time, bleeding time, and clotting time remain essentially within normal limits.

In pregnancy, there is a progressive inhibition of fibrinolysis. Although the plasminogen level itself remains unchanged, the activity of plasminogen activator decreases and that of the inhibitors (antiplasmin and macroglobulin) increases, thus leading to a delayed fibrinolysis, especially in late pregnancy. A hypercoagulable state is indicated by the presence of increased fibrin-fibrinogen complexes, which are detected by chromatographic elution experiments (see Chapter 16, Thromboembolism). The hypercoagulable state predisposes to thromboembolism, especially in the postpartum period.[24] Pregnancy induced changes in coagulation factors are summarized in Table 2–3.[23]

RENAL FUNCTION AND SODIUM AND WATER BALANCE

The dilation of the renal pelvis and calices together with the ureters is probably caused by progesterone. The dilatation starts early in pregnancy and may persist as late as 12 weeks after delivery. The glomerular filtration rate (GFR) and renal plasma flow (RPF) increases 60% and 30%, respectively, with the result that blood urea nitrogen (BUN) and creatinine decrease.[25] The normal values for BUN (6 to 8 mg/dl) and creatinine (0.4 to 0.6 mg/dl) are lower in pregnant women than in nonpregnant subjects. The tubular reabsorptive capacity for glucose, histidine, creatine, uric acid, and other solutes is decreased.[25] Because glycosuria may occur even at normal blood glucose levels, one must use caution in using urine glucose levels (sliding scale) as a guideline for insulin therapy in pregnant diabetics.

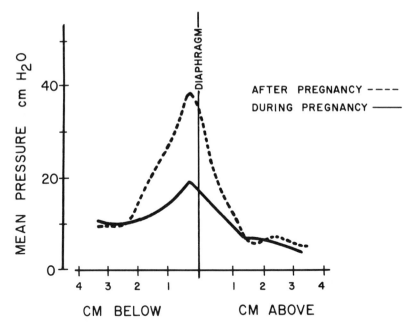

FIG. 2–9. A graph of trans-sphincteric pressure across the gastroesophageal junction in a pregnant woman with severe heart burn compared with pressure recorded in the same patient six weeks after delivery. CM below and above represent distance in centimeters below and above diaphragm. (Originally published in *Canadian Medical Association Journal, 98*:571, March 23, 1968. *In*: Lind JF, Smith AM, Coopland AJ, and Crispin JS: Heartburn in pregnancy–A manometric study).

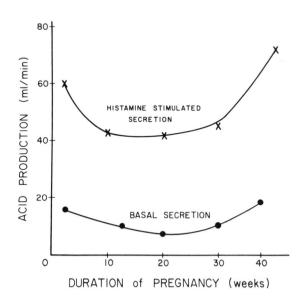

FIG. 2–10.   Gastric acid production in pregnancy. Note the reduction in acid production in the middle weeks of pregnancy and a rise above controls towards term. (From Erskine JP, and Fielding J: Gastric secretion in pregnancy. Br J Obstet Gynecol *64*:373, 1957.)

BODY FLUIDS AND INTRAVENOUS FLUID THERAPY

Plasma osmolality (P-osm) decreases 8 to 10 mosm/kg during pregnancy. Only a small fraction of this reduction results from reduced blood urea levels. Pregnant patients maintain their P-osm in a relatively narrow range (Fig. 2–11) In nonpregnant subjects, even a small reduction in P-osm (of this magnitude) will induce diuresis. Polyuria does not occur in pregnant subjects,

Table 2–3.   Coagulation Changes in Late Pregnancy

Fibrinogen	4.0–6.5 g/l
Factor II	100–125%
Factor V	100–150%
Factor VII	150–250%
Factor VIII	200–500%
Factor IX	100–150%
Factor X	150–250%
Factor XI	50–100%
Factor XII	100–200%
Factor XIII	35–75%
Antithrombin III	75–100%
Antifactor Xa	75–100%
Plasminogen activator	reduced
Plasminogen inhibitor	increased

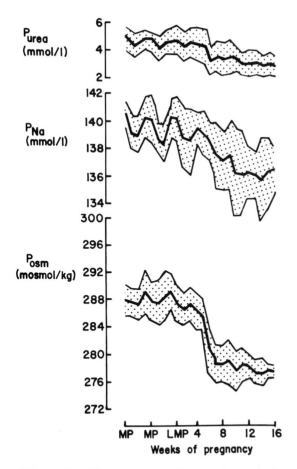

FIG. 2–11. Plasma urea, sodium, and osmolarity (P-osm) in nonpregnant and pregnant states: MP: menstrual period; LMP: last menstrual period. Shaded area represents 1SD. (From Davison JM, Valotton MB, and Lindheimer MD: Plasma osmolality and urinary concentration and dilution during and after pregnancy: evidence that lateral recumbency inhibits maximal urinary concentrating ability. Br J Obstet Gynaecol, *88*:472, 1981.)

thus it is likely that the osmotic threshold for both thirst and vasopressin release are set at levels 10 mosm lower than in nonpregnant subjects.[5,6] Given a liter of water to drink, the pregnant patient will reduce her osmolarity by 10 mosmol/L just like a nonpregnant patient, but will return her osmolarity to the baseline value within 2 hours.[5,6] In the first trimester, the excess water is eliminated by increased diuresis. During the third trimester, however, the volume of urine produced in response to hydration is reduced. Despite this, the osmolarity is still returned to prehydration level in the third trimester. It is believed that the excess water

migrates into the extravascular compartment, thereafter to be excreted (perhaps more slowly) by the kidneys.[25] The water-induced diuresis is reduced especially in the supine position (vide infra).

The hemodilution of pregnancy affects the concentration of many substances. The serum total protein and albumin concentrations and the plasma oncotic pressure (POP) decrease (Fig. 2–12).[26] Intravenous infusion of 1 to 1.2 liters of crystalloid solution will further reduce plasma oncotic pressure. Concomitant administration of at least 50 g of albumin is necessary in order to prevent this fall in plasma oncotic pressure; however, the acute reduction of POP is not usually associated with serious pulmonary complications in healthy gravidas.[26]

Ringer's lactate (RL) solution has been used extensively for hydration and has been found to be safe. Despite the lactate content (28 mMol/L), RL infusion does not cause increased lactate levels in the mother or the fetus.[27] Plasmalyte A solution contains no lactate, but does contain acetate, which is associated with increased fetal lactate levels. This may be the result of inhibition of placental glycolysis by the acetate ions.[27] Plasmalyte A solution should therefore be used with caution in pregnant patients. Rapid infusion of normal saline solution may decrease maternal arterial blood pH, and should probably be avoided.[27]

SODIUM BALANCE IN PREGNANCY

The increase in glomerular filtration rate and renal plasma flow causes increased natriuresis in pregnancy.[5,6] Increased concentrations of progesterone, arginine-vasopressin (AVP), melanocyte stimulating hormone (MSH), and prostaglandins produce further natriuresis. Thus approximately, 20,000 to 30,000 mmols of sodium may be filtered through the kidneys of a pregnant patient. If all the filtered sodium is allowed to be excreted in the urine, the pregnant subject may rapidly develop circulatory collapse. All of the filtered sodium must therefore be absorbed in the renal tubules. Indeed the pregnant patient gains 4 to 6 mmols of sodium per day to be stored in the fetal and maternal compartments. The increase in renal tubular reabsorption of sodium is perhaps the single

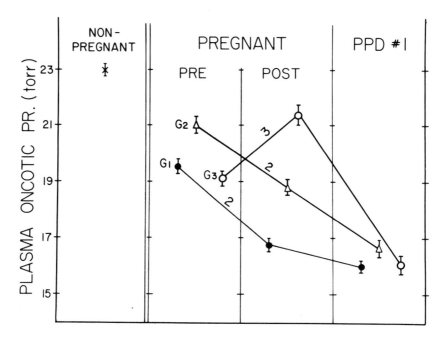

FIG. 2–12. Plasma oncotic pressure values in non-pregnant and term-pregnant patients. G₁, G₂ and G₃ represent groups 1, 2, and 3, respectively. G₁ received 1200 ml of Ringer's Lactate (RL) solution, G₂ received 700 ml of RL plus 500 ml of 5% albumin (albumin 25 g) and G₃1000 ml of RL plus 200 ml of 25% albumin (albumin 50g). "Pre" and "post" signify values before and after infusion. PPD#1 = first postpartum day. Statistical significance: 2, p <0.0001 and 3, p <0.01. (Reprinted with permissin from the International Anesthesia Research Society, from: Maternal and fetus effects of prophylactic hydration with crystalloids or colloids before epidural anesthesia, by Ramanathan S., et al. Anesth Analg 62:673, 1983.)

most important adjustment of renal function in pregnancy.[6]

What are the mechanisms for increased renal absorption of sodium in pregnancy? Two types of factors are at play: hormonal and physical.

Hormonal Factors

Aldosterone production increases during pregnancy. Increased aldosterone levels are believed to serve a homeostatic function during pregnancy, as they do in nonpregnant states. Although blood volume increases in pregnancy, the increase is inadequate to fill the overdilated vascular bed, thus creating a relative hypovolemia. The dilation of the vascular bed is caused by the prostaglandins. The increased aldosterone level is really in response to this "functional" hypovolemia. The increased aldosterone levels play only a minor role in augmenting renal reabsorption of sodium.

The deoxycorticosterone (DOC) level is also increased in pregnancy. DOC is produced in the mother and plays a major role in renal sodium reabsorption.

Prostaglandins produce vasodilation, resulting in stimulation of the renin-angiotensin system, which in turn causes increased sodium retention. Prostaglandins may also directly stimulate the renin-angiotensin system.

Estrogens cause sodium retention by stimulating the renin-angiotensin system. The renin-angio-tensin system activity may also increase on its own right without being stimulated by prostaglandins or estrogens. Plasma renin substrate and angiotensin II may be synthesized by the myometrium and chorion.

Physical Factors

The upright and supine postures have an antidiuretic effect in pregnant subjects independent of changes in renal plasma flow.[5] Therefore the reduction in urine flow that occurs when a pregnant subject assumes a supine or upright position may not be caused simply by the reduction of renal blood flow. Lateral decubitus is known to mobilize large volumes of fluid in pregnant subjects. In the upright position, the absorption rate increases in the proximal nephron. Marked increases in ureteral pressures have been noted in pregnant patients who assume upright or supine positions. Increased ureteral arteriopressure is known to be associated with reduced urine formation. The uteroplacental blood flow acts as an arterio-venous communication. Vascular communications are known to cause an antinatriuretic effect in experimental animals. The factors that cause increased sodium filtration or reabsorption are shown in Table 2–4.

ENDOCRINOLOGY

Pregnancy causes major changes in the endocrine function of the woman.

NONPLACENTAL HORMONES

The anterior pituitary enlarges and secretes more ACTH, TSH, prolactin and β-endorphins.[24] Although the posterior lobe does undergo hypertrophy, its secretory activity is not increased. The levels of free and bound plasma cortisol, androgen, aldosterone, and deoxycorticosterone levels increase without clinical evidence of hypercortism. In addition, the activity of the renin-angiotensin system is augmented.

Pregnancy also causes increased levels of total thyroxine, and triiodothyronin, and thyroxin-binding globulin. However, the effective levels of the thyroxine and triiodothyronine do not increase, which results in the patient becoming clinically euthyroid. Radioiodine uptake is markedly elevated and there may be slight thyroid enlargement. Thyroid function in pregnancy is more fully discussed in Chapter 13, Endocrine

Diseases. Serum β-endorphin levels have been noted to increase in pregnancy. There is further elevation during labor.[28,29] Beta endorphin is released from the pituitary in many stressful conditions (see Chapter 6, Spinal Opioids).

PLACENTAL HORMONES

The placenta synthesizes many important hormones.

Human Chorionic Gonadotropin (HCG)

Starting in early gestation, the placental syncytiotrophoblasts produce human chorionic gonadotropin (hCG). The hCG has an α and a β subunit. The synthesis of the two subunits is regulated by two separate messenger RNA molecules. The most apparent function of hCG is to maintain the function of the corpus luteum, a function similar to that of the luteinizing hormone (LH) of the pituitary. The presence of antibodies for the β-subunit of hCG forms the basis of early pregnancy tests. Antibodies against α-subunit are not useful in this regard because the subunit is not structurally distinguishable from its counterpart of the LH. The concentration of hCG starts waning after the 12th week of gestation (Fig. 2–13).

Human Placental Lactogen (HPL)

The human placental lactogen (HPL, human somatomammotropin, hCS),[30] has a single polypeptide chain and is biologically and immunologically similar to the growth hormone. The hormone increases lipolysis, inhibits gluconeogenesis and prevents glucose uptake by maternal tissues (anti-insulin action). The hormone is believed to play a role in causing the accelerated fed and starved states of pregnancy, which fa-

Table 2–4. Sodium Balance in Pregnancy

Factors increasing Na+ filtration	Factors increasing Na+ reabsorption
Renal plasma flow	Aldosterone
Glomerular filtration	Deoxycorticosterone
Progesterone	Prostaglandin (vasodilation)
Prostaglandin	Renin-angiotensin system
Arginine-vasopressin	Increased ureteral pressure
Melanocyte stimulating hormone	Supine-upright posture
	Prolactin, estrogen

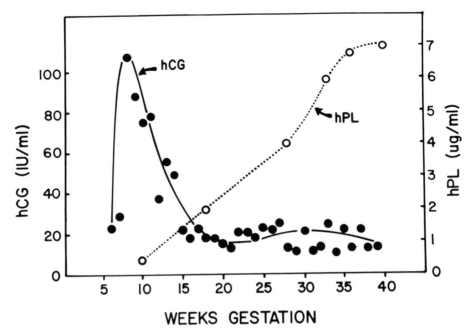

FIG. 2–13.   Chorionic gonadotropin (hCG) and human placental lactogen (hPL) in pregnancy. (From Pritchard JA, McDonald PC, and Gant NF: The placental hormones. *In* Williams Obstetrics. 17th Edition. Norwalk, Appleton-Century-Crofts, 1985.)

cilitate maximum supply of nutrients to the fetus[30] (see Chapter 14, Diabetes Mellitus).

Estrogens

Placenta is the source of the enormous amounts of estrogen.[24] In pregnancy, 85 to 95% of estrogen is estriol. The placenta uses the 16-α-hydroxylated C_{19} steroids as the precursor for the synthesis of estriol. The placenta cannot use C_{21} steroids as it lacks the hydroxylase activity. The major C_{19} precursor is the dehydroepiandrosterone sulfate (DHEAS). The DHEAS may originate either from the maternal or from the fetal adrenal gland. Most of the fetal DHEAS is hydroxlated to 16-α-OH-DHEAS in the fetal liver.[24] This compound is the precursor of 90% of estriol in the mother.[31] The fetal adrenal gland is similar to adult adrenal gland in size but secretes 10 times more steroids than the adult gland. More than 85% of the fetal adrenal gland is composed of the specialized fetal zone that is absent in the adult organ.[24] A decrease in maternal urinary estriol excretion indicates defective adrenal function rather than impaired placental sythesis. The measurement of urinary estriol is used as an index of antepartum fetal well-being.[24] The fetal adrenal gland utilizes low density lipoprotein (LDL) cholesterol for the synthesis of DHEAS. Progesterone is necessary for maintaining a quiescent uterus during gestation. Although the corpus luteum secretes progesterone in early pregnancy, the placenta assumes this function in mammals with a long gestational period. The progesterone levels increase a hundred-fold in pregnancy. Unlike estrogens, the progesterones are not dependent on fetal precursors. Progesterone is synthesized by the placenta from LDL cholesterol.

METABOLISM

The basal metabolic rate increases 15% because of the demands from the conceptus. Pregnancy affects the metabolism of many nutrients, minerals, and water. The changes in water and Na^+ handling have been discussed previously. Pregnancy is a potentially diabetogenic state because of the presence of both steroidal hormones and placental insulinase. When a pregnant patient starves, she develops ketosis more rapidly than a nonpregnant patient (accelerated starvation). When she ingests a meal, the levels of insulin and nutrients reach a higher peak (accelerated fed state). These changes are generally attributed to HPL. For a more detailed description of changes in metabolism, see Chapter 14, Diabetes Mellitus. Pregnancy also causes an increase in total lipids, total cholesterol, phospholipids, and free fatty acids in the serum.[24] Serum alkaline phosphatase level almost doubles because of placental production.[24]

SERUM CHOLINESTERASE ACTIVITY

During pregnancy, a suppression of serum cholinesterase activity starts soon after the 10th week of gestation (Fig. 2–14). It remains suppressed throughout pregnancy and reaches a nadir on the third postpartum day.[32] Despite this reduction, dibucaine, fluoride, and chloride numbers remain within normal limits. Although succinylcholine has caused prolonged apnea in some pregnant patients, the majority of pregnant patients respond normally to it.[33] Since rapid intubation is preferred in pregnant patients, anesthesiologists should use a full paralyzing dose of succinylcholine. Reduction in the

dosage, in view of the possibly decreased enzyme level, may lead to unsatisfactory conditions for tracheal intubation and possible aspiration of gastric contents.

CHANGES IN THE NERVOUS SYSTEM

Pregnancy may induce a 20 to 30% reduction in MAC (minimum alveolar concentration)[34] which is attributed to increased β-endorphin and progesterone levels. The epidural veins (the valveless veins of Bateson) form the collaterals when the inferior vena cava is compressed by the gravid uterus. The distended veins may reduce the compliance of the epidural and the subdural spaces. In pregnant patients, the pressure in the epidural space is usually $+1$ cm H_2O. In the lateral decubitus, the epidural pressures may reach 4 to 10 cm H_2O during labor. The pressure in the epidural space is usually higher in the supine position because of increased distention of the epidural veins. During uterine contractions, further increases may occur in epidural pressures.[35] The cerebrospinal fluid (CSF)

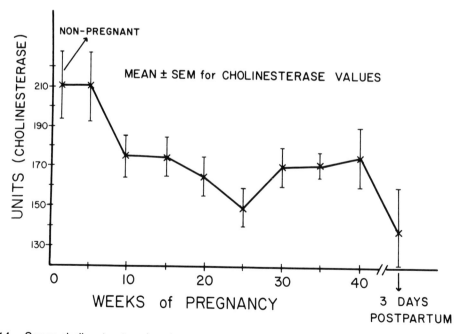

FIG. 2–14.   Serum cholinesterate values in pregnant and nonpregnant patients. The graph was constructed using the data of Robertson GS: (Serum cholinesterase deficiency II: Pregnancy. Brit J Anaesth 38:361, 1966.) and Shnider SM: (Serum cholinesterase activity during pregnancy, labor and the puerperium. Anesthesiology 50:524, 1979.)

pressure is normal in uncomplicated pregnancy. The CSF pressure may rise 3 cm H_2O during an uterine contraction. It has been noted that the increases in both epidural and CSF pressures are higher when the patient moves in bed in response to pain.[35]

These facts are clinically relevant. Because of the absence of subatmospheric pressure in a patient near term, the "hanging drop" method may not be suitable for identifying the epidural space. If possible, the epidural space must be entered during the interval between contractions to avoid "wet taps" and "bloody taps". The epidural catheter may migrate into a distended vein easily during the course of labor, therefore careful aspiration of the catheter and administration of a test dose is recommended before a bigger dose of local anesthetic is administered. The reduced compliance of the epidural and spinal spaces may *not* contribute to the reduced dose requirement for the local anesthetic noticed in pregnancy. This aspect is more fully covered under epidural and spinal anesthesia.

REFERENCES

1. Bonica JJ: Obstet Analg Anesth. 2d Ed. Amsterdam, World Federation of Societies of Anesthesiologists. 1980.
2. Lang RM, and Borrow KM: Pregnancy and heart disease. Clin. Perinatol. *12*:551, 1985.
3. Pirani BBK, Campbell DM, and MacGillivray I: Plasma volume in normal first pregnancy. Br J Obstet Gynaecol, *80*:884, 1973.
4. MacGillivray I: Pre-eclampsia: the hypertensive disease of pregnancy. London, WB Saunders, 1983.
5. Barron WM, and Lindheimer MD: Renal sodium and water handling in pregnancy. *In* Obstetric Gynecology Manual (Edited by Wynn R) *13*:36, 1984.
6. Davison JM: Renal haemodynamics and volume homeostasis in pregnancy. Scand J Clin Lab Invest (44 Suppl)*169*:15, 1984.
7. Kerr, MG, Scott DB, and Samuel E: Studies of the inferior vena cava in late pregnancy. Br Med J *1*:532, 1964.
8. Abitbol MM: Aortic compression by pregnant uterus. NY State J Med *76*:1470, 1976.
9. Scott DB: Inferior vena cava occlusion in late pregnancy and its importance in anesthesia. Br J Anesth *40*:120, 1968.
10. Bienarz J, Maqueda E, and Caldeyro-Barcia R: Compression of the aorta by the uterus in late human pregnancy. Am J Obstet Gynecol *95*:781, 1966.
11. Eckstein KL, and Marx GF: Aortocaval compression and uterine displacement. Anesthesiology *40*:92, 1974.
12. Weinberger SE, et al.: Pregnancy and the lung. Am Rev Resp Disease, *21*:559, 1980.
13. Craig DB, and Toole MA: Airway closure in pregnancy. Can Anesth Soc J 22:665, 1975.
14. Ramanathan S, et al.: Oxygen transfer from mother to fetus during cesarean section under epidural anesthesia. Anesth Analg *61*:576, 1982.
15. Templeton A, and Kelman GR: Maternal blood gases, (PA_{O_2} to Pa_{O_2}), Physiological shunt and VD/VT in normal pregnancy. Br J Anaesth, *48*:1001, 1976.
16. Baldwin GB, Moorthi DS, Whelton JA, and MacDonnel KF: New lung functions and pregnancy. Am J Obstet Gynecol *127*:235, 1977.
17. Archer GW, Marx GF: Arterial oxygen tension during apnoea in parturient women. Br J Anaesth *46*:358, 1974.
18. Holdsworth JD: Mixing of antacids with stomach contents. Anaesthesia 35:641, 1980.
19. Lind JF, Smith AM, Coopland AT, and Crispin JS: Heartburn in pregnancy—A manometric study. Can Med Assoc J *98*:571, 1968.
20. Wald A: Effects of pregnancy on gastrointestinal tract. Dig Dis Sci 27:1015, 1982.
21. Davidson JM, Davison MC, and Hay DM: Gastric emptying time in late pregnancy and labour. Br J Obstet Gynaecol 77:37, 1970.
22. Murray FA, Erskine JP, and Fielding J: Gastric secretion in pregnancy. Br J Obstet Gynaecol *64*:373, 1957.
23. Romero R: The management of acquired hemostatic failure in pregnancy. Crit Care Obstet Patient (Edited by Berkowitz RL) New York Churchill-Livingstone, 1983.
24. Pritchard JA, McDonald PC, and Gant NF: The placental hormones. *In* Williams Obstetrics. 17th Edition. Norwalk, Appleton-Century-Crofts, 1985.
25. Lind T: Fluid balance during labor: A review. J Soc Med 76:870, 1983.
26. Ramanathan S, et al.: Maternal and fetal effects of prophylactic hydration with crystalloids or colloids before epidural anesthesia. Anesth Analg 62:673, 1983.
27. Ramanathan S, et al.: Concentration of lactate and pyruvate in maternal and neonatal blood with different intravenous fluids used for prehydration before epidural anesthesia. Anesth Analg 63:69, 1984.
28. Browning AJF, et al.: Maternal and cord plasma concentrations of B lipotrophin, B endorphin, and Y lipotrophin at delivery; effect of analgesia. Br J Obstet Gynaecol *90*:1152, 1983a.
29. Browning AJF, Butt WR, Lynch SS, and Shakespear RA: Maternal plasma concentrations of B endorphin and Y lipotrophin throughout pregnancy. Br J Obstet Gynaecol *90*:1147, 1983b.
30. Hollingsworth DR: Alternations of maternal metabolism in normal and diabetic pregnancies. Differences in insulin-dependent, non-insulin dependent, and gestational diabetes. Am J Obstet Gynecol *146*:417, 1983.
31. Bardin CW: Fertilization, pregnancy, and lactation. *In* Best and Taylor's Physiological Basis of Medical Practice. (Edited by West JB) Baltimore, Williams & Wilkins, 1985.
32. Shnider SM: Serum cholinesterase activity during pregnancy, labor and the puerperium. Anesthesiology 50:524, 1979.

33. Blitt CD, Petty WC, and Alberternst EE: Correlation of plasma cholisterase activity and duration of action of succinylcholine during pregnancy. Anesth Analg 56:78, 1977.

34. Palahniuk RJ, and Shnider SM: Maternal and fetal cardiovascular acid-base changes during halothane and isoflurane anesthesia in the pregnant ewe. Anesthesiology 41:462, 1974.

35. Marx GF, and Bassell GM: Physiologic considerations of the mother. *In* Obstetric Analgesia and Anaesthesia. (Edited by Marx GF and Bassell GM) New York. Elsevier, 1980.

RESPIRATORY FUNCTION OF THE PLACENTA

The placenta is the vital link between the mother and the fetus. The major functions of the placenta include the following: exchanging respiratory gases between the mother and the fetus; supplying metabolic hormones; providing nutrients to the fetus; and protecting the fetus immunologically. The hormonal function has been discussed in Chapter 2, Maternal Adaptation to Pregnancy.

The placenta and the fetus are foreign proteins to the mother and it is still presently not known why the mother does not reject the fetal allograft.[1,2] According to a recent hypothesis, this failure to reject is suspected to be caused by the presence of some common markers on the lymphocytes of the mother and fetus. The placenta also transfers IgG antibodies to the fetus, affording it some protection against diphtheria, chickenpox, and measles. The maternal antibodies are believed to be engulfed by the syncytiotrophoblast before they are transferred to the fetal capillaries (pinocytosis). The fetal chorionic syncytiotrophoblasts are the only layer of cells separating the mother and the fetus,[3,4] an arrangement called the hemomonochorial arrangement.

MATERNAL COMPONENT OF THE PLACENTA

The placenta consists of maternal and fetal components. The maternal portion is called the decidua (L, deciduous, falling off). That portion of the decidua forming the placental bed is called the decidua basalis; the part overlying the fetus is the decidua capsularis, and the rest is called the decidua parietalis (Fig. 3–1). The decidual cells provide nutritive support to the fetus until the intervillous circulation is adequately established. The decidua also secretes both prolactin, which enters the amniotic fluid, and several polyamines, which are required for the growth of the gravid uterus. The decidua is also a source of diamine oxidase (histaminase), which catalyzes the breakdown of the polyamines.[1]

FETAL COMPONENT OF THE PLACENTA

Following fertilization, the blastocyst firmly anchors itself to the endometrium with the help of the trophoblast. The trophoblast rapidly proliferates into an inner and outer layer. The inner layer is more cellular (cytotrophoblast) and the outer layer is a true syncytium (syncytiotrophoblast). The syncytiotrophoblast is invasive, ingestive, and digestive and it is responsible for drawing nutritive materials for the fetus from the endometrium. Although the decidual chorion arborizes extensively, the remaining chorion is compressed by the growing fetus and becomes smooth (chorion laeve, Fig. 3–1).

A space appears between the developing em-

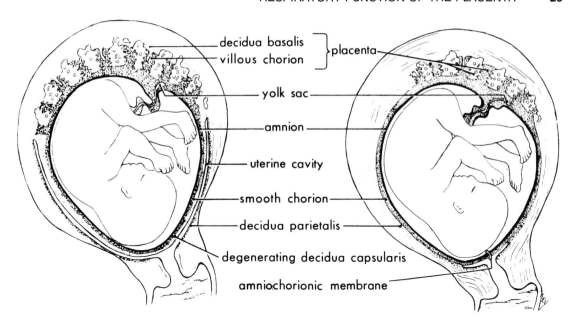

FIG. 3–1.   The chorion and the amnion. The placental villi persist only where the chorion is in contact with the decidua basalis. The pressure of the fetus causes the villi to degenerate in the rest of the amniotic sac, giving it a smooth appearance (the smooth chorion). The decidua parietalis fuses with the amnion to form the amniochorionic membrane that ruptures during labor. (From Moore KL: The fetal membranes and the placenta. *In* The Developing Human. 3rd Edition. Philadelphia, WB Saunders, 1982.)

bryo and the cytotrophoblasts and soon becomes the amniotic cavity. The amniotic cavity slowly engulfs the fetus (Fig. 3–1). The amnion along with the smooth chorion is believed to be capable of steroid hormone metabolism and prostaglandin production.

The amniotic fluid provides buoyancy to the fetus. At 36 weeks of gestation, the volume of amniotic fluid reaches 1 L, after which it slightly decreases in quantity. In early pregnancy, the composition of the amniotic fluid resembles that of the plasma. As pregnancy advances, phospholipids are added from the fetal lungs. Desquamated fetal cells, lanugo hair and vernix caseosa are added. Late in pregnancy, the fetal urine contributes to the total amount of amniotic fluid. Because the fetal urine is hypotonic, the amniotic fluid becomes increasingly hyposmolar. The fusion of the smooth chorion with the amnion forms the amniochorionic membrane, which ruptures at the onset of labor.

The invading chorionic villi breaks into lacunae containing endometrial blood vessels and glands. The lacunae form the future intervillous space. All villi arise from the chorionic plate (Fig. 3–1) and project into the intervillous space. Some villi function as anchors; most villi, how-

ever, branch repeatedly into finer villi. Two or more main stem villi with their subdivisions may be contained in a separate district called the cotyledon, which are separated from each other by placental septa. The septa do not reach the chorionic plate, resulting in confluency of the intervillous space. The villi are bathed by the maternal arterial blood arriving via the spiral arteries. The villi, which contain branches of fetal vein and artery, are thus exposed to maternal circulation (Fig. 3–2).

The placental membrane, which intervenes between the maternal and fetal circulation, consists mainly of the syncytiotrophoblasts, the connective tissue core of the villus, and the endothelium of the fetal capillary (cytotrophoblasts may also be a part of the membrane before the 20th week of pregnancy). The syncytiotrophoblast cells have specialized microvilli on their surface, which give them the brush-border appearance (Fig. 3–3). The presence of microvilli greatly enhances the surface area for transfer of gases and other substances. Often a fibrinoid layer (Nitabuch's layer) is deposited on the surface of the syncytiotrophoblasts. The pattern of invasion of the syncytiotrophoblasts into the maternal arteries is described in greater detail in

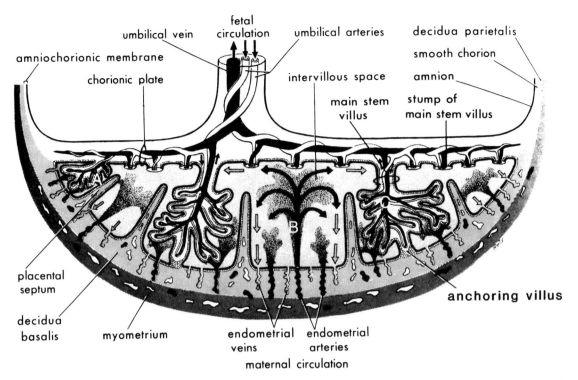

FIG. 3–2.   Schematic diagram of blood flow through the placenta. Note (A) the cotyledons are separated from each other by the decidual septa, which stop short of the chorionic plate causing the entire intervillous space to become confluent; (B) spurts of arterial blood escaping from the maternal endometrial spiral arteries; (C) the arborization of the fetal villi with the fetal capillaries contained in them. (From Moore KL: The fetal membranes and the placenta. *In* The Developing Human: Clinically Oriented Embryology. 3rd Ed, 1982. Courtesy of WB Saunders, Philadelphia.)

Chapter 10, Hypertensive Disorders of Pregnancy.

THE FETAL-MATERNAL CIRCULATION

The maternal driving pressure forces blood into the intervillous space through the 80 to 100 spiral arteries. The arterial blood is pushed up into the intervillous space where exchange occurs between the fetal and maternal villi (Figs. 3–2, 3–4). The respiratory gas exchange between the mother and fetus is governed by the laws of diffusion. The maternal blood does not exit as a homogeneous pool around the fetal villi but flows successively past a large number of villi in the intervillous space. Although maternal P_{O_2} will be uniform around any particular villus, the blood P_{O_2} in the fetal capillaries near the spiral arteries will be greater than the P_{O_2} in capillaries near the chorionic plate. This is be-

cause the maternal blood P_{O_2} progressively decreases during the passage through the intervillous space because of the oxygen extraction by the villi. This makes the oxygen content of the intervillous pool inhomogeneous.

FETAL-MATERNAL GAS TRANSFER

The direction of fetal blood flow seems to be at right angles to that of the maternal blood flow. Such an exchange system is called a multivillous crosscurrent system.[4,5] This vascular geometry is a less efficient exchange system than a countercurrent system, but it is more efficient than a concurrent or a homogeneous pool system.[5] In the pool system, multiple villi extract oxygen from a static maternal pool of blood. The gas exchange in the placenta is flow limited. This happens because despite the availability of sufficient diffusion gradient, (maternal arterial P_{O_2} − fetal arterial P_{O_2} = 85 mm Hg) the fetal blood

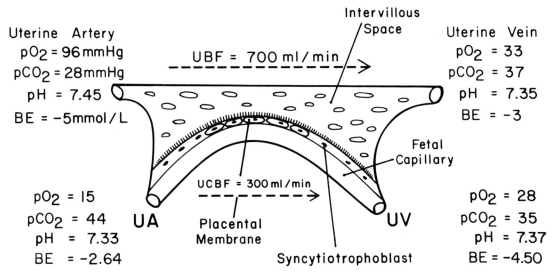

Uterine Artery

Uterine Artery
$pO_2 = 96$ mmHg
$pCO_2 = 28$ mmHg
pH = 7.45
BE = −5 mmol/L

UBF = 700 ml/min

Intervillous Space

Uterine Vein
$pO_2 = 33$
$pCO_2 = 37$
pH = 7.35
BE = −3

Fetal Capillary

$pO_2 = 15$
$pCO_2 = 44$
pH = 7.33
BE = −2.64

UA

UCBF = 300 ml/min

Placental Membrane

Syncytiotrophoblast

UV

$pO_2 = 28$
$pCO_2 = 35$
pH = 7.37
BE = −4.50

FIG. 3–3. Schematic representation of the double-Bohr and the double-Haldane effect in the placenta. The CO_2, reaching the mother from the fetus, causes a rightward shift of the maternal oxyhemoglobin dissociation curve and a leftward shift of the fetal curve (the double-Bohr effect). The oxygen affinity of maternal hemoglobin decreases and that of the fetal hemoglobin increases, facilitating transfer. Note the widening of the crevice of the alpha chain of hemoglobin, permitting more oxygen entry into the heme molecule. Because of the Haldane effect, the oxygenated fetal hemoglobin will release the CO_2 and the mother's reduced hemoglobin will be in a state of readiness to receive the incoming CO_2 (the double-Haldane effect). P_{O_2} and P_{CO_2} tension gradients across the placental membrane are also shown. Refer to the text for a description of chloride shift.

gains only 10 mm Hg during its passage through the placenta (Fig. 3–3). Thus the gas transfer appears not to be limited by the diffusion gradient. The limiting factor appears to be the transport capacity of fetal circulation (umbilical blood flow × fetal hemoglobin oxygen carrying capacity per 100 ml of blood). The limited oxygen transfer in fact protects the fetus from too much oxygen. If, for instance, the transfer of oxygen occurs with relative ease (as in the case of the lungs), the fetal P_{O_2} may approach the maternal P_{O_2}, which could result in the premature closure of the fetal ductus arteriosus. However, because of the limited exchange, maternal hyperoxia will never lead to the closure of the fetal ductus.[6]

The fetal hemoglobin (HbF) which consists of two alpha and two gamma chains has a higher affinity for oxygen than the mother's. For a given P_{O_2}, the oxygen saturation of fetal hemoglobin is greater than that of the mother's. The P_{50} of fetal and maternal hemoglobin are 20 and 27 mm Hg, respectively. A complete replacement of the

fetal RBC with adult ones will not alter the fetal P_{O_2} but will reduce its oxygen supply by 60% because of the decrease in oxygen saturation of hemoglobin.[7] The leftward shift of the fetal oxyhemoglobin dissociation curve is partially caused by the diminished binding of 2-3, diphosphoglyceraldehyde (2-3, DPG) with the gamma chain of the HbF. The 2-3, DPG molecule has 5 titratable acid groups.[8] It lowers the affinity of hemoglobin for oxygen by lowering the intra RBC pH relative to plasma.[9] A change of 4.3×10^{-8} M in 2-3, DPG content will change the P_{O_2} by 1 mm Hg.

The four chains of the hemoglobin molecule lie like a crumpled necklace within the RBC. Figure 3–5 shows a section of the alpha chain. The heme lies in the crevice bound by the two histidine residues at the 58th and 87th positions on the side of the Fe^{++} ions in the center. The crevice arrangement controls the access of oxygen into the heme.[9] The unique configuration of the hemoglobin molecule is believed to form the basis of both the Bohr and the Haldane ef-

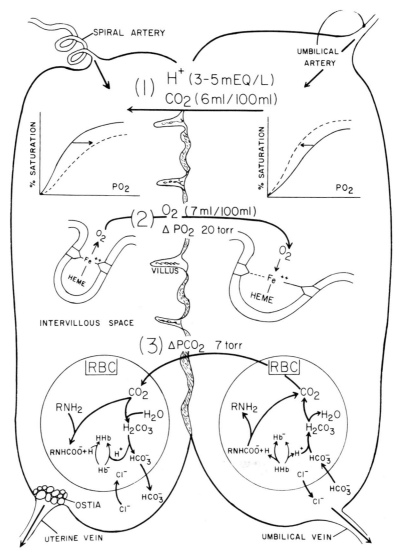

FIG. 3–4.   Gas transfer across the placental membrane. Note the microvilli brush border on the syncytiotrophoblasts. UBF = uterine blood flow; UCBF = umbilical cord blood flow. Blood pH and gas tensions were measured in patients undergoing elective cesarean section. Maternal F_{IO_2} = 0.21. Note the small negative base excess values in the umbilical vein (UV) and the umbilical artery (UA).

fects. The two histidine amino acids bind CO_2 as carbamino compounds. Increased H^+ ion concentration or binding of CO_2 to the histidine residues closes the crevice by strengthening the bond between Fe^{++} and the sentinel histidines, thus limiting entry of oxygen into the crevice.[10] This decreases the affinity of heme for oxygen (Bohr effect). When the heme becomes oxygenated, it becomes more acidic (Fig. 3–4) along with the histidine residues. This releases CO_2, thus explaining why oxygenated blood cannot carry CO_2 as effectively as deoxygenated blood (Haldane effect).[10]

In the placenta, oxygen diffuses from the intervillous space into the fetal circulation while CO_2 diffuses in the reverse direction (Fig. 3–4). When the mother breathes normal room air, the oxygen diffusion gradient between the maternal artery and the fetal umbilical artery (UA) blood is 85 mm Hg.[4] The diffusion gradient for CO_2 is approximately 22 mm Hg. The fetal UA blood contains more H^+ than does the maternal blood because of increased P_{CO_2}. The fetal CO_2 entering the intervillous space decreases the maternal blood pH. The maternal oxyhemoglobin dissociation curve shifts to the right and the fetal

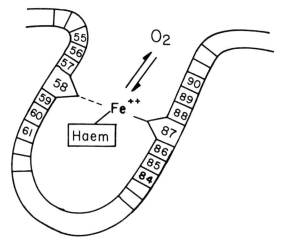

FIG. 3–5. A section of the alpha chain of hemoglobin. Heme lies in the crevice enclosed by the histidine amino acids at the 87th and 58th positions and by the Fe^{++} ion. The CO_2 is bound to the histidine amino acids, which facilitates the double-Bohr and the double-Haldane effect (see text). (From Nunn JF: Oxygen. *In* Applied Respiratory Physiology. Boston, Butterworths, 1977.)

oxyhemoglobin dissociation curve is caused by a reduced CO_2 content. Thus, the transplacental oxygen transfer is regulated by a change in the oxygen affinity of the maternal and fetal hemoglobin caused by altered H^+ concentrations (and CO_2 contents) on both sides (double-Bohr effect). In order to achieve the same degree of efficiency without the Bohr effect, the diffusion gradient should be greater or the uteroplacental blood flow should increase considerably.[5] The relationship between maternal and fetal P_{O_2} is discussed below.

CO_2 transfer is regulated by the diffusion gradient, and the double-Haldane effect. Although CO_2 diffuses readily across membranes, a continuous supply of CO_2 must be available at the placental site for diffusion. This is provided by the HCO_3^- which enters the RBC from the plasma. In order to maintain ionic equilibrium within the RBC when HCO_3^- enters the cell, Cl^- must leave the RBC (Chloride shift or the Hamburger phenomenon) (Fig. 3–4). Because the fetal hemoglobin has now gained H^+ from increased oxygenation, the CO_2 is driven out of the histidine amino acids, which further augments the diffusion gradient across the placental membrane. On the maternal side, the deoxygenated alkaline blood will now more readily accept the incoming CO_2. The HCO_3^- will leave the maternal RBC in exchange of Cl^-. Because the CO_2 affinity is affected by the change in the degree of oxygenation on the maternal and the fetal side, a double-Haldane effect regulates the CO_2 transfer across the placental membrane (Fig. 3–4).

NORMAL BIOCHEMICAL ENVIRONMENT OF A WELL-OXYGENATED FETUS

It was originally thought that the fetus lived in a hypoxic and acidotic environment. Rooth and Sjostedt[11] reported a base excess (BE) value of -9.4 for the umbilical artery (UA) and -6.2 for the umbilical vein. They showed that the net H^+ transfer from the fetus to mother was 3.6 mEQ, of which 3.0 mEQ were fixed acids and the balance were volatile acid. In other words, the Bohr shift of the maternal hemoglobin was mainly caused by the transplacental fixed acid transfer. In this study, however, the BE measurements were made on patients who were in labor. Labor is a condition that predisposes to fetal and maternal acidosis. For this reason, even scalp samples are of limited value in defining the acid-base environment of the unborn fetus. It is generally accepted that in a nonasphyxiated fetus, the main source of H^+ is the metabolically produced CO_2[12] and not increased fixed acid content.

Measurements made on normal term neonates during uncomplicated elective cesarean section are more representative of normal fetal environment. These measurements have shown that the undisturbed fetus does not live in an acidotic or hypoxic environment.[12–14] Blood pH and gas tensions, HCO_3^-, BE, and indices of anaerobic metabolism show that the lower pH in the fetus is repiratory in origin. For instance, the HCO_3^- and BE values are highest in the fetal UA, lowest in the maternal artery, and have intermediate values seen in the fetal UV blood (Fig. 3–3, Table 3–1). Thus, the fetal UA blood, which is in equilibrium with the fetal tissues, does not show any evidence of a greater degree of metabolic acidosis than that of maternal blood. Therefore, the H^+ ions necessary for causing the Bohr shift of the maternal oxyhemoglobin curve are derived from transplacental CO_2 transfer.

Table 3–1.   Acid-Base Parameters in the Mother and Fetus

Measurement	MA/MV	UV	UA
P_{O_2} (mm Hg)	238(7)	32(1)	20(1)
P_{CO_2} (mm Hg)	29(1)	40(2)	48(1)
pH	7.42(0.01)	7.35(0.01)	7.3(0.01)
Glucose (mg%)	104(4)	88(3)	77(3)
Lactate (mM/L)	1.48(0.1)	1.45(0.1)	1.53(0.1)
Pyruvate (mM/L)	0.1(0.01)	0.08(0.01)	0.08(0.01)
L/P ratio	17(1)	22(1)	21(1)
XL (mM/L)	0.5(0.1)	0.7(0.1)	0.7(0.1)
HCO_3^- (mM/L)	18(0.4)	21.4(0.4)	23(0.4)
BE (mM/L)	-6(0.3)	-3.5(0.3)	-2.8(0.3)

Data are mean ± 1SE (figures within parentheses). Measurements were made at uncomplicated cesarean delivery with the mother breathing 50% oxygen. MA = maternal artery; MV = maternal vein; UV and UA = fetal umbilical artery and vein. Note that the maternal blood pH and gas tensions, HCO_3^- and BE are obtained on the radial artery blood. Maternal glucose, lactate, and pyruvate are measured in venous blood. The UV blood HCO_3^- and BE were significantly greater than the corresponding maternal artery values. Both UA blood values are significantly greater than the UV and MA value. This shows that the lowered blood pH in the fetal UA is caused by respiratory acidosis and not by metabolic acidosis. XL = excess lactate, a derived value, representing that portion of the measured lactate that cannot be accounted for by the amount of measured pyruvate. (From Ramanathan S: The biochemical profile of a well-oxygenated human fetus. Anesthesiology, 61:A397, 1984.)

The mother is in a state of moderate respiratory alkalosis and compensatory metabolic acidosis, while the fetus is in a state of mild respiratory and metabolic acidosis.

In animal fetuses, the UV blood lactate is greater than the UA blood lactate. This has led to the speculation that animal fetuses may perhaps utilize lactate as an aerobic fuel. However, in the human fetus, the UA blood lactate concentration is greater than the UV lactate, making it unlikely that the human fetus utilizes this substrate under normal conditions (Table 3–1). The human fetus mainly utilizes glucose as an aerobic fuel as evidenced by a UV-UA gradient of 11 mg/dl. Glucose homeostasis is more completely discussed in Chapter 14, Diabetes Mellitus. The lactate in the fetal blood (Table 3–1) is caused by basal production unrelated to anaerobic metabolism. This is evidenced by the fact that lactate levels obtained from normoxic fetuses do not correlate with the H^+ concentration (Fig. 3–6). Lactate produced under basal conditions is usually intracellularly buffered and therefore will affect neither the extracellular fluid pH nor the BE. However, during overwhelming anaerobic metabolism, the lactate levels will rise along with the extracellular H^+ concentration.[12,15]

OXYGEN DEPRIVED FETUS

A well-oxygenated fetus utilizes up to 40% of its oxygen supply for growth and the remaining

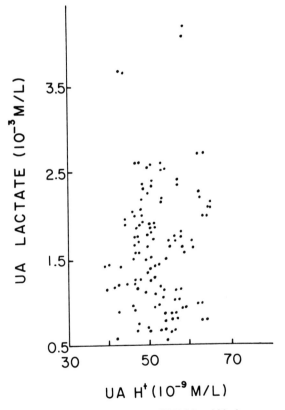

FIG. 3–6. Umbilical artery (UA) blood H^+ ion concentration is plotted against the lactate correlation. The lack of correlation between the two variables, signifying that in the normoxic fetus the lactate level represents only the basal production.

60% for acute vital cellular function. Thus the fetus may lose up to 40% of its oxygen supply without resorting to anaerobic metabolism.[16] Oxygen supply to the fetus may be curtailed by the following factors: maternal hypoxia, reduction in uterine blood flow, and interruption in umbilical cord blood flow. Whereas the anesthesiologist may influence the first two factors, he may not be in a position to control the third factor. Regardless of the cause of the hypoxia, the fetus sets in motion a series of compensatory mechanisms to preserve oxygen supply to the vital organs.

INCREASED CATECHOLAMINE SECRETION

Even a 10 to 20% reduction in uterine blood flow (UBF) will cause an increase in fetal catecholamine secretion, with no other signs of hypoxia being evident[15] (Fig. 3–7). The greater the degree of UBF reduction, the higher the cate-

cholamine level in the fetal blood will be. Catecholamines not only augment the cardiac stroke volume of the fetus, which determines the umbilical cord blood flow, but also decrease perfusion to skin and muscle, which extract 40% of fetal oxygen supply.[7]

BRADYCARDIA

When the UBF is reduced to 30 to 35% of control, fetal arterial pressure will rise and the heart rate will fall in the first 10 minutes. After that period, the heart rate will rise above control values. The fetal P_{O_2} will decrease. Hypoxic bradycardia caused by a reduction in UBF is caused by aortic and carotid body chemoreceptor stimulation. The efferent pathway is via the vagus. Thus in early phases of hypoxemia, bradycardia will be evident regardless of whether tissue hypoxia is present or not. Umbilical cord compression will cause fetal hypertension because of out-

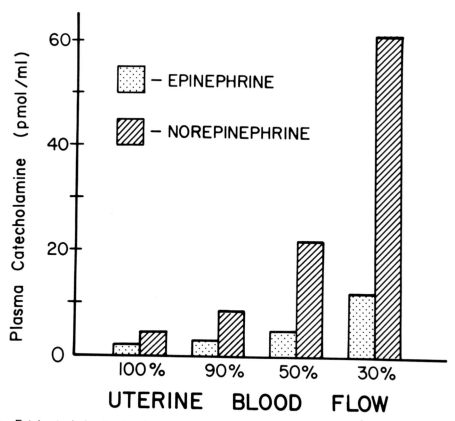

FIG. 3–7. Fetal catecholamine level at different degrees of reduction in uterine blood flow (UBF). Even a 10% reduction in UBF is sensed by the fetus, resulting in increased catecholamine levels. (The histogram is based on data from Gu W, Jones CT, and Parer JT: Metabolic and cardiovascular effects on fetal sheep of sustained reduction of uterine blood flow. J Physiol 368:109, 1985.)

flow obstruction. The resultant baroceptor stimulation will cause bradycardia. Chemoreceptor stimulation will come into play if the cord compression is severe enough to decrease the fetal P_{O_2}.[16]

REDUCTION IN OXYGEN CONSUMPTION

Until the oxygen supply decreases 40%, the fetus will not decrease its oxygen consumption ($\dot{V}_{O_2}$). When the supply decreases further, the oxygen consumption will decrease to a similar degree (regardless of the etiology of hypoxia) and the fetus will develop intense anaerobic metabolism[15-17] (Fig. 3–8). In lamb fetuses, the critical level of oxygen delivery below which a decrease in $\dot{V}_{O_2}$ occurs is 12 ml/min/Kg.[16,17] When a sudden reduction in oxygen supply occurs, the fetus attempts to supply glucose to the placenta by not only reducing its own glucose consumption, but by mobilizing its glycogen stores. Subsequently, the fetus will produce enough lactate to support its own needs and the needs of the placenta as well. During severe hypoxia, the placental oxygen consumption will remain unchanged while the fetal oxygen consumption will decrease considerably.[15]

REARRANGEMENT OF BLOOD FLOW

When oxygen availability is limited, the fetus redistributes its blood flow so that the vital organs such as the brain, the heart, and the adrenals preferentially receive blood supply over nonvital organs such as the intestines, skin, muscle, and lungs. Because the oxygen supply needed for growth is only minimal in the vital organs, they lack significant oxygen stores. During hypoxia, the ductus venosus blood is channeled preferentially across the foramen ovale and the blood from the distal inferior vena cava is channeled through the tricuspid valve. The left hepatic venous blood, which has a higher oxygen content than the right is also channeled across the foramen ovale.[7] This streamlining of blood within the thoracic portion of the inferior vena cava of the fetus enables the fetus to maximize oxygen supply to the vital organs during the hypoxia. There will be widespread vasoconstriction in the splanchnic bed, the liver, the skin, and the lungs (hypoxic pulmonary vasoconstriction). Cardiac output, umbilical cord blood flow, and organ blood flow changes during hypoxia are summarized in Table 3–2.[18] The fetal blood P_{CO_2} invariably rises during fetal asphyxia because the transplacental exchange of the gas is decreased and the neutralization of H^+ ions

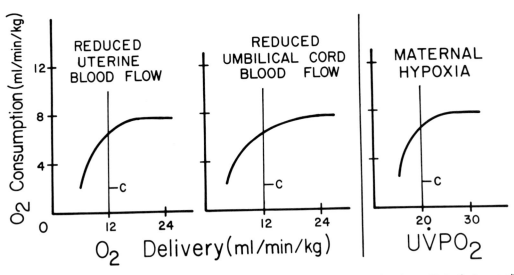

FIG. 3–8.   Fetal oxygen consumption with hypoxia produced by different mechanisms. Note that regardless of the mechanism of hypoxia, the fetal $\dot{V}_{O_2}$ starts decreasing only when the oxygen delivery falls below the critical value of 12 ml/min/kg, represented by the vertical line C. (Based on data from Gu W, Jones CT, ad Parker T: Metabolic and cardiovascular effects on fetal sheep of sustained reduction of uterine blood flow. J Physiol *368*:109, 1985.)

Table 3–2.   Effects of Fetal Asphyxia

Parameter		Change (%)
	Cardiac output	−25
	Stroke volume	+8
	Total body flow	−48
	Umbilical blood flow	+8
Organ blood flow	Gut	−50
	Spleen	−82
	Kidneys	−50
	Carcass	−60
	Lungs	−60
	Heart	+240
	Brain	+150
	Adrenals	+280

Note the increase in blood flow to the heart, brain and adrenals.
(Derived from Cohn HE, et al.: Cardiovascular responses to hypoxemia and acidemia in fetal lambs. Am J Obstet Gynecol, *120*:817, 1974.)

with the HCO_3^- causes liberation of CO_2. The increased P_{CO_2} may further increase cerebral blood flow.

DRUG DISPOSITION IN AN ACIDOTIC FETUS (TABLE 3–3)

The distribution, metabolism, and elimination of drugs may be affected by fetal acidosis.[19] The acidosis decreases protein-binding[19] of the drug and increases the ionized fraction of the local anesthetic. This causes the fetal artery to maternal artery concentration ratio of the local anesthetics to increase (Fig. 3–9).[20] Because of the circulatory adaptations, the brain and the heart will receive a maximum amount of the drug, increasing the likelihood of toxicity. In addition, decreased hepatic blood flow will diminish the ability of the fetus to metabolize any drug contained in the UV blood.

Table 3–3.   Drug Disposition in an Acidotic Fetus

Affect of acidosis	Results
Decreased pH	Increased ionized fraction of the drug
	Ion trapping in the fetus
	Decreased protein binding
	Decreased placental clearance (reduced umbilical cord blood flow)
Modified circulation	Decreased hepatic metabolism (reduced hepatic blood flow)
	Greater drug delivery to brain and heart (increased cerebral, coronary blood flows)

OPTIMIZATION OF TRANSPLACENTAL RESPIRATORY GAS EXCHANGE

The fetus is precariously dependent on its mother for its oxygen needs. Even a slight reduction in uterine blood flow causes stress in the fetus. The anesthesiologist must take some precautions to optimize transplacental gas exchange.

AVOIDING SYSTEMIC HYPOTENSION

Whenever the systolic blood pressure is reduced below 100 mm Hg because of spinal or epidural anesthesia, the UBF may be reduced. The simplest and most effective way to avoid this problem is to administer 1 to 1.5 L of Ringer's lactate solution to the mother before the regional anesthetic is administered. The anesthetic must only be administered in increments and the effect of each increment on the systemic blood pressure must be assessed before further injections are made. Aortocaval compression must be avoided. The patient should be instructed to lie on her side; the fetal heart tones are not heard well if the mother is in the lateral decubitus. With patients who receive epidural labor analgesia, it is recommended that an internal fetal scalp electrode be used for monitoring the fetal heart rate. The internal method is not affected by the lateral position. After the induction of epidural anesthesia or after each time a reinforcing dose is administered, the blood pressure must be measured at least once

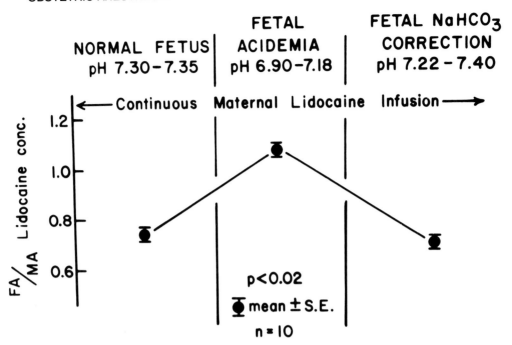

FIG. 3–9.   The increased fetal artery to maternal artery (FA/MA) ratio of lidocaine during fetal acidemia (p <0.02). (From Biehl D, Shnider SM, Levinson G, and Callender K: Placental transfer of lidocaine. Anesthesiology, *48*:409, 1978.)

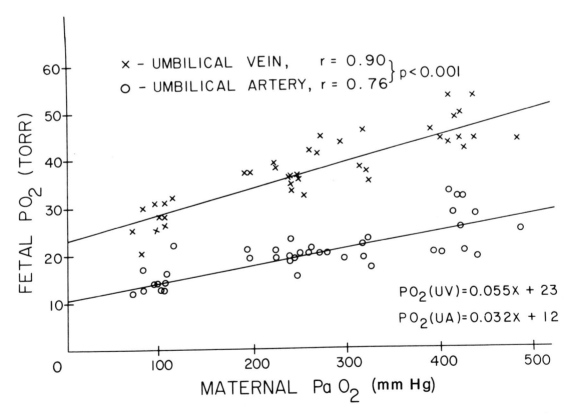

FIG. 3–10.   The relationship between maternal and fetal Pa_{O_2}. (From Ramanathan S, et al.: Oxygen transfer from the mother to fetus during cesarean section under epidural anesthesia. Anesth Analg *63*:69–74, 1982.)

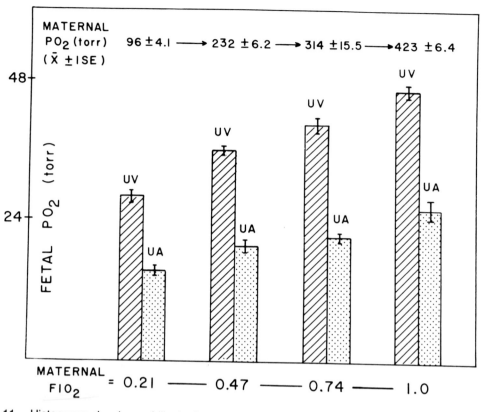

FIG. 3–11. Histograms showing umbilical vein (UV) and umbilical artery (UA) P_{O_2} levels at different maternal F_{IO_2}'s. The maternal P_{O_2} is shown at the top. Note that even at an F_{IO_2} of 1.0, the maternal P_{O_2} reaches only 423 mm Hg ($\dot{V}/\dot{Q}$ mismatch in the lung). (From Ramanathan S, et al.: Oxygen transfer from the mother to fetus during cesarean section under epidural anesthesia. Anesth Analg 63:69, 1982.)

every minute and systemic hypotension corrected by administration of 5 mg intravenous injections of ephedrine. The treatment of systemic hypotension is more fully discussed in Chapter 7, Regional Blocks.

INCREASING MATERNAL Pa_{O_2}

Several studies have shown that increasing maternal Pa_{O_2} will increase the P_{O_2} of both fetal UV and fetal UA (Figs. 3–10 and 3–11).[6] Because of the limited flow exchange in the placenta, a given increase in maternal Pa_{O_2} does not produce an increase of equal magnitude in fetal P_{O_2}. However, even a small increase in fetal P_{O_2} will considerably increase the oxygen saturation because of the shape of the oxyhemoglobin dissociation curve,[6] which increases fetal oxygen stores. When mothers are allowed to breathe the room air before delivery during cesarean section, both the mother and the newborn have

increased base deficit at birth (Fig. 3–12).[6] Thus administering at least 50% oxygen to the mother before delivery optimizes maternal and fetal oxygenation and acid-base status.

AVOIDING MATERNAL HYPOCARBIA

Active or passive hyperventilation will lead to a reduction in fetal oxygenation because of the leftward shift of the maternal oxyhemoglobin dissociation curve (Fig. 3–13). The maternal hemoglobin will not readily liberate the oxygen.[21] Active hyperventilation occurs whenever the patient is in pain. Passive hyperventilation may be produced by improper ventilator settings during controlled mechanical ventilation. Ventilatory response to labor pains are more fully discussed in Chapter 8, Labor Analgesia. Although the increased intrathoracic pressure of mechanical ventilation reduces cardiac output (and therefore the UBF), the respiratory alka-

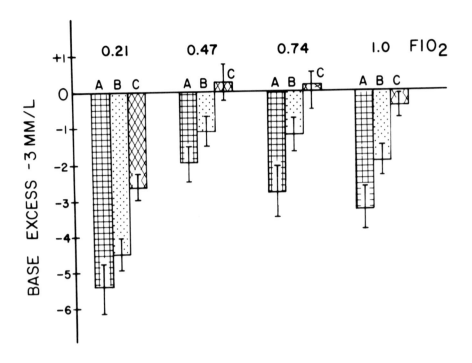

FIG. 3–12. Increased maternal and fetal acidosis (larger negative base excess, BE) at a maternal F_{IO_2} of 0.21. The BE either in the mother or in the fetus did not significantly differ among the three hyperoxic F_{IO_2}'s. A = maternal artery; B = fetal umbilical vein; C = umbilical artery. (From Ramanathan S, et al.: Oxygen transfer from the mother to the fetus during cesarean section under epidural anesthesia. Anesth Analg *63*:69, 1982.)

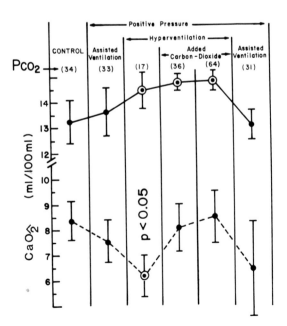

FIG. 3–13. Effects of maternal hyperventilation on fetal blood oxygen content (CaO_2, Y-axis). When the maternal Pa_{CO_2} is reduced by hyperventilation, the fetal CaO_2 decreases, however, when the maternal Pa_{CO_2} is increased by adding CO_2 to the inspired gas, the fetal CaO_2 increases despite the fact that the same respiratory minute volume is being used. (From Levinson G, Shnider SM, de Lorimer AA, and Steffenson JL: Effects of maternal hyperventilation on uterine blood flow and fetal oxygenation and acid-base status. Anesthesiology *40*:340, 1974.)

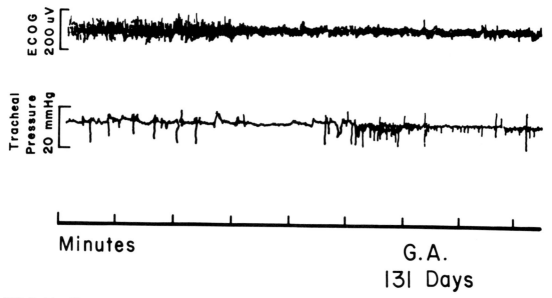

FIG. 3–14. Electrocortical activity and tracheal pressure tracing in fetal lambs. Note the increase in breathing activity during low-voltage activity. The low-voltage activity is decreased when the mother is starved. (Modified from Richardson B, Hohimer Ar, Muegler B, and Bissonette J: Effects of concentration on fetal breathing movements and electrocortical activity in fetal lambs. Am J Obstet Gynecol *142*:678, 1982.)

losis is actually a more important factor in reducing fetal oxygenation than is the reduction in maternal cardiac output. In compromised pregnancies, however, both factors may play a role. Judicious use of analgesia will decrease hyperventilation caused by labor pains. Metabolic alkalosis ($NaHCO_3$ administration) also diminishes fetal oxygenation by the same mechanism as does respiratory alkalosis.[22]

AVOIDING STRESS

Labor pains are a formidable cause for increased stress. Animal experiments show that increased stress causes an increase in maternal blood levels of catecholamines, which diminish UBF.[23] The beneficial effects of lumbar epidural analgesia on the stress of labor is discussed in Chapter 8, Labor Analgesia.

AVOIDING ACID-BASE CHANGES IN THE FETUS

In addition to the above-mentioned factors, administration of excessive amounts of glucose or acetate containing solutions to the mother, maternal hypoglycemia, and the presence of abnormal fetal hemoglobins may interfere with the fetal acid-base status and/or the fetal well-being.

Maternal hyperglycemia causes fetal hyperglycemia, which is associated with increased fetal levels of lactate and decreased fetal blood pH. Large volumes of intravenous fluids are administered to prevent systemic hypotension caused by regional anesthesia. Nonglucose containing crystalloid solution must be used for this purpose. Should glucose administration become necessary, the rate of glucose administration must not exceed 20 g/hour.[24,25]

Maternal hypoglycemia may also interfere with fetal breathing movements by diminishing the low-voltage cerebral electrical activity (Fig. 3–14). Fetal breathing movements are considered a reliable index of fetal well-being.[26] (For further discussion of this topic see Chapter 24, Fetal Monitoring.) Thus it becomes necessary to maintain the maternal blood sugar level between 80 to 120 mg/dL. The use of acetate-containing solutions (Plasmalyte-A) may be associated with increased lactate levels in the fetus because acetate ions are potent inhibitors of glycolysis.

Maternal cigarette smoking increases the carboxyhemoglobin level in the fetus.[27] The fetal hemoglobin has a higher affinity for CO than does maternal hemoglobin. The use of excessive amounts of prilocaine may cause methhemoglobin production in the mother and fetus[19] (see Local Anesthetics, Chapter 5). The presence of abnormal hemoglobins interferes with fetal oxygen carrying capacity.

REFERENCES

1. Pritchard JA, MacDonald PC, and Gant NF: The placenta and fetal membranes. *In* Williams Obstetrics. 17th Edition. Norwalk, Appleton-Century-Crofts, 1985.

2. Finn R, Davis JC, St. Hill CA, and Hilpkin LJ: Feto-maternal bidirectional mixed lymphocyte reaction and survival of fetal allograft. Lancet 1:200, 1977.

3. Moore KL: The fetal membranes and the placenta. *In* The Developing Human. 3rd Ed. Philadelphia, WB Saunders, 1982.

4. Reynolds FJM: The fetus and the placenta. *In* A Practice of Anaesthesia. (Edited by Churchill-Davidson HC) Chicago, Year Book Medical Publishers, 1984.

5. Metcalfe J, Bartels H, and Moll W: Gas exchange in the pregnant uterus. Physiol Rev 47:782, 1967.

6. Ramanathan S: The biochemical profile of a well-oxygenated human fetus. Anesthesiology 61:A397, 1984.

7. Rudolif AM: Oxygenation in the fetus and the neonate—A perspective. Semin Perinatol 8:158, 1984.

8. Rapaport SI: The red blood cell. *In* Best and Taylor's Physiologic Basis of Medical Practice. (Edited by West JB) Baltimore, Williams and Wilkins, 1985.

9. Sacks LM, Delivoria-Papadopoulos M: Hemoglobin–oxygen interactions. Semin Perinatol 8:168, 1984.

10. Nunn JF: Oxygen. *In* Applied Respiratory Physiology. Boston, Butterworths, 1977.

11. Rooth G, and Sjostedt S: The placental transfer of gases and fixed acids. Arch Dis Child 37:366, 1966.

12. Rooth G: Fetal homeostasis. *In* Clinical Perinatology. (Edited by Aldajem S, Brown AK, and Sureau C) St. Louis, CV Mosby, 1980.

13. Ramanathan S, et al: Oxygen transfer from the mother to fetus during cesarean section under epidural anesthesia. Anesth Analg 63:69, 1982.

14. Thalme B: Electrolyte and acid-base balance in midterm pregnancy women and their fetuses. Acta Obstet Gynecol Scand 45(Suppl 8):55, 1967.

15. Gu W, Jones CT, Parer JT: Metabolic and cardiovascular effects on fetal sheep of sustained reduction of uterine blood flow. J Physiol 368:109, 1985.

16. Edelstone DI: Fetal compensatory responses to reduced oxygen delivery. Semin Perinatol 8:184, 1984.

17. Itskovitz J, LaGamma EF, and Rudolf AM: The effect of reducing umbilical blood flow on fetal oxygenation. Am J Obstet Gynecol 145:813, 1983.

18. Cohn HE, et al.: Cardiovascular responses to hypoxemia and acidemia in fetal lambs. Am J Obstet Gynecol 120:817, 1974.

19. Ralston DH, and Shnider SM: The fetal and neonatal effects of regional anesthesia in obstetrics. Anesthesiology 48:34, 1978.

20. Biehl D, Shnider SM, Levinson G, and Callender K: Placental transfer of lidocaine. Anesthesiology 48:409, 1978.

21. Levinson G, Shnider SM, De Lorimer AA, and Steffenson JL: Effects of maternal hyperventilation on uterine blood flow and fetal oxygenation and acid-base status. Anesthesiology 40:340, 1974.

22. Ralston DH, Shnider SM, and De Lorimer AA: Uterine blood flow and acid-base changes after bicarbonate administration to the pregnant ewe. Anesthesiology 40:348, 1974.

23. Shnider SM, et al: Uterine blood flow and plasma norepinephrine changes during maternal stress in the pregnant ewe. Anesthesiology 50:524, 1979.

24. Ramanathan S, et al: Concentrations of lactate and pyruvate in maternal and neonatal blood with different intravenous fluids used for prehydration before epidural anesthesia. Anesth Analg 63:69, 1984.

25. Mendiola J, Graylock LJ, and Scanlon JW: Effects of intrapartum glucose infusion on normal fetus and the newborn. Anesth Analg 61:32, 1982.

26. Richardson B, Hohimer AR, Muegler B, and Bissonette J: Effects of concentration on fetal breathing movements and electrocortical activity in fetal lambs. Am J Obstet Gynecol 142:678, 1982.

27. Burea MA, Monette J, and Shapcott D: Carboxyhemoglobin concentration in fetal cord blood of mothers who smoked during labor. Pediatrics 69:371, 1982.

4

PERINATAL PHARMACOLOGY AND SYSTEMIC MEDICATION

Many anesthetic and nonanesthetic drugs used on obstetric patients readily cross the placenta and may produce both short and long-term effects in the fetus and the neonate. The long-term teratogenic effects are discussed in Chapter 18. This chapter will focus on factors that influence the transfer of drugs across the placenta as well as the fetal uptake, distribution, and metabolism of commonly used drugs. Also discussed are the neonatal effects of these drugs with special emphasis on the central nervous system.

General Characteristics and Effects of Perinatal Medication

FACTORS REGULATING PLACENTAL TRANSFER OF DRUGS

Anesthetic drugs and respiratory gases are transferred across the placenta mainly by passive diffusion, regulated by physical and chemical properties of the drug, and physiologic factors relating to the feto-placental unit.

DRUG FACTORS

Increased Lipid Solubility. Increased lipid solubility increases the rate of transfer across the placenta.

Degree of Ionization. The degree of ionization is determined by the pH of the biophase and the pKa of the drug. The relationship between pKa and pH is governed by the Henderson-Hasselbach equation (see Chapter 5). Only the un-ionized form of the drug can cross biologic membranes. Muscle relaxants such as succinylcholine and d-tubocurarine, which are greatly ionized at body pH, undergo only limited placental transfer.

Molecular Weight. Placenta is generally impermeable to substances with molecular weight >1000 and quite permeable to substances with MW <600. The diffusion rate across any membranes varies inversely as the square root of the MW (Graham's law). Most of the local anesthetics have MW <400 and are therefore expected to cross the placenta.

Concentration Gradient. The greater the concentration gradient of free drug across the placenta, the greater is the diffusion across the placenta (Fick's law).

Protein Binding. Many drugs are bound to maternal plasma proteins. It is generally assumed that only the free unbound drug in the maternal circulation is available for transfer. Protein binding is less important for highly lipophilic compounds in preventing placental transfer.[1] For instance, bupivacaine is many times more lipid soluble and protein bound than is lidocaine. The total amounts of the two compounds reaching the fetus from the mother may be the same. Since the local anesthetics may be taken up by the fetal tissues, fetal blood/maternal blood concentration ratio alone may not be a reliable index of transfer across the placenta. Measuring tissue concentration in (animal) models is a more rational approach to quantify placental transfer. Measurement of metabolites in the neonatal urine may also serve as an indirect means of quantifying the net transfer of the drug transferred.[2]

Metabolism in the Mother. Rapid metabolic degradation of the substance in the maternal plasma limits its fetal transfer across the placenta. The classical example is 2-chloroprocaine, which is rapidly hydrolyzed by the maternal plasma limiting its placental transfer.

PLACENTAL FACTORS

The greater the blood flow to the placenta, the greater is the amount of drug delivered to the fetus. More than 75% of uterine blood flow is distributed to the intervillous space from where drugs diffuse across the placenta to the fetus. A reduction in intervillous flow (IVF) may decrease placental transfer of drugs (but at the same time interfere with fetal oxygenation). The reduction in IVF that occurs during a uterine contraction may be used beneficially to limit placental passage of pentothal, meperidine, and diazepam (vide infra). The drug may be intentionally injected at the onset of uterine contraction when the patient is being induced for an emergency cesarean section.[3] Other factors such as thickness of placental membrane and metabolism of the drug by the placental enzymes are not clinically relevant. Barbiturates are degraded by the placenta.[4] The process, however, is readily saturable and offers little or no protection to the fetus. Placental insulinase may limit the transfer of insulin across the placenta.[5]

FETAL UPTAKE OF DRUGS

The distribution of drugs is slightly different in the fetus than it is in the mother. The fetal liver is strategically located in the fetal circulation (see Fig. 25–1). A portion of the drugs reaching the fetus via the umbilical vein may be metabolized by the liver before they are distributed throughout the body. At any given time, the fetal liver will contain a maximum amount of the administered drug, whereas in the adult it accumlates in the kidney.[6]

The fetal plasma contains less α-1 acid glycoprotein, which limits protein-binding[7] and increases the unbound fraction of the local anesthetic.

The fetal blood pH and intracellular pH may be slightly more acidic than the mother's which increases ionized fraction of the drug in the fetal tissues (see Fig. 5–10).

In an asphyxiated fetus the distribution of drugs is considerably different from that in a normal fetus (see Fig. 5–11). These differences, discussed briefly here, are discussed in greater detail in Chapters 3 and 5. Since hypoxia rearranges fetal circulation to maximize blood supply to the brain, the umbilical venous blood flow bypasses the liver resulting in decreased hepatic metabolism. The decreased pH will favor increased formation and trapping of the ionized form of the local anesthetic in the fetal tissues.

The mother and her fetus are exposed to myriads of xenobiotics and environmental toxins every day. Primate fetuses (including humans) have enzymes necessary for biotransformation of many drugs. Sizeable quantities of P-450 have been found in human fetal liver from early gestation.[8] The fetus, however, may lack specific enzyme systems required for efficient handling of certain drugs. For instance, the lack of hydroxylating pathway is probably responsible for the prolonged half-life of mepivacaine in the fetus.

NEUROBEHAVIORAL EFFECTS OF ANESTHETIC AND ADJUVANT DRUGS

The neurobehavior testing procedures are used to elicit subtle CNS depressant effects of anesthetic drugs. Apgar scores are not sensitive enough to detect these changes. Brazelton pioneered the investigation of this area. The Brazelton Neonatal Assessment Scale has formed the basis of many other neonatal neurobehavior assessment systems such as the Early Neonatal Neurobehavioral Scale (ENNS, Scanlon) and the Neurologic and Adaptive Capacity Score (NACS) (Amiel-Tyson Barrier and Shnider).

THE ENNS SYSTEM

In 1974, Scanlon published his report on the effects of local anesthetic drugs on neonatal neurobehavior.[9] This probably acted as a catalyst for the innumerable number of publications that followed on the subject. The ENNS system is mainly based on the infant's ability to adapt to his environmental stimuli. For instance, an infant who receives a light pinprick in the foot withdraws this foot. When the stimulus is repeated again the degree of withdrawal decreases, and continues to decrease with each pinprick, until there is no longer a response to this stimulus. The decremental response (habituation) to the stimulus indicates that the infant is capable of differentiating between benign and harmful stimuli and suitably tailoring responses. The ENNS also includes assessment of reflex responses, muscle tone, and alertness. The examiner must have received special instruction in the scoring system and his evaluation of neonates must yield scores comparable to those obtained by other trained observers. The Early Neonatal Neurobehavioral Scale (ENNS) is comprised of a number of individual observations. The following list describes some of the basic components:

1. Habituation to pinprick, sound, and shining light in the eyes. Score: the higher the number of stimulations before the adaptation occurs, the lower the score is.
2. Reflexes: Rooting, sucking, Moro response.
3. Muscle tone: Resistance against passive motion, pulling to sitting position; arm recoil; truncal tone; general tone.
4. Placing: Flexion of the leg and placing of the foot when a part of the baby's foot is stimulated in the upright position.
5. Alertness: Turning of the head towards the direction of stimulus, widening of eyes, and bright-looking face.
6. General assessment (abnormal, borderline, normal, or superior).

The state of wakefulness must be noted before each individual test is performed. Compared to the Brazelton scoring system, the ENNS puts more emphasis on muscle tone.

NACS

The Neurological and Adaptive Capacity Scores (NACS) were introduced to assess the effects of obstetric medication, perinatal asphyxia, and birth trauma.[10] The specific tests, believed to be useful for this purpose, are those that assess muscle tone in the upper and lower parts of the body. The presence of unilateral or upper body hypotonia may indicate birth trauma or asphyxia rather than drug effect, which produces generalized motor depression. Increased tone in the extensor muscles of the neck may indicate intracranial hypertension. The NACS does not utilize the strongly aversive pinprick stimulus. The Neurologic and Adaptive Capacity Scores (NACS) include the following types of observations:

1. Response and habituation to sound, light, and consolability.
2. Passive tone: Scarf sign, recoil of elbows, popliteal angle, recoil of lower limbs.
3. Active tone: Active contraction of neck flexors and extensors from the leaning-forward position, Palmar grasp, response to traction with the palm grasped, supporting reaction in upright position.
4. Primary reflex: Automatic walking, Moro reflex, sucking.
5. General assessment: Alertness, crying, motor activity.

MATERNAL MEDICATION AND INFANT'S NEUROBEHAVIOR

The effects of maternal medication on infant's neurobehavior has been the subject of innumerable publications in the last 15 years. The results of these studies are conflicting in many instances.[11] The choice of a particular drug for use during regional or general anesthesia must be based on obstetric and anesthetic factors and not solely on the agent's effect on the infant's neurobehavior.

Regional Anesthesia

Scanlon, et al.[9] first reported that maternal epidural anesthesia with lidocaine or mepivacaine reduced neurobehavior scores whereas bupivacaine did not. However, several recent reports have failed to disclose any major difference between the commonly used anesthetics. The report by Scanlon may however have been indirectly responsible for the tremendous increase in popularity of bupivacaine for obstetric anesthesia. The subsequent indiscriminate use of bupivacaine resulted in several maternal deaths (see Chapter 5, Local Anesthetics). Perinatal asphyxia resulting from complications of epidural anesthesia will impair neurobehavior regardless of the local anesthetic being used. Therefore the anesthesiologist must concentrate on optimizing the cardiovascular status of the mother during epidural anesthesia rather than worrying about minor drug effects on the neonate.

Because of the small amount of local anesthetic used, properly conducted spinal anesthesia produces little or no impairment in the neurobehavior scores. Paracervical block, however, is falling into disfavor because of the increased risk of fetal bradycardia. Pudendal block produces smaller blood levels of local anesthetic in the fetus and is therefore not associated with impaired neurobehavior scores.

The use of intrathecal and epidural narcotics alone or in combination with local anesthetics is currently being investigated. Earlier reports have shown that epidural and spinal administration of morphine does not adversely affect neurobehavior scores. At present, however, the experience with these methods is limited. Narcotics are rapidly absorbed into the maternal systemic circulation from where they easily reach the fetus. It is therefore logical to conclude that at comparable maternal systemic blood levels, narcotics will produce the same degree of impairment in neurobehavior, regardless of the route of administration.

General Anesthesia

In contrast to epidural anesthesia, general anesthesia administered for cesarean section or for vaginal delivery is associated with decreased neurobehavior scores in the first 24 hours. Thiopental readily crosses the placenta and may produce impaired neurobehavior. Even the use of N_2O has been implicated in causing a reduction in the neurobehavior scores.[12] Thiopental-N_2O combination causes a greater reduction in neurobehavior scores than does ketamine-N_2O combination.[13] Surprisingly, when halothane, isoflurane, or enflurane were used for supplementing N_2O during cesarean section or vaginal delivery no reduction was found in the Apgar or the neurobehavior scores.[14,15] The use of a halogenated agent probably allows a smaller concentration of N_2O to be used for anesthesia.

Systemic Medication

Depressant drugs such as barbiturates cause a transient decrease in neurobehavior scores. Meperidine alone or in combination with a phenothiazine is commonly used for producing analgesia during labor. Meperidine use is associated with low neurobehavior scores even on the first postpartum day.[16] The combination generally produces lower scores than does meperidine alone.[17] Butorphanol produces similar scores as does meperidine.[18] The maternal use of 5 to 10 mg of diazepam may be associated with decreased muscle tone for a short period of time following delivery. The effects of excessive doses of diazepam are discussed later in the chapter.

CRITIQUE OF NEUROBEHAVIOR SCORING SYSTEMS

In the last 10 to 15 years, numerous reports have been published on the effects of obstetric medication on infant neurobehavior. There are several problems with these studies.

Method. The methods used for evaluating neurobehavior may be somewhat subjective. For instance, in the NACS system, one test item calls for consolability of the infant. In the ENNS system, the general assessment test requires that the examiner conclude how the infant fared (i.e., abnormal, borderline, normal, or superior). Both the ENNS and the NACS systems are simplifications of the original more elaborate Brazelton scoring system, which comprehensively assesses the infant's behavior.

Design. The designs of many of these studies are faulty; many of them lack unmedicated control groups. There is little provision for standardization for obstetric history, perinatal events, and the stress of labor.

Inconclusive Long-term Data. It is currently difficult to speculate if the transient CNS depression produced by obstetric medication has a lasting effect on child development. Ounsted, Scott, and Molar have reported that drugs used for pain relief do not affect mental and physical growth of the baby. Perinatal asphyxia, however, does have a noticeable effect on child development.[19,20]

Systemic Analgesia

A wide variety of substances are used on obstetric patients to produce labor analgesia and anesthesia for delivery. In addition, several drugs, such as antiarrhythmics, antihypertensives, antinauseants, anxiolytics, and other therapeutic drugs are prescribed during pregnancy and labor. The maternal and fetal effects of many of these drugs are discussed in the section on abnormal pregnancy. This section will focus on medications administered in the peripartum period.

SPECIFIC SYSTEMIC DRUGS USED DURING LABOR

Both narcotic analgesics and anxiolytics are used for producing labor analgesia. Narcotics, especially meperidine, are particularly popular as analgesics during labor. They may be used alone or in combination with a phenothiazine or benzodiazepines. Important clinical and physico-chemical properties of narcotics and sedatives used in obstetric patients are summarized in Table 4–1.

MEPERIDINE

Meperidine is safe for the mother and the fetus and is used extensively for labor analgesia world-wide. The dose may have to be repeated systemically every 3 to 4 hours during labor. Epidural use of meperidine is discussed in Chapter 6. Following intravenous administration, the drug is detectable in the fetus in seconds, while maternal and fetal blood concentrations reach equilibrium within 6 minutes. Following intravenous injection of the drug, the maternal plasma level falls rapidly. The peak levels are higher with i.v. administration than with i.m. administration, thus the i.v. route often re-

sults in a greater fetal brain concentration of meperidine than the i.m. route. An effective way of minimizing fetal uptake is to start the injection at the onset of uterine contraction and to then administer the dose over a 2 to 3 minute period.[21,22]

Meperidine is N-dealkylated in the liver to form normeperidine, which is more toxic than the parent compound. Accumulation of normeperidine may cause twitching, especially in patients with renal failure.[23] The neonate also produces a significant amount of normeperidine from maternally administered meperidine[24,25] (Fig. 4–1). In the fetus, the half-life of meperidine and normeperidine are approximately 20 and 60 hours, respectively.[26] Meperidine produces several fetal effects. It may cause diminished baseline variability of the fetal heart rate, or it may affect the fetal electroencephalogram (EEG) and diminish infant neurobehavior scores (vide supra). The EEG effects include an increase in θ waves and burst suppression. These effects may last up to 60 minutes following administration of meperidine.[27] In most instances, these effects are not clinically significant and it is unlikely that 50 to 100 mg of meperidine administered for labor analgesia will produce long-term effects in the baby.[28]

The time interval between administration of meperidine to the mother and delivery of the baby has been shown to influence neonatal Apgar scores.[29] When the baby is born within an hour after i.m. administration of meperidine to the mother, neonatal depression is less likely to occur than if the interval is greater than 2 hours. Although the reason for this is not known, it is likely that when the interval increases, the fetal uptake of meperidine also increases, leading to neonatal depression. This is evidenced by the following facts: (1) as the time interval between injection and delivery increases the umbilical artery blood level of meperidine will equal or exceed that in the umbilical vein, indicating high tissue levels in the fetus (the UA blood is in equilibrium with fetal tissues); and (2) the neonate excretes the maximum amount of meperidine and normeperidine in the tissue when the injection-delivery interval is between 2 to 3 hours.[25]

Morphine

Morphine is no longer used for producing labor analgesia. Although equianalgesic doses of

Table 4–1. Maternal and Fetal Effects of Drugs Used in Obstetric Anesthesia

Drug	Part. coeff	Protein binding	Dose		Onset		Duration		Metabolites		Fetal effects	Remarks
			IM	IV	IM	IV	IM	IV	Mother	Fetus/Neonate		
Narcotics												
Meperidine	38.8	58%	50 mg	25 mg	45 min	10 min	3 hrs	2 hrs	Normeperidine	Normeperidine	Prolonged effect on neurobehavior	Extensively used. Fetal depression likely if delivery occurs 2 hours after injection.
Morphine	1.42	35%	10 mg	3–5 mg	1 hr	30 min	5 hrs	4 hrs	Glucuronide	Glucuronide	More potent depressant than meperidine	Rarely used
Oxymorphone	—	—	1 mg	0.5 mg	1 hr	30 min	4 hrs	4 hrs	Glucuronide	Glucuronide	More potent depressant than meperidine	Rarely used
Alphaprodine	—	—	30 mg	15 mg	—	5 min	—	2 hrs	Normeperidine	Normeperidine	Potent depressant	Maternal apnea
Fentanyl	813	60%	100 μg	50 μg	10 min	5 min	1 hr	30 min	Hepatic degradation	Hepatic degradation		May be used for sedation before the birth of the baby during cesarean section.
Butorphanol	100	80%	2 mg	1 mg	10 min	5 min	4 hrs	3 hrs	Norbutorphanol Hydroxybutorphanol			Maternal drowsiness
Sedatives												
Diazepam	—	99%	NR	5 mg	—	5 min	—	45 min	Desmethyldiazepam	Desmethyldiazepam	Neonatal hypotonia and impaired thermogenesis in high doses.	
Promethazine	High	83%	50 mg	25 mg	20 min	20 min	5 hrs	5 hrs	Hydroxylation and conjugation leading to sulphoxide formation.	—	Safe	Maternal hypotension. Widely used in combination with meperidine.
Hydroxyzine	High	—	50	NR	30 min	—	4 hrs	—	—	—	No major effects	May be used for maternal sedation
Thiopental	High	80%	—	4 mg/kg	—	Immediate	—	5 min	Liver	Liver	No major effect in clinical doses.	Induction agent for general anesthesia
Ketamine (Analgesia)				15 mg increments	—	1 min	—	5 min	N-demethylation in the liver	N-demethylation in the liver	No major effects	
Ketamine (Anesthesia)				1 mg/kg	—	1–2 min	—	5 min			No major effects; high doses may produce neonatal hypertonia.	Psychotomimetic side effects in excessive doses.

NR: Not recommended.

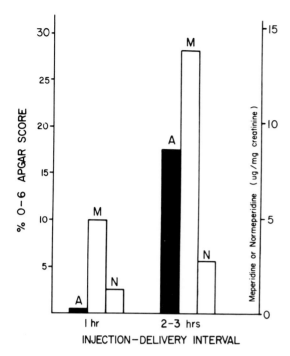

FIG. 4–1. Percentage of neonates with low Apgar scores (A) and neonatal blood meperidine (M) and normeperidine (N) levels at different injection-delivery intervals.[20,21,25]

Fentanyl

Fentanyl is a highly lipid soluble phenylpiperidine derivative (similar to meperidine). It has a rapid onset and a short duration of action. It crosses the placenta rapidly and attains a fetal-maternal ratio of approximately 0.4.[31] However, in doses of 1 μg/Kg, it does not affect the neonatal Apgar or neurobehavior scores significantly. The possible uses of these drugs in pregnant patients includes the sedation during regional anesthesia before the infant is delivered, and the production of analgesia in patients with renal impairment. The drug is rapidly metabolized by the liver and only 10% appears unchanged in the urine.[32] Unlike meperidine, fentanyl has little or no potential for cumulative toxicity in patients with renal disease. In addition, even high doses have little effect on renal function. Fentanyl may be particularly useful in patients with cardiac disease in whom the use of thiopental for induction of obstetric anesthesia may be hazardous. Fentanyl is also useful for sedating patients with cardiac disease before the infant is delivered.

different narcotics produce similar effects on the CO_2 response curve, neonates are more depressed with maternal morphine administration than with meperidine administration. The difference is perhaps related to the prolonged duration of action of morphine.[28] The delayed onset of action following i.v. injection makes it difficult to precisely adjust the dose.

Alphaprodine and Anileridine

These two phenylpiperidines are meperidine congeners. The onset of action of alphaprodine (Nisentil) is faster and its duration of action shorter than that of meperidine. Because of unpredictable absorption, the i.m. route is not recommended. The drug may cause apnea even in clinical doses. A sinusoidal fetal heart rate pattern has been associated with this agent.[30] Anileridine, another congener of meperidine, is 2.5 times more potent than meperidine. The agent is believed to produce more fetal CNS depression than meperidine.

Butorphanol (Stadol)

Unlike the metabolites of meperidine, butorphanol's metabolites (norbutorphanol and hydroxybutorphanol) are pharmacologically inactive. In addition, when used for producing labor analgesia, the incidence of nausea and vomiting is less with the use of this agent than with meperidine.[18] However, the drug causes significant drowsiness, which may limit its use in obstetric patients. One mg of butorphanol possesses the same analgesic activity as 40 mg of meperidine. Butorphanol crosses the placenta readily and produces similar neonatal effects as does meperidine.[33] Butorphanol has a ceiling effect on the CO_2 response curve. Increasing the dose beyond 4 mg is not necessarily associated with increasing respiratory depression.[34] This may be caused by the antagonistic action of butorphanol on the μ-opioid receptors (see Chapter 6). Thus, its use is contraindicated in narcotic addicts. The ceiling effect has little practical use in obstetrics because of the possible ceiling effect on analgesia as well.

Pentazocine

Pentazocine is a potent benzomorphone which stimulates κ- and σ-receptors but slightly antagonizes the action of the μ-receptors. Its use must therefore be avoided in narcotic addicts (see Table 6–1). Pentazocine is three times less potent than morphine. Pentazocine has no definite advantages over meperidine and closely resembles meperidine in its ability to cause maternal and neonatal CNS depression. The drug readily crosses the placenta and was never widely used in obstetrics.

Nalbuphine

Nalbuphine (Nubaine) is a new synthetic narcotic with agonist-antagonist properties. It stimulates κ- and σ-receptors and antagonizes the μ-receptor activity. It is chemically related to naloxone and oxymorphone. Like butorphanol, its tendency to respiratory depression is limited by a ceiling effect, which is especially apparent in increasing doses.[35] Its potency and dosage requirements are similar to that of morphine. There are very few studies available on the use of nalbuphine in obstetrics.

NARCOTIC ANTAGONISTS

Naloxone

In contrast to nalorphine, naloxone is a pure antagonist without agonistic properties. The duration of action of naloxone is only 30 to 60 min. Most potent narcotics will last longer than naloxone, thus resulting in possible redevelopment of respiratory depression, following a seemingly successful reversal with naloxone. The agent crosses the placenta and is detectable within minutes in the infant. Administration of naloxone to the babies exposed to narcotics in utero has been shown to reverse subclinical respiratory depression.[36]

It has been recommended that naloxone be prophylactically administered to the mother (5 to 8 μg/Kg) to antagonize fetal effects of narcotic administered to the mother during labor.[37] However, such a practice is associated with disadvantages. Naloxone reverses maternal analgesia rapidly rendering the patient uncooperative. Should general anesthesia become necessary for vaginal delivery, the anesthesiologist may not be able to use a narcotic and will be forced to use an inhalational agent. Not all the babies are depressed following the maternal administration of meperidine. Sudden reversal of narcotic depression with naloxone may lead to vomiting, hypertension, ventricular arrhythmias, and even pulmonary edema.[38] Fetal β-endorphin levels increase during hypoxic distress.[39] Reversal of the respiratory depressant effects of β-endorphins with naloxone may lead to increased fetal breathing movements and increased chances of fetal intrauterine pulmonary aspiration. Because naloxone has a short duration of action, the newborn may develop either signs of respiratory depression and/or impaired neurobehavior in the second hour after birth, thus prophylactic administration of naloxone to the mother seems unwarranted. A more rational approach is to administer naloxone to the neonate only when it seems to require it.

TRANQUILIZERS

Tranquilizers include benzodiazepines, phenothiazines, hydroxyzines, and certain barbiturates.

Benzodiazepines

The benodiazepines to be discussed here are diazepam, midazolam, lorazepam.

Diazepam. Diazepam is used for producing sedation in the mother. The drug is also an anticonvulsant and produces some skeletal muscle relaxation. The presence of a specific central nervous system (CNS) benzodiazepine receptor has been postulated. The mechanism of action of all benzodiazepines is believed to be related to their ability to facilitate the action of inhibitory neurotransmitters in the brain, which are γ-aminobutyric acid (GABA) and glycine. Facilitation of glycine action produces skeletal muscle relaxation, whereas facilitation of GABA action produces anticonvulsant and sedative activity.

Diazepam crosses the placenta rapidly and accumulates in the fetus. Both diazepam and its metabolite desmethyldiazepam may persist in the neonate for days.[40] Although doses less than 10 mg are readily metabolized, doses greater than 30 mg, which are administered over several hours, cause accumulation of the drug in the fetus. This produces the following problems: loss of baseline variability of the fetal heart rate; neonatal hypotonia; poor feeding; impaired neonatal thermogenesis in response to cold stress; a decrease in the respiratory quotient signifying fat metabolism; neonatal hypotonia; and neonatal hypothermia[41] (Fig. 4–2).

Diazepam may be useful when sedating an apprehensive patient who will be undergoing a cesarean section that is performed under regional anesthesia. Diazepam, used in moderate amounts (<5 mg), for this purpose, is unlikely to produce any serious maternal or neonatal side effects. Diazepam is particularly useful during induction of general anesthesia in patients with severe cardiac disease, since the drug only minimally depresses the cardiovascular system. In comparison, the use of thiopental may lead to cardiovascular collapse under these circumstances. Diazepam may also be combined with fen-

tanyl for a safe induction in such patients (see Chapter 12). In contrast to prolonged administration lasting several hours, a single injection of diazepam (0.3 mg/kg) just prior to the delivery of the infant is less likely to cause neonatal problems.[42] This may be related to the smaller neonatal/maternal blood ratio (0.5) and the decreased likelihood for accumulation of desmethyldiazepam in the neonate when diazepam is administered as a single bolus. It is, however, advisable to carefully monitor the body temperature of the neonates of mothers who received diazepam prior to delivery and also to institute remedial measures for hypothermia, as well.

Midazolam. Midazolam is more water soluble than diazepam and is therefore less likely to produce phlebitis. The drug is rapidly absorbed following intravenous or intramuscular administration and produces little irritation at the site of

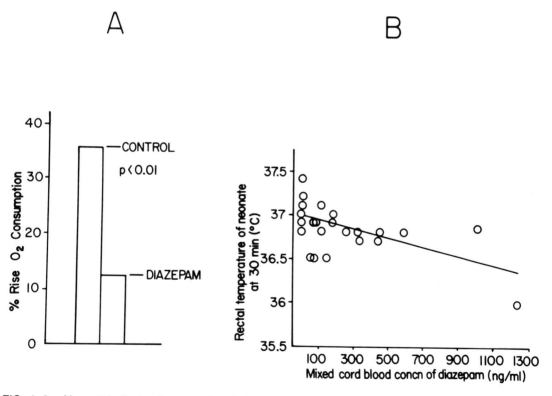

FIG. 4–2. Neonatal effects of maternally administered diazepam. A: The effect of diazepam on neonatal thermogenesis in response to cold. Note diminished thermogenesis in babies whose mothers received diazepam (Source Cree IE, Myer J, and Hailey DM: Diazepam in labour. Its metabolism and effect on the clinical condition and thermogenesis of the newborn. Br Med J *IV*:251, 1973.) B: The influence of blood diazepam levels on the neonate's body temperature. P = statistical significance. (Modified from McAllister CB: Placental transfer and neonatal effects of diazepam when administered to women just before delivery. Br J Anaesth *52*:423, 1980.)

injection. The experience of using this drug with obstetric patients is limited. When administered to patients undergoing cesarean section under epidural anesthesia, the drug produces profound sedation.[43]

Lorazepam. Lorazepam produces excellent sedation and minimal cardiorespiratory depression, thus it may be useful in sedating patients with cardiac disease. Its half-life is shorter than diazepam and is conjugated to glucuronide before elimination.[44] Although the drug rapidly crosses the placenta, it has little tendency to accumulate in the fetus.[44] However, the drug has been implicated in producing feeding problems and neonatal respiratory depression.[45] It offers no specific advantage over diazepam.

Phenothiazines

These drugs have significant H-1 antihistaminic action and possess anxiolytic, antiemetic, and atropine-like activity. Phenothiazines like prochlorperazine, chlorpromazine, and promazine (Sparine) may also produce systemic hypotension because of their weak α-adrenolytic activity. Phenothiazines have been administered to a large number of pregnant patients without any adverse fetal or neonatal effects.[46]

Promethazine (Phenergan) is believed to stimulate respiration.[28] It is used in combination with meperidine for labor analgesia and has been found to reduce meperidine dose requirement. Promethazine by itself, however, has mild antianalgesia action and should therefore not be administered alone to patients in pain.[47] The side effects of promethazine include aching limbs, ataxia, and dry mouth. Prochlorperazine (Compazine) and diphenhydramine (Benadryl) are used to treat nausea in postpartum patients. The promethazine-meperidine combination produces greater impairment in the neonatal score than meperidine alone. Promethazine crosses the placenta rapidly, causing maternal-fetal equilibrium to occur within 15 minutes.[28]

Hydroxyzine (Vistaril)

Although not a phenothiazine, this drug does have antihistaminic properties. It is useful for relieving anxiety in pregnant patients. Because of its irritant properties, the drug must not be used intravenously, which has made it somewhat unpopular. The usual i.m. dose is 50 mg and at this dose it does not produce any adverse fetal effects. Unlike promethazine the drug does not have antianalgesic properties. Used with meperidine the drug produces excellent maternal sedation without increasing fetal depression.[28]

Barbiturates

The barbiturates have enjoyed great popularity as sedative-hypnotic agents. They are, however, rapidly being replaced by benzodiazepines. The use of short and intermediate acting barbiturates (pentobarbital, amobarbital, secobarbital) are no longer popular because of their depressant effects on mother and fetus. The addition of a narcotic to barbiturates further increases the risk of maternal and fetal depression. High doses of barbiturates are associated with prolonged fetal depression lasting 2 to 3 days. Barbiturates when administered to patients with pain may produce excitation. Extremely short-acting barbiturates, such as pentothal, are still used for induction of general anesthesia in pregnant patients.

Barbiturates are weak acids with a pKa equal to or slightly higher than body pH and they readily cross the placenta. The protein binding of barbiturates is more extensive in the mother (98%) than in the fetus (87%). Highly lipid-soluble barbiturates (such as pentothal) reach equilibrium with fetal tissues much earlier than the less lipid soluble ones (such as pentobarbital). Following a single intravenous administration to the mother, pentothal is detectable in the umbilical vein blood within 30 seconds and its peak level may be reached within a minute (Fig. 4–3). Christensen and his colleagues, found that the UV blood concentration at delivery was approximately equal to maternal venous blood concentration.[48] They also noted that the fetal concentration fell much slower than the maternal venous concentration (Fig. 4–4).

Although pentothal crosses the placenta rapidly, it does not produce significant fetal CNS depression if the total dose used does not exceed 4 mg/Kg. Since the UV blood levels rapidly attain equilibrium with maternal levels, it is impossible to deliver the baby before barbiturates have crossed in amounts that significantly affect the baby. Although the UV blood levels decrease rapidly, the fetal tissue levels may continue to

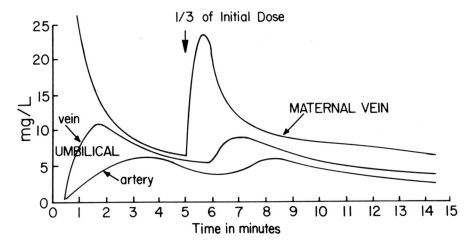

FIG. 4–3.   Maternal and fetal blood levels of thiobarbiturates. Fetal blood levels reach peak within 2 to 3 minutes following maternal administration. Note that a repeat injection of one third of the initial dose causes the blood level to rise to the original level in the mother and the fetus. (Modified from Kosaka Y et al.: Intravenous thiobarbiturate anesthesia for cesarean section. Anesthesiology 31:489, 1969.)

rise for up to 40 minutes.[49] Following maternal administration, the fetal capillary blood (tissue)/maternal venous concentration ratio may reach 0.8 at 2 hours. The injection-delivery interval may influence the MV/UV ratio in the fetus (Fig. 4–5). The longer the injection-delivery interval, the higher the neonatal/maternal ratio will be, which suggests an ongoing net transfer of drug to the fetus in utero.[42] However, if the total dose does not exceed 4 mg/kg, no serious fetal effects

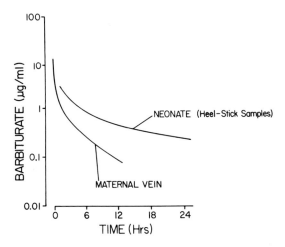

FIG. 4–4.   The thiobarbiturate level declines in the maternal and fetal blood following maternal injection. Note the slower fall of concentration in the neonate. (Modified from Christensen JH, et al.: Pharmacokinetics of thiopental in cesarean section. Acta Anesth Scand, 25:174, 1981.)

may occur. Repeated doses of pentothal, however, may lead to neonatal depression. One third of the original dose is sufficient to increase the fetal level, returning it to normal.[50] When used in equipotent doses, there is little difference between methohexital and pentothal, with respect to their neonatal effects.[51]

Barbiturates with high lipid solubility, such as thiopental, are metabolized by the liver. Thiopental may also undergo biotransformation in the brain, lung, and other tissues; oxybarbiturates, however, undergo only hepatic degradation. The process of awakening from thiopental effect, however, is not caused by metabolism of the drug but by the rapid redistribution to body tissues which results in reduction of the concentration of the agent in the brain. Side chain oxidation, the most important degradation pathway, terminates the biologic activity of the very short-acting barbiturate.[52] Less lipid soluble agents, such as phenobarbital, may be excreted by the kidneys unchanged. Alkalinization of the urine may hasten their excretion.

Ketamine

This phencyclidine derivative has gained limited popularity as an analgesic during vaginal delivery and also as an inducing agent during general anesthesia for cesarean section. Ketamine may be particularly suitable for induction in patients who are hypovolemic or in those with

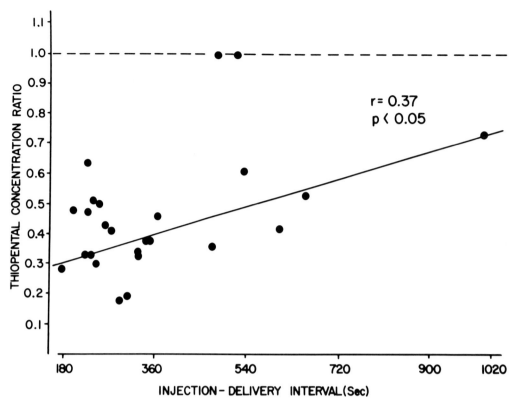

FIG. 4–5. Neonatal/maternal thiopental blood concentration ratio following maternal injection. (From Bakke OM, Haram K, and Wallem G: Comparison of the placental transfer of thiopental and diazepam in caesarean section. Eur J Clin Pharmacol, *21*:221, 1981.)

a history of asthma (see Chapter 15). Thiopental may cause severe hypotension in patients who are hypovolemic, whereas ketamine may not cause such a drastic reduction in blood pressure in these patients. Ketamine may, however, lead to tissue lactic acidosis by causing peripheral vasoconstriction.[53] Thus, the use of ketamine does not replace the need for optimization of circulating volume in hypovolemic patients. The analgesic dose is usually 0.25 mg/kg and the induction dose is 1 mg/kg.[54] Although ketamine increases the blood pressure it does not appreciably alter uterine blood flow.[55] Ketamine should be avoided in patients with preeclampsia. In early pregnancy, ketamine increases the uterine tone, but such an effect is not seen in doses up to 2 mg/kg when pregnancy is close to term.[56] After the baby is born, the uterus becomes more sensitive to the stimulating action of the drug.[57] Ketamine crosses the placenta but does not produce neonatal depression unless the total dose exceeds 1 to 1.5 mg/kg.[58] At higher doses, low Apgar scores, neonatal depression, and muscular hypertonicity may be seen.

When used for producing labor analgesia, ketamine is injected in 10 to 15 mg increments (total dose <100 mg) until the patient is comfortable.[59] When ketamine is carefully titrated, the mother does not lose consciousness. Laryngeal reflexes remain active. Troublesome side effects such as dreams and hallucinations are usually not a problem. When used for cesarean section, the neonatal neurobehavior scores are slightly higher than those obtained with pentothal.[13] It is unlikely that ketamine will replace thiopental as an inducing agent because of the high incidence of side-effects (hallucinations, dreams).

Ketamine has been recommended to be used for supplementing "spotty" regional anesthesia. Such a practice may be associated with risks because when the regional block is inadequate it may be necessary to exceed the 1 mg/kg dose of ketamine to produce ideal operating conditions. At this dose, one can no longer be sure that laryngeal protective reflexes are intact. In addition, the incidence of hallucinatory side-effects and neonatal depression may increase. The safest method of managing a spotty block is to either readminister the block (if time permits) or to administer endotracheal general anesthesia. Mental illness complicates 1:1000 pregnancies, mainly in the form of puerperal psychoses. Fear, anxiety, and the subconscious rejection of the pregnancy predispose to this condition. The precipitating factor, which tilts the mental balance toward psychoses, is the birth of the infant. The use of a psychotomimetic drug, such as ketamine, must be used with great caution in pregnant patients who seem emotionally unstable.

MUSCLE RELAXANTS

Muscle relaxants (Table 4–2) are quaternary ammonium compounds and are therefore fully ionized at body pH, which limits their placental transfer. Other factors, which limit the placental transfer of muscle relaxants, are protein binding and low lipid solubility. When administered in clinically useful doses to the mother, the muscle relaxants do not cause any significant muscle paralysis in the newborn. However, when large doses are used over a prolonged period of time, the fetus may be paralyzed in utero and develop contracture of the limbs, or arthrogryposis (see Chapter 17).

Succinylcholine

Of the currently available muscle relaxants, succinylcholine provides excellent conditions for tracheal intubation in the shortest period of time, which makes it an ideal agent for rapid sequence induction in obstetric patients. The drug is administered in 1 to 1.5 mg/kg bolus to facilitate tracheal intubation. A continuous infusion of succinylcholine may be employed to maintain paralysis throughout the procedure. Pregnancy reduces plasma pseudocholinesterase concentrations. However, the enzyme is qualitatively normal and the dibucaine number is within normal range. Thus, in most patients, degradation of the drug proceeds at a normal rate.[60] In patients with atypical pseudocholinesterase, the drug may lead to maternal and neonatal skeletal muscle impairment.[61]

Continuous infusion of succinylcholine has been popular for maintenance of paralysis during cesarean section. An electrical nerve stimulator must be used not only to carefully titrate the infusion rate, but also for the early detection of phase-II block. Phase-II block occurs with increased frequency in those with pseudocholinesterase deficiency. The nerve stimulator may also be used to ensure sufficient recovery of the neuromuscular junction from depolarizing block before a nondepolarizing agent is administered. Monitoring of the neuromuscular junction is more fully discussed in Chapter 10.

Succinylcholine does cross the placenta but not in quantities sufficient to cause neonatal problems.[62] The rapid hydrolysis of the drug in the maternal plasma probably limits the transfer. The neonatal concentration is only 4% of peak maternal concentration.[62] The injection-delivery time does not prolong the fetal uptake.[62]

d-Tubocurarine (dTC)

This nondepolarizing blocker is used (3 mg) for minimizing succinylcholine fasciculations

Table 4–2. Muscle Relaxants in Obstetric Anesthesia

Drug	Dose (mg/kg)	Plasma concentration (μg/ml)			I-D interval and fetal uptake	Paralyzing concentration
		MV	UV	UA		
Succinylcholine	1–1.5	1	0.6		No effect	2.0
d-tubocurarine*	0.2–0.3	1.92	0.24	0.11	Increases	
Gallamine	1.5	5.1	1.8		Not known	
Pancuronium	0.07	0.34	0.27	0.05	Increases	1.3
Vecuronium	0.06	0.16	0.02	0.01	No effect	1.4
Atracurium	0.3	1.32	0.11		? no effect	0.29
Fazadinium	1.0	1.81	0.32	0.23	No effect	2.0

*—values given are for [14c]dimethyltubocurarine. Plasma concentrations in maternal vein (V), neonatal umbilical vein (UV), and umbilical artery (UA), obtained at the time of delivery approximately 6 minutes after injection. Note that plasma concentrations in the UA are lower than that required to cause muscle paralysis.

and for producing muscle relaxation during general anesthesia for cesarean section (9–15 mg). The d-tubocurarine crosses the placenta (Table 4–2) slowly. Following maternal injection, the drug may not be detectable in fetal plasma at 6 minutes, and at 9 minutes it may reach 10 to 15% of maternal concentration. It does not, however, produce any neonatal problems as long as the maternal dose does not exceed 15 mg. Unlike pancuronium, the drug does not cause tachycardia. General anesthesia is usually maintained in light planes not only to avoid fetal depression but to minimize uterine relaxation. Since light anesthesia is often associated with tachycardia, use of d-tubocurarine is particularly suitable in obstetric patients. The dimethyl ether of d-tubocurarine (metocurine), which is 2.5 times more potent than dTC has been used in obstetric patients. It is believed to cause less histamine release than the dTC. The drug achieves a fetal/maternal ratio of 0.12 following maternal administration.[63]

Pancuronium

Pancuronium may be used for maintaining muscle paralysis. It may also be used for facili-tating intubation in patients in whom succinyl-choline may be contraindicated (burns, neuro-muscular disease). Succinylcholine, however, is a more reliable agent for tracheal intubation than pancuronium because of its faster onset. Pancuronium crosses the placenta (Table 4–2), but when used in clinical doses, fetal blood concentrations are insufficient to produce muscle paralysis in the infant.[64] Neonatal/maternal concentration ratios of pancuronium increase with increasing injection-delivery interval, suggesting a continuing placental transfer of the agent (Fig. 4–6).[64] The uptake of pancuronium by the fetal liver limits its accumulation in the other fetal tissues.[64]

Vecuronium

Vecuronium (Org NC 45): This nondepolarizing relaxant may also be used in obstetric patients. Since it causes minimum cardiovascular effects, it is particularly suitable for use in cardiac patients. It has potential advantages in patients with renal failure which are discussed in Chapter 22. The drug readily crosses the placenta,[65] but at maternal clinical doses, it does

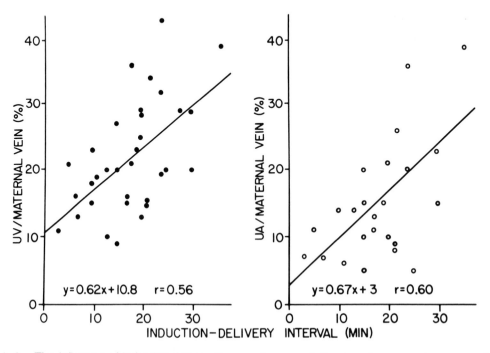

FIG. 4–6. The influence of induction-delivery time on the neonatal/maternal pancuronium concentration ratio. UV = umbilical vein; UA = umbilical artery. (From Duvaldstein M, et al.: The placental transfer of pancuronium and its pharmacokinetics during cesarean section. Acta Anaesth Scand, 22:327, 1978.)

not cause neonatal neuromuscular blockade problems. Unlike pancuronium, the injection-delivery time does not seem to increase the fetal/maternal concentration ratio.

Atracurium

This muscle relaxant has been used in obstetric patients.[66] Since it undergoes rapid Hoffman hydrolysis in the plasma, it may be useful in patients with myasthenia gravis (see Chapter 17), renal disease (see Chapter 22), or pseudocholinesterase deficiency. The drug crosses the placenta (Table 4–2), but at clinical maternal doses, it does not produce neonatal sequelae.

Other Muscle Relaxants

Fazadinium is a nondepolarizing muscle relaxant with a rapid onset and a duration of 30 minutes. Although it does not cause systemic hypotension, it may produce significant vagal blockade and tachycardia. It offers no specific advantages over the newer muscle relaxants. The agent crosses the placenta and achieves a fetal/maternal ratio of approximately 0.2. The fetal drug concentration does not increase with the injection-delivery interval.[67]

ANTICHOLINESTERASES AND ANTICHOLINERGICS

Neostigmine is the most commonly used anticholinesterase for reversing muscle relaxants. Atropine and glycopyrrolate are used for minimizing their muscarinic side effects. Atropine crosses the placental barrier readily and crosses transient fetal tachycardia. The fetal/maternal ratio attains 0.93 at 5 minutes reaching equilibrium at 10 minutes.[68,69] Glycopyrrolate attains a fetal/maternal ratio of only 0.13. Neostigmine, which is fully ionized at body pH, crosses the placenta poorly. Since both glycopyrrolate and neostigmine cross the placenta poorly, a mixture of both agents may be used for reversing the muscle relaxants in patients who undergo nonobstetric surgery (see Chapter 21). Scopolamine, which was once popular for sedating patients during labor, is no longer used because of severe delirium that accompanies its use. Physostigmine is used for treating scopolamine induced delirium. Physostigmine has also been used to reverse the effects of diazepam, droperidol, and ketamine.

When administered to the mother, both scopolamine and atropine produce loss of baseline variability of the fetal heart rate. Physostigmine administration to the mother can restore the baseline variability to normal. Since neostigmine crosses the placental barrier poorly, it is ineffective in this regard.

INHALATION AGENTS

Volatile anesthetics, such as halothane, enflurane, isoflurane, methoxyflurane, diethyl ether, trichlorethylene, and chloroform have been used in obstetrical patients (Table 4–3). Those agents currently being used are halothane, enflurane, and isoflurane. Nitrous oxide has been used widely. By suitably adjusting the inhaled concentration, the anesthetics may be used for producing analgesia or anesthesia (Table 4–3). Analgesic concentrations are usually smaller than anesthetic concentrations. An increase in cardiac output associated with pregnancy retards anesthetic uptake rate from the alveoli, however, the reduction in FRC and the increase in minute ventilation overrides the effect of cardiac output, resulting in an increased anesthetic uptake rate in pregnancy (see Chapter 2). In addition, minimum alveolar concentration (MAC) is reduced 20 to 30% in pregnancy, possibly because of elevated plasma levels of β-endorphin and/or progesterone, which both have sedative effects.

Analgesia

An acceptable and safe degree of analgesia may be produced during the first and second stage of labor with judicious use of analgesic concentrations of these agents. This form of analgesia has always been more popular in the United Kingdom than in the United States. Since the patient does not lose consciousness, the presence of an anesthesiologist or other trained personnel is not necessary. In addition, this method of analgesia is useful in patients who refuse regional anesthesia or in situations where regional anesthesia may be contraindicated (i.e., coagulopathy, anatomic abnormalities of the lumbodorsal spine). However, this method is becoming outmoded because of the increasing

Table 4–3.   Inhalation Anesthesias for Obstetrics

Agent	MW	Solubility Coefficients		% Inhaled	
		Blood/gas	Oil/gas	Analgesia	Anesthesia
Nitrous oxide	44	0.47	1.4	50.0	60.0
Cyclopropane	42	0.42	11.2	5.0	10.0
Isoflurane	185	1.4	99.0	0.5	1.0
Enflurane	185	1.8	99.0	0.5	1.0
Halothane	200	2.3	224.0	—	0.5
Methoxyflurane	165	13.0	825.0	0.35	0.4
Diethyl ether	74	12.1	65.0	1.0	2.5

Concentrations are percent inspired. Anesthetic concentrations for volatile agents are based on concomitant N_2O-oxygen use.

popularity of regional analgesic techniques; the possibility of increased environmental pollution; the risk of abuse by the patient, which may lead to overdose; and the need for availability of properly calibrated equipment for self-administration. The actual use of inhalational analgesia for labor is described in Chapter 8.

Anesthesia

Because of the possible risk of aspiration, inhalation anesthesia must always be delivered via an endotracheal tube. The proper use of inhalation anesthesia for vaginal or cesarean births is described in Chapter 8.

Fetal Effects of Inhalation Agents

Because of their high lipid solubility and low molecular weight, inhalation agents rapidly cross the placenta and accumulate in the fetal brain and other tissues. In analgesic concentrations, they are devoid of major fetal problems because the concentrations used are small.[70] However, when used in anesthetic concentrations, especially for a prolonged period of time, they may produce fetal depression. Fetal effects are negligible when the duration of exposure is 10 minutes or less, and the total MAC (volatile agent + N_2O) does not exceed approximately 1%.[14] The use of a volatile agent in the anesthetic mixture not only helps minimize intraoperative recall but permits the use of greater FIO_2 in the anesthetic mixture. With prolonged administration, the fetal blood concentration increases and approaches maternal blood concentration (Fig. 4–7).

Fetal MAC is less than that of the mother.[71]

Depending on the concentration administered to the mother, the anesthetics may also cause fetal cardiovascular effects. Prolonged anesthesia with halothane or isoflurane may lead to reduction in fetal blood pressure. However, halothane anesthetic will not affect fetal cardiac output or fetal regional blood flow in normoxic neonates.[72] Even when maternal anesthesia lasts 90 minutes, halothane administration does not result in fetal acidosis.[72] However, the use of isoflurane for 1 hour may cause fetal acidosis, probably because of depressed myocardial function.[73]

In order to maximize and maintain oxygen delivery to the brain, the asphyxiated fetus de-

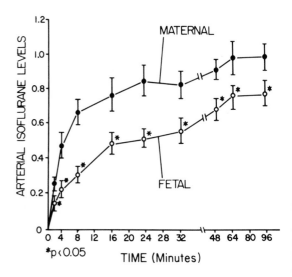

FIG. 4–7.   Time versus increase in fetal blood anesthetic concentration during maternal administration. (From Biehl DR, et al.: The uptake of isoflurane in the fetal lamb in utero: Effect on regional blood flow. Can Anaesth Soc J, *30*:581, 1983.)

velops hypertension and increases its cerebral blood flow (see Chapter 3). Since general anesthesia is often used for cesarean section for fetal distress, it is important to know the effects of general anesthetics on the fetal hypoxic circulatory adaptations. Exposure of the asphyxiated fetus to halothane will usually abolish the fetal hypertensive response to asphyxia without significantly altering the cardiac output so long as the total duration of exposure does not exceed 15 minutes.[7] Halothane and N_2O exposure does not interfere with the increase in cerebral blood flow caused by asphyxia.[75] The use of N_2O prior to delivery of a distressed fetus may however reduce the maternal F_{IO_2}, thereby further interfering with fetal oxygenation.

Inhalation Agents and Uterine Contractility

Nitrous oxide and cyclopropane do not affect myometrial contractility significantly. Halogenated volatile agents are potent myometrial depressants. Equipotent concentrations of halothane, enflurane, and isoflurane produce equal degrees of myometrial depression.[76] However, significant myometrial depression is seen only when the concentration exceeds one MAC in oxygen. The use of 0.5% halothane, 1% enflurane and 0.75% isoflurane in combination with N_2O is usually not associated with increased intraoperative bleeding from the uterus.[14] At these concentrations, the myometrium will respond to exogenously administered oxytocin.[77] Only at excessive concentrations of halothane (1.6%) and of enflurane (3%) is myometrial response to oxytocin diminished. Thus the use of high concentrations of halogenated hydrocarbons may lead to postpartum hemorrhage.

Specific Indications for Volatile Agents in Obstetrics

Although halogenated anesthetics may be employed routinely for cesarean section without fear of adverse fetal or neonatal effects, there are situations where their ability to relax the myometrium may be specially taken advantage of. These situations include the following: anesthesia for the delivery of the entrapped head during a breech delivery; manual removal of the placenta; performing internal version of the second twin after the first one has already been born; and uterine tetany (see Chapter 19). Halogenated agents are also useful in patients with asthma (see Chapter 15).

Individual Agents

Important data with respect to clinical use of inhalation agents are listed in Table 4–3.

Nitrous Oxide. Nitrous oxide may be used for labor analgesia and for anesthesia for cesarean section or vaginal delivery. Because of its low blood gas solubility, its brain concentration rises rapidly. Recovery from the effects of N_2O is faster than recovery from agents with higher solubility. The disadvantage of N_2O is that it is a weak anesthetic requiring at least 50% concentration for labor analgesia and 60 to 70% for anesthesia during cesarean section, which limits the F_{IO_2} in the anesthetic mixture. The incidence of maternal awareness is 5 to 20% when N_2O alone is used for general anesthesia. The agent crosses the placenta rapidly and the fetal tissue concentration reaches 87% of maternal concentration in 20 minutes.[78] In animal experiments, the use of N_2O has been shown to result in the death of a severely asphyxiated fetus.[75] Caution is therefore advised in administering this agent for anesthesia or for delivery of a distressed fetus.

Another theoretical problem with the maternal use of N_2O is its rapid elimination from the neonatal lungs at birth. Although neonatal diffusion hypoxia has never been reported, neonates must be closely watched for cyanosis after birth.

Cyclopropane. Once popular in obstetrics, this agent is no longer used because it is flammable and produces cardiac arrhythmias, nausea, vomiting, and fetal depression, even when the administration lasts only five minutes. When anesthetic concentration is used, 70% of neonates may be depressed if the administration lasts 20 minutes before delivery.[79]

Trichlorethylene. This potent agent produces excellent analgesia and was once popular for obstetric analgesia and anesthesia. It is no longer available in this country because it produces toxic products when used with soda lime, and it may cause cardiac arrhythmias.

Methoxyflurane. This highly lipid-soluble agent was very popular in obstetric anesthesia because of its excellent analgesic properties. The agent is extensively metabolized to inorganic fluoride ion, which is implicated in causing high output renal failure. Although renal failure has not been reported in obstetric patients, serum inorganic fluoride (F⁻) levels may reach potentially nephrotoxic levels in some patients.[80] (The effects of inhalation agents on renal function are discussed in Chapter 22.) Following maternal methoxyflurane anesthesia, neonates also excrete increased concentrations of F⁻ in the urine.[81] Because of the availability of better inhalation agents, methoxyflurane application is currently very limited in obstetrics.

Halothane. Since halothane does not possess analgesic properties at subanesthetic concentrations, it is not suitable for use for producing inhalation analgesia during labor. However, it may be combined with N_2O for producing anesthesia (0.5%) for cesarean section. Concentrations higher than 0.8% may not only produce maternal systemic hypotension but may also result in uterine atony. Halothane may be used in early pregnancy for cerclage procedures. The lack of any adverse fetal effects of halothane even following prolonged administration has been discussed previously.

Enflurane and Isoflurane. This agent has been used for obstetric analgesia and anesthesia. It may be used in 0.5% concentration for producing analgesia and up to 1–2% for cesarean section anesthesia to diminish awareness. Although enflurane releases F⁻, the potential for nephrotoxicity is negligible in patients with normal kidney function. The metabolism of enflurane is more fully discussed in Chapter 22. The experience with isoflurane is limited in obstetric patients. It has been used in a 0.75% inhaled concentration in combination with N_2O for cesarean section anesthesia.[14] Its possible fetal adverse effects have been discussed before.

Oxytocics. Historically, ergot alkaloids were the first agents to be used for initiating or accelerating labor. However, oxytocin has become the drug of choice for this purpose. Ergot preparations are mainly used to augment postpartum or postabortal uterine contractions. Prostaglandins are mainly used to induce labor or abortion and also to treat postpartum uterine atony.

Oxytocin

Currently, all commercial preparations of oxytocin are synthetically prepared. Endogenous oxytocin is mainly synthesized by the supraoptic paraventricular nuclei of the hypothalamus that are distinct from ADH containing neurons.[82] It is formed from a precursor (oxytocin-neurophysin), which contains a sequence of amino acids that is identical with a part of ADH-neurophysin. The two neurophysins can bind either ADH or oxytocin. Sensory stimuli from the vagina and cervix initiate secretion of oxytocin from posterior pituitary. Breast stimulation also results in secretion of oxytocin. The secretion of both ADH and oxytocin is stimulated by increases in osmolarity and inhibited by ethanol.[82]

Oxytocin stimulates contractility of myometrium that has been primed by estrogen. The immature uterus is resistant to its action. The responsiveness of the uterus to oxytocin is directly related to the increase in the frequency of Braxton-Hicks contractions that occur in the third trimester. However, a definite relationship between plasma oxytocin level and human parturition has been difficult to prove. Excitatory receptors to oxytocin have been demonstrated in the human uterus.[82] The sensitivity and the total number of these receptors increase as pregnancy advances. Oxytocin may produce systemic hypotension by directly inhibiting the adult vasculature smooth muscle, an effect more noticeable with bolus injections than with infusion of dilute oxytocin solution.[83] Oxytocin is a powerful constrictor of fetal umbilical arteries and veins.[84] Thus, they have a possible role in causing their closure at birth. In clinical doses, oxytocin does not have any ADH-like activity. However, when excessive doses are used along with large volumes of electrolyte-free intravenous solutions, water intoxication may ensue.[85] An infusion rate of 40 milliunits per minute has been shown to cause a definite reduction in urine flow. The half-life of exogenous oxytocin is 20 minutes in human females.

Oxytocin has been used for inducing and augmenting labor and for minimizing postpartum hemorrhage following delivery. The dosage guidelines are shown in Table 4–4.[86,87] Uterine tetany is a serious complication associated with the use of oxytocin for augmenting or inducing labor. A close watch must be kept on the uterine activity and the fetal heart rate, when oxytocin is being used.

Table 4–4. Oxytocic Drugs

Agent	For induction	For stimulation	Postpartum use
Oxytocin	Start 0.5 mU/min; double the rate every 30 min. until satisfactory uterine activity is obtained. Maximum 30 mU/min.	Start 1 mU/min; increase rate every 30 min. until a maximum of 10 mU/min is achieved.	100–200 mU/min after delivery of the placenta until uterus is firmly contracted and maintain 10–20 mU/min × 24 hours.
Ergonovine Methyl ergonovine	Not used	Not used	0.2–0.4 mg i.v., i.m. or PO
Prostaglandins PGF$_{2\alpha}$	i.v.: 6 μg/min.* May increase up to 50 μg/min.		Direct injection into the myometrium
PGE$_2$	i.v.: 250 mg/min.; may double in 30 min.* Oral: 1 mg hourly for 10 hours Vaginal: 3 mg pessary Extra-amniotic paste: 350 μg Intravaginal paste: 5 mg		PGE$_2$: oral tablets

Source: References 75, 76, 79, and 80.
*—used only for induction for fetal demise.

Ergonovine and Methyl Ergonovine

Ergonovine maleate (Ergotrate) and methyl ergonovine maleate (Methergine) are alkaloids derived from a fungus called claviceps purpurea that grows on rye. They are derivatives of d-lysergic acid. From a pharmacologic comparison, little difference exists between the actions of the two agents. Ergot preparations are powerful stimulants of uterine activity, which may be administered parenterally or orally. The sensitivity of pregnant uterus is so great that an injection of 0.1 mg may result in uterine tetany.

Ergot preparations possess serious cardiovascular side effects. The nonuterine pharmacologic effects of ergot preparations are complex and varied. They stimulate and antagonize, in various degrees, the activities of tryptaminergic, dopaminergic, and α-1 adrenergic receptors. Both ergonovine and methyl ergonovine stimulate human umbilical blood vessels and placental blood vessels (tryptaminergic receptor). They may slightly antagonize dopaminergic receptors in certain blood vessels and in certain other vascular beds they may stimulate α-1 adrenoceptors.[82] Unlike other members of the ergot family, ergonovines do not possess significant α-blockade activity. The drug must perhaps be avoided in patients who have received a long-acting α-vasoconstrictor for the treatment of spinal hypotension. Used parenterally, they may occasionally result in hypertensive crisis.[88] They also cause transient increase in pulmonary artery blood pressure.[83] The incidence of nausea and vomiting following their parenteral use may reach 20%. Ergonovines must be avoided in patients with cardiac disease and in patients who are hypertensive.

Prostaglandins

Prostaglandins E and F are locally synthesized hormones that occur abundantly in the uterus, amniotic fluid, and fetal membranes. The two prostaglandins that have been used extensively in obstetrics are prostaglandin E$_2$ (PGE$_2$) and prostaglandin F$_{2\alpha}$ (PGF$_{2\alpha}$) (Table 4–4). Administered in the last two trimesters of pregnancy, both agents can initiate uterine contractions leading to expulsion of the fetus. They are mainly used for inducing midtrimester abortions and inducing labor. The agents have also been used to ripen the cervix, prior to facilitating the onset of spontaneous or induced labor. Intracervical applications of PGE$_2$-gel can induce cervical ripening within 5 hours without inducing myometrial contraction. One unit of oxytocin equals in potency approximately 85 μg of PGE$_2$.

PGE_2 is 8 times more potent than $PGF_{2\alpha}$. PGE_2 acts mainly on the cervix, whereas $PGF_{2\alpha}$ acts mainly on the uterus.[89]

Prostaglandins may be administered intravenously, orally, or locally (intracervical or intravaginal).[89,90] Intravenous administration is associated with increased incidence of nausea, diarrhea, flushing, and abdominal cramps. Uterine hyperstimulation may be minimized by carefully titrating the dose. Oral administration is associated with severe gastrointestinal side effects. Properly used, prostaglandins provide a safe means of inducing labor with an efficacy that approaches that of oxytocin. Other nongastrointestinal side effects include the possibility of precipitating bronchial spasm in asthmatics, pyrexia (possibly due to the action of the agent on the hypothalamus), and raised intraocular pressure and uterine hypertonicity.[91] Direct injection of prostaglandin into the myometrium has been recommended for the treatment of postpartum uterine atony.[90]

BREAST FEEDING

Many of the commonly used anesthetics and adjunct drugs pass easily into the breast milk. Their passage from the maternal plasma into the milk are governed by the same factors that govern their transplacental transfer.[92] However, they do not produce appreciable fetal effects. General anesthesia for cesarean section does not contraindicate breast feeding. Narcotics given for pain relief during labor supplementing regional or general anesthesia will not produce significant fetal effects. Following maternal administration, the concentration of the drug in the breast milk reaches a peak within 30 minutes to 2 hours.[92] The avoiding of breast feeding during this time will decrease fetal drug exposure. However, chronic use of excessive amounts of sedatives and narcotics may cause drowsiness in the breast-fed baby. Breast feeding is contraindicated when mothers receive immunosuppressants and cytotoxics that may produce bone marrow depression in the baby.

REFERENCES

1. Rajchgot P, and MacLeod S: Perinatal pharmacology. *In* Developmental Pharmacology. New York, Alan R Liss, 1983.

2. Kuhnert PM, Kunhart BR, Stitts JM, and Gross TL: The use of a selective ion monitoring technique to study the disposition of bupivacaine in mother, fetus, and neonate following epidural anesthesia for cesarean section. Anesthesiology 55:611, 1981.

3. Finster M, et al: Plasma thiopental concentration in the newborn following delivery under thiopental-nitrous oxide anesthesia. Am J Obstet Gynecol 95:621, 1986.

4. Kyegombe D, Franklin C, and Turner P: Drug metabolizing enzymes in the human placenta, their induction, and repression. Lancet 1:405, 1966.

5. Pritchard JA, McDonald PC, and Gant NF: Williams Obstetrics. 17th Edition. Norwalk, Appleton-Century-Crofts, 1985.

6. Covino BG and Vassallo HG: Local Anesthetics: Mechanisms of Action and Clinical Use. New York, Grune and Stratton, 1976.

7. Wood M and Wood AJJ: Changes in plasma drug binding an α 1-acid glycoprotein in mother and newborn infants. Clin Pharmacol Ther 29:522, 1981.

8. Pelkonen O: Biotransformation of xenobiotics in the fetus. Pharmacol Ther 10:261, 1980.

9. Scanlon JW, Brown WU, Weiss JB, and Alper MH: Neurobehavioral responses of newborn infants after maternal epidural anesthesia. Anesthesiology 40:121, 1974.

10. Amiel-Tison C, et al: A new neurologic and adaptive capacity scoring system for evaluating obstetric medications in full-term newborns. Anesthesiology 56:340, 1982.

11. Sepkosky CM: Neonatal neurobehavior I: Development and its relation to obstetric medication. Clin Anaesth 4:209, 1986.

12. Palahniuk RH, et al: Evaluation of methoxyflurane, nitrous oxide and lumbar epidural anesthesia for elective cesarean section. Can Anaesth Soc J 24:586, 1977.

13. Hodgkinson R, et al: Neonatal neurobehavioral tests following vaginal delivery under ketamine, thiopental and extradural analgesia. Anesth Analg 56:548, 1977.

14. Warren TM, et al: Comparison of the maternal and neonatal effects of halothane, enflurane, and isoflurane for cesarean delivery. Anesth Analg 62:516, 1983.

15. Stefani SJ, et al: Neonatal neurobehavioral effects of inhalation analgesia for delivery. Anesthesiology, 56:351, 1982.

16. Hodgkinson R, Bhatt M, and Wang CN: Double blind comparison neurobehavior of neonates following different doses of meperidine to the mother. Can Anaesth Soc J 25:405, 1978.

17. Corke BC: Neonatal neurobehaviour II: Current clinical status. Clin Anaesth 4:209, 1986.

18. Hodgkinson R, et al: Double blind comparison of maternal analgesia and neonatal neurobehaviour following intravenous butorphanol and meperidine. J Int Med Res 7:224, 1979.

19. Ounsted M: Pain relief during child birth and development at 4 years. J R Soc Med 74:629, 1981.

20. Ounsted M, Scott A, and Molar A: Delivery and development. To what extent can one associate cause and effect? J R Soc Med 73:786, 1980.

21. Shier RW: Placental transfer of meperidine HCl: Part II. Am J Obstet Gynecol 115:557, 1973.

22. Szeto HH: Brain uptake of meperidine in the fetal lamb. Am J Obstet Gynecol 138:528, 1980.

23. Weir PHC and Chung FF: Anaesthesia for patients with chronic renal disease. Can Anaesth Soc J 31:468, 1984.

24. Kuhnert PR, et al: Meperidine, normeperidine levels following meperidine administration during labor II. Fetus and neonate. Am J Obstet Gynecol 133:909, 1979.

25. Kuhnert P, et al.: Meperidine and normeperidine levels following meperidine adminstration during labor. Am J Obstet Gynecol 133:904, 1979.

26. Caldwell J, et al: Maternal and neonatal disposition of pethidine in child birth. A study using gas chromatograph-mass spectrometry. Life Sci 22:589, 1978.

27. Rosen MG, Scibetta JJ, and Hochberg CJ: Human fetal electroencephalogram. 3. Pattern changes in presence of fetal heart rate alterations and after use of maternal medications. Obstet Gynecol 36:132, 1970.

28. Clark RB, and Seifen AB: Systemic medication during labor and delivery. Obstet Gynecol Annu 12:165, 1983.

29. Shnider SM, and Moya F: Effects of meperidine on the newborn infant. Am J Obstet Gynecol 89:1009, 1964.

30. Modanlou HD and Freeman RK: Sinusoidal fetal heart rate pattern: Its definition and clinical significance. Am J Obstet Gynecol 142:1033, 1982.

31. Eisele JH, Wright R, and Rogge P: Newborn and maternal fentanyl levels at cesarean section. Anesth Analg 61:179, 1982.

32. Monks PS, and Lumeley J: Anesthetic aspects of renal transplantation. Ann R Coll Surg Engl 50:354, 1978.

33. Maduska AL, and Hajgassemali M: Double blind comparison of butorphanol and meperidine in labor. Maternal pain relief and the effect on the newborn. Can Anaesth Soc J 25:398, 1978.

34. Nagashima H, et al: Respiratory and circulatory effects of intravenous butorphanol and morphine. Clin Pharmacol Ther 19:738, 1976.

35. Romognoli A, Keats AS: Ceiling effect of respiratory depression by nalbuphine. Clin Pharmacol Ther 27:478, 1980.

36. Gerhardt T, et al: Use of naloxone to reverse narcotic respiratory depression in the newborn infant. J Pediatrics 90:1009, 1977.

37. Clark RB: Transplacental reversal of meperidine depression in the fetus by naloxone. J Arkansas Med Soc 68:128, 1971.

38. Andree RA: Sudden death following naloxone administration. Anesth Analg 59:789, 1980.

39. Goebelsmann U, Abboud TK, Hoffman TI, and Hung TT: Beta-endorphin in pregnancy. Europ J Obstet Gynecol Reprod Biol 17:77, 1984.

40. Cree IE, Myer J, and Hailey DM: Diazepam in labour. Its metabolism and effect on the clinical condition and thermogenesis of the newborn. Br Med J IV:251, 1973.

41. McAllister CB: Placental transfer and neonatal effects of diazepam when administered to women just before delivery. Br J Anaesth 52:423, 1980.

42. Bakke OM, Haram K, Lygre T, and Wallem G: Comparison of the placental transfer of thiopental and diazepam in caesarean section. Eur J Clin Pharmacol 21:221, 1981.

43. Kanto J, et al.: Pharmacokinetics and sedative effects of midazolam in connection with cesarean section performed under epidural anesthesia. Acta Anaesthesiol Scand 28:116, 1984.

44. Kanto J, et al: Transfer of lorazepam and its conjugate across the human placenta. Acta Pharmacol et Toxicol 47:130, 1980.

45. McAuley DM, et al: Lorazepam premedication in labor. Br J Obstet Gynaecol 89:149, 1982.

46. Slone D, et al.: Antenatal exposure to the phenothiazines in relation to congenital malformations, perinatal mortality rate, birth weight, and intelligence quotient score. Am J Obstet Gynecol 128:486, 1977.

47. Smith SE: Psychotropic agents and anti-emetics. In A Practice of Anaesthesia. 5th Edition (Edited by Churchill-Davidson HC) Chicago, Year Book Medical Publishers, 1984.

48. Christensen JH, Andreasen F, and Jansen JA: Pharmacokinetics of thiopental in caesarean section. Acta Anaesthesiol Scand 25:174, 1981.

49. Dawes GS: Theory of fetal drug equilibration. In Fetal Pharmacology (Edited by Boreus L) New York, Raven Press, 1973.

50. Kosaka Y, Takahashi T, and Mark LC: Intravenous thiobarbiturate anesthesia for cesarean section. Anesthesiology 31:489, 1969.

51. Morgan B: Comparison of thiopentone and methohexitone as induction agents for cesarean section. Anaesth Intensive Care 8:431, 1980.

52. Harvey SC: Hypnotics and sedatives. In The Pharmacological Basis of Therapeutics. (Edited by Gilman AG, Goodman LS, Rall TW, and Murad F) New York, McMillan Publishing, 1985.

53. Wiskopf RB, Bogetz MZ, Roizen MF, and Reid IA: Cardiovascular and metabolic sequelae inducing anesthesia with ketamine or thiopental in hypovolemic swine. Anesthesiology 60:214, 1984.

54. Little B, et al: A study of ketamine as an obstetric agent. Am J Obstet Gynecol 113:247, 1972.

55. Craft JB Jr, et al: Ketamine, catecholamines and uterine tone in pregnant ewes. Am J Obstet Gynecol 146:429, 1983.

56. Oats JN, Vasey DP, and Waldron BA: Effects of ketamine on the pregnant uterus. Br J Anaesth 51:1163, 1979.

57. Marx GF, Hwang HS, and Chantra P: Postpartum uterine pressures with different doses of ketamine. Anesthesiology 50:163, 1979.

58. Janeczko GF, El Etr AA, and Younes S: Low-dose ketamine anesthesia for obstetrical delivery. Anesth Analg 53:828, 1974.

59. Akamatsu TJ, et al: Experiences with the use of ketamine for parturition. I. Primary anesthetic for vaginal delivery. Anesth Analg 53:828, 1974.

60. Blitt CD, Petty WC, and Alberternst EE: Correlation of plasma cholisterase activity and duration of action of succinylcholine during pregnancy. Anesth Analg 56:78, 1977.

61. Aagesen G, and Ronquist G: Prolonged succinylcholine induced paralysis in connection with the caesarean section: A case report. Acta Anaesthesiol Scand 21:379, 1977.

62. Drabkova J, Crul JF, and Kleijn V: Placental transfer 14C labelled succinylcholine in near-term macaca mulatta monkeys. Br J Anaesth 45:1087, 1973.

63. Kivalo I, and Saarikoski S: Placental transfer of ^{14}C-dimethyltubocurarine in cesarean section. Br J Anaesth 48:239, 1976.

64. Duvaldestin P, et al: The placental transfer of pancuronium and its pharmacokinetics during caesarian section. Acta Anaesth Scand 22:327, 1978.

65. Demetriou M, et al: Placental transfer of Org NC 45 in women undergoing caesarean section. Br J Anaesth 54:643, 1982.

66. Flynn PJ, Frank M, and Hughes R: Use of atracurium in caesarean section. Br J Anaesth 56:599, 1984.

67. Bertrand JC, et al: Quantitative assessment of placental transfer of fazadinium in obstetric anaesthesia. Acta Anaesth Scand 24:133, 1980.

68. Kivalo I, and Saarikoski I: Placental transfer of atropine at full term pregnancy. Br J Anaesth 49:1017, 1977.

69. Kanto J, et al: Placental transfer and pharmacokinetics of atropine after a single maternal intravenous and intramuscular injection. Acta Anaesth Scand 25:85, 1981.

70. Abboud TK, et al: Enflurane analgesia in obstetrics. Anesth Analg 60:133, 1981.

71. Gregory GA, et al: Fetal anesthetic requirement. Anesth Analg 62:9, 1983.

72. Biehl DR, et al: Effect of halothane on cardiac output and regional blood flow in the fetal lamb in utero. Anesth Analg 62:489, 1983.

73. Biehl DR, et al: The uptake of isoflurane in the fetal lamb in utero: Effect on regional blood flow. Can Anaesth Soc J 30:581, 1983.

74. Yarnell R, et al: The effect of halothane anesthesia on the asphyxiated foetal lamb in utero. Can Anaesth Soc J 30:474, 1983.

75. Swartz J, et al: The effect of general anesthesia on the asphyxiated fetal lamb in utero. Can Anaesth Soc J 32:577, 1985.

76. Munson ES, and Embro WJ: Enflurane, isoflurane and halothane and isolated human uterine muscle. Anesthesiology 46:11, 1977.

77. Marx GF, et al: Postpartum uterine pressures under halothane and enflurane anesthesia. Obstet Gynecol 51:695, 1978.

78. Marx CF, Joshi CW, and Orkin LR: Placental transmission of nitrous oxide. Anesthesiology 32:429, 1970.

79. Bassell GM, Belonsky BL, and Marx GF: Systemic anesthetic methods. *In* Obstetric Anaesthesia and Anaesthesia. (Edited by Marx GF and Bassell GM) New York, Elsevier, 1980.

80. Palahniuk RJ and Cumming M: Plasma fluoride levels following obstetrical use of methoxyflurane. Can Anaesth Soc J, 22:291, 1975.

81. Clark RB: Renal function in newborns and mothers exposed to methoxyflurane analgesia for labor and delivery. Anesthesiology 51:464, 1979.

82. Rall TW and Schliefer LS: Oxytocin, prostaglandin, and tocolytic agents. *In* The Pharmacological Basis of Therapeutics. (Edited by Gilman AG, Goodman LS, Rall TW, and Murad F) New York, McMillian Publishing, 1985.

83. Secher NJ, Arnsbo P, and Wallin L: Hemodynamic effects of oxytocin (syntocinon) and methyl ergometrine on the sytemic and pulmonary circulations of pregnant anesthetized women. Acta Obstet Gynecol Scand 57:97, 1978.

84. Altura BM, and Altura BT: Actions of vasopressin, oxytocin, and synthetic analogs on vascular smooth muscle. Fed Proc 43:80, 1984.

85. Eggers TR, and Fliegner JR: Water intoxication and syntocinon infusion. Aust NZ J Obstet Gynaecol 125:310, 1976.

86. Pritchard JA, McDonald PC, and Gant NF: Williams Obstetrics. 17th Edition. Norwalk, Appleton-Century-Crofts, 1985.

87. Petrie RH: The pharmacology and use of oxytocin. Clin Perinatol 8:45, 1981.

88. Browning DJ: Serious side effects of ergometrine and its routine use in obstetric practice. Med J Aust 1:957, 1974.

89. Shepard JH, and Knuppel RA: The role of prostaglandins in ripening the cervix and inducing labor. Clin Perinatol 8:49, 1981.

90. Andersson KE, Forman A, and Ulmsten U: Pharmacology of labor. Clinical Obstet Gynecol 26:56, 1983.

91. Stirrat GM, and Thomas TA: Prescribing for labor. Clin Obstet Gynaecol 13:215, 1986.

92. Beeley L: Drugs and breast feeding. Clin Obstet Gynaecol 13:247, 1986.

5

LOCAL ANESTHETIC

The inhabitants of the Peruvian Andes who chewed the leaves of Erythroxylum coca to diminish fatigue, noted that these leaves caused the tongue to become numb. Von Anrep, in 1880, noted that subcutaneous infiltration of the plant extract rendered the skin numb. In Europe, Sigmund Freud used cocaine to treat morphine addiction. Carl Koller introduced cocaine into ophthalmic surgery in 1884. R.J. Hall used cocaine in dentistry and within a short period of time William Halstead performed the first nerve block using cocaine.[1] In 1905, Alfred Einhorn synthesized procaine. In 1940, lidocaine was synthesized which marked a great milestone in the history of local anesthetics.

Local anesthetics produce a reversible blockade of neural conduction. Their molecular structure consists of an aromatic ring, a linking chain, and a carbon chain bearing an amino group (Fig. 5–1).[2] Although it is composed of only a few atoms, the linking chain is important because it determines whether a given local anesthetic belongs to the ester or the amide class of substances. The linking chain of the esters generally have the "COO" (ester linkage) configuration, whereas the amides have the "NH-CO" configuration. Esters are hydrolyzed by plasma pseudocholinesterase, while amide compounds are metabolized by the liver.

BASIC PHYSICOCHEMICAL PROPERTIES OF THE LOCAL ANESTHETICS

Molecular Weight. The molecular weights of clinically useful local anesthetics range between 220 and 300, and therefore, cross the placenta.

pK$_a$. The pK$_a$ of a compound is the pH at which the ratio between the dissociated and the undissociated fractions of the compound is one. Table 5–1 gives a list of local anesthetic agents and their important physico-chemical properties. The pK$_a$ of the local anesthetic determines the degree of ionization at a given pH (Fig. 5–2). Local anesthetic substances are basic substances. Generally speaking, the higher the pK$_a$, the higher will be the degree of ionization for the local anesthetic. For a given local anesthetic, the higher the pH of the medium, the higher will be the percentage of the nonionized base (Table 5–2). The relationship between the undissociated (base form, unionized form) and the dissociated (charged form, ionized form, cation) is governed by the Henderson-Hasselbalch equation:

$$pH = pK_a + base/cation.$$

Lipid Solubility. As in the case of the general anesthetics, the potency of the local anesthetics is determined by their lipid solubility. Increased lipid solubility of the local anesthetic enables the agent to easily penetrate the neural membrane, which contains 42% lipids in its structure. The other constituents of cell membranes include proteins (55%) and carbohydrates (3%).[3] The lipid solubility of local anesthetics is measured in terms of their partition coefficients. Etidocaine and bupivacaine have much higher partition coefficients than does lidocaine. The other advantage of increased lipid solubility is the increased duration of action. Obviously, the price

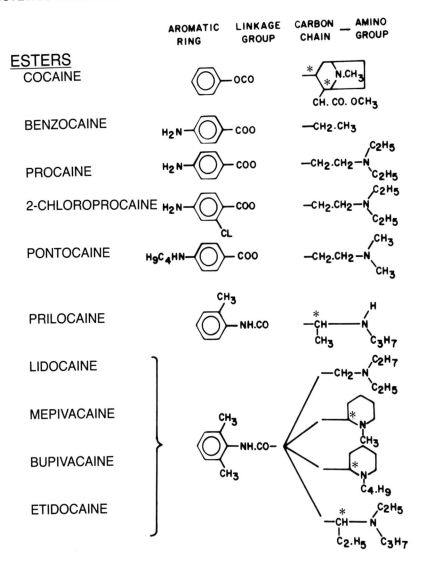

FIG. 5–1.   Chemical structure of clinically useful anesthetics. The * indicates an asymmetric carbon atom and therefore the existence of stereoisomers. (Reproduced from Tucker GT: Pharmacokinetics of local anesthetic drugs. *In* Practical Regional Anaesthesia. (Edited by Henderson JJ, and Nimmo WS. Boston, Blackwell Scientific, 1983.)

one pays for increased potency is the increase in potential for toxicity.

Protein Binding. Because of the high molecular weight of protein, cell membranes contain more protein-mass than they do lipid-mass. However, because of the low molecular weight of lipids, the membranes contain a lot more lipid molecules than protein molecules. Protein-binding confers on the local anesthetic molecule increased potency and increased duration of action. The local anesthetics are also bound to plasma proteins. Diminished plasma protein concentration therefore results in an increase in the concentration of free drug, thus potentiating toxic side effects. The basic physico-chemical properties of the commonly used local anesthetic agents are summarized in Table 5–1.

THE MECHANISM OF NEURAL BLOCKADE

There are a number of different aspects involved in the mechanism of neural blockade.

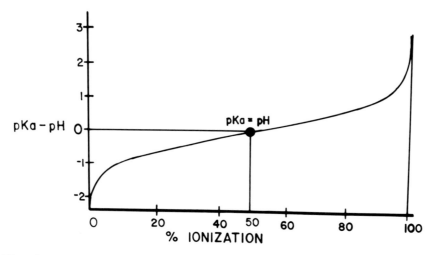

FIG. 5–2.   The relationship between the pK$_a$-pH difference and the degree of ionization of local anesthetics. Note that when pK$_a$ = pH the local anesthetic is ionized 50%. (From Bromage PR: Epidural Analgesia. Philadelphia, WB Saunders, 1978.)

Table 5–1.   Physico-Chemical Properties of Local Anesthetics

Agent	MW	Potency rating	pKa 25°C	Partial coefficient	Protein binding %	Toxic dose (mg/kg)	*CC/CNS ratio
Esters							
Procaine	272	1	9.0	0.02	5.8	15.0	
2-chloroprocaine	302	1	8.7	0.14		20.0	
Tetracaine	300	8	8.3	4.10	76.0	1.0	
Amides							
Lidocaine	234	2	7.9	2.9	64.0	7.0	7.1
Mepivacaine	246	2	7.7	0.8	77.0	7.0	
Prilocaine	220	2	7.9	0.9	55.0	10.0	
Bupivacaine	325	8	8.1	28.0	95.0	2.0	3.7
Etidocaine	276	6	7.7	41.0	94.0	3.0	4.4

*CC/CNS ratio indicates the ratio between the dose that produces cardiovascular failure and the dose that causes convulsion

THE CELL MEMBRANE

The local anesthetics must overcome several diffusion barriers before they can reach the receptor site where they are believed to block sodium conductance through the cell wall. The first obstacle the local anesthetic encounters is the cell membrane. The cell membrane consists of a bimolecular lipid layer in which carbohydrate and protein molecules are interspersed (Fig. 5–3).

The proteins are of two types: the peripheral proteins that are attached to the surface of the bilayer; and integral proteins that penetrate through the thickness of the membrane. The integral proteins provide the structural pores or channels along which different substances can diffuse into and out of the cell. Two types of channels transport Na$^+$ and K$^+$ into and out of the cell. They are the leak-channels, which are much more permeable to K$^+$ than to Na$^+$; and the voltage-gated channels, which are important in building the action-potential. The voltage-gated channels may be opened and closed by special gate-like extensions of the membrane

Table 5–2.   The pH and Dissociation of Lidocaine (pKa 7.8)

Tissue pH	Percentage cation	Percentage base
7.4	74%	26%
7.6	64%	36%
7.2	82%	18%

Note when the tissue pH decreases the cationic form increases.

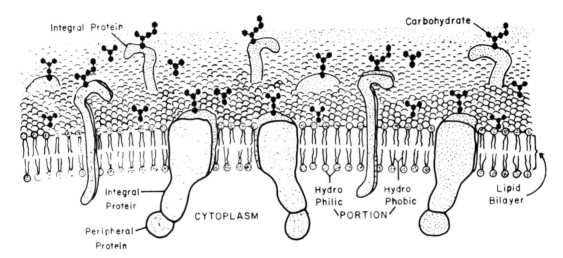

FIG. 5–3.   Structure of cell membrane. Note the organization of the bimolecular lipid-bilayer and the presence of protein and carbohydrate molecules in the cell membrane. (From Guyton AC: The Cell and its Function. *In* Textbook of Medical Physiology. Philadelphia, W.B. Saunders, 1986.)

proteins. The transport of Na^+ and K^+ ions across the cell membrane is also regulated by the Na^+-K^+ pump, which depends on active participation by carrier proteins.

ACTION POTENTIAL (AP)

The cell-membrane resting potential is -90 mV because the inside of the cell carries more negative charges. The origin of the negative cell-membrane potential is attributed to the constant activity of the Na^+-K^+ electrogenic pump, which pumps out 3 Na^+ atoms for every 2 K^+ atoms that it pumps into the interior of the cell and the constant leakage of K^+ through the leakage channels. Nerve impulses are transmitted by action potentials (AP).[4]

In the resting state, both activation and inactivation gates of the Na^+ channels are closed. The action potential causes the membrane potential to become positive. The activation gates of Na^+ channels open, allowing entry of the Na^+ ions into the cell, causing depolarization of the membrane. Conformational changes in the protein gates are believed to open the gates (Fig. 5–4). This is called the activated state. When the inside voltage reaches a certain critical level (the threshold potential), the depolarization process quickens. Soon, the Na^+ inactivation gates close (Fig. 5–4), which starts the repolarization process of the cell membrane. The inactivation gates will remain closed until the cell

membrane is fully repolarized. Nearly coinciding with the inactivation of the Na^+ channels, the K^+-gated channels start allowing passage of K^+ to the exterior, accelerating the repolarization process. The depolarization occupies 30% of the action potential and repolarization process the remaining 70%.[5] The sequence of events occurring during an action process is depicted in Fig. 5–5. The AP spreads along a myelinated nerve by jumping from one node of Ranvier to the next. Local anesthetics are thought to block the depolarization and repolarization process mainly by inhibiting the Na^+ permeability of the cell membrane.

ACTIVE FORM OF THE LOCAL ANESTHETIC

The undissociated (base) form will penetrate the neural membrane barriers, but the charged (cation) form is ultimately responsible for binding with the receptor in the sodium channel. Thus, both the charged and uncharged moieties are essential for neural blockade to occur. Even when applied externally to a nerve, the local anesthetic must cross the membrane in the undissociated form. In acidic axoplasm, a more cationic form occurs that blocks the sodium channel from the inside.

RECEPTOR CONCEPT

Hille[6] has developed a single receptor concept to explain the mechanism of action of local an-

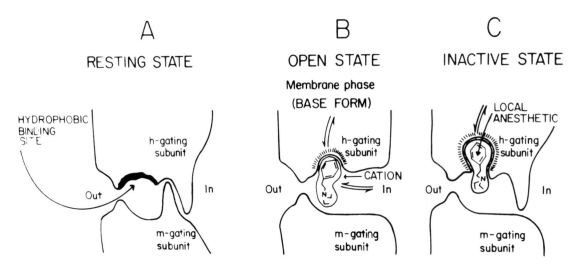

FIG. 5–4. Local anesthetic receptor in the sodium channel. The m-gate activates the Na+ channel and h-gate deactivates Na+ channel. In the resting state (panel A), both gates are closed. In the open state (panel B), both gates are open; and in the inactive state (panel C), the h-gates are closed. Note the location of the receptor within the sodium channel and the augmenting effect of closure of the h-gate on the binding of the local anesthetic to the receptor. (From Tucker GT: Chemistry and pharmacology of local anesthetic drugs. *In* Practical Regional Anaesthesia. (Edited by Henderson JJ, and Nimmo WS). Boston, Blackwell Scientific Publications, 1983.)

esthetic. He believes that the receptor is situated in the sodium channel and that the local anesthetic blocks sodium permeability by binding with this receptor (Fig. 5–4). Both nonionized and ionized moieties may reach the receptor from the axoplasm, if both activation and inactivation gates are open. Because of its high lipid solubility, the base form may reach the receptor through the membrane matrix, regardless of whether the gates are open or closed. For the hydrophilic cation to reach the sodium channel, the inactivation gates must be open (Fig. 5–4). The receptor theory helps explain the frequency-dependent block, wherein the increased frequency of nerve stimulation enhances the block. Since rapid stimulation of the membrane will tend to keep the activation and inactivation gates open, the increased amount of local anesthetic will reach the receptor site. A practical demonstration of this phenomenon may be seen in the labor ward. Following an epidural block, pain relief will often be noticeable before sensory anesthesia is detected because of the earlier blockade pain fibers.

BUPIVACAINE CARDIOTOXICITY

Another aspect of local anesthetic action that the receptor concept is applicable to is the car-diotoxicity of bupivacaine. The drug binds with the sodium channel during the systole (open state), and during the inactivated state that immediately follows the open state. It dissociates itself from the channel during diastole (resting state). Because of its highly lipophilic nature of bupivacaine, the dissociation process is slower than the binding process (fast in–slow out) leading to incomplete dissociation. In other words, increasing heart rate will produce an increase in the number of occupied channels, thus resulting in the decrease of the action potential velocity (V_{MAX}, Fig. 5–6). However, lidocaine, a weakly lipid soluble agent, dissociates rapidly from the binding sites (fast-in and fast-out) (Fig. 5–6).[7] In many animal experiments, lidocaine has been shown to be less cardiotoxic than bupivacaine.

The local anesthetic modifies the electrophysiological events that happen during action potential (Fig. 5–7). Neither the resting potential nor the threshold potential is significantly altered after exposure to lidocaine. The depolarization phase, however, is inhibited. Local anesthetics also produce changes in the ionic fluxes in the cardiac cell. The normally occurring slow diastolic depolarization (phase IV depolarization) is caused by the decrease in K^+ efflux, occurring during this period. At antiarrhythmic

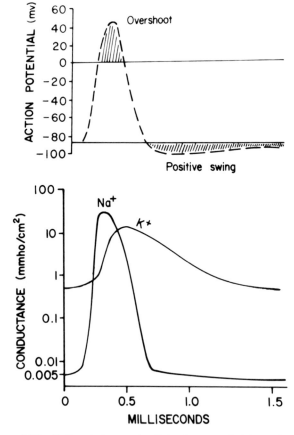

FIG. 5–5. Action potential of an excitable cell membrane. Note the negative resting potential and the sudden change to positive potential following stimulation. The bottom panel shows rapid change in Na+ and K+ conductance. The change in Na+ conductance precedes the change in the K+ conductance. (From Guyton AC: The Cell and its Function. *In* Textbook of Medical Physiology. Philadelphia, WB Saunders, 1986.)

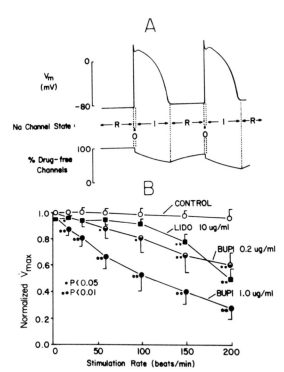

FIG. 5–6. (A) Binding of bupivacaine to sodium channel in the myocardium. V_m = action potential; R = resting state of the sodium channel (systole); O = open state; I = inactive state (diastole). Note that the incomplete dissociation of bupivacaine during diastole causes the percentage of drug-free channels to decrease with each contraction. (B) V_{max} = maximum upstroke velocity. Note with increasing heart rate bupivacaine produces a dose dependent inhibition of V_{max}, an effect not noticeable with very high concentration of lidocaine. * = $p < 0.05$; ** = $p < 0.01$. (Reproduced from Clarkson CW, and Hondeghem LM: Mechanism for bupivacaine depression of cardiac conduction. Anesthesiology *62*:396, 1985.)

doses, lidocaine causes an increase in the efflux of K+ ions, thus abolishing the phase IV depolarization in the Purkinje fibers. Toxic doses of lidocaine will, however, inhibit phase 0 depolarization probably through its action on Na+ permeability in the cardiac muscle (Fig. 5–7). The action potential amplitude will decrease, thereby diminishing cardiac contractility.[5]

CLASSIFICATION OF NERVE FIBERS

The nerve fibers are classified into A, B, and C types based on the type of impulses they transmit, the presence of myelin, and their size (Table 5–3). The A group has four minor subdivisions.

Within the same major group, the small slow-conducting fibers are more readily blocked by the local anesthetic than are larger fast-conducting fibers. For instance, A-δ fiber are more readily blocked than A-α fibers (Table 5–3). However, this principle does not apply when two different major groups of fibers are being compared. For instance, the fast conducting myelinated preganglionic B fibers tend to get blocked much more easily than the slower non-myelinated C fibers.[8] The preganglionic sympathetic B fibers are probably the most sensitive of all major and minor fiber types, which explains the rapid onset of hypotension following

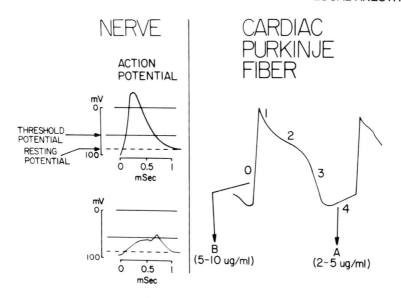

FIG. 5–7. Effect of local anesthetic on action potential of a nerve membrane (left) and a cardiac Purkinje fiber (right). Note that the anesthetic has no affect on either the resting potential or the threshold potential of the neural membrane. It does, however, prevent the development of the action potential (see bottom left). Phase 4 depolarization of the Purkinje fiber is affected by the local anesthetic at low concentration; however, at high concentration, phase 0 is also affected. When phase 0 is affected, myocardial depression is usually evident. (From Covino BG, and Vassallo HG: Local Anesthetics: Mechanisms of Action and Clinical Use. New York, Grune and Stratton, 1976.)

epidural anesthesia. Sensory A-α fibers are more sensitive than motor A-α fibers because the former conduct at higher frequency (frequency-dependent block).[9]

ABSORPTION, RATE, AND EXCRETION

No matter which nerve block is performed, local anesthetics are readily absorbed into systemic circulation. The rate of rise of local an-esthetic concentration, however, is dependent on the type of nerve block performed. Intercostal nerve blocks probably produce the highest blood level of local anesthetic. Among the nerve blocks performed in obstetrical patients the site of injection influences the blood level in the following order: paracervial block,[10] caudal block, lumbar epidural block, and subarachnoid block.[5] Within minutes of performing an epidural block, local anesthetic will be detectable in maternal and fetal plasma. Obviously, the blood level depends on the total amount of local anesthetic

Table 5–3.   Type of Nerve Fibers and the Sequence of Blockade

Fiber	Sensory function	Motor function	Diameter (μM)	Speed (m/sec)	Sequence of blockade
A-α	Proprioception	Somatic	12–20	70–120	3/5*
A-β	Touch, pressure	————	5–12	30–70	4
A-γ	————	Muscle spindle	3–6	15–30	
A-δ	Pain, temperature	————	2–5	12–30	2†
B	————	Preganglionic	<3	3–15	1
C	Pain–reflex	Postganglionic	0.3–1.3	0.3–2.3	2

Note that A and B fibers are myelinated.
*A-α sensory fibers are the third type fibers to be blocked, whereas A-α motor fibers are the fifth fibers to be blocked.
†A-δ fibers and C fibers are the second type of fibers to be blocked, but A-δ fibers will get blocked before the C fibers probably because of the frequency-dependent block.

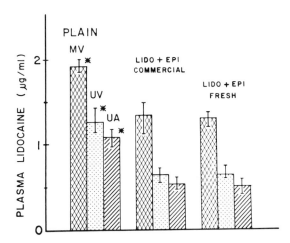

FIG. 5–8. A bar graph showing different levels of lidocaine in the blood from a maternal vein (MV) and a fetal umbilical vein (UV) and an umbilical artery (UA) with plain lidocaine, with commercial lidocaine-epinephrine mixture (lido + epi) and with fresh lidocaine-epinephrine mixture. * = p <0.01. (Source: Ramanathan S, Dursztman M, and Turndorf H: Local anesthetics with freshly added epinephrine produce longer obstetrical analgesia. Anesthesiology 63:3A, 1985.)

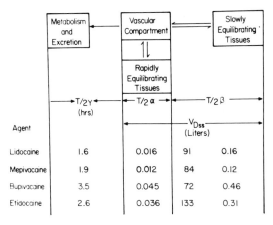

FIG. 5–9. Pharmacokinetic properties of different local anesthetic agents. $V_{D_{SS}}$ = volume distribution in liters. Other figures are in hours. (From Covino BG, and Vassallo HG: Local Anesthetics: Mechanisms of Action and Clinical Use. New York, Grune and Stratton, 1976.)

used (mg). Addition of a vasoconstrictor, such as epinephrine, will decrease the maternal and fetal blood levels of local anesthetic. For instance, addition of epinephrine to local anesthetic will reduce the maternal and fetal levels by approximately 50%[11] (Fig. 5–8).

The local anesthetics are significantly bound to plasma proteins (Table 5–1). The binding sites may easily become saturated, and as the total plasma concentration of the drug increases, the ratio of the unbound to bound fraction will also increase.[12] There are two binding sites available: α_1-acid glycoprotein sites that have a high affinity but low capacity, and albumin sites that have a low affinity but large capacity. The concentration of α_1-glycoprotein differs considerably from patient to patient, which explains the individual variation in local anesthetic toxicity. Local anesthetics are distributed throughout the body water. The initial rapid disappearance (Tα) from the blood results from the uptake by rapidly equilibrating tissues. This is followed by a slower phase of disappearance (Tβ) resulting from the distribution to poorly perfused tissues and from the metabolism and excretion of the drug. Generally speaking, the Tα values and Tβ are longer

for the potent anesthetics, such as bupivacaine and etidocaine than they are for lidocaine.[5]

The volume of distribution of a drug at steady state ($V_{D_{SS}}$) is a derived parameter, which indicates the total volume of the body water reservoir in which the drug appears to be distributed. Volume of distribution gives us an idea about the penetrability of the drug. Agents with greater lipid solubility will have a greater distribution, and therefore a greater $V_{D_{SS}}$ (compare lidocaine with etidocaine) Fig. 5–9. The $V_{D_{SS}}$ may be calculated using total blood concentration of the local anesthetic or the unbound concentration. The $V_{D_{SS}}$ that is calculated by using total concentration shows only a two-fold variability among different local anesthetics, whereas the $V_{D_{SS}}$ calculated using an unbound fraction displays a wider variability among the different agents;[5,13] also, the potent agents, bupivacaine and etidocaine, will have a much higher $V_{D_{SS}}$ than lidocaine. Values for $V_{D_{SS}}$ are modified in certain disease states. For lidocaine, in liver disease, the $V_{D_{SS}}$ is higher and the clearance rate is smaller than in normal patients (Table 5–4).[14] This may result from decreased levels of α_1-acid glycoprotein.[15] In heart failure, the $V_{D_{SS}}$ and clearance are reduced, probably because of poor distribution and diminished hepatic blood blow, respectively. In renal disease, the clearance of lidocaine may not be appreciably affected in the absence of significant liver disease (Table 5–4).

Table 5–4. Lidocaine Pharmacokinetics in Various Disease States

State	VD$_{ss}$ (l/kg)	Cl (ml/min/kg^{-1})	T1/2 (h)
Normal	1.32	10.0	1.8
Heart failure	0.88	6.3	1.9
Liver disease	2.31	6.0	4.9
Renal disease	1.2	13.7	1.3

VD$_{ss}$—volume of distribution at steady state; Cl—clearance
T1/2—termination elimination half-life

Following systemic absorption, the lung is exposed to the local anesthetic first. The lung sequestrates a large quantity of the drug, thus protecting the heart and the brain.[16] Injection of even a small quantity of local anesthetic into a carotid or vertebral artery, rapidly results in convulsion because of the lack of buffering effect of the lung. Patients with increased anatomic or physiologic vascular shunts (pneumonia or adult respiratory distress syndrome) may be similarly exposed to greater risk of local anesthetic toxicity.[16]

METABOLISM AND ELIMINATION OF LOCAL ANESTHETICS

Amide local anesthetics are metabolized in the liver through the following pathways: (1) N-dealkylation of the tertiary amine produces a more water-soluble, secondary amine, which then undergoes amide hydrolysis; (2) hydroxylation of the aromatic nucleus. Ring-hydroxylation is inefficient in the fetus and the neonate.[17] However, the rate of N-dealkylation seems to be comparable to that of the adult. Monoethylglycinexylidide (MEGX) is a metabolic by-product of lidocaine formed by N-dealkylation. Further dealkylation of MEGX leads to the formation of glycine xylidide (GX).[5] Both, MEGX and GX share some of the local anesthetic properties of the parent compound.[18] The fetus metabolizes lidocaine in a manner similar to that of the adult but at a lower rate.[17]

The major metabolic product of bupivacaine in the mother and fetus is 2-6 pipecoloxylidine (PPX) and is formed by N-dealkylation. Metabolism of prilocaine results in the formation of O-toluidine, which may produce methemoglobinemia in the mother and fetus.[19] Prilocaine is no longer recommended for obstetrical patients. Mepivacaine mainly depends on ring hydroxylation for metabolism, a metabolic pathway that

is quite inefficient in the fetus.[17] Consequently, mepivacaine has prolonged half-life in the fetus and the neonate (>9 hours).

Clearance rates of amide local anesthetic agents is identical to their hepatic metabolic rate as renal elimination of the unchanged compound accounts for only 1 to 5% of elimination.[13] Clearance rate of the commonly used amide local anesthetics is listed in Table 5–5. Bupivacaine has the least clearance rate and prilocaine the highest. In normal patients, the terminal half-lives of elimination for many local anesthetic agents following i.v. administration is 2 to 3 hours. Clearance rates of amide local anesthetic agents is slowed in patients with heart or liver disease (Table 5–4).

Ester type local anesthetic agents are rapidly hydrolyzed by pseudocholinesterase. The speed of hydrolysis of ester compounds is striking. For instance 2-chloroprocaine (2-CP) has an in vitro half-life of approximately 1 minute in maternal and fetal plasma. The hydrolysis products of 2-chloroprocaine are 2-chloroaminobenzoic acid (CABA) and 2-diethylaminoethanol. Following epidural administration, both mother and fetus excrete 2-chloroprocaine and CABA in the urine for 2 to 3 days.[20] However, the total amount of unchanged 2-chloroprocaine and CABA is much less in the neonate, signifying only a limited placental transfer of 2-chloroprocaine. Different ester compounds undergo different rates of hydrolysis. Pontocaine hydrolysis rate is one fifth

Table 5–5. Blood Clearance of Amide Type Local Anesthetics

Drug	Clearance (l/min)
Bupivacaine	0.58
Mepivacaine	0.78
Lidocaine	0.95
Etidocaine	1.11
Prilocaine	2.37

of procaine hydrolysis.[21] Cocaine is *not* hydrolyzed by plasma chlolinesterase.

PLACENTAL TRANSFER AND FETAL DISPOSITION OF LOCAL ANESTHETICS

Following injection into the epidural space, the local anesthetic attains peak levels in the mother and fetus within minutes. Local anesthetics cross the placenta mainly by passive diffusion, which results in the maternal and fetal blood concentrations attaining equilibrium quickly.[22] The degree of protein-binding of a given local anesthetic agent will determine the rate of placental transfer. However, the total amount of the injected drug that can be recovered from the fetus is not influenced by protein binding. For instance, the fetal to maternal blood ratios of lidocaine and etidocaine are 0.56 and 0.17, respectively, although, the total amounts of the two drugs recovered from the fetal tissues are similar to each other.[23] This is probably caused by the increased tissue binding of etidocaine, which decreases its fetal plasma levels. A local anesthetic such as 2-chloroprocaine that undergoes rapid hydrolysis in the maternal plasma will undergo negligible placental transfer.

The tissue distribution of local anesthetic in the fetus differs slightly from that of the mother. The maternal kidney will contain a maximum amount of the injected drug, whereas in the fetus, the drug will be concentrated in the liver.[5] This perhaps reflects the strategic location of the liver in fetal circulation (Table 5–6, Fig. 5–10). The fetal liver can metabolize the local anesthetic and the metabolites may be excreted in the urine into the amniotic fluid.[17] The binding of local anesthetic by fetal proteins is less efficient because of reduced concentrations of α_1-acid glycoproteins in the fetus,[24] and slightly increased H^+ concentration in the fetal tissues. The increased H^+ concentration will favor the formation of more ionized moiety in the tissues.

Fetal asphyxia modifies the distribution of local anesthetics (Fig. 5–11). Since asphyxia induced circulatory adaptations will maximize blood supply to the brain and heart at the expense of muscles and liver, the local anesthetics will be preferentially distributed to vital organs. In addition, the diminished protein binding and ion-trapping (see Fig. 3–9) that is caused by acidosis will increase the likelihood of CNS and cardiovascular toxicity in the neonate. The convulsive dose and the blood level at which CNS toxicity occurs are 2.5 to 3 times less in the asphyxiated fetuses compared to corresponding figures in normal fetuses.[25]

PHARMACOLOGIC ACTIONS OF LOCAL ANESTHETICS

The pharmacologic effects of local anesthetics are caused by systemic absorption. As the blood concentration rises, a series of systemic pharmacologic effects are seen (Fig. 5–12). The central nervous system (CNS) and cardiovascular system are mainly affected because they contain highly excitable tissues.

CENTRAL NERVOUS SYTEM EFFECTS

The most serious CNS side-effect is convulsion, which results from an excessive dose of the local anesthetic agent or by accidental intravenous injection. Numbness of the tongue and lips are early warning signs, followed by lightheadedness, dizziness, and tinnitus. Facial twitching, which may follow these effects often precedes convulsion, thus the physician must always observe the face of the patient while injecting a

Table 5–6. Maternal and Fetal Tissue Concentrations of Lidocaine in a Guinea Pig

Tissue	Peak maternal level	Peak fetal level
Blood (μg/ml)	7.6	3.6
Myocardium (μg/g)	17.2	8.9
Brain	31.9	9.7
Kidney	42.3	5.8
Liver	7.8	22.9

(Reproduced from Covino BG, and Vassallo HG: Local Anesthetics: Mechanisms of Action and Clinical Use. New York, Grune and Stratton, 1976.)

MOTHER   FETUS

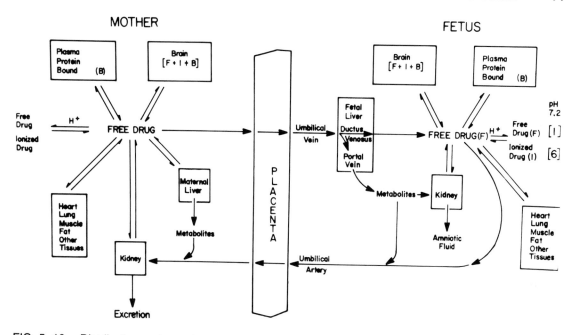

FIG. 5–10. Distribution and metabolism of local anesthetics in the mother and fetus. F = free drug; I = ionized; B = plasma-protein bound. Note the decreased plasma-protein binding in the fetal unit. (From DeFazio CA: Metabolism of local anesthetics in the fetus, newborn and adult. Br J Anaesth 51:29S, 1979.)

local anesthetic to produce a nerve block. Preconvulsive warning signs, such as the dizziness and loss of consciousness that occur with lidocaine,[26] may be absent with other more potent amide analgesics.[5] At subconvulsive doses, lidocaine produces a characteristic EEG pattern in the amygdala. This pattern is described as rhythmic spindling[27] and is a property that is not shared by bupivacaine or etidocaine. With these other agents, convulsions may occur without any clinical or EGG warning signs.

Potent local anesthetics, such as bupivacaine, have lower convulsive threshold dosages than

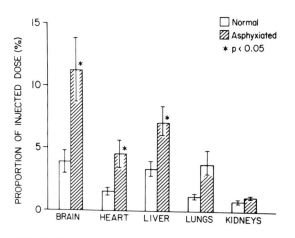

FIG. 5–11. Mean (± standard error) ratios of lidocaine in different organs in normal and hypoxic baboon fetuses. * = significantly different from the normal group. (From Morishima HO, and Covino BG: Toxicity and distribution of lidocaine in nonasphyxiated and asphyxiated baboon fetuses. Anesthesiology 54:182, 1981.

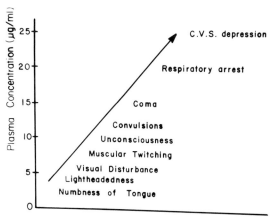

FIG. 5–12. Toxicity with increasing local anesthetic concentration. (Adapted from Scott DB, and Cousins MJ: Clinical Pharmacology of Local Anesthetic Agents. In Neural Blockade in Clinical Anesthesia and Pain Management. Edited by MJ Cousins and PO Bridenbaugh. Philadelphia, JB Lippincott, 1980.)

do less potent local anesthetics. For a given agent, the convulsive threshold dose decreases when the $PaCO_2$ increases (Fig. 5–13). When blood levels increase further, CNS excitation gives way to depression, leading to life-threatening respiratory depression. For the treatment of local anesthetic induced convulsions see the section in this chapter on bupivacaine.

CARDIOVASCULAR EFFECTS

Increased systemic absorption or accidental i.v. administration may produce profound cardiovascular effects. Local anesthetics may affect the myocardium as well as the vascular smooth muscle. The electrophysiologic effects of local anesthetics on cardiac tissues have been previously described in this chapter (Fig. 5–6, Fig. 5–7). Lidocaine exerts antiarrhythmic activity at blood levels that do not affect cardiac ionotropicity.[5] The antiarrhythmic property of lidocaine results from its ability to decrease phase 4 depolarization, although at higher blood concentrations, it also inhibits Phase 0 depolarization. The PR interval of the EKG increases and the QRS complex widens. Extremely high concentrations of lidocaine will arrest spontaneous sinus activity. In addition to the electrophysiologic alterations, local anesthetics may directly affect cardiac contractility.[28]

The ability to depress cardiac contractility correlates directly with the intrinsic anesthetic potency of the agent (Fig. 5–14). Generally speaking, potent local anesthetic agents such as bupivacaine, tetracaine, and etidocaine produce a more profound effect on the myocardium than does the less potent lidocaine or 2-CP.[28] The potent anesthetics produce 25% inhibition of contractility at a serum level of 1 to 1.5 μg/ml. With less potent agents such as lidocaine, mepivacaine, and prilocaine, the serum concentrations must be 10 times higher to produce the same effect.[29] The ability to depress the cardiac output also correlates roughly with anesthetic potency (Fig. 5–14).[30,31] A 50% reduction in cardiac output may be seen in intact animals at a dose of 5 to 10 mg/kg of bupivacaine or etidocaine. With lidocaine, a dose of at least 10 to 30 mg is needed to produce the same effect.[29]

Recently, bupivacaine has been implicated in several cardiac arrests. The increased cardiac toxicity of bupivacaine may be related to its increased potency. A more detailed description of bupivacaine cardiotoxicity appears in this chapter under bupivacaine.

PERIPHERAL VASCULAR EFFECTS

Local anesthetics have a biphasic action on the vascular smooth muscle. In concentrations

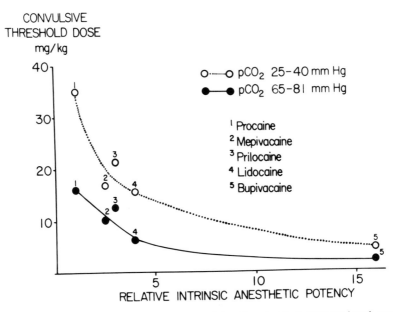

FIG. 5–13. The relationship between $PaCO_2$ and convulsive threshold of different local anesthetics. (From Covino BG, and Vassallo HG: Local Anesthetics: Mechanism of Action and Clinical Use. New York, Grune and Stratton, 1976.)

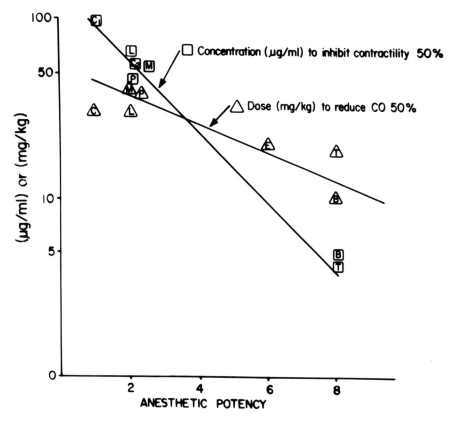

FIG. 5–14. In vivo anesthetic potency of different anesthetics and their potential to produce cardiac toxicity. C1 = chloroprocaine; C2 = cocaine; M = mepivacaine; L = lidocaine; P = prilocaine; E = etidocaine; B = bupivacaine; T = tetracaine.

up to 1 mg/ml, lidocaine produces vasoconstriction; in concentrations in the range of 10 mg/ml, lidocaine will result in vasodilatation.[32] For instance, when injected intra-arterially, local anesthetics may decrease the blood flow in the forearm by constricting the capacitance blood vessels.[33] When the concentration increases, vasoconstriction gives way to vasodilatation.[33] The pulmonary vasculature is affected the most by the vasoconstrictive effect of the local anesthetics. Both ester and amide type local anesthetic agents produce an increase in pulmonary vascular resistance (PVR).[30,31] At 3 mg/kg dose, both bupivacaine and etidocaine markedly increase the PVR. All local anesthetics except cocaine exert this biphasic effect on the vascular smooth muscle. Cocaine produces vasoconstriction at almost all doses because of its ability to inhibit the reuptake of norepinephrine into sympathetic nerve endings.

DIFFERENT TISSUE REACTIONS TO LOCAL ANESTHESIA

Local anesthesia results in a number of different tissue reactions.

Allergy

True anaphylactic reactions to local anesthetics are rare. Clinical manifestations of hypersensitivity include urticaria, angioneurotic edema, and anaphylactic reaction.[34] In many instances, alleged anaphylactoid reactions to local anesthetics are difficult to verify and indeed may instead be a toxic reaction to either the anesthetic or epinephrine. Although local tissue reactions occur with both esters and amides, esters are implicated more frequently. The ester-type of local anesthetics contain p-amino benzoic acid (PABA), a common ingredient found in sun screen lotions. Ester local anesthetics are also implicated in causing contact dermatitis of the hand in dentistry personnel. Previous exposure to antihemorrhoidal preparations or ointments used for minor skin irritation may also cause delayed hypersensitivity reactions.[34] Amide local anesthetic may contain a preservative called methyl paraben, which chemically resembles PABA and thus may cause a reaction in those who are allergic to PABA or ester-type local anesthetic agents.[34]

Local Tissue Reaction

Clinical concentrations of local anesthetic agents do not produce direct neural damage (with the possible exception of 2-chloroprocaine). However, local anesthetic agents may produce muscle damage. In general, the greater the potency of the local anesthetic agent, the greater is the degree of damage to the muscle. The damage heals usually within 2 to 3 weeks.[5] Intramuscular administration of lidocaine may result in an increase in creatine phosphokinase (CPK).[5] A recent study found neither direct muscular damage nor any increase in indices of muscle damage (CPK and lactic dehydrogenase) following intravenous regional anesthesia (Bier block) with bupivacaine.[35] When used for Bier block 2-chloroprocaine produces phlebitis.[2]

Maternal-Fetal Toxicity

In pregnant sheep, signs of CNS toxicity occur at lidocaine blood levels of 5 to 10 μg/ml. The concentrations required to produce CNS toxicity in a normal newborn is 10 to 20 μg/ml. The corresponding figure in the normal fetus is 40 μg/ml. This suggests that the fetus and the newborn may be somewhat less susceptible to the toxic effects of local anesthetic agents than are adults.[36,37] However, acidosis and asphyxia markedly decreases the toxic threshold in the fetus.

INDIVIDUAL ANESTHETIC AGENTS

ESTERS

The esters include cocaine, procaine, 2-chloroprocaine, and tetracaine.

Cocaine

This agent produces vasoconstriction by blocking the reuptake of norepinephrine into the sympathetic nerve endings. A 10% solution is used for topical anesthesia of nose and throat. Because of a low ratio of toxic effect versus therapeutic effect, it is not used for nerve blocks. Its CNS effects are described in Chapter 23 Drug Abuse.

Procaine

This agent has a high pK$_a$ and is therefore highly ionized at body pH. It is not useful as a topical anesthetic. Its duration of action is approximately half that of lidocaine. Procaine penetrates tissue barriers poorly, thus the incidence of unsuccessful nerve blocks is high. The agent has been superseded by other local anesthetics.

Tetracaine (Pontocaine)

Tetracaine produces effective surface analgesia of mucous membranes at 1 to 2% concentration. At 0.2 to 0.5% concentration, it may be used for epidural anesthesia and other nerve blocks. It is an excellent agent for spinal anesthesia (see Chapter 7). Tetracaine is hydrolyzed by plasma cholinesterase.

2-Chloroprocaine (2-CP)

Many (theoretical) benefits have been attributed to this agent. It is rapidly metabolized by the pseudocholinesterase, which limits its placental transfer,[20] and it does not impair neonatal neurobehavior. Given these theoretical considerations, many anesthesiologists came to prefer 2-CP over other agents for obstetric anesthesia. Thus, use of 2-CP escalated throughout the country in the last decade. The widespread use of 2-chloroprocaine helped disclose a major problem of potential neurotoxicity that is associated with use of the drug. Several cases of permanent paraplegia were reported that implicated 2-CP in the neurotoxicity. In many of these cases, large volumes of 2-chloroprocaine were accidentally injected into the intrathecal space during an attempted epidural anesthetic. Several animal studies attempted to determine whether 2-CP or the antioxidant contained in 2-CP was the neurotoxin.[38,39] Nesacaine the commercial preparation of 2-CP contains 0.2% sodium bisulfite (SBS) as an antioxidant to prevent spontaneous oxidation of the ester compound in solution. In an acidic medium, the compound releases SO_2, which penetrates the nerve and forms the neurotoxic sulfurous acid. In animal experiments, neurologic damage only occurred when the total dose of SBS exceeded approximately 0.6 mg/kg.[38] There is, however, no consensus of opinion about the exact mechanism of neurotoxicity caused by 2-CP. Some still believe that 2-CP itself is a neurotoxin.[40]

Caution must be exercised in applying data from animal experiments to clinical situations. Isolated nerve preparations are not representative of the sequence of events that may follow total spinal anesthesia. Total spinal anesthesia will reduce systemic perfusion pressure and will consequently reduce perfusion to the spinal cord. Injecting a large volume of local anesthetic into a closed space is likely to increase the cerebrospinal fluid pressure and further reduce spinal cord perfusion.[41] Some have suggested removing a large volume of cerebrospinal fluid in an attempt to clear the intrathecal space of 2-CP. Even a cisternal puncture was advocated to establish a continuous wash-out of the CSF.[42] Because of total spinal anesthesia in a pregnant patient requires immediate attention to failing ventilation and circulation to prevent death, it may not be possible to promptly institute CSF wash-out procedures.

Should the anesthesiologist feel a compelling urge to use 2-CP in obstetric patients, he must observe some precautions to avoid the serious neurologic complication. He must use a preparation containing the minimum possible concentration of SBS. (A preparation containing 0.07% of SBS is now available in the market.*) He must always administer a test dose to ascertain that the epidural needle or the catheter has not entered the subarachnoid space, and he must avoid injecting a large volume of 2-CP into the intrathecal space as a single bolus. It is necessary to administer the agent in divided doses, allowing sufficient time between injections.

*Astra Pharmaceuticals

AMIDES

Bupivacaine (Marcaine, Sensorcaine)

Bupivacaine is extensively used for labor analgesia and for cesarean section anesthesia. For labor analgesia, it may be used at 0.125% and 0.25% concentrations. At these concentrations, it produces excellent analgesia for labor with little or no motor impairment. A more detailed discussion of its use for labor may be found in Chapter 8. Intermittent injection or continuous infusion may be used for labor analgesia. For cesarean section, anesthesia of a 0.5% concentration may be used. Bupivacaine has also been used for spinal anesthesia (see Chapter 8).

Although a 0.75% concentration of bupivacaine was once popular for cesarean section anesthesia, it is no longer recommended because of the possibility of increased cardiovascular toxicity. Both, the Federal Drug Administration Agency (FDA) and the manufacturers have advised against the use of this concentration in obstetric patients. Several studies published in the last decade claimed that bupivacaine did not have significant effects on infant neurobehavior.[43] This was attributed to its binding to maternal plasma proteins that limited its placental passage; also, many of these studies were based on a small number of patients. It is now known that although protein-binding may diminish the fetal-maternal blood concentration ratio, it may not alter the total amount of drug crossing the placenta. Neonates excrete both 2-6 pipecoloxylidine (PPX) and unmetabolized bupivacaine for prolonged periods of time following maternal epidural anesthesia.[44] As in the case of 2-CP, a minor theoretical advantage propelled bupivacaine into widespread popularity. The issue of possible maternal toxicity that is likely to be caused by a potent local anesthetic such as bupivacaine was not addressed; consequently, many cases of cardiac arrests were reported with the indiscriminate use of bupivacaine.

Albright[45] has collected information on a number of cases of alleged cardiac arrests following the use of potent local anesthetics such as bupivacaine and etidocaine. Although more likely to occur with a concentration of 0.75% than with 0.5% concentration, the occurrence of cardiac arrest is still possible with the weaker concentration. I know of an obstetric patient who developed convulsions and cardiac arrest following accidental intravascular injection of 0.5% bupivacaine. Intracardiac injection of epinephrine restored cardiac rhythm in this patient. I also know of at least 5 cases of CNS toxicity associated with the use of 0.5% bupivacaine in the New York metropolitan area.

Animal experiments have conclusively shown that bupivacaine is more toxic to the CNS and the myocardium than is lidocaine. Of those patients who sustain cardiac arrest following intravascular administration of bupivacaine, many need prolonged cardiorespiratory resuscitation and multiple attempts at electrical defibrillation. It is tempting to postulate that obstetric patients may be prone to cardiac toxicity because of diminished protein binding and the direct access of bupivacaine to the myocardium via the azygos system. However it is doubtful that these factors put the obstetric patients at increased risk for toxicity. The most likely reason for increased frequency of cardiac toxicity of bupivacaine in obstetric patients is related to the widespread use of the agent.

Intractable ventricular arrhythmias and cardiac arrest are hallmarks of bupivacaine cardiac toxicity. The slow diffusion of bupivacaine from the sodium channel in the myocardial cell membrane is probably responsible for the intense cardiac toxicity of the agent. Acidosis and hypoxia may further compound the problem of toxicity. Another problem with bupivacaine is that cardiotoxicity and CNS toxicity may occur simultaneously. Even when CNS toxicity occurs, it may begin acutely without any prodromal signs (see the section on "Central Nervous System Effects" which was discussed previously in this chapter). Bupivacaine may also possess an arrhythmogenic property at subconvulsant doses.[46] However, with the less potent lidocaine, CNS toxicity usually precedes cardiovascular toxicity (Fig. 5–15). Even in doses of lidocaine that far exceed the convulsive threshold, cardiac arrhythmias do not occur (Fig. 5–15). Experiments on animals have shown that bupivacaine may also induce cardiac arrhythmais by a neurogenic mechanism. Administration of 300 μg of bupivacaine into the lateral ventricle of the brain induces severe cardiac dysrhythmias in the cat. The mechanism of neurogenic dysrhythmia is unknown and is believed to be caused by increased catecholamine turnover in the brain.[47]

Systemic toxicity caused by bupivacaine must be treated promptly because hypoxia and acidosis rapidly ensue, further intensifying the toxic effects of the drug.[48] An anticonvulsant such as pentothal or diazepam must be used to control seizures. Endotracheal intubation must be performed without delay to prevent aspiration. Succinylcholine may be required to facilitate endotracheal intubation. If cardiovascular collapse occurs, cardiopulmonary resuscitation must be performed immediately. Prolonged external cardiac massage may be needed to restore cardiac action, and in those patients who do not respond, open chest cardiac massage may be needed. Circulation must be supported by vasopressors. Left uterine displacement must be performed, using a sand bag wedged under the right hip.

The fetal heart rate must be monitored. In severe cases, immediate delivery of the baby by cesarean section must be considered. Even in less serious cases, persistent fetal bradycardia is an indication for immediate cesarean section. Immediate delivery of the baby not only removes the baby from the toxic environment but helps relieve maternal aortocaval compression.

To avoid massive intravascular injections of potent local anesthetics such as bupivacaine or etidocaine, one must observe some simple precautions. A 3 ml test dose of local anesthetic solution containing epinephrine solution 5 μg/ml must be used to detect inadvertent intravenous injection. The patient will often complain of palpitation or "a funny feeling in the chest" when epinephrine is injected intravenously. I have often found such a test dose helpful in preventing accidental intravenous injection. A test dose of bupivacaine or lidocaine containing no epinephrine is not reliable at all. The inducing dose must be injected intermittently, in increments, allowing sufficient time between injections.

Bupivacaine produces excellent analgesia for labor and abdominal delivery. When toxic reactions occur, it is almost always the fault of the anesthesiologist's failure to observe these simple rules. Some centers still use the No. 20 gauge Lutz needle for performing single-shot epidural anesthesia. This blunt-tipped needle has a sidehole and its use allegedly decreases the inci-

LIDOCAINE

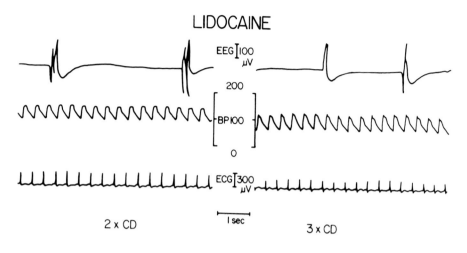

2 x CD   I sec   3 x CD

BUPIVACAINE

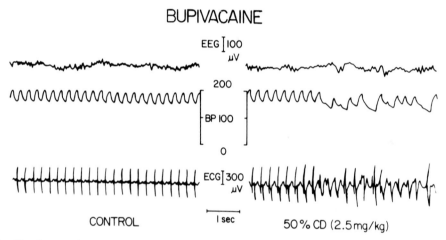

CONTROL   I sec   50% CD (2.5 mg/kg)

FIG. 5–15. Cardiovascular effects of convulsant and supraconvulsant doses of local anesthetics. Even at 3× the convulsive dose (CD), the lidocaine does not induce cardiac arrhythmias. Bupivacaine produces arrhythmias at 0.5 CD. (Reprinted with permission from the International Anesthesia Research Society from De Jong RH, Ronfeld RA, and De Rosa RA: Cardiovascular effects of convulsant doses of amide local anesthetics. Anesth Analg *61*:3, 1982.)

dence of dural punctures. However, I have noted that use of this needle has been associated with several intravascular and intrathecal injections of bupivacaine that resulted in serious maternal, and in some instances, fetal complications. The side-port may lie against the vessel wall causing a false-negative aspiration test.

Lidocaine

Lidocaine is used in obstetric patients both for spinal and epidural anesthesia. For labor analgesia, a 1 or 1.5% solution may be used, and for cesarean section, a 1.5 or 2% may be used. A 5% solution is used for spinal anesthesia. Even at 1.5% concentration plain lidocaine may not produce a satisfactory block for labor analgesia or for cesarean section. Addition of epinephrine to lidocaine in 1:200,000 concentration improves both the quality and the duration of the block. The commercially available local anesthetic-epinephrine mixture has a pH of 4[11] because it contains citric acid, which is added to stabilize epinephrine. The commercial solution also contains sodium metabisulphite. Commercially available licocaine-epinephrine mixtures contain

0.5 mg/ml of sodium metabisulfite (SMBS), which also results in the formation of SBS. The concentration of SMBS may be reduced by preparing a plain lidocaine-epinephrine mixture just before use. Plain lidocaine does not contain SMBS and epinephrine (1:1000, Parke-Davis) contains 0.15 mg per ml of SBS. However, in the final mixture, which contains 1:200,000 concentration of epinephrine, SBS is diluted 200 times. The pH of the freshly mixed solution is 6.5, and consequently, the base form of the drug increases. Since the base form penetrates the neural barriers, the freshly made mixture has a longer duration of action.[11]

Use of lidocaine in obstetric patients drastically decreased in the late seventies following reports that it affected neonatal neurobehavior.[43] However, studies done by Abboud, et al.[49] have shown that lidocaine has little or no effect on neonatal neurobavior. Even assuming that lidocaine does affect neurobehavior, it is doubtful that the transient drug effect alone will have any major impact on the subsequent growth and development of the newborn.

At the New York University Medical Center, my colleagues and I have used lidocaine with epinephrine in over 15,000 cases for labor analgesia and for anesthesia for cesarean section without any serious cardiac or neurotoxicity. If one believes in the dictum "primum non nocere" (or "First of all, do no harm") then lidocaine becomes the automatic choice for obstetric anesthesia, especially when a large volume of local anesthetic is needed.

EPINEPHRINE IN OBSTETRIC ANESTHESIA

Epinephrine is added to local anesthetic solution to decrease the systemic absorption of the local anesthetic and to prolong the duration of action. Epinephrine may also potentiate the action of local anesthetic by suppressing activity of wide dynamic range neurons (WDR neurons) in the dorsal horn.[50] The WDR neurons are cells of origin of the spinothalamic tract, which transmits pain. The use of epinephrine in obstetrics has long been controversial. Many animal experiments have shown that epinephrine because of its β-mimetic action decreases uterine blood flow. Epinephrine is absorbed into the systemic circulation and consequently produces several cardiovascular effects.[51] Earlier studies also showed that the use of epinephrine may prolong labor.

Although β-mimetic effects are likely to cause deleterious side-effects in patients with preclampsia or thyrotoxicosis, they are not likely to be harmful in a healthy parturient. We have used lidocaine with epinephrine for several years and have not noticed any prolongation of labor.[11] A recent study by Abboud T.K., et al. reported a similar finding.[52] The use of epinephrine may also decrease the number of injections and the total dose of lidocaine required during labor.[11] The reduction in the number of injections may reduce the incidence of tachyphylaxis. Tachyphylaxis to lidocaine may become clinically noticeable after the third dose. Tachyphylaxis decreases the number of segments blocked and the duration of anesthesia produced by a given dose of local anesthetic. At the New York University Medical Center, the neonatal acid-base status at birth has been satisfactory in those who received lidocaine-epinephrine mixture,[53] which signifies adequate uteroplacental perfusion. Thus, advantages associated with the use of epinephrine tend to outweigh the disadvantages.

CARBONATED LOCAL ANESTHETIC AGENTS

Bromage has studied the action of a carbonated form of lidocaine. Lidocaine carbonate has a shorter latency than does lidocaine hydrochloride. The enhanced effect of carbonate is believed to be caused by the following factors: the carbonate solution has a higher pH that increases the base form of the drug; and the CO_2 liberated from the compound will diffuse across the cell membrane and decrease the intracellular pH. This increases the cation form within the cell, which intensifies the nerve block. Rapid formation of cation within the cell increases the diffusion gradient for the base into the cell.[54] Other investigators have noted that although carbonation improves the quality of the block, it does not decrease latency.[55] Carbonated lidocaine is not available for general use in the United States.

REFERENCES

1. Ritchie JM, and Greene NM: Local anesthetics. *In* Goodman and Gilman's The Pharmacological Basis of

Therapeutics. 7th Edition. New York, Macmillan Publishing, 1985.

2. Tucker GT.: Chemistry and pharmacology of local anesthetic drugs. *In* Practical Regional Anaesthesia. (Edited by Henderson JJ and Nimmo W). Boston, Blackwell Scientific, 1983.

3. Guyton AC: The Cell and Its Function. *In* Textbook of Medical Physiology. 7th Edition. Philadelphia, W. B. Saunders, 1986.

4. Guyton AC.: Membrane Potentials and Action Potentials. *In* Textbook of Medical Physiology. 7th Ed. W.B. Saunders, 1986.

5. Covino BG, and Vassallo HG.: Local Anesthetics: Mechanisms of Action and Clinical Use. New York, Grune & Stratton, 1976.

6. Hille B.: Local anesthetics: Hydrophilic and hydrophobic pathways for the drug-receptor reaction. J Gen Physiol 69:497, 1977.

7. Clarkson CW and Hondeghem LM.: Mechanism for bupivacaine depression of cardiac conduction: Fast block of sodium channels during the action potential with slow recovery from block during diastole. Anesthesiology 62:396, 1985.

8. Heavner JE, and De Jong RH.: Lidocaine blocking concentrations for B- and C-nerve fibers. Anesthesiology 40:228, 1974.

9. Franz DN and Perry RS.: Mechanisms for differential block among single myelinated and non-myelinated axons by procaine. J Physiol (London) 236:193, 1974.

10. Evans JA, Chastain GM, and Phillips JM.: The use of local anesthetic agents in obstetrics. South Med J 62:519, 1969.

11. Ramanathan S, Dursztman M, and Turndorf H.: Local anesthetics with freshly added epinephrine produce longer obstetrical analagesia. Anesthesiology 63:3A, 1985.

12. Tucker GT, Boyes RN, Bridenbaugh PO, and Moore DC.: Binding of anilide-type local anesthetics in human plasma. I: Relationships between binding physiochemical properties and anesthetic activity. Anesthesiology 33:287, 1970.

13. Tucker GT, and Mather LE.: Clinical Pharmacokinetics of local anesthetics. Clin Pharmacokinet 4:241, 1979.

14. Tucker GT.: Pharmacokinetics of local anesthetic drugs. *In* Practical Regional Anaesthesia. (Edited by Henderson JJ, and Nimmo WS). Boston, Blackwell Scientific, 1983. pp. 1–25.

15. Huet PM, Arsene D, and Richer D.: The volume of distribution of lidocaine in chronic hepatitis: Relationship with serum α-1 acid glycoprotein and serum protein binding. Clinical Pharmacology and Therapeutics 29:252, 1981.

16. Lofstrom B.: Tissue distribution of local anesthetics with special reference to the lung. Int Anesthesiol Clin 16:53, 1978.

17. DiFazio CA.: Metabolism of local anesthetics in the fetus, newborn and adult. Br J Anaesth 51:29S, 1979.

18. Inoue R, et al.: Plasma concentrations of lidocaine and its principal metabolites during intermittent epidural anesthesia. Anesthesiology 63:304, 1985.

19. Tucker GT: Pharmacokinetics of local anesthetic drugs. *In* Practical Regional Anaesthesia. (Edited by Henderson JJ, and Nimmo WS). Boston, Blackwell Scientific, 1983. pp. 25–47.

20. Kuhnert BR, Kuhnert PM, Prochasta AL, and Gross TL.: Plasma levels of 2-chloroprocaine in obstetric patients and their neonates after epidural anesthesia. Anesthesiology 53:21, 1980.

21. de Jong RH.: Biotransformation of local anesthetics: General concepts. Int Anesthesiol Clin 13:1, 1975.

22. Yurth DA.: Placental transfer of local anesthetics. Clin Perinatol 9:13, 1982.

23. Finster M.: Toxicity of local anesthetics in the fetus and the newborn. Bull NY Acad Med 52:222, 1976.

24. Wood M, and Wood AJJ.: Changes in plasma drug binding an αα 1-acid glycoprotein in mother and newborn infant. Clin Pharmacol Ther 29:522, 1981.

25. Morishima HO, and Covino BG.: Toxicity and distribution of lidocaine in nonasphyxiated and asphyxiated baboon fetuses. Anesthesiology 54:182, 1981.

26. Eriksson E, and Persson A.: The effect of intravenously administered prilocaine and lidocaine on the human electroencephalogram studied by automatic frequency analysis. Acta Chir Scand (Suppl) 358:37, 1966.

27. Munson ES, Gutnik MJ, and Wagman IH.: Local anesthetic drug-induced seizures in rhesus monkeys. Anesth Analg 49:986, 1970.

28. Feldman HS, Covino BM, and Sage DJ: Direct chronotropic and inotropic effects of local anesthetic agents in isolated guinea pig atria. Reg Anaesth 7:149, 1982.

29. Covino BG.: Toxicity of local anesthetics. Advances in Anesthesia. (Edited by Stoelting RK, Barash PG, and Gallagher) Chicago, Year Book Medical Publishers, 1986.

30. Lui PL, et al.: Acute cardiovascular toxicity of procaine, chloroprocaine, and tetracaine in anesthetized ventilated dogs. Reg Anaesth, 7:14, 1982.

31. Lui PL, et al.: Acute cardiovascular toxicity of intravenous amide local anesthetics in anesthetized ventilated dogs. Anesth Analg 61:317, 1982.

32. Blair MR.: Cardiovascular pharmacology of local anesthetics. Br J Anaesth 47:247, 1975.

33. Jortfeldt L, et al.: The effect of mepivacaine and lidocaine on forearm resistance and capacitance vessels in man. Acta Anaesthesiol Scand 14:183, 1970.

34. Curley RK, Macfarlane AW, and King CM.: Contact sensitivity to the amide anesthetics lidocaine, prilocaine, and mepivacaine. Arch Dermatol 122:924, 1986.

35. Kalso EA, et al.: Evaluation of the myotoxicity of bupivacaine in bier blocks–A biochemical and electron microscopic study. Anesth Analg 62:796, 1983.

36. Lund PC, and Covino BG.: Distribution of local anesthetics in man following peridural anesthesia. J Clin Pharmacol 7:324, 1967.

37. Morishima HO, et al.: Toxicity of lidocaine in the adult, newborn and fetal sheep. Anesthesiology 55:57, 1981.

38. Wang BC, Hillman DE, Spielholz NI, and Turndorf H.: Chronic neurological deficits and nesacaine-CE–An effect of the anesthetic, 2-chloroprocaine, or the antioxidant, sodium bisulfite? Anesth Analg 63:445, 1984.

39. Gissen AJ, Datta S, and Lambert D.: The chloroprocaine controversy. II. Is chloroprocaine neurotoxic? Reg Anaesth 9:135, 1984.

40. Myers RR, Kalichman MW, Reisner LS, and Powell

HC.: Neurotoxicity of local anesthetics: Altered peri-neurial permeability, edema and nerve fiber injury. Anesthesiology 64:29, 1986.

41. Gissen AJ, Datta S, and Lambert D: The chloroprocaine controversy. A hypothesis to explain the neural complications of chloroprocaine epidural. Reg Anaesth 9:124, 1984.

42. Covino BG, et al.: Prolonged sensory/motor deficits following inadvertent spinal anesthesia. Anesth Analg 59:399, 1980.

43. Scanlon JW, Brown WU, Weiss JB, and Alper MH: Neurobehavioral responses of newborn infants after maternal epidural anesthesia. Anesthesiology 40:121–128, 1974.

44. Kuhnert PM, Kunhart BR, Stitts JM, and Gross TL: The use of selective ion monitoring technique to study the disposition of bupivacaine in mother, fetus, and neonate following epidural anesthesia for cesarean section. Anesthesiology 55:611, 1981.

45. Albright AA, Ferguson JE, Joyce TH, and Stevenson DK: Anesthesia in Obstetrics Maternal, Fetal, and Neonatal Aspects. Boston, Butterworths, 1986.

46. de Jong RH, Ronfeld RA, and DeRosa RA: Cardiovascular effects of convulsant and supraconvulsant doses of amide local anesthetics. Anesth Analg 61:3, 1982.

47. Heavner JE: Cardiac dysrhythmias induced by infusion of local anesthetics into the lateral cerebral ventricle of cats. Anesth Analg 65:133, 1986.

48. Moore DC, et al.: Severe hypoxia and acidosis following local-anesthetic-induced convulsions. Anesthesiology 53:259, 1980.

49. Abboud TK, et al.: Lack of adverse neonatal neurobehavioral effects of lidocaine. Anesth Analg 62:473, 1983.

50. Collins JG, et al.: Spinally administered epinephrine suppresses noxiously evoked activity of WDR neurons in the dorsal horn of the spinal cord. Anesthesiology 60:269, 1984.

51. Bonica JJ, et al.: Circulatory effects of peridural block. Anesthesiology 34:514, 1971.

52. Abboud TK, et al.: Maternal, fetal, and neonatal effects of lidocaine with and without epinephrine for epidural anesthesia in obstetrics. Anesth Analg 63:973, 1984.

53. Ramanathan S, Arismendy J, and Turndorf H: The biochemical profile of a well-oxygenated human fetus. Anesthesiology 61:A397, 1984.

54. Catchlove RFH: The influence of CO_2 and pH on local anesthetic action. J Pharmacol Exp Ther 181:298, 1972.

55. Morrison DH: A double blind comparison of carbonated lidocaine and lidocaine hydrochloride in epidural anaesthesia. Can J Anaesth 28:387, 1981.

6

SPINAL OPIOIDS

The practice of injecting opiates into the epidural and intrathecal or epidural space to produce selective spinal analgesia is a recent development. When injected, these opiates gain access to the special receptor sites located in the dorsal horn of the spinal cord.[1] The existence of endogenous substances that possess opiate-like characteristics has been suspected for at least 20 years. In 1973, Pert and Snyder first demonstrated the presence of opiate receptors in the brain.[2] The discovery of the receptor prompted a furious search for an endogenous opiate ligand. The first endogenous opioid-like peptides, methionine enkephalin (met-enkephalin) and leucine enkephalin (leu-enkephalin), were isolated by Hughes. This was soon followed by the identification of the second endogenous opioid peptide, β-endorphin, by Li and Chung.

OPIOID RECEPTORS

There are three types of opioid receptors: sensory; limbic; and neuroendocrine.[2] The sensory opioid receptors diminish transmission of noxious impulses in the spinal cord, but they will not modify transmission of vibration, position, and light touch sensations. The sensory opioid receptors also occur in relation to the central terminals of the vagus nerve. Opioid receptors, located in the area postrema of the medulla, may explain the nausea and vomiting caused by the spinal opiates. The limbic system opioid receptors are found in the amygdala and the basal ganglia. The limbic system activity affects mood and behavior. The neuroendocrine opioid receptors are found in the posterior pituitary and/or the hypothalamic nuclei. These receptors probably play a role in the release of hormones from the anterior and posterior pituitary. They may also influence catecholamine release, temperature regulation, and diurnal function.

Opiate receptors are also found outside the central nervous system where they mainly exhibit an inhibitory effect on neuronal function. Opiate receptors occurring in the adrenal glands cause diminished release of catecholamine. Opiate receptors are also located in the sympathetic ganglia, myenteric plexus of the intestines (decreased gut motility), and throughout the peripheral autonomic nervous system.[2]

The spinal opiate receptors have been the subject of intense investigation. The ability of a given opioid drug to precipitate or diminish opiate withdrawal symptoms has been used to study the different receptors.[3] The opioid receptors have been classified into subgroups μ, δ, κ and σ based on the type of opioid agonist that binds with them. The μ-receptors mediate analgesia, respiratory depression, euphoria, and physical dependence caused by opioids. In addition, they bind β-endorphins. The δ-receptors mediate epileptic, behavioral, and sedative effects of opioids, and they bind enkephalins more avidly than they do β-endorphin.[3] The κ- and σ-receptors bind special opiate compounds namely ketocyclozocine and N-allylnormetazocine, respectively.[4] The κ-receptor mediates analgesia, miosis and sedation, and the σ-receptors mediate dysphoria, hallucinations, as well as respiratory and vasomotor stimulation. The phencyclidine (PCP, a derivative of which is ketamine) binds with the σ-receptors. The antagonist naloxone is more effective in reversing the effects mediated by the μ-receptor than it is against the effects of κ- and σ-receptors.[3] Naloxone antagonizes very few effects of PCP. The characteristics of the opiate receptors are summarized in Table 6–1.

ENDOGENOUS OPIOID PEPTIDES

There are three distinct families of opioid peptides secreted by the central nervous system: enkephalins, endorphins, and dynorphin. The opioid peptides are believed to exert their effects not only in the central nervous system, but throughout the body.[2,3,5] The peptides occur in relation to the opiate receptors described in the preceding section. Each precursor polypeptide yields a variety of compounds (Table 6–2) that bind differentially with the opiate receptors (Table 6–1). The opioid peptides seem to function as neurotransmitters, modulators of neurotransmission, or neurohormones. Their physiologic role has not been completely understood.

ENKEPHALINS

Enkephalins occur in globus pallidus, periaqueductal gray matter, and in the basal ganglia and amygdala. In the spinal cord, enkephalins occur in relation to substantia gelatinosa and the intermediolateral horn. Enkephalins are also

Table 6–1.   Opiate Receptors

	MU	Delta	Kappa	Sigma
Effect	Analgesia Respiratory depression Euphoria Addiction	Analgesia Seizure Mood Behavior	Analgesia Miosis Sedation	Dysphoria Hallucination Stimulation
Agonists	Dihydromorphine Morphine Buprenorphine Propiram	Morphine* Dihydromorphine*	Morphine Butorphanol Nalbuphine Nalorphine Pentazocine Ketocyclazocine	Pentazocine Butorphanol Nalbuphine Nalorphine N-allylnormetozocine
Antagonists	Naloxone Pentazocine Nalbuphine Nalorphine	Naloxone*	Naloxone*	Not known

Distribution	Cerebral cortex
	  (Laminae I, IV)
	Thalamus
	Hypothalamus
	Periaqueductal
	  gray matter
	Median raphe
		Cortex (Laminae
		  II, III, V)
		Corpus striatum
		Amygdala
		Adrenals
		Peripheral auto-
		  nomic nervous
		  system
		Myenteric plexus
		
		Tractus solitarius
		Lamina VI (cortex)
		Vagal fibers
		Trigeminal nerve
		Substantia gelatinosa
			Cerebral cortex	Cerebral cortex

Endogenous
  Peptides
	β-endorphin
	Met-enkephalin
	Dynorphin A, B
		β-endorphin
		Met-enkephalin
		Dynorphin A, B
		Leu-enkephalin
			Prodynorphin
			  peptides
				Not known

*Low affinity.

Table 6–2.   Opiate Polypeptides

Precursor polypeptide	Active substance
Pro-opiomelanocortin (POMC)	Melanocyte stimulating hormone ACTH Beta-endorphin
Proenkephalin	Met-enkephalin Leu-enkephalin
Prodynorphin	Leu-enkephalin Alpha and beta neoendorphin Dynorphin A and B

found in the sympathetic ganglia and the adrenal gland. The enkephalin that occurs in relation to the sympathetic nervous system is believed to be responsible for the cardiovascular effects of the opioids. The adrenal enkephalin is formed from a precursor molecule proenkephalin (Proenkephalin A). The hypothalamic enkephalin is formed from prodynorphin (proenkephalin B), which also releases dynorphin.

β-ENDORPHIN

The β-endorphin mainly occurs in the pituitary gland and in the hypothalamus. The β-endorphin precursor, which is released from the anterior pituitary, also releases melanocyte-stimulating hormone and ACTH. The β-endorphin has 31 amino acids in its molecular structure. Hypothalamic β-endorphin, occurring in relation to hypothalamus, may also influence cardiovascular function through neural connections of the hypothalamic neuclei with brain stem and vagal nuclei.

DYNORPHIN

Although found in minute quantities, dynorphin is an extremely potent endogenous opioid. It binds with its own receptor. It has 13 amino acids in its structure and it has been isolated from the pituitary extracts. As already mentioned, dynorphin is released as a part of the prodynorphin. (Table 6–2). Dynorphin is further fragmented into dynorphins A and B.

THE DORSAL HORN

The afferent sensory impulses are carried to the dorsal horn of the spinal cord by the myelinated and the unmyelinated afferents. The myelinated afferents (A-β-fibers) conduct fine touch sensations requiring a high degree of localization and vibration, motion, and pressure modalities.[6] The β afferents mainly enter the dorsal columns, with some fibers connecting with laminae III to VI of the dorsal horn (Fig 6–1). The smaller unmyelinated afferents (Aδ- and C-fibers) conduct from the periphery the modalities of pain, temperature, crude touch, tickle, and itch, together with sexual sensations. The Aδ-fibers conduct the acute pain and the C-fibers conduct slow pain. The impulses carried in the myelinated fibers travel upward or downward two or three segments in the tract of Lissauer. The Aδ-fibers terminate at laminae I and IV and the C-fibers in laminae II and III (substantia gelatinosa). Visceral pain impulses that are carried along the sympathetic C-fibers are processed in the substantia gelatinosa of the dorsal horn. The spinal opioids bind with the specific receptors situated in the substantia gelatinosa, thus diminishing pain sensation. The impulses processed at the substantia gelatinosa cross over to the opposite side and ascend in the anterolateral spinothalamic tracts.

THE DESCENDING PAIN CONTROL SYSTEM

The nociceptive impulses, arriving at the spinal cord via the unmyelinated afferents, release neurotransmitters including substance-P. The neurotransmitters facilitate conduction of the impulses into the spinothalamic system. The nervous system is capable of inhibiting pain impulses at several crucial points.[1] The impulses may be inhibited at the dorsal horn by binding of enkephalins with the opioid receptors. The activity of enkephalins is just not limited to the dorsal horn.[1] A descending anti-nociceptive

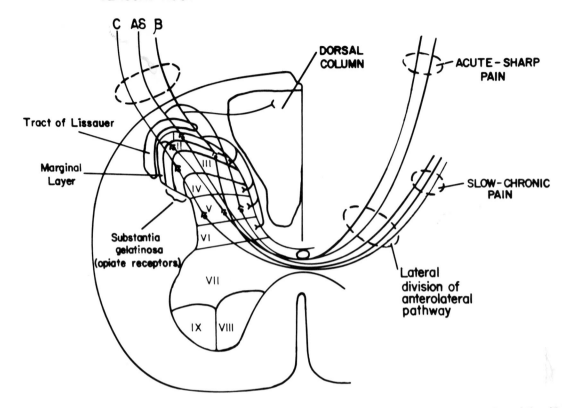

FIG. 6–1. The laminae in the dorsal and ventral horns of the spinal cord. Note the synapsing of the Aδ and C fibers in the substantia gelatinosa of the spinal cord. The myelinated β afferents connect with both the dorsal column and the laminae of the gray matter. (Original source: Guyton AC: Somatic sensations. I and II sensations. *In* Textbook of Medical Physiology. 7th Ed. Philadelphia, WB Saunders, 1986.)

tract, which takes origin from the periaqueductal gray matter (Fig. 6–2) is known to modulate pain at the spinal segment level. This system uses enkephalin and serotonin as neurotransmitters (Fig. 6–2).[6] Norepinephrine and 5-hydroxytryptamine are also believed to play a role in activating the descending anti-nociceptive system.[1]

SPINAL OPIATES IN OBSTETRICS

In 1979, Wang, et al.[1] showed that a subarachnoid injection of morphine will produce long lasting analgesia in patients with cancer. Several opiates (Table 6–3) have since then been used in obstetrics for the purposes of producing both labor analgesia and post-operative pain relief. Morphine has received extensive clinical trial. Many nonopiate substances, such as ke-

tamine, have also been used in the epidural space to produce analgesia.[7] The site of action of these drugs is believed to be the specific receptors located in the substantia gelatinosa of the spinal cord. The opiates may be injected into the epidural space or into the subarachnoid space. The dose required for epidural injection is (as in the case of the local anesthetic) greater than that required in the subarachnoid space. Epidural injection must be made only after ascertaining that the needle or the catheter has not been inadvertently placed in the subarachnoid space. This may be done either by careful aspiration of the catheter or by administering a test dose of local anesthetic before administering the opiate.

UPTAKE AND DISTRIBUTION

The higher the lipid solubility of the agent, the greater is the speed of onset (Table 6–3, Fig.

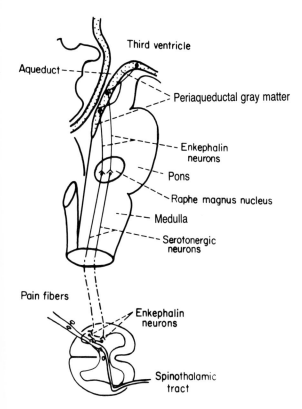

Third ventricle

Aqueduct

Periaqueductal gray matter

Enkephalin neurons

Pons

Raphe magnus nucleus

Medulla

Serotonergic neurons

Pain fibers

Enkephalin neurons

Spinothalamic tract

FIG. 6–2.   The anti-nociceptive system of the brain stem and the spinal cord. Note the location of the enkephalin neurons in the midbrain, and in the spinal cord in relation to the substantia gelatinosa. (From Guyton AC: Somatic sensations. I and II Sensations. *In* Textbook of Medical Physiology. 7th Ed. Philadelphia, WB Saunders, 1986.)

6–3).[8] For instance, morphine with a lipid solubility coefficient of 1.42 has a latency of 30 to 60 minutes and fentanyl (partition coefficient 800) has a latency of only 5 minutes. In general those agents with a lower partition coefficient will also have a longer duration of action (Table 6–3). Epidural injections will have a slower onset than will intrathecal injections. The opiate injected into the epidural space may reach the subarachnoid space by diffusing across the dura matter or by being carried in the perforating spinal arteries.[1] The undissociated form of the drug (lipophilic moiety) is required to penetrate the dura. The ratio between the concentrations of the uncharged and the charged moieties will depend on the pK_a of the opiate and the pH of the CSF. The molecular weight and the pK_a of the commonly used opiates are similar to those of local anesthetics (Table 6–3). Once in the

CSF, the undissociated form may enter the dorsal horn and bind with the receptor. At the receptor, there is redissociation to form the charged moiety, which ultimately produces the receptor blockade. As in the case of the local anesthetics, the undissociated form also undergoes rapid vascular absorption into the epidural veins. The epidural veins drain into the azygos vein, and basivertebral venous plexus, which connect with the cerebral venous sinuses. A simplified summary of the uptake of the opiate from the epidural space is presented in Fig. 6–4. The dissociated form is also believed to ascend rostrally and produce various side effects.[1] In the case of a poorly lipid soluble substance such as morphine, the vascular clearance is slow causing the CSF to contain a large concentration of the opiate for a long time. This increases the chances of rostral spread.[1] On the other hand, substances that are highly lipid soluble have less risk for cephalad spread when compared to morphine.

The opiates are readily absorbed into the systemic circulation from the epidural and subarachnoid spaces.[9,10] The rate of absorption is faster from the epidural space than from the subarachnoid space because the subarachnoid space is less vascular than the epidural space, and because only a small opiate dose is used for producing analgesia. Subarachnoid injections also produce lower plasma levels than do epidural injections (Fig. 6–5). The rate and degree of absorption from the epidural space, however, are quite rapid, almost equalling those seen with intramuscular injection (Fig. 6–5). The unconjugated morphine will attain peak plasma concentration within a half hour after epidural injection. The morphine that enters the vascular compartment will be conjugated with glucuronide immediately after its entry into the intravascular compartment. Although the addition of epinephrine to the opiate solution may diminish vascular uptake, it may also facilitate uptake by the spinal cord with the result that the side effects related to receptor binding (nausea, vomiting, itching) may increase in frequency and intensity.[11]

Even an amount as small as 0.25 mg of morphine injected into the subarachnoid space will result in a large concentration of morphine in the CSF (Fig. 6–6).[9] With epidural administration, the dose of morphine required to produce a given concentration in the CSF is approxi-

Table 6–3. Characteristics of Spinal Opioids

Agent	MW	Partition Coefficient	pKa	Dose	Onset (min.)	Duration (hours)
Morphine	285	1.42	7.9	3–5 mg	30–60	16–24
Meperidine	247	38.8	8.5	30–100 mg	12–30	6–8
Methadone	309	116	9.3	5 mg	15–20	6–8
Fentanyl	336	813	8.4	50–100 μg	6–9	3–5
Lofentanil	408	1450	7.8	1–5 μg	2–5	8–10
Sufentanil	386	1778	8.0	15–50 mg	2–8	4–6
Butorphanol	270	100		2–4 mg	10–15	6–12
Hydromorphone				1 mg		6–8

Note: Ketamine and pentazocine have also been used for this purpose. Doses are for epidural administration.

mately 20 times greater than that required with intrathecal administration. Intramuscular administration of morphine does not result in a significant CSF level of morphine. Morphine will persist for up to 20 to 24 hours in the subarachnoid space (Fig. 6–6), thus explaining the long duration of action. Spinal opiates have been used for labor analgesia and for postoperative analgesia in obstetric patients.[12–19]

LABOR ANALGESIA

The use of spinal opiates may offer some theoretic advantages over the use of local anesthetics. The spinal opiates do not cause hypotension or impair motor power. In addition, they provide prolonged pain relief. The clinical trials, however, have yielded generally disappointing results. Even with an epidural injection of 7.5 mg of morphine, 50% of patients may not experience complete pain relief.[18] The incidence of annoying side effects, such as nausea and itching is high. The delayed onset of action is another disadvantage. The onset time may be shortened by using more lipid soluble opiates, such as meperidine and fentanyl, although they also fail to produce adequate analgesia. In general, the pain relief may be better during first stage than during second stage. Subarachnoid injections produce better results than do epidural injections. β-endorphins have also been used to produce labor analgesia. The drug must

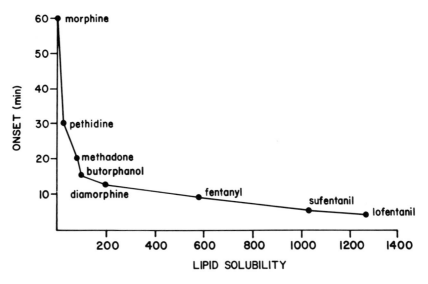

FIG. 6–3. Onset of spinal analgesia in relation to lipid solubility. (From Naulty JS: Intraspinal narcotics. Clinics in Anaesthesiology, 4:145, 1986.)

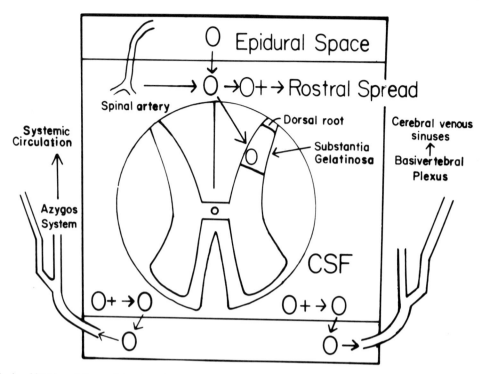

FIG. 6–4. Uptake of the opiate drug from the epidural space. O represents the undissociated form of the drug and O+ the dissociated form. Note the uptake into the substantia gelatinosa and the epidural vasculature.

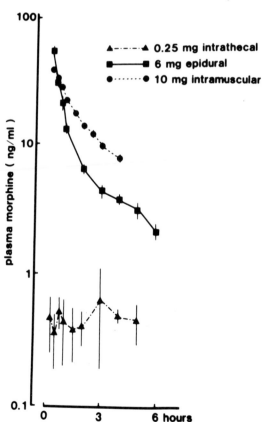

FIG. 6–5. Plasma concentrations of morphine after intrathecal, epidural, and intramuscular injections. (From Nordberg G: Pharmacokinetic aspects of spinal morphine analgesia. Acta Anaesthesiol Scand Suppl. 28, 79:1, 1984.)

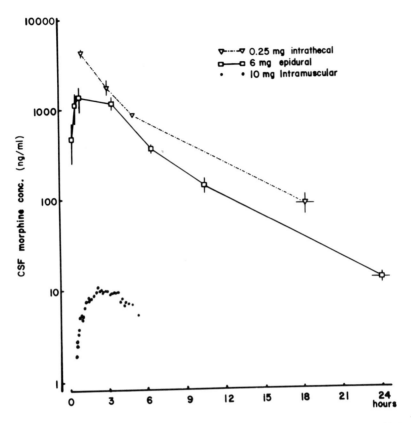

FIG. 6–6.   Cerebrospinal fluid morphine concentrations after intramuscular, epidural, and intrathecal administration. Note the persistent level of morphine in the CSF after intrathecal and epidural administration. (From Nordberg G: Pharmacokinetic aspects of spinal morphine analgesia. Acta Anaesthesiol Scand 27, 79:1, 1984.)

be injected intrathecally because it will not penetrate the dura mater because of its large molecular weight.[20] It does not cross the blood brain barrier, and therefore may not depress the fetal CNS. There have been only a few clinical trials, however, and the cost is prohibitive.

In order to improve the success rate of labor pain relief with spinal opiates, some recommend using the narcotic in combination with a dilute solution of local anesthetic (0.125% bupivacaine with fentanyl 50 to 100 μg). Until more studies become available, the routine use of the combination is not recommended because the combination is always more potent than the individual agent in producing both beneficial as well as adverse effects. The use of spinal opioid may carry some advantages in parturients with severe pulmonary hypertension of severe aortic stenosis in whom a rapid sympathetic denervation caused by the local anesthetic may not be desirable.[21]

CESAREAN SECTION

The use of spinal opiates for providing postoperative analgesia after cesarean section has been successful. Morphine, fentanyl, meperidine, or other narcotics may be used (Table 6–3). Epidural injection of 5 mg of morphine will produce analgesia lasting 24 hours. In the vast majority of cases, no other parenteral narcotic administration is required in the first 24 hours. The dosages and duration of action of the other opioids is summarized in Table 6–3. The use of more fat soluble opiates necessitates more than one injection because of their shorter duration of action. When such agents are being used, the epidural catheter must be left in place for at least 24 hours. The spinal opiates when used for postoperative analgesia offers the following advantages: (1) the mother is usually pain-free, which may permit early ambulation and minimize the risk of deep vein thrombosis; (2) nursing be-

tatonia and dysphoric mood changes (probably a result of δ-receptor activation in the limbic system).[27]

REFERENCES

1. Cousins MJ, and Mather LE: Intratracheal and epidural administration of opioids. Anesthesiology 61:276, 1984.

2. Lagamma EF: Endogenous opiates and cardiopulmonary function. Adv Pediatr 31:1, 1984.

3. Jaffe JH, and Martin WR: Opioid analgesics and antagonists. In The Pharmacologic Basis of Therapeutics. (Edited by Gilman AG, Goodman LS, Rall TW, and Murad F). New York, Macmillan Publishing, 1985.

4. Wolozin BL, Nishimura S, and Pasternak GW: The binding of κ and σ opiates in the rat brain. J Neurosci 2:708, 1982.

5. Akil S, et al.: Endogenous opioids: biology and function. Annu Rev Neurosci 223, 1984.

6. Guyton AC: Somatic sensations. I and II sensations. In Textbook of Medical Physiology. 7th Ed. Philadelphia, WB Saunders, 1986.

7. Mankowitz E, Brock-Utne JG, Cosnett JE and Green-Thompson R: Epidural ketamine: A preliminary report. S Afr Med J 61:441, 1982.

8. Naulty JS: Intraspinal narcotics. Clinics in Anaesthesiology 4:145, 1986.

9. Nordberg G: Pharmacokinetic aspects of spinal morphine analgesia. Acta Anaesthesiol Scand Suppl. 79 28:1, 1984.

10. Kafer ER, et al.: Biphasic depression of ventilatory responses to CO_2 following epidural morphine. Anesthesiology 58:418, 1983.

11. Bromage PR, Camporesi EM, Durant PA, and Nielsen CH: Influence of epinephrine as an adjuvant to epidural morphine. Anesthesiology 58:257, 1983.

12. Gustafsson LL, Schildt B, and Jacobsen K: Adverse effects of extradural and intrathecal opiates: Report of nationwide survey in Sweden. Br J Anaesth 54:479, 1982.

13. Writer WDR, et al.: Epidural morphine prophylaxis of postoperative pain. Canad Anaesth Soc J 32:330, 1985.

14. Stensheth R, Sellevold O, and Breivik H: Epidural morphine for postoperative pain: Experience with 1085 patients. Acta Anaesthesiol Scand 29:148, 1985.

15A. Kotelko DM, et al.: Epidural morphine analgesia after cesarean delivery. Obstet Gynecol 63:409, 1984.

15B. Dailey PA, et al.: The effects of naloxane associated with the intrathecal use of morphine in labor. Anesth Analg 64:658, 1985.

16. Cohen SE, and Woods WA: The role of epidural morphine in postcesarean patient: Efficacy and effects on bonding. Anesthesiology 58:500, 1983.

17. Daily PA, et al.: The effects of naloxone associated with the intrathecal use of morphine in labor. Anesth Analg 64:658, 1985.

18. Hughes SC, et al.: Maternal and neonatal effects of epidural morphine for labor and delivery. Anesth Analg 63:319, 1984.

19. Thind GS, et al.: The effects of continuous intravenous naloxone on epidural morphine analgesia. Anaesthesia 41:582, 1986.

20. Oyama T, et al.: Beta-endorphin in obstetric analgesia. Am J Obstet Gynecol 137:613, 1980.

21. Abboud TK, Raya J, Noueihed R, and Daniel J: Intrathecal morphine for relief of labor pain in a parturient with severe pulmonary hypertension. Anesthesiology 59:477, 1983.

22. Rawal N, et al.: Comparison of intramuscular and epidural morphine for postoperative analgesia in the grossly obese: Influence on postoperative ambulation and pulmonary function. Anesth Analg 63:583, 1984.

23. Camporesi EM, Nielsen CH, Bromage PR, and Durant PAC: Ventilatory CO_2 sensitivity after intravenous and epidural morphine. Anesth Analg 62:633, 1983.

24. Cohen SE, Tothblatt AJ, and Albright GA: Early respiratory depression with epidural narcotic and intravenous droperidol. Anesthesiology 59:559, 1983.

25. Ramanathan S, Horn R, Parker F, and Turndorf H: Naloxone infusion is ineffective in preventing the side-effects of epidural morphine in post-cesarean section patients. Anesthesiology 65 (in press).

26. Rawal N. et al.: An experimental study of urodynamic effects of epidural morphine and of naloxone reversal. Anesth Analg 62:641, 1983.

27. Engquist A, Jorgensen BC, and Andersen HB: Catatonia after epidural morphine. Acta Anaesth Scand 25:445, 1981.

CHAPTER 7

REGIONAL BLOCKS

Of all the branches of anesthesia, it is in obstetric anesthesia where regional nerve blocks offer the greatest advantage over general anesthesia. Regional blocks, when safely performed, not only enable the mother to remain awake during delivery of her infant, but they also avoid the fetal CNS depression that is likely to be caused by inhalational agents. In addition, the aspiration of gastric contents and other serious complications of general anesthesia are avoided.

EPIDURAL ANESTHESIA

Epidural anesthesia is a very popular technique for producing labor analgesia, an anesthesia for either vaginal delivery or cesarean section. In 1901, Sicard and Cathelin used the caudal approach to epidural injection. By 1920, caudal epidural anesthetic was being used extensively. Pagès described the lumbar approach to epidural anesthesia in 1921, but it was Dogliotti who popularized the technique. The next important milestone in the history of epidural anesthesia was the adaptation of Tuohy's spinal needle for epidural anesthesia. The use of epidural anesthesia in obstetric patients became popular in the 1950's. The lumbar approach to epidural anesthesia was soon being preferred to the caudal approach because with the caudal approach, not only were larger doses of local anesthetics needed, but the segmental blockade that was necessary for labor analgesia was difficult to achieve.

ANATOMY OF THE LUMBAR EPIDURAL SPACE

Ligaments

A basic knowledge of the spinal ligaments is essential to understanding the anatomy of the epidural space.[1] The anterior and posterior longitudinal ligaments run between the anterior and posterior aspects to the vertebral bodies, respectively. The supraspinous ligament stretches from the 7th cervical vertebra to the sacrum, acquiring maximum thickness in the lumbar area. The interspinous ligament is dense in the lumbar area. The ligamentum flavum, which consists of yellow elastic fibers, runs from the anterior and inferior aspects of the vertebral lamina to the posterior and superior aspects of the lamina below (Fig. 7–1). The ligamentum flavum is a paired structure. The left and the right ligamenta flava are connected to each other in the midline by fibrous strands. The ligamentum flavum is most dense in the lumbar area (3 to 3.5 mm). The distance between the ligamentum flavum and the dura is 4 to 6 mm. The epidural needle perforates the lower and medial portion of the ligamentum flavum[1] (Fig. 7–1).

Epidural Space Boundaries

The epidural, or the extradural space, is a potential space outside the dural canal. It stretches from the base of the skull to the sacral hiatus. The term epidural is a misnomer because

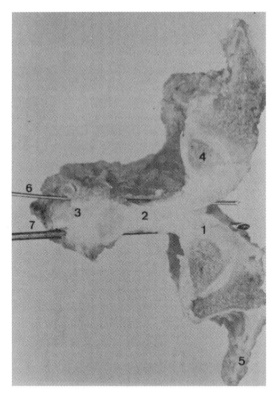

FIG. 7–1. The ligamentum flavum in relation to the bevel of the needle. (1) ligamentum flavum; (2) interspinous ligament; (3) supraspinous ligament; (4) articular process; (5) transverse process; both (6) and (7) are epidural needles. (Reprinted with permission from the International Anesthesia Research Society from Zarzur E: Anatomic studies of the human lumbar ligamentum flavum. Anesth Analg 63:499, 1984.)

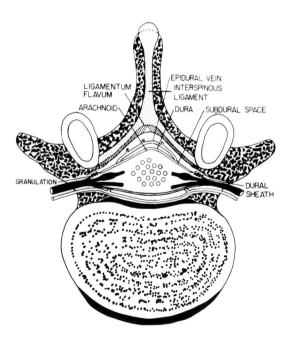

FIG. 7–2. Transverse section through the lumbar spinal column. Note the venous plexus in the epidural space together with prolongation of the dura arachnoid over the mixed spinal nerve (dural cuff area). Note the location of arachnoid granulations near the cuff area. Also note the subdural space between the dura and the arachnoid mater.

the space is really situated between the two layers of the dura mater. The spinal dura mater consists of two layers: an outer periosteal layer and the inner investing layer. The periosteal layer blends with the periosteum of the vertebrae, and the inner layer invests the spinal cord. The epidural space is situated between these two layers. The two layers of the spinal dura are firmly adherent to each other, and to the base of the skull at the foramen magnum. Thus, local anesthetic solutions injected into the spinal epidural space cannot spread directly into the cranial epidural space. Both the anterior and the posterior roots emerging from the spinal cord are ensheathed in a dural extension (dural cuff), which forms the epineurium of the mixed spinal nerve (Fig. 7–2). The subdural space lies between the dura matter and the arachnoid membrane. This space is continuous with the corresponding intracranial space.

Thus, the boundaries of the epidural space are as follows: anteriorly the investing layer of the spinal dura; posteriorly, the periosteal layer of the dura mater (which almost imperceptibly merges with the ligamentum flavum); laterally, the dural cuff area; superiorly, the foramen magnum (where the two layers of the dura fuse with each other); and inferiorly, the sacrococcygeal hiatus. The epidural space contains the nerve roots, fibrous tissue, fat blood vessels, and lymphatics. Epidural venous plexus, which are part of the vertebral plexus, run vertically. The plexus are arranged into two or three main masses (one on each side) and are found on the sides of the epidural space. There are interconnections between the two sides completing a vascular ring at each level (Fig. 7–2). The veins are valveless (valveless veins of Batson) and help establish communication between the pelvic and the intracranial venous sinuses[2] connecting with vertebral, azygos, and lumbar veins. The epidural veins are likely to be engorged in a pregnant patient because they form important collaterals when the inferior vena cava is obstructed by the gravid uterus (see Chapter 2).

Blood Supply of the Spinal Cord

The arterial blood supply of the spinal cord is somewhat precarious. The posterior spinal arteries (one or two) supply portions of the posterior columns and the posterior horns. A single anterior spinal artery supplies the ventral horn and the pyramidal tracts. The posterior spinal artery, which originates from the posterior inferior cerebellar arteries, receives reinforcements at several levels from the regional arteries. In addition, several surface vessels also supply the spinal cord. The anterior spinal artery extends along the entire length of the anterior median fissure and receives reinforcements from several regional arteries such as the cervical and intercostal arteries. In the lumbosacral area, a single named blood vessel (artery of Adamkiewicz) is a major feeder of the anterior spinal artery. This artery arises in a majority of instances from one of the intercostal or lumbar arteries between T8 and L3.[2,3] The spinal cord viens are arranged into an anterior group and a posterior group of plexus, both of which drain into the epidural vein (Fig. 7–2).

The epidural space is not a closed space. It freely communicates with the paravertebral spaces through the intervertebral foramina. In young individuals, radiographic contrast media that is injected into the epidural space readily reach the paravertebral areas. In older subjects, fibrous tissue may cause narrowing of the intervertebral foramen, which limits communication between the two spaces. The epidural space contains the anterior (motor) and the posterior nerve roots (sensory). Cervical and sacral roots are larger than the lumbodorsal roots. Sacral roots 1, 2, and 3 are bulkier than the lumbar roots, which perhaps explains the difficulty occasionally encountered in obtaining adequate perineal anesthesia with a lumbar epidural anesthetic.

Sympathetic Outflow

The sympathetic fibers are also contained in the spinal roots emerging from the spinal cord.[4] It must be remembered that the sympathetic outflow starts only in the dorsal area. The preganglionic sympathetic fibers arise from the intermediolateral horn of the spinal cord and exit in the ventral roots and reach the vertebral ganglia along the white rami communicantes (Fig. 7–3). The gray rami, which arise from the sympathetic ganglia (mnemonic: ganglion gives gray) convey postganglionic fibers back to the spinal roots for distribution to sweat glands and pilomotor muscles as well as to blood vessels of skeletal muscle and skin. However, most of the preganlionic fibers arising from the 5th to 12th dorsal segments pass through the vertebral ganglia without synapsing to form the splanchnic nerves. Most splanchnic fibers have their first synapse at the celiac ganglion. The postganglionic fibers leaving the celiac ganglion supply the splanchnic blood vessels and the abdominal viscera. The visceral afferent sympathetic fibers also conduct pain sensations from the uterus (for a detailed discussion of pain pathways from the uterus, see Chapter 8).

The sympathetic innervation of the head and neck is carried along the postganglionic fibers of the cervical ganglia. The sympathetic supply reaches the trunk and the limbs along the respective spinal nerves. Many of the upper thoracic sympathetic fibers form the cardiac, pulmonary, and esophageal plexus. The adrenal medulla is in all respects homologous to a sympathetic ganglion and its chromaffin cells are innervated by preganglionic fibers.

It is thus seen that the sympathetic outflow is inseparably linked to somatic outflow from the spinal cord. The preganglionic sympathetic fibers are very susceptible to blockade by local anesthetics. Blockade of splanchnic outflow will result in splanchnic vasodilation and denervation of the adrenal medulla, thus explaining hypotension that sometimes complicates epidural anesthesia. A high level of spinal or epidural anesthesia will cause blockade of the preganglionic fibers that form the cardiac and pulmonary plexus.

The dura mater is penetrated by numerous arachnoid villi that are especially concentrated around the dural cuff area. The arachnoid villi may remain in contact with one of the spinal veins, they may penetrate the dura and reach the epidural space, or they may open into an epidural vein.[5] The spinal arachnoid villi, which structurally resembles the cranial arachnoid

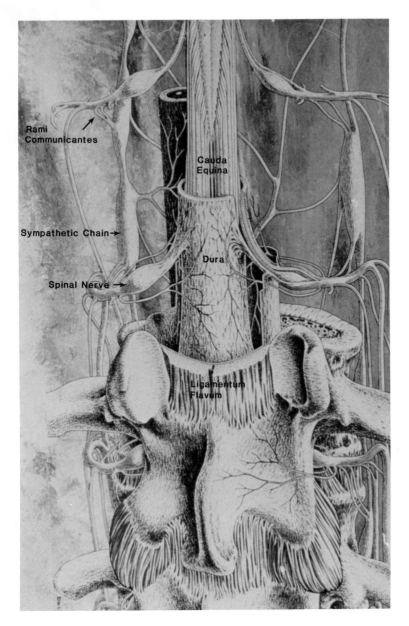

FIG. 7–3. Spinal roots emerging from the spinal cord and exiting through the intervertebral foramina. The mixed spinal nerve and the rami communicantes are shown. Also note the lower end of the spinal cord. Reproduced with kind permission from Astra Pharmaceuticals.

villi, not only help reabsorb CSF, but aid in removal of unwanted particulate matter from the intrathecal space. The pia mater and the arachnoid mater fuse at the junction between the dorsal and ventral roots to form the perineural epithelium, which extends over the mixed spinal nerve.[2] The perineural membrane is also a fenestrated structure. Thus, the dura mater forms the epineurium, and the pia-arachnoid form the perineurium of the mixed spinal nerve. Both perineurium and epineurium are weak diffusion barriers, especially at the dural cuff area, which makes it possible for the local anesthetics to reach the nerve roots from the epidural space.

The Sites of Action of Epidural Anesthesia

The mechanism and site of action of epidural anesthesia is poorly understood at this time. It has been known for a long time that local anesthetics injected into the epidural space reach CSF within a short period of time and that they will also be taken up into the neural tissues.

Following extradural injection, the concentration of local anesthetic found in the intra- and extradural portions of the nerve roots have been noted to be similar to each other. At doses that produce similar levels of anesthesia, spinal and epidural injections cause the same degree of local anesthetic uptake into the spinal roots and the spinal cord.[6-9] Bromage feels that the local anesthetics first reach the intradural nerve roots by diffusing across the dural cuff region, and that this diffusion process is aided by the presence of arachnoid granulations, which perforate the dura. During the late phases of the block, portions of the spinal cord also become anesthetized. The contribution of a paravertebral block or block of the dorsal root ganglia appears to be negligible to the total neural blockade.[6]

TECHNIQUE OF IDENTIFYING THE EPIDURAL SPACE

At least one dozen methods have been described to aid in the detection of epidural space.[2] Although the epidural pressure may be subatmospheric in nonpregnant subjects, in pregnant women, negative pressure cannot be consistently demonstrated, thus the hanging-drop method of identifying the epidural space is of little value in pregnant patients. A parturient in labor can hardly be expected to cooperate during the administration of an epidural anesthesia, thus the clinician must master at least one technique of identifying the epidural space. The loss-of-resistance technique, using and air-containing syringe, is simple and reliable. Many commercially available epidural kits provide a glass syringe for this purpose. The physician must verify that there is no friction between the barrel and the piston of the syringe. Lubricating the piston with local anesthetic or with saline will reduce friction. The epidural catheter bears external markings to facilitate proper positioning in the epidural space. The operator must be familiar with the markings and must make a particularly careful note of the marking that represents the length of the needle, because this helps in accurately positioning the catheter. If a marked catheter is not available, a sterile marker must be used to mark off the length of the needle

on the catheter and two other marks 5 cm apart from the first mark (Fig. 7-4).

Inserting the Needle

The procedure may be performed either in the sitting position or in the lateral decubitus. The sitting position is preferable with obese patients in whom bony landmarks or the midline cannot be satisfactorily ascertained. When the epidural anesthetic is being performed in this position, it is important to instruct the patient to arch her lower back outward in an attempt to widen the intervertebral gaps. Leaning forward alone will not accomplish this. Under sterile precautions, a local anesthetic skin wheel is raised with a No. 25-gauge needle. Next, deeper tissues are infiltrated for a depth of 2 to 3 cm with a No. 21-gauge needle. When deeper tissues are not anesthetized, some patients experience discomfort when the epidural needle is inserted. In addition, the No. 21-gauge also acts as a pathfinder. The epidural needle must be inserted at the lower pole of the intervertebral space and angled slightly cephalad. The epidural needle is then inserted until a slight resistance is encountered, which signifies that the needle has entered the interspinous ligament. The well-lubricated glass syringe is then attached to the epidural needle and the air bounce is elicited. The operator holds the needle-syringe unit as shown in the photograph (Fig. 7-5). The right hand (of a right-handed person) is used to advance the needle and the left hand, which rests on the patient's back, is used to hold the needle back to prevent uncontrolled movement of the needle. The needle should not be advanced more than 2 to 3 mm each time, and after each advancement, the right hand is used to elicit bounce while the left hand steadies the needle-syringe unit (Fig. 7-5).

Inserting and Positioning the Catheter

When loss of resistance is detected, the epidural catheter is inserted 5 to 8 cm (Fig. 7-4). Before inserting the catheter, the patient must be warned of the possibility of paraesthesia, which may be caused by the catheter making contact with a nerve root. The needle is then removed and the catheter is withdrawn so that the 9 or 10 cm mark on the catheter lies at the

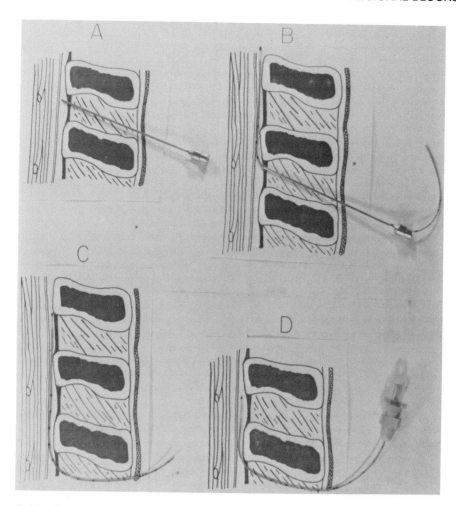

FIG. 7–4. Epidural catheter and the needle. (A) The epidural needle has entered the epidural space. (B) The epidural catheter is inserted 18 cm into the needle (the 18 cm mark is at the hub). (C) The needle has been withdrawn and the 15 cm mark lies opposite the skin. (D) The catheter is pulled out until the 10 cm mark lies opposite the skin. This method assures that at least 3 to 4 cm of the catheter lies within the epidural space. Note that many commerical catheters have exit holes located 1 to 1.5 cm from the tip. Therefore, at least 2 cm of the catheters must be in the epidural space to facilitate easy injection.

level of the skin. In the majority of patients, this method will ensure that approximately 3 to 4 cm of catheter remain in the epidural space (Fig. 7–4). In thinner subjects the catheter may be withdrawn to the 8 cm mark; in obese patients, the length to be withdrawn is determined by the distance between the skin and the epidural space. The length of the needle that is projecting outside the skin (when the needle tip is in the epidural space) is approximately equal to the length of the catheter remaining in the epidural space. For instance, when only 1 cm of the needle lies outside the skin, only 1 cm of the catheter will remain in the space, if the catheter is withdrawn to the 10 cm mark. In this case,

the catheter must be withdrawn only to the 12 cm mark. This will leave behind 3 cm of catheter in the epidural space.

In the method described above, the final length of the catheter that is left in place is adjusted during withdrawal of the extra length of the catheter that was inserted through the needle. Advancing more catheter than one needs offers the following advantages: (1) when 10 to 15 cm of the catheter advances freely, it assures the operator that the epidural catheter did indeed enter the space in the midline and not an intervertebral foramen, (2) inserting the extra length minimizes the chances of the accidental removal of the cathether from the epi-

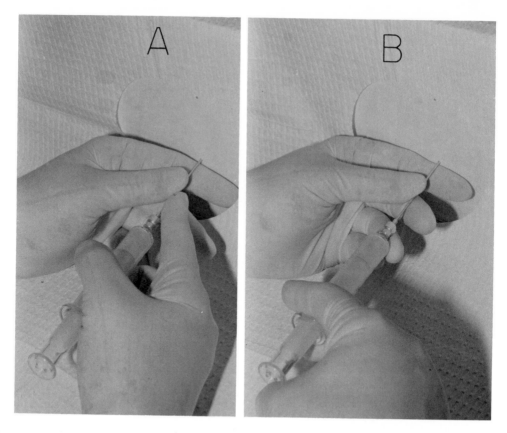

FIG. 7–5.   Photograph showing the method of holding the epidural needle-syringe assembly: (A) the needle is advanced by the right hand while the left hand (resting on the patient's back) steadies the needle to prevent uncontrolled motion; (B) after each advancement, the right hand is used to verify the presence of bounce.

dural space when the needle is being withdrawn.

After the catheter is withdrawn to the desired length, it must be aspirated to detect the presence of CSF or blood. Holding the outer tip of the catheter below the level of the lumbar area will facilitate flow of CSF or blood. A test dose of 3 ml of 1.5 or 2% lidocaine with epinephrine is injected into the catheter. The lidocaine detects accidental entry of the catheter into the subarachnoid space, in which case the patient will complain of extensive numbness of the lower extremities and loss of motor power. Intravascular injection of epinephrine contained in the test dose mixture will produce tachycardia, and the patient will complain of palpitations. Although the reliability of heart rate changes has been questioned in patients in labor, in our experience, it has avoided several mishaps. When the catheter is correctly placed in the epidural space, no major motor or sensory deficits will

be noticed. At least 3 to 5 minutes must be allowed for signs of spinal anesthesia to appear. Signs of intravascular reactions usually develop promptly. Even with a negative test dose it is a good practice to administer the dose in fractions. It must also be remembered that in a pregnant patient, the dose of local anesthetic required to produce a given degree of block is 30 to 50% of the dose needed in nonpregnant subjects. The reduction in dose requirement is noticeable even in early pregnancy. The reason for this is unknown. The use of epidural anesthesia for definitive obstetric procedures is further discussed in Chapters 8 and 9.

Should the epidural needle accidentlly perforate the meninges, the needle is withdrawn and the procedure is repeated in a different intervertebral space. If the catheter enters the CSF or if the test discloses spinal placement, the catheter is removed and the procedure is repeated in a different intervertebral space. The presence of a dural hole may cause increased spread of the anesthetic if the procedure is repeated in the same space. If the aspiration of the catheter reveals blood, the catheter is withdrawn and the procedure may be repeated in the same intervertebral space.

PHYSIOLOGIC EFFECTS OF EPIDURAL ANESTHESIA

The physiologic effects of epidural anesthesia may be related to neural blockade or to the effects of local anesthetics that are absorbed from the epidural space. When toxic thresholds for local anesthetics are not exceeded, the effects produced by neural blockade predominate.

Neural Blockade

The cardiovascular effects of epidural anesthesia are mainly caused by blockade of sympathetic fibers. Sympathetic blockade leads to dilatation of the resistance and capacitance blood vessels. Blood pooling occurs in the lower extremities and the splanchnic bed. The venous return to the heart decreases and systemic hypotension rapidly ensues. In pregnancy, this problem is further compounded by the increased likelihood of obstruction of the inferior cava by the gravid uterus. When the sympathetic block is below T5, the perfusion pressure may be somewhat restored by the following compensatory mechanisms: (1) vasoconstriction in the resistance and capacitance bed in the unblocked areas, and (2) increased heart rate. Both these responses are mediated by the baroceptor activity. However, when the block extends above T5, both these compensatory mechanisms may be impaired not only because of defective vasoconstriction in the upper part of the body but also because of the blockade of cardiac accelerator fibers. The blockade of adrenal sympathetics further impairs compensatory mechanisms. Systemic hypotension affects the hemodynamics of a pregnant patient by increasing the heart rate and decreasing the cardiac output. Systemic hypotension will also slightly decrease the ejection fraction, which is a measure of cardiac contractility, and it will decrease end-diastolic volume of the ventricle.[10,11] All these changes point to the reduced cardiac venous return caused by venous pooling. Administration of a vasopressor will reverse all of these changes probably improving venous return by constricting the capacitance bed (Fig. 7–6). Epinephrine added to local anesthetic solutions gets absorbed into the systemic circulation and produces systemic effects such as tachycardia, increased cardiac contractility, and decreased central venous pressure caused by its β-mimetic activity.[12] The controversy surrounding the use of epinephrine in obstetric patients is more fully discussed in Chapter 5.

Two simple precautions that are effective in minimizing the cardiovascular sequelae of epidural block are the intravenous administration of 1 to 1.5 L of crystalloid solution before the epidural block is administered, and the instituting of left uterine displacement. If these two simple precautions are not followed, catastrophic hypotension that is unresponsive to treatment may develop following regional block in pregnant patients.

Drug Effect

The blood level that is obtained following epidural injection is approximately 15% of that resulting from direct intravascular injection. For instance, a blood concentration of 2 to 3 μg/ml is seen following epidural administration of 300 mg of lidocaine. At this blood concentration lidocaine may exert only antiarrhythmic activity with no other apparent serious cardiovascular impairment. However, when large doses are injected directly into an epidural vein, serious cardiovascular sequelae ensue (see Chapter 5).

Other Effects of Epidural Anesthesia

The effects of epidural anesthesia on respiratory muscle activity is not clinically significant. For instance, even at a T3 sensory level the motor block extends only up to T8. This is not accompanied by any change in the vital capacity. Even with a T1 level, phrenic nerve paralysis is not likely to occur. Apnea from a high epidural block is not caused by direct blockade of phrenic nerve but by the diminished perfusion of the medullary centers caused by systemic hypotension. A total spinal anesthesia, however, will affect the respiratory center as well as the respiratory muscles. When the sensory block reaches a high level, patients may complain of dyspnea

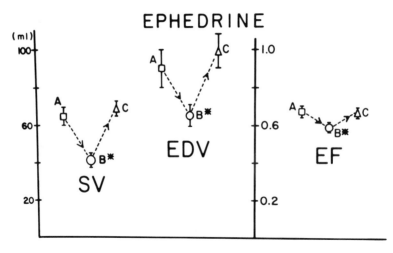

FIG. 7–6. Maternal hemodynamic changes following treatment of hypotension (caused by epidural anesthesia) with ephedrine. A = Baseline value; B = values obtained during hypotension; C = values obtained after therapy with ephedrine. SV = stroke volume; EDV = end-diastolic volume and EF = ejection fraction. Increase in EDV following ephedrine therapy suggests an increase in venous return. (Reprinted with permission from The International Anesthesia Research Society from Ramanathan S, Grant G, and Turndorf H: Cardiac preload changes with ephedrine therapy for hypotension in obstetrical patients. Anesth Analg 65:S1, 1986.

because of lack of sensory input from the intercostal muscles. Patients must be reassured that such a feeling is to be expected. Asking them to take a breath will often reduce anxiety.

When the intercostal muscles are paralyzed by a high epidural block, lateral flaring of the chest wall will be absent during deep inspiration. Only vertical excursions of the diaphragm will be noticeable. This sign may be used to rule out a high motor block with epidural anesthesia.

The effects of regional anesthesia on renal function is discussed in Chapter 22. The role of anesthesia on the release of stress hormones is discussed in Chapters 8 and 13.

DOSAGE GUIDELINES

Since the dose requirement and spread of local anesthetic is unpredictable in pregnancy, no definite recommendations may be made with respect to dosages. Single-shot injections of a large volume of local anesthetic may produce exaggerated levels. Single-shot injections are reserved for urgent situations (fetal distress) or for when inserting a catheter is technically difficult. When an epidural catheter is used the dose must be injected through the catheter in 3 to 5 ml increments. The conduct of epidural anesthesia for labor, delivery, and cesarean section is dis-

cussed in Chapters 8 and 9. Posture has noticeable effect on the spread of epidural anesthesia. Injecting the dose in a patient in the sitting position favors the rapid onset of anesthesia at the sacral segments. Left uterine displacement achieved with a sand bag wedged under the right hip may slightly delay the spread of anesthesia to the top segments, but with time the block will become symmetrical.

COMPLICATIONS OF EPIDURAL ANESTHESIA

Systemic Hypotension

The most common complication of epidural anesthesia is systemic hypotension. The cause and prevention of systemic hypotension has been discussed previously. If the preanesthesia systolic pressure was greater than 100 mm Hg any reduction in blood systolic pressure to less than 100 mm Hg must be treated. In those who have a starting systolic pressure of less than 100 mm Hg, a 10% reduction may indicate treatment. Tachycardia, nausea, and light-headedness are the other signs of hypotension. Since maternal hypotension will result in reduced placental perfusion, prompt treatment of hypotension is necessary. Hypotension may be treated with 5 to 10 mg increments of ephedrine, administration of oxygen, lateral positioning (if the patient is not already in that position), and further fluid administration. If hypotension remains unresponsive to ephedrine administration, phenylephrine injections may be tried in 100 μg increments. Used in small amounts, both phenylephrine and ephedrine constrict the venous capacitance bed and augment the cardiac venous return.

Total Spinal Anesthesia

Inadvertent injection of a large volume of local anesthetic into the CSF will result in rapid cardiovascular and respiratory collapse. This complication is a direct result of failure to follow proper technique, by either failing to administer a test dose before administering the definitive dose, or by injecting the entire dose as a single bolus. In this regard, it must be noted that the use of bupivacaine is unreliable for a test dose. When total spinal anesthesia occurs, the patient's voice is reduced to a whisper because of the lack of adequate vital capacity. If prompt treatment is not instituted, severe hypotension and apnea will follow. Untreated hypoxia will result in cardiac arrest. The treatment consists of endotracheal intubation and ventilation, support of circulation with vasopressors, and relieving aortocaval compression. The fetal heart must be closely monitored. If there is evidence of fetal bradycardia or the maternal resuscitation is impossible, the baby must be immediately delivered.

Occasionally, the epidural needle or the catheter may enter the subdural space located between the dura and the arachnoid membranes[13] (Fig. 7-2). This results in extensive spread of the local anesthetic. Since the subdural space is continuous with the cranial cavity, the cranial nerves may also be affected. The subdural spread affects the dorsal roots more than it does the anterior roots.[13]

Intravenous Injection

When the epidural space is entered too far laterally the chances of venepuncture increase. Intravenous injection of a large volume of local anesthetic into the epidural vein may lead to convulsion, cardiac toxicity, and respiratory arrest. The prevention and treatment of this problem is fully discussed under bupivacaine toxicity (Chapter 5). Careful aspiration of the catheter and judicious use of a test dose are required to prevent this complication.

Perforation of the Meninges

Accidental perforation of the dura mater is a disquieting complication during epidural anesthesia. Wet taps occur even in experienced hands. The dural hole produces spinal fluid leakage, which leads to a severe headache. The headache may appear soon after the puncture is made, but in many instances it is delayed for 24 hours. In the majority of instances, it lasts 7 to 10 days but it may persist for a month.

The spinal headache is typically postural. The patient is usually asymptomatic when lying flat in bed. The semirecumbent or upright postures, however, cause a severe headache. In severe cases, photophobia and diplopia (traction on the abducent nerve) may also occur. Several methods have been used for the treatment of postspinal headache. These include intermittent injection of saline into the epidural space, continuous infusion of saline[14] into the epidural space, parenteral administration of caffeine, administration of ergot preparations, bed rest with intravenous hydration, and an epidural blood patch. An epidural blood patch and saline infusion are commonly used in obstetric patients.

Blood patches must be performed 24 hours after the spinal tap is done. Blood patches performed within the first 24 hours are associated with a high failure rate.[15] The epidural space is preferably entered in the same intervertebral space where the spinal tap occurred. An assistant draws 10 to 15 ml of the patient's blood under sterile precautions, following which the blood is injected by the operator into the epidural space. The pateint is asked to remain in bed for 30 to 60 minutes before she is allowed to move about. The mechanism of action of a blood patch is not understood and is generally believed to be caused by formation of a gelatinous seal at the site of the dural hole. A blood patch provides an immediate cure in 90% of patients. Occasionally, headaches may recur, requiring that repeated blood patches be performed. In patients who develop neurologic symptoms such as diplopia or paresis of the fifth cranial nerve[16] tinnitus or deafness,[17] following a wet tap, a blood patch must be performed without delay to prevent permanent damage. Blood patches have been used successfully for treating focal neurologic signs caused by CSF leakage and to treat CSF cutaneous fistula resulting from CSF drainage procedures.

The blood injected into the epidural space spreads more cephalad than it does caudad. A 15 ml dose has been shown to spread 9 segments,[18] thus a 10 ml dose will usually suffice in most instances. Therefore, when confronted with two dural rents in two different spaces, the lower space must be chosen for performing the block. The epidural blood patch is free of any chronic sequelae. A patient may complain of pain in the back and lower extremities probably because of radicular pressure. Back pain and lower extremity pain may last for a few days following the procedure. If the dura is perforated accidently, the blood patch may be performed in the intervertebral space below. The volume of blood injected may be increased to 15 ml in this instance. Subarachnoid injection must be avoided because it may produce chronic neurologic sequelae. Blood patches must not be performed in the presence of local or generalized sepsis.

Headaches that do not respond to repeated blood patches may respond to epidural infusion of saline (15 to 30 ml/hour, total volume <700 ml).[19] Crawford[14] has used up to 1.5 to 2 L of saline in a 24 hour period. Not all headaches occurring after a wet tap are caused by CSF leakage. Occasionally, the patient may develop an intracranial subdural hematoma in the postpartum period. It is not known whether the low CSF pressure itself may result in the accumulation of such hematoma. Intracranial hematomas are characterized by constant nonpostural headaches. The possibility of an intracranial space-occupying lesion must be considered in those whose spinal headaches do not respond to epidural blood patches or when the headache lacks the typical postural relationship.

Backache

Even atraumatic epidural procedure is associated with backache. The incidence of backache is higher in obstetric patients. The backache is usually mild and subsides after a few days.

Isolated Nerve Injuries

Mild transient paresthesias that often occur during the insertion of the epidural catheter do not produce any chronic impairment. However, severe paresthesias caused by forceful attempts to insert the catheter may cause sensory impairment along the distribution of the affected nerve root. The symptoms usually improve with time. When severe paresthesias occur, the needle and the catheter must be withdrawn and the procedure repeated in another intervertebral space. When the local anesthetic is injected close to the intervertebral foramen, prolonged block of the mixed spinal nerve may ensue, which may last up to 24 hours.[20]

Many isolated nerve injuries occur as a result of factors unrelated to epidural anesthesia (Table 7–1).[21] For instance, the fetal head may cause compression injury of the lumbosacral trunk. Improper positioning of the patient causes compression of the common peroneal nerve against the stirrups leading to foot drop. When evaluating patients with nerve trauma, hypesthetic cutaneous areas must be carefully noted. An attempt must be made to determine whether the injury involves the peripheral nerve or the spinal roots. Electromyography (EMG) is useful in the evaluation of nerve injury.[22] The EMG is used to detect fibrillation potentials in the denervated muscles. Fibrillations start appearing 2 to 3 weeks following nerve injury. If the root is injured, the paraspinal muscles will also be affected because they are also ennervated by the posterior primary ramus. Paraspinal muscles are not affected when only the peripheral nerve is affected. Because freshly denervated muscles do not exhibit denervation potentials the EMG is also useful in ascertaining if the injury is an old one or occurred during anesthesia.

Arachnoiditis

This extremely rare complication results in chronic paraplegia with loss of bladder and bowel sphincter tone. Recently, subarachnoid injection of large volumes of 2-chloroprocaine has been implicated in causing arachnoiditis. The antioxidant sodium bisulfite contained in the local anesthetic solution is thought to be responsible. A full discussion of 2-chloroprocaine neurotoxicity appears in Chapter 5.

Table 7–1. Peripheral Nerve Injuries in Obstetric Patients

Nerve	Root value	Mechanism of injury	Clinical picture
Lumbosacral trunk	L4,5,S1	Forceps Fetal head	Foot drop Quadriceps and Hip Adductors affected.
Femoral nerve	L2,L3,L4	Fetal head Retractor	Quadriceps weakness Weak hip flexion Absent patellar reflex Hypalgesia in thigh and calf
Lateral cutaneous nerve	L2,L3	Stirrups	Hypalgesia in the front thigh
Common peroneal nerve	L4–S2	Stirrups	Foot drop Hypasthesia in the lateral calf
Obturator nerve	L2–L4	Fetal head	Weakness of thigh adduction Hypasthesia in the medial aspect of thigh

The nerve may be compressed by the fetal head, or by the stirrups because of improper positioning.

Anterior Spinal Artery Syndrome

Epinephrine contained in the local anesthetic solution is implicated in causing prolonged vasoconstriction of the anterior spinal artery. The use of too high a concentration of epinephrine, especially in the elderly, is allegedly associated with this complication.[2,23] This complication is unlikely to occur with the judicious use of epinephrine in a concentration of 1:200,000 in healthy obstetric patients.

Other Complications

Epidural Hematoma. Epidural hematoma may occur in patients with bleeding diathesis or in patients who are on anticoagulant therapy. Epidural abscess may occur in septicemic and debilitated individuals. With the availability of modern disposable equipment, this complication should become a rarity.

Shivering. Shivering is another annoying side effect of epidural anesthesia. The degree of shivering is proportional to the total volume of local anesthetic used. Patients who receive labor analgesia tend to shiver less than those who receive a larger dose of local anesthetic for cesarean section. The cause of shivering is not fully understood. Fractionating the total dose seems to produce less shivering than a single large dose. Should the shivering become annoying, a small dose of meperidine or of phenothiazine may be used to control it.

Broken Catheter. The modern epidural catheters are durable and difficult to break. Catheters get sheared off if one tries to withdraw the catheter through the needle when the latter is still in situ. If the catheter fails to advance, both the needle and the catheter must be removed simultaneously. If the catheter happens to break at the level of the skin, it may be removed through a small incision. If a segment of the catheter is left behind in the spinal canal, however, removal is not advised because it entails a major laminectomy. The catheters are made out of inert material and cause no long-term ill effects. The patient must be notified of the mishap and a note to that effect must be made in the hospital records. A neurosurgeon's opinion may be reassuring to the patient.

Contraindications for Epidural Anesthesia

Patient refusal, skin sepsis over the lumbar region and the presence of severe coagulopathy are contraindications for epidural anesthesia. Epidural anesthesia has been used in patients with spinal fusion and Harrington rod.[24] Many other conditions such as preexisting neurologic disease or lumbosacral discopathy[25] or the presence of genital herpes,[26] do not medically contraindicate the procedure. When selecting epidural anesthesia in patients with neurologic disease, the anesthesiologist must carefully explain the pros and cons of regional anesthesia and leave the final decision to the patient. For a complete discussion of the use of regional anesthesia in patients with neurologic disease, refer to Chapter 17.

CAUDAL EPIDURAL ANESTHESIA

The epidural space can be entered through the sacral hiatus also. The sacrum is formed by the fusion of the five sacral vertebrae. The expanded lateral portions of the sacrum are called the ala and represent fused elements representing costal articulations and the transverse processes. The sacrum in its dorsal surface has a median crest. On either side of the crest are found the sacral tubercles, which are formed by the fusion of the articular processes of the five vertebrae. The inferior articular processes of the 5th vertebra are prolonged downward and are called the sacral cornu (Fig. 7–7). The cornu form the lateral boundaries of the sacral hiatus, which is covered by the sacrococcygeal membrane. The sacrococcygeal hiatus provides access to the caudal canal in which lie the lumbar plexus (L1 to L4 and a branch of T12), the sacral plexus (L4, L5, S1 to S3) and coccygeal plexus (S4, S5).[27] There are four sacral foramina situated on either side through which the posterior primary rami of the sacral roots emerge. On the ventral surface are located anterior sacral foramina through which the anterior primary rami exit. These foramina allow easy escape of local anesthetic, resulting in an unpredictable vertical spread of the agent. In addition, the spacious sacral canal itself leads to increased dose requirement.

Pregnancy reduces the capacity of the sacral canal because of engorgement of the venous plexus. During pregnancy, a 30% reduction occurs in the dose requirement of local anesthetic.[2,28] Local anesthetic injected into the caudal space in moderate volumes is known to cause Horner's syndrome in pregnant patients.[29]

Technique for Administering Caudal Epidural Anesthesia

The patient is placed in one of the following positions: lateral decubitus, prone position with a bolster under the thighs (with the toes turned inward), or in the knee-elbow position. The sacral hiatus is identified by using one of the following techniques. Either one of the sacral

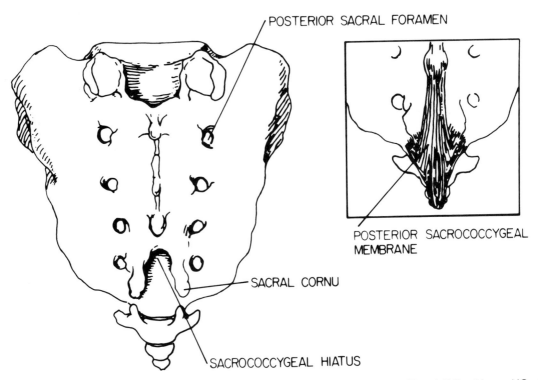

POSTERIOR SACRAL FORAMEN

POSTERIOR SACROCOCCYGEAL MEMBRANE

SACRAL CORNU

SACROCOCCYGEAL HIATUS

FIG. 7–7. The anatomy of sacrum and sacrococcygeal membrane. (From Churchill-Davidson, HC: A Practice of Anesthesia. 5th Edition. Chicago, Year Book Medical Publishers, 1984.)

cornua may be used as a landmark for identifying the hiatus, or when the tip of the index finger rests on the free tip of the coccyx, the proximal interphalangeal joint will lie opposite to the hiatus (Galley's technique).[30]

Performing a Single Dose Caudal Injection. One of the following needles may be used to perform a single dose caudal injection: A No. 20-gauge 3-inch spinal needle; a Crawford-tip special caudal needle; or a No. 22-gauge hypodermic needle. A skin wheel is first raised over the hiatus following which the sacrococcygeal membrane is punctured with the caudal needle at right angles to the surface. The hub of the needle is depressed to about a 35° angle (to the surface of the skin) to facilitate entry into the caudal canal (Fig. 7–8). The needle is turned so that its beval faces downward and is advanced 2 to 3 cm into the sacral canal. An air injection test may then be performed to ensure that the needle is not placed in the subcutaneous tissue. Injecting 5 ml of air forcefully into the caudal needle should not produce a midline crepitus, if the needle tip is inside the caudal canal. Patients may complain of discomfort in the posterior aspects of the thighs during air injection.

Because the subarachnoid space extends down to the S2 level, the needle must not be advanced above the S2 foramina (Fig. 7–8). A line may be drawn between the two second sacral foramina with an indelible marker before starting the procedure to serve as a visual guide. The S2 foramen lies medial and inferior to the sacral dimple in which lies the posterior superior iliac spines (Fig. 7–8).

Inserting a Catheter. To insert a catheter into the sacral canal one of the following needles may be used.

No. 18-gauge thin-walled spinal needle. This needle may be used for introducing a catheter into the caudal space. The catheter is usually inserted 3 to 4 cm into the caudal space. Some authorities insert the catheter approximately 13 to 15 cm into the caudal canal. In this case, the catheter tip is expected to lie opposite the S1 vertebra and therefore may be used for producing low lumbar epidural anesthesia. The problems with this technique are the unpredictable course of the catheter in the sacral canal and the increased chances of entering a sacral foramen or the dural sac.

Huber-tipped Tuony needle. This needle

may be used to enter the caudal space. The needle is inserted with the bevel facing upward. After the sacrococcygeal membrane is perforated, it is rotated so that the bevel faces anteriorly before it is advanced 2 to 3 cm. An epidural catheter is inserted 2 to 3 cm beyond the tip of the needle.[2]

No. 16-gauge I.V. indwelling (over-the-needle) teflon cannula. This device may be used for entering the caudal space.[31] The needle with the cannula is inserted 2 cm into the caudal space. The stylet is withdrawn 0.5 cm into the cannula, and the whole unit is further advanced by 3 cm. Withdrawing the needle into the cannula facilitates advancement of the blunt atraumatic cannula tip into the caudal space. The needle is then withdrawn and an epidural catheter is inserted 2 to 3 cm beyond the tip of the teflon cannula. Advancing the teflon cannula is difficult if the cannula is placed subcutaneously or subperiosteally in the sacral canal.

USE OF CAUDAL ANESTHESIA IN OBSTETRICS

The caudal approach to the epidural space is associated with a decreased incidence of dural puncture. In addition, caudal epidural anesthesia produces perineal analgesia more reliably than does the lumbar approach, which makes it particularly suitable for anesthesia for vaginal delivery. However, caudal anesthesia presents many problems. The failure rate is high because of the increased incidence of anatomic variations of the sacral canal. There is also an increased likelihood of intravascular injection, and an increased dose requirement for local anesthetic. In addition, if the needle is advanced past the S2 foramen, dural puncture may also occur. An additional serious potential hazard is the perforation of the fetal presenting part with the caudal needle, which may inadvertently be inserted through the thin anterior plate of the sacrum. The massive injection of local anesthetic into the head of the fetus has occurred accidentally during caudal anesthesia.[32] For these reasons, lumbar epidural anesthesia has in the most part superseded the caudal approach. The caudal approach may be useful in patients with anatomic abnormalities of the lumbar vertebrae or the surgical fusion of the lumbar spine.

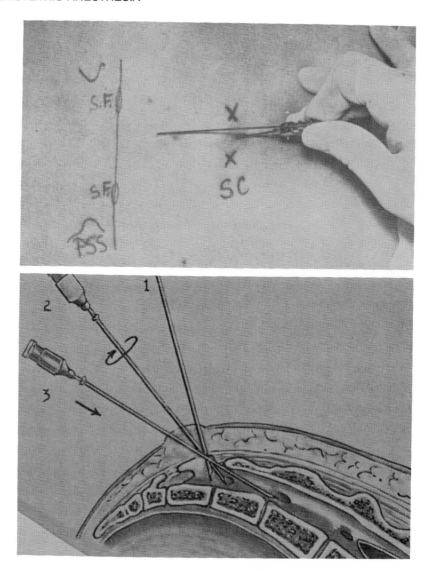

FIG. 7–8.   Surface land marks and needle positions during caudal anesthesia. Top: SF = second sacral foramen; PSS = posterior superior iliac spine lying in the sacral dimple; SC = sacral cornua. Bottom: Note (1) the starting needle position; (2) rotation to bevel-down position; and (3) advancement. (From Moore DC: Regional Block. 1971. Courtesy of Charles C Thomas Publisher, Springfield, Illinois.)

A test dose of 3 to 5 ml of lidocaine containing a 1:200,000 concentration of epinephrine must be used to ensure that the catheter has not perforated the meninges or entered a blood vessel. Both these complications have occurred during clinical anesthesia. To produce analgesia during the first stage of labor 20 to 25 ml of anesthetic solution (1% lidocaine, 2% chloroprocaine, or 0.25% bupivacaine) is initially required; for top-ups, 75% of the original dose is needed. All injections must be made in the lateral position because the supine position may cause exaggerated spread (engorged caudal veins). Anesthesia for forceps delivery may require a higher concentration of the local anesthetic. When the presenting part is at station zero or below, the likelihood of fetal injection increases. Some advise doing a rectal examination to ascertain that the needle has not perforated the rectum (or the fetal head) before injecting the dose. Using a teflon cannula to insert the catheter in the caudal space will also minimize this complication. A saddle block is a much safer technique in situations where delivery is imminent.

Table 7–2. Dermatomes in Spinal or Epidural
Anesthesia

Landmarks	Importance	
Angle of Louis	T4	
Xiphoid process	T6	
Umbilicus	T10	
Sacral dimple	S2	(dural sac ends)
Shoulder	C5	
Thumb	C6	
Little finger	C8	
Inguinal ligament	L1	

SPINAL ANESTHESIA

Bier introduced spinal anesthesia in clinical practice in 1899. Spinal anesthesia is used for producing anesthesia for vaginal delivery for cesarean section. The occurrence of post-spinal headache, the unpredictable spread of the local anesthetic in pregnancy, increased risk of hypotension and the recent advances made in the use of lumbar epidural anesthesia in obstetrics have somewhat diminished the popularity of spinal anesthesia. However, the ease with which spinal anesthesia may be induced and its rapid onset makes this method an attractive choice in many difficult obstetric situations. Surface landmarks for important dermatomal innervation are listed in Table 7–2.

ANATOMY OF SPINAL ANESTHESIA

The anatomy of the intervertebral ligaments has been reviewed in the section on epidural anesthesia. The spinal cord ends at the level of the first lumbar vertebra (Fig. 7–3). Occasionally, it may extend to the second or even third lumbar vertebra. In the newborn, the spinal cord ends at the 3rd lumbar vertebra. The growth of the spinal cord does not, however, keep pace with that of the spinal column with the result that the spinal roots take a downward course (Fig. 7–3) to their exit points at the intervertebral foramina (Fig. 7–9). Below the L1 level, the spinal canal is occupied by a leash of nerve roots called the cauda equina (Fig. 7–9). The disparity between the vertebral level at which a given spinal segment is represented in the cord and the actual intervertebral foramen from which the root escapes must be remembered when blocking neural roots for chronic pain. For instance, the 12th thoracic nerve, which exits through the T12-L1 foramen, orig-

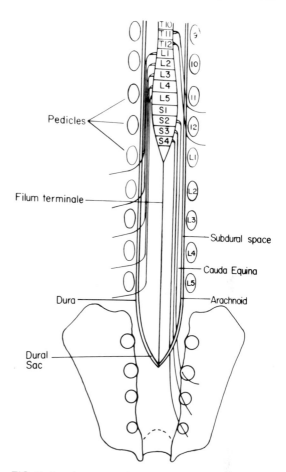

FIG. 7–9. Anatomy of the contents of the vertebral canal. Note the end of spinal cord at L1 and the end of dural sac at S2. Also note the disparity between the level at which the spinal segment is represented in the cord and the vertebral level at which the roots emerge.

inates from the T12 spinal segment located near the T9 vertebra. The disparity between the cord segment and the vertebral body is listed in Table 7–3.

The dura and arachnoid extend up to the second sacral vertebra (Fig. 7–8). A strand of tissue called the filum terminale interna extends from the lower end of the spinal cord to the S2 vertebra where it pierces the dura-arachnoid and extends as the filum terminale externa to the coccyx. There are 31 pairs of spinal roots (Table 7–3), which emerge at the respective intervertebral or sacral foramina. The cord has two enlargements, the cervical and lumbar, which coincide with the nerve supply of the upper and lower limbs, respectively.

The subarachnoid space contains CSF. The

Table 7–3. Disparity Between Cord Segment and Vertebral Body

Cord segment	Vertebral body	Nerve roots	
C8	C7	Cervical-	8
T6	T4	Thoracic-	12
T12	T9	Lumbar-	5
L5	T12	Sacral-	5
Sacral	T12–L1	Coccygeal-	1
		Total	31 pairs

Note the increasing disparity between location of the cord segment and the level at which the respective roots emerge.

average volume of CSF in the adult is 135 ml, of which 35 ml is found within the ventricles; 25 ml is found in the intracranial subarachnoid space; and 75 ml is found in the spinal subarachnoid space. It is secreted by the choroid plexus at a rate of 0.3 to 0.4 ml/min. The normal protein content of CSF is 27 mg%, with equal amounts of albumin and globulin. In pregnancy this may be reduced because of hypoproteinemia.[33] The decreased protein binding is one of the reasons for diminished requirements for local anesthetics for producing spinal anesthesia in pregnant patients.[33] The specific gravity of CSF at 37°C compared to that of water at the same temperature is 1.007.[34] Most of the hyperbaric local anesthetic solutions containing 5 or 10% dextrose have a specific gravity of 1.02 to 1.034, which makes them heavier than CSF. Hyperbaric solutions settle towards the lower roots in the sitting position. The spread of isobaric solutions is not influenced by gravity; the only factor which determines their spread is the total volume used. Hypobaric solutions spread upward in the CSF and are not useful in obstetric anesthesia.

DRUGS USED FOR OBSTETRIC SPINAL ANESTHESIA

Tetracaine, lidocaine, and bupivacaine are used in obstetric patients. All the local anesthetic solutions may be made hyperbaric by adding 5 to 10% dextrose solution. Epinephrine or phenylephrine may be added to the local anesthetic solution to prolong the duration of action. The duration of operative anesthesia is more important than how long the motor and sensory deficits last in the lower extremities. For instance, it is not unusual for patients to complain of discomfort during abdominal surgery when the lower extremities have a significant degree of motor block. A tetracaine-epinephrine

mixture prolongs the total duration of a block in the lower segments, but does not appreciably increase the duration of clinically useful anesthesia. A tetracaine-phenylephrine mixture provides both.[35] Bupivacaine action is not affected by either one of the vasopressors. Lidocaine action is prolonged by phenylephrine and not by epinephrine.[36,37] The effects of local anesthetic-vasoconstrictor action on the duration of spinal anesthesia is summarized in Table 7–4.

The ability of a given vasoconstrictor to affect the duration of spinal anesthesia is dependent not only on the type of vasoconstrictor but also on the local anesthetic with which it is used. For instance, the action of bupivacaine, which decreases the spinal cord blood flow on its own, may not be appreciably prolonged by the addition of a vasopressor. Tetracaine, which has been shown to increase cord blood flow in animals, will be significantly prolonged by vasoconstrictors.[36] The lack of effect of epinephrine on lidocaine action may be caused by its transient action in the subarachnoid space. Epinephrine injected into the subarachnoid space reduces spinal cord blood flow only in the first 15 minutes. During this time, however, the removal of lidocaine from the intrathecal space is only minimal. Absorption of lidocaine from the intrathecal space increases in the next 15 minutes, when the spinal cord flow has returned to normal, following the use of epinephrine.[36] This perhaps explains the lack of effect of epinephrine on lidocaine action. However, the duration of action of phenylephrine has a lasting effect on the spinal cord blood flow, and consequently, it is effective in prolonging the duration of lidocaine spinal anesthesia. Unlike epidural anesthesia, the vasoconstrictor that is added to the local anesthetic solution used for spinal anesthesia has only negligible effect on the absorption and systemic levels of the local anesthetic.[38,39]

Table 7–4. Effects of Vasopressor on the Duration of Spinal Anesthesia

Anesthetic	Epinephrine	Phenylephrine
Lidocaine	No	Yes
Tetracaine	Yes*	Yes
Bupivacaine	No	No

*Total duration is prolonged but not the duration of clinically useful anesthesia.[33–35]

The local anesthetics injected into the CSF may reach the deeper portions of the cord either by slow diffusion across the pia mater or by fast diffusion along the Virchow-Robin spaces, which are perivascular extensions of the arachnoid space into the substance of the cord.[38] Following spinal injection, the lateral and posterior columns take up the maximum amount of local anesthetic injected into the CSF. The lowest concentration is found in the dorsal root ganglia and in the anterior gray matter (Table 7–5). The increased myelin content of the posterolateral columns accounts for their increased local anesthetic content. The diminished local anesthetic content in the anterior cord is probably explained by its diminished myelin content; the greater blood supply per unit mass of tissue (which facilitates removal of the local anesthetic) and/or the greater diffusion distance from the site of injection, which is usually near the dorsal roots.

The degree of uptake alone does not influence a given spinal cord component's sensitivity to blockade by local anesthetics. For instance, the posterolateral columns (pressure and proprioception), which take up the maximum amount of local and anesthetic, are the last to be affected during clinical spinal anesthesia. This perhaps reflects the differential sensitivity of nerve fibers to local anesthetics (see Chapter 5). The preganglionic sympathetic fibers are blocked first, followed by pain, temperature, touch, proprioception, and pressure sensations, in that order. Motor fibers are affected last.

The epidural fat has been shown to contain a significant amount of local anesthetic when it is injected intrathecally (Table 7–5), which indicates that the local anesthetics freely diffuse across the dura. The local anesthetics are removed from the CSF in the following manner: they diffuse across the dura into the epidural space from where they are absorbed into (1) the epidural veins; (2) the blood vessels of the pia mater; and (3) the blood vessels of the cord itself. Following administration of 75 mg of lidocaine, the blood level of lidocaine increases more slowly in the first 5 minutes with intrathecal injection than with epidural injection. After this period, however, the blood level starts rising rapidly with the result that the final blood peak concentration occurs within 15 minutes. Neither the time to peak concentration nor the actual

Table 7–5. Procaine or Lidocaine Concentrations in Spinal Cord

Spinal cord component	Concentration (mean) μg/mg tissue	SE
Lateral column	1.38	0.12
Posterior column	1.36	0.18
Dura mater	0.98	0.3
Dorsal root	0.87	0.2
Anterior columns	0.73	0.24
Posterior horn	0.53	0.09
Whole gray matter	0.34	0.13
Ventral root	0.32	0.1
Whole cord	0.27	0.1
Extradural fat	0.25	0.1
Anterior horn	0.21	0.08
Dorsal root ganglion	0.16	
CSF	0.83	0.15

(Modified from Greene NM: Uptake and elimination of local anesthetics during spinal anesthesia. Anesth Analg 62:1013, 1983.)

peak concentration itself is different from those seen with epidural injections.[39] However, during clinical epidural anesthesia, more local anesthetic is needed to produce a given sensory level with the result maternal and fetal levels of the local anesthetic will be higher than with spinal anesthesia (Fig. 7–10).[40]

USES OF SPINAL ANESTHESIA

Because spinal anesthesia produces intense blockade it is not suitable for producing labor analgesia. However, it produces excellent anesthesia for spontaneous and instrumental vaginal delivery, for a Shirodkar operation, for manual removal of placenta, and for cesarean section. The onset of sympathetic, sensory, and motor blocks is faster, and the blocks last longer in pregnant patients.[41] A T10 level will suffice for vaginal delivery and Shirodkar procedures, whereas a T6–T4 level is required for cesarean delivery. Because of the risk of rapid sympathetic blockade, spinal anesthesia must be used with great caution (or not at all) in patients with severe preeclampsia or in those in whom rapid sympathectomy will lead to severe cardiovascular compromise (i.e, patients with aortic stenosis). Even in normal patients, spinal anesthesia may produce severe systemic hypotension if patients are not prophylactically hydrated with 1.5 to 2.0 L of crystalloid solution and if aortocaval compression is not avoided.

TECHNIQUE

A No. 25-gauge or No. 26-gauge needle may be used to perform the spinal puncture through

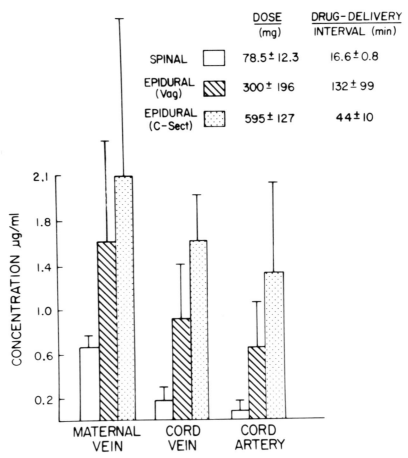

FIG. 7–10. Lidocaine levels of blood in the maternal vein and in the neonatal umbilical vein and artery following maternal epidural and spinal anesthesia. (Reprinted with permission from The International Anesthesia Research Society from Kuhnert BR, et al.: Lidocaine disposition in mother, fetus, and neonate after spinal anesthesia. Anesth Analg 65:139, 1986.)

a median, lateral, or a paramedian approach at L3–L4 or L2–L3 intervertebral space. A No. 21-gauge introducer needle may be used to facilitate the passage of the thin spinal needle, although the spinal puncture may be performed without the aid of the introducer. The lateral approach avoids the passage of the needle through the interspinous ligament; therefore the patient does not have to flex her back. During lateral approach, the skin wheel is raised 1 cm lateral to the midpoint of the chosen intervertebral space. The spinal needle is inserted without the introducer at an angle of 5 to 10 degrees from the midline and advanced in a straight line without cephalad or caudad deviation until the ligamentum flavum is reached. Should the needle make contact with the bone, it should be "walked-off" the bone in a cephalad direction to reach the ligamentum flavum. In the paramedian approach, the needle is inserted 1 cm lateral to the spinous process and directed toward the ligamentum flavum inward (5 to 10°) and cephalad (30 to 40°). Both lateral and paramedian approaches are useful in patients who have narrow intervertebral spaces or in those who are unable to flex their backs. Selective anesthesia of the saddle area (S2-S4) and the lower dorsolumbar (T10-S5) area may be produced by injecting the drug in the sitting position and maintaining that position at least 2 to 3 minutes. Saddle block and low spinal block are discussed in Chapter 8.

COMPLICATIONS OF SPINAL ANESTHESIA

Hypotension

The mechanism of hypotension in spinal anesthesia is similar to that in epidural anesthesia. Hypotension occurs much more frequently and rapidly with spinal anesthesia than with epidural anesthesia. Management of hypotension is discussed under epidural anesthesia. When severe hypotension occurs, the medullary perfusion may decrease, leading to severe nausea and repeated yawning. The immediate reaction on the part of the novice is to raise the head-end of the patient to prevent further cephalad spread of the agent. It should, however, be appreciated that when the sensory level has reached the T4 level, one may safely assume that a total sympathectomy has occurred. Raising the head is therefore useless and will lead to apnea by further decreasing medually perfusion. Faced with a severe hypotensive episode, the anesthesiologist must concentrate on improving perfusion pressure with fluids, diminishing inferior vena cava compression, and by judicious use of a vasopressor.

Headache

Headache is an annoying complication that follows spinal anesthesia. Even with a No. 25-gauge needle the spinal headache may reach 5 to 10% in obstetric patients. The treatment of spinal headache is discussed under epidural anesthesia.

Nausea

Nausea, which is probably related to decreased medullary perfusion, often complicates spinal anesthesia. The incidence of nausea may be minimized by administering oxygen to the mother and administering vasopressor as soon as a fall in blood pressure is noticed.[42] If the blood pressure is allowed to fall to low levels (80 or 70 mm Hg systolic) before treatment is instituted, nausea and vomiting will be disturbingly high despite restoration of blood pressure.

Other Complications

With the availability of disposable spinal anesthesia equipment, neurologic complications are practically unknown.

Contraindications

Contraindications for spinal anesthesia are the same as those for epidural anesthesia (vide supra). Extreme caution is advised in using spinal anesthesia in preeclamptic patients.

LUMBAR SYMPATHETIC BLOCK

The sympathetic trunk in the lumbar region consists of four ganglions and their connecting fibers. The chain lies on the anterolateral aspect of the body of the vertebra immediately medial to the psoas muscle, which fills the triangular space between the transverse process and the vertebral bodies. The block is performed at the level of the L2 vertebra. The patient lies prone. A horizontal line is drawn through the middle of the spine of L2 vertebra. A vertical line is drawn connecting the tips of the transverse processes. The point of intersection between the two lines should lie in the center of the space between L2 and L3 transverse processes. A No. 22-gauge 10 cm spinal needle is inserted through the point of intersection at 45° cephalad inclination and advanced cephalad until the transverse process is contacted (4 cm). The needle is then withdrawn and directed caudad, making an 85° angle with the skin to make it slip past the bone. It is advanced an additional 5 cm to the anterolateral surface of the vertebra (Fig. 7–11). Ten ml of 0.5% bupivacaine injected into each side will block the entire lumbar sympathetic chain and will produce 2 to 3 hours of analgesia during the first stage of labor. Before the local anesthetic is injected, the needle must be aspirated to exclude the possibility of intravascular

or subarachnoid placement of the needle. There is some evidence to suggest that the lumbar sympathetic block may accelerate the first stage of labor.[43] Its use is therefore best avoided in a patient with a hyperirritable uterus. Lumbar sympathetic block may also produce systemic hypotension.

PARACERVICAL BLOCK

Paracervical block was first described by Gellert in 1926. Its use, however, was first described in North America only in 1945 by Rosenfeld. It became very popular in the 1950's and 1960's, but soon, occurrence of fetal bradycardia and fetal hypoxia were reported. The visceral afferent sympathetic fibers that transmit labor pains lie in the paracervical area where they are known as Frankenhausers's plexus (see Fig. 8–1). Paracervical block produces excellent analgesia for the first stage, does not impair mo-

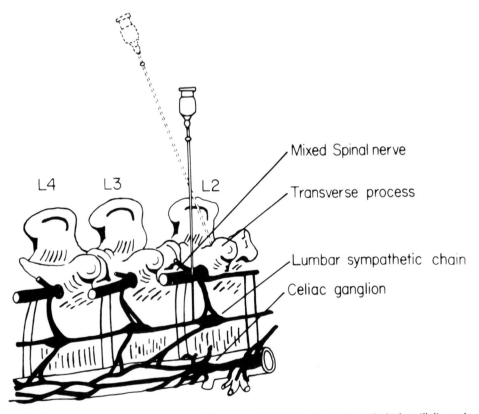

FIG. 7–11. The lumbar sympathetic block. The needle is first directed cephalad until it contacts the transverse process. After withdrawing the needle, the angle is changed in order that the needle may slip past the transverse process to reach the sympathetic ganglia. (Modified from Moore DC: Regional Block, 1971. Courtesy of Charles C Thomas Publisher, Springfield, Illinois.)

tor power required for effective bearing-down efforts, and does not cause systemic hypotension.

The block is performed in the lithotomy position. A needle guide, such as an Iowa trumpet, is used to facilitate injection. The needle guide is placed in the lateral fornix of the vagina at the 4 o'clock position. The needle is inserted into the needle guide not more than 0.5 cm to pierce the fornix. After careful aspiration, 3 to 5 ml of 1% lidocaine or 2% chloroprocaine is injected. The injection site is shifted to the 5 o'clock position. The effect of these two injections on the fetal heart rate is assessed during the next 5 minutes. If no fetal bradycardia is observed, two more injections are made at the 8 and 7 o'clock positions on the opposite side.[44] The duration of action of lidocaine is approximately 60 minutes and that of 2-chloroprocaine less than 45 minutes. Mepivacaine has a prolonged half-life in the fetus (see Chapter 5) and therefore its use is not recommended for this purpose. The use of mepivacaine and bupivacaine has resulted in severe fetal bradycardia and neonatal deaths.[45,46] The concentration of bupivacaine should not exceed 0.25%. Addition of epinephrine to local anesthetic solution is not recommended as it might further increase the incidence of fetal bradycardia.

Complications

Toxic reactions to local anesthetics may occur if the local anesthetic is injected intravascularly. The most serious side effect of a paracervical block remains the high incidence of fetal bradycardia. The fetal heart rate changes occur within 2 to 10 minutes following the block. The degree and duration of fetal bradycardia correlate with fetal hypoxia and acidosis. Bradycardia induced by paracervical block starts as a fixed rate bradycardia, followed by late deceleration. The recovery is marked by tachycardia.[47] Several mechanisms have been proposed to explain fetal bradycardia. It may result from excessive absorption of local anesthetic into the fetal circulation, which causes fetal myocardial depression (the fetal heart systolic time intervals have been shown to increase after paracervical block).[48] Fetal bradycardia might also result either from uterine artery vasoconstriction or from an increase in uterine tonus, both of which are caused

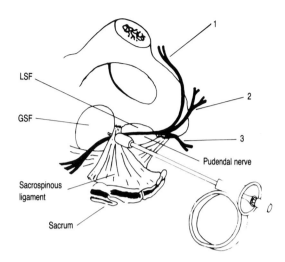

FIG. 7–12. Anatomy of the pudendal nerve: (1) Dorsal nerve of the clitoris; (2) perineal nerve; (3) inferior hemorrhoidal nerve. GSF = greater sciatic foramen; LSF = lesser sciatic foramen. Note the location of the main trunk of the pudendal nerve beneath the sacrospinous ligament.

by a high concentration of the local anesthetic. Because of these factors, paracervical block also causes a reduction in fetal tissue PO_2.[49] Prolonged fetal bradycardia will result in severe fetal acidosis, and possibly, in neonatal death.

The ideal agent for a paracervical block is 2-chloroprocaine because it is rapidly metabolized in the maternal plasma with the result that only limited placental transfer of the agent occurs. A paracervical block should be used only with continuous fetal monitoring and its use is perhaps better avoided in high-risk pregnancies.

PUDENDAL BLOCK

The pudendal nerve (S2, S3 and S4) is a branch of the sacral plexus. It leaves the pelvis through the greater sciatic foramen, passes behind the ischial spine, and reenters the pelvis through the lesser sciatic foramen behind the sacrospinous ligament (Fig. 7–12). It traverses the ischiorectal fossa where it is contained in a tubular prolongation of the obturator fascia called the Alcock's canal. The internal pudendal artery and the pudendal vein accompany the nerve. The branches of the nerve are the inferior hemmorhoidal nerve, the perineal nerve, and the dorsal nerve of the clitoris (or the penis). In addition to the pudendal nerve, the perineal area is supplied by the branches of ilioinguinal, genitofemoral, and inferior pudendal nerve (a branch of posterior femoral cutaneous nerve of the thigh.[44]

The pudendal nerve block is performed to relieve pain produced by the second stage of labor and to provide anesthesia for episiotomy and low forceps delivery. A pudendal nerve block is not adequate for midforceps rotations and extractions. A transvaginal or a perineal route may be used, but the transvaginal route is more practical than the perineal route in the obstetric patients. The ischial spine is first located and the sacrospinous ligament is traced 1 cm posteromedial to the tip of the spine. The needle guide (Iowa trumpet) is held in against this point and the needle is inserted 1 cm beyond the tip of the guide. The needle will pierce the ligament with a "pop" and lie next to the nerve. After careful aspiration, 10 ml of lidocaine or 2-chloroprocaine is injected. The procedure is repeated on the opposite side. The block has a latency of 5 minutes and has a duration of approximately 45 minutes. Maternal complications include toxic reaction to the local anesthetic, hematoma resulting from puncture of the internal pudendal artery, and retropsoas and subgluteal abscesses. Disposable equipment is now available for performing pudendal nerve blocks.

REFERENCES

1. Zarzur E.: Anatomic studies of the human lumbar ligamentum flavum. Anesth Analg 63:499, 1984.
2. Bromage PR: Epidural Analgesia. Philadelphia, WB Saunders, 1978. p. 68.
3. Cousins MJ: Epidural Neural Blockade. In Neural Blockade. (Edited by Cousins MJ and Bridenbaugh PO). Philadelphia, Lippincott, 1980.
4. Weiner N., and Taylor P.: Neurohumoral transmission: The autonomic and somatic motor nervous systems. In Goodman and Gilman's The Pharmacological Basis of Therapeutics. (Edited by Gilman AG, Goodman LS, Rall TW, and Murad F). New York, Macmillan Publishing, 1985.
5. Shantha TR, and Evans JA: The relationship of epidural anesthesia to neural membranes and arachnoid villi. Anesthesiology, 37:543, 1968.
6. Cohen EN: Distribution of local anesthetic agents in the neuraxis of the dog. Anesthesiology, 29:1002, 1968.
7. Bromage PR, Joyal AC, and Binney JC: Local anesthetic drugs: Penetration from the spinal extradural space into the neuraxis. Science 140:392, 1963.
8. Bromage PR, and Burfoot MF: Further studies in the distribution and site of action of extradural local anesthetic drugs using 14-C labeled lidocaine in dogs. 3rd Congress Mund Anaesth. Sao Paulo, Tom. 1:371, 1964.
9. Bromage PR: Spread of analgesic solutions in the epidural space and their site of action: A statistical study. Br J Anaesth 34:161, 1962.
10. Ramanathan S, Grant G, and Turndorf H: Cardiac preload changes with ephedrine therapy for hypotension in obstetrical patients. Anesth Analg 65:S125, 1986.
11. Grant GJ, Ramanathan S, and Turndorf H: Maternal hemodynamic effects of ephedrine and phenylephrine. Anesth Analg 66:S73, 1987.
12. Bonica JJ, et al.: Circulatory effects of peridural block. Anesthesiology, 34:514, 1971.
13. Hatrick CT, et al.: Subdural migration of an epidural catheter. Anesth Analg 64:175, 1985.
14. Crawford JS.: Headache after lumbar puncture, correspondence. Lancet 2:418, 1981.
15. Loeser EA, Hill GE, Bennett GM, and Sederberg JH: Time vs. success rate for epidural blood patch. Anesthesiology 49:2, 1978.
16. Lee JJ, and Roberts RB: Paresis of the fifth cranial nerve following spinal anesthesia. Anesthesiology 49:217, 1978.
17. Lee CM, and Peachman FA: Unilateral hearing loss after spinal anesthesia treated with epidural blood patch. Anesth Analg 65:312, 1986.
18. Szeinfeld M, et al.: Epidural blood patch: Evaluation of the volume and spread of blood injected into the epidural space. Anesthesiology, 64:820, 1986.
19. Baysinger CL, Menk EJ, Harte E, and Middaugh R: The successful treatment of dural puncture headache after failed epidural blood patch. Anesth Analg 65:1242, 1986.
20. Ramanathan S, et al.: Prolonged spinal nerve involvement after epidural anesthesia with etidocaine. Anesth Analg 57:361, 1978.
21. Noronha A: Neurologic disorders during pregnancy and the puerperium. Clin Perinatol 12:695, 1985.
22. Goodgolds J, and Eberstein A: Electrodiagnosis of neuromuscular diseases. Baltimore, Williams and Wilkins, 1977.
23. Usubiaga JE: Neurological complications following epidural anesthesia. Int Anaesthesiol Clin, 13:2, 1975.
24. Feldstein G, and Ramanathan S: Obstetrical lumbar epidural anesthesia in patients with previous posterior spinal fusion for kyphoscoliosis. Anesth Analg 64:83, 1985.
25. Crawford JS, et al.: Regional analgesia for patients with chronic neurological disease and similar conditions. Anaesthesia 36:821, 1981.
26. Ramanathan S, Sheth R, and Turndorf H: Anesthesia for cesarean in patients with genital herpes. Anesthesiology, 64:806, 1986.
27. Moore DC: Regional Block. Springfield, Charles C Thomas, 1971.
28. Crawford OB, and Chester RV: Caudal anesthesia in obstetrics. A combined procaine-pontocaine single injection technic. Anesthesiology 10:473, 1949.
29. Mohan J, and Potter JM: Pupillary constriction and ptosis following caudal epidural analgesia. Anaesthesia 30:769, 1975.

30. Galley AH: Continuous caudal analgesia in obstetrics. Anaesthesia 4:154, 1949.

31. Owens WD, Slater EM, and Batit GE: A new technic of caudal anesthesia. Anesthesiology 39:451, 1973.

32. Sinclair JC, Fox HA, and Lentz JF: Intoxication of fetus by a local anesthetic. A newly recognized complication of maternal caudal anesthesia. New Engl J Med 273:1173, 1975.

33. Sheth AP, Dautenhahn DL, and Fagraeus L: Decreased CSF protein during pregnancy as a mechanism facilitating the spread of spinal anesthesia. Anesth Analg 64:280, 1985.

34. Levin E, Muravchick S, and Gold MI: Density of normal human cerebrospinal fluid and tetracaine solutions. Anesth Analg 60:814, 1981.

35. Armstrong IR, Littlewood DG, and Chambers WA: Spinal anesthesia with tetracaine-effect of added vasoconstrictors. Anesth Analg 62:793, 1983.

36. Vaida GT, Moss P, Capan LM, and Turndorf H: Prolongation of lidocaine spinal anesthesia with phenylephrine. Anesth Analg 65:781, 1986.

37. Chambers WA, Littlewood DG, Logan MR, and Scott DB: The effect of added epinephrine on spinal anesthesia with lidocaine. Anesth Analg 60:417, 1981.

38. Greene NM: Uptake and elimination of local anesthetics during spinal anesthesia. Anesth Analg 62:1013, 1983.

39. Giasi RM, D'Agostino E, and Covino BG: Absorption of lidocaine following subarachnoid and epidural administration. Anesth Analg 58:360, 1971.

40. Kuhnert BR, et al.: Lidocaine disposition in mother, fetus, and neonate after spinal anesthesia. Anesth Analg 65:139, 1986.

41. Marx GF, and Bassell GM: Physiologic considerations of the mother. In Obstetric Analgesia and Anaesthesia. (Edited by Marx GF, and Bassell GM). New York, Elsevier, 1983.

42. Datta S, Alper MH, Ostheimer GW, and Weiss JB: Method of ephedrine administration and nausea and hypotension during spinal anesthesia for cesarean section. Anesthesiology 56:68, 1982.

43. Hunter CA, Jr: Uterine motility studies during labor. Observations on bilateral sympathetic nerve block in the normal and abnormal first stage of labor. Am J Obstet Gynecol 85:681, 1983.

44. King JC, and Sherline DM: Paracervical and pudendal block. Clin Obstet Gynecol. 24:587, 1981.

45. Rosefsky JB, and Petersiel ME: Perinatal deaths associated with mepivacaine paracervical-block anesthesia in labor. New Engl J Med 278:530, 1968.

46. Cibils LA, and Santonja-Lucas JJ: Clinical significance of fetal heart rate patterns during labour. III. Effect of paracervical block anesthesia. Am J Obstet Gynecol 170:73, 1978.

47. Parev JT: Handbook of fetal heart monitoring. Philadelphia, WB Saunders, 1983.

48. Jenssen H: Fetal systolic time intervals after paracervical block during labor. Acta Obstet Gynecol Scand 59:115, 1980.

49. Baxi LV, Petri RH, and James LS: Human fetal oxygenation following paracervical block. Am J Obstet Gynecol 135:1109, 1979.

8

LABOR ANALGESIA

LABOR PAIN, REAL OR IMAGINARY?

Contrary to views held by some proponents of natural child birth, the labor pain is real and can produce mental and physical anguish in the parturient. All women do not react to pain in the same manner. It is possible that some women with a high pain threshold do not require any form of pain relief; this, however, is an exception rather than the rule. According to Melzak and colleagues,[1] pain of parturition is one of the worst types of pain that may be experienced by a human being, including pathologic pain. Although the preparatory courses reduce the intensity of pain, they are by no means a clear substitute for artificial analgesia.

Childbirth preparatory courses, which have become quite commonplace, must act as a source of reliable information to the mother. The course instructor should give an honest description of all methods of pain relief that are available and let the mother choose a method of pain relief that is best suited for her. She should be told that she may switch at any time during the course of labor from one form of analgesia to another without any danger to herself, or to her baby. Above all, it must be appreciated by every one concerned that pain of labor is not imaginary; pain of parturition is universal and is experienced by women from all cultures, races, civilizations, and socioeconomic and intellectual backgrounds.[2] Although cultural influences may modify overt behavioral response to pain, they will not diminish the degree of pain actually ex-

perienced by the patient. An interesting study by Nettelbladt[3] reported that health care professionals believed 80% of their patients had only mild labor pain, while 72% of these women (when directly interviewed) reported that they experienced excruciating pain. The degree of pain actually experienced by the patient cannot be properly assessed by the presence, absence, and intensity of overt behavioral responses. This is quite apparent to anyone observing a busy labor floor at a medical facility. Women who have received regional blocks for labor are perhaps the most appreciative patients that the anesthesiologist may work with.

PAIN PATHWAYS IN LABOR

CENTRAL PROCESSING

The Aδ and C fibers conduct pain sensations from the uterus and the spinal cord (for further discussion of nerve fiber types see Chapter 5), along with nociceptive information.[2] The pain of parturition is mainly a visceral pain and therefore is conducted in the Aδ and C fibers to the spinal cord. The Aδ fibers conduct acute pain, and the C fibers conduct slow pain. These fibers make contact with lamina I, II, and V (Fig. 6–1). The convergence of cutaneous and visceral fibers in lamina V is believed to form the basis of referred pain. For instance, the patient who is in labor will complain of pain in cutaneous areas, which receive innervation from those segments processing the visceral afferent fibers. A more detailed description of the processing of signals in the dorsal horn may be found in Chapter 6.

From the spinal cord the pain signals are transmitted to the brain via the spinothalamic system, which is divided into a lateral and a medial system. At the spinal level, the lateral system includes the neospinothalamic tract. The neospinothalamic tract is responsible for rapid conduction of phasic discriminative information to the somatosensory cortex about the pain so that remedial action may be taken without delay. The slower conducting medial system consists (at the spinal level) of the paleospinothalamic tract, which projects to the reticular formation, the periaqueductal gray matter, the hypothalamus, and the limbic system. The lateral system brings about higher responses such as fear, anxiety, and also helps initiate an appropriate course of action, whereas the medial system is mainly involved with the primitive responses to pain, which include the neuroendocrine responses (catecholamine, β-endorphin, and ACTH secretion), and hyperventilation. A schematic description of the organization and the function of the lateral and medial systems is presented in Figure 8–1.

In recent years, a wealth of information has been accumulated regarding the body's ability to modulate pain perception. The nociceptive transmission is affected in the spinal cord by the interaction between the local neurons at the spinal segment and the neurons of the descending anti-nociceptive tract. The impulses streaming down in this tract end in the interneurons of the substantia gelatinosa at each segmental level. These impulses probably liberate enkephalins, which prevent the release of substance P responsible for pain transmission. A more detailed description of the descending anti-nociceptive tract is given in Figure 6–2. Emotional, affective, and motivational factors facilitate or inhibit pain perception by the brain.

PERIPHERAL TRANSMISSION

The pain of the first stage of labor is caused by dilatation of the cervix and the lower uterine segment. The pain impulses arising from the uterus and cervix (visceral afferent impulses) are carried in the Aδ and C fibers, which travel along the sympathetics. The sympathetic fibers that

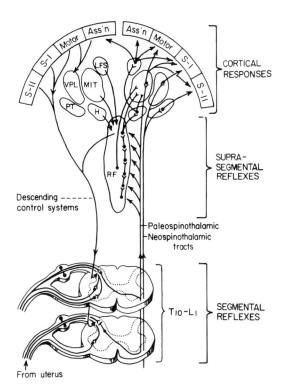

FIG. 8–1.   Organization of lateral (neo) and anterior (paleo) spinothalamic tracts. SI and SII = sensory cortex; LFS = limbic forebrain structures; VPL = ventral posterolateral thalamus; MIT = medial and intralaminar thalamic nuclei; PT = posterior thalamus; H = hypothalamus; RF = reticular formation. The areas responsible for cortical, suprasegmental, and segmental responses to pain are shown on the right. The reflexes are described in Table 8–1. (From Bonica JJ: Pain of Parturition. Clin Anaesth 4:1, 1986.)

travel upward are given different names, depending on their location: pelvic (inferior hypogastric), superior hypogastric plexus, and the lumbar sympathetic chain. From the lumbar sympathetic chain they are connected with the somatic mixed spinal nerves through the rami communicantes at T10, T11, T12 and L1 (Fig. 8–2). The pain impulses then reach the dorsal horn via the dorsal root. In early labor, only T11 and T12 roots are active with the other two being recruited as labor progresses. The cutaneous distribution of these dermatomes overlies the lower lumbar and sacral areas. This perhpas explains why the parturient often complains of pain in these cutaneous areas (Fig. 8–3)

After the cervix is fully dilated, the intensity of pain decreases. However, uterine contrac-

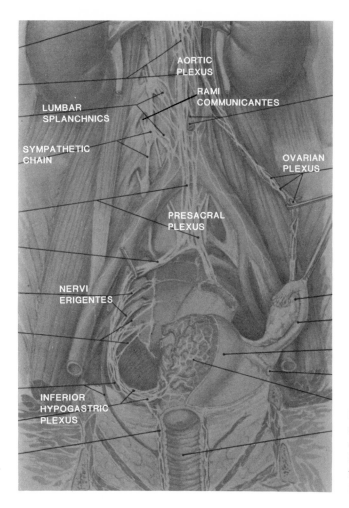

FIG. 8–2. Pain pathways during first stage of labor. (From Bonica JJ: An Atlas on Mechanisms and Pathways Pain in Labor "What's New" No. 217, 1960. Courtesy: Abbot Laboratories, North Chicago, IL).

tions and distention of the uterine lower segment continue to cause significant discomfort in the same areas of cutaneous distribution. In addition, stretching and tearing of the pelvic ligaments and musculature by the presenting part add to the nociceptive stimulation. The pain may actually be referred to the upper thighs. The pain impulses caused by the second stage travel along both the sympathetic fibers (uterine and cervical impulses) and the pudendal nerves (S2, S3, and S4; impulses of the pelvis and the perineum). Pain impulses produced by the distention of the vagina and perineum just before delivery (crowning) are conducted along the genitofemoral (L1, L2), ilioinguinal (L1), and posterior cutaneous nerve of the thighs (S2, S3). Figure 8–3 summarizes the peripheral pathways of labor pains during the first and second stages.

MATERNAL AND FETAL SEQUELAE OF UNCONTROLLED LABOR PAIN

When pain of parturition is not adequately treated, several maternal and fetal sequelae ensue because of widespread maternal sympathetic activation (Table 8–1); this leads to hormonal and metabolic disturbances in the mother. These responses may be classified into cortical, suprasegmental, and segmental effects. Women usually hyperventilate in response to pain, which shifts the maternal oxyhemoglobin dissociation curve to the left, thus interfering with fetal oxygenation. Hyperventilation is soon followed by hypoventilation during the interval between contractions, which leads to apnea in some women (Fig. 8–4). Maternal hypoventilation, combined with a decrease in uterine blood flow

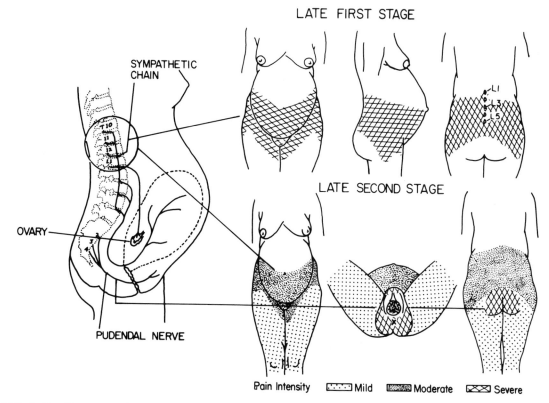

LATE FIRST STAGE

SYMPATHETIC CHAIN

OVARY

PUDENDAL NERVE

LATE SECOND STAGE

Pain Intensity ⬜ Mild ▨ Moderate ⊠ Severe

FIG. 8–3.   Summary of pain pathways in labor (left) and the cutaneous areas in which pain is felt during first and second stage of labor (right). (From Bonica JJ; Obstetric Analgesia and Anesthesia. 2nd Edition. [Edited by Bonica JJ.] World Federation of Societies of Anesthesiologists. Amsterdam, 1980.)

caused by catecholamines may lead to fetal hypoxemia.[4] A judiciously performed epidural block will eliminate the cyclical decreases in fetal oxygenation. The cyclical increase in the sympathetic activity also causes an increase in cardiac output, blood pressure and the pulse rate of the mother.

Although transient respiratory alkalosis occurs with each uterine contraction, the overall tendency is toward acidosis because of the increased production of lactic acid (skeletal muscle movement) and free fatty acid (sympathetic activation). During the course of labor, the base excess concentration will fall[5] and the plasma lactate levels will rise. Fear and anxiety, combined with decreased gastrointestinal motility caused by sympathetic activity, will delay the gastric emptying time.

It is thus seen that uncontrolled pain produces widespread systemic sequelae some of which affect fetal well-being also. Although the use of systemic medication may somewhat reduce the intensity of these effects, epidural anesthesia is unsurpassed in its ability to protect the mother and the fetus from the undesirable endocrine effects.[2,5,6] Lumbar epidural analgesia for labor decreases maternal catecholamine levels.[6]

PAIN RELIEF METHODS IN LABOR

A number of methods are available for providing analgesic during labor.
1. Regional blocks:
   A. Epidural block
   B. Subarachnoid block
   C. Paravertebral block
   D. Lumbar sympathetic block
   E. Paracervical block
   F. Pudendal block (second stage).
2. Systemic medication.
3. Inhalation analgesia.
4. Psychoprophylaxis
   A. Natural childbirth
   B. Jacobsen
   C. Lamaze

Table 8–1.   Maternal and Fetal Consequences of Labor Pain

Cortical	Suprasegmental	Segmental
Fear	Hyperventilation (tetany); Shift of maternal O_2 dissociation curve to the left; fetal hypoxemia	Increased sympathetic tone leading to decreased GI motility; delayed gastric emptying. Ileus, nausea, vomiting
Anxiety		
Verbalization		
Increased skeletal muscle activity leading to lactic acid production	Increased catecholamine production, hypertension, tachycardia, increased lactic acid and free fatty acid production, hyperglycemia, increased oxygen consumption. Decreased uterine blood flow, impaired uterine contraction	
	Increased production of corticosteroids, β-endorphins	

Cortical effects are mediated by impulses arriving in the somatosensory cortex via the neospinothalamic tract. The suprasegmental reflexes are mediated by the connections of the paleospinothalamic tract with the reticular formation. Local neuronal connections at the spinal dermatome are responsible for the segmental effects.

D. Bradley

E. Laboyer.

5. Transcutaneous electrical stimulation.

6. Hypnosis.

7. Acupuncture.

REGIONAL BLOCKS

Regional blocks have the advantage of producing less fetal CNS depression than do systemic or inhalation analgesics. Of all the regional blocks available for this purpose epidural block is the most practical one.

LABOR ANALGESIA WITH EPIDURAL BLOCK

The anatomy, physiology, the technique, and complications of epidural anesthesia have been discussed in Chapter 7. In this chapter we will discuss the use of the block for the purpose of producing labor analgesia. Controversy surrounds the effects of epidural analgesia on the obstetric care of the patient. This controversy includes questions about the following: whether epidural analgesia prolongs the duration of first or the second stage of labor; whether epidural analgesia increases the incidence of operative deliveries; whether epidural analgesia increases

the incidence of instrumental deliveries; and what the effect of epidural anesthesia is on uterine activity. Given the escalating number of law suits and the cost of malpractice insurance premium rates, these issues assume paramount importance and directly influence the physician's

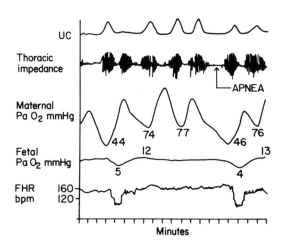

FIG. 8–4.   Maternal Pa_{O_2} and fetal Pa_{O_2} during uterine contraction (UC). Note marked maternal hyperventilation during uterine contraction (as indicated by the impedance tracing) followed by apnea. The fetal Pa_{O_2} falls during maternal apnea. (From Bonica JJ: Pain of parturition. Clin Anaesth, 4:1, 1986.)

decisions about patient care. For example, although it is well known that low-forceps deliveries do not harm babies, many obstetricians will at all costs avoid instrumental deliveries.

Many obstetricians believe that epidural analgesia administered prior to well established labor may be followed by desultory labor.[7] In addition, many believe that when complete analgesia is provided for second stage labor that the incidence of instrumental deliveries may increase.[8] This they attribute to interference with maternal expulsive efforts caused by weakness of the lower abdominal muscles and failure on the part of the mother to feel the perineal distention by the presenting part. Epidural anesthesia is also believed to interfere with an oxytocin surge that is normally caused by an active second stage of labor.[9]

The literature is riddled with conflicting findings on all these issues. For instance, Gal, et al.[10] reported that, when complete second stage anesthesia was provided, the low-forceps delivery rate doubled. Willedeck-Lund and colleagues,[11] and Hoult and colleagues[12] reported a 4 to 5 fold increase in instrumental deliveries. However, Jouppila, et al.[13] reported no difference in the duration of labor, malpositions, and the incidence of instrumental deliveries between patients who received continuous low dose epidural anesthesia and those who received conventional types of analgesia. Other authors have also reported findings similar to those of Jouppila, et al.[14] Epidural anesthesia is also implicated in diminishing uterine activity. The slowing is noticeable in the first 30 minutes, especially when epinephrine is added to the local anesthetic. However, uterine contractions are restored within 30 minutes following the administration of the block. In those patients with an abnormally low uterine activity before the administration of the block, it may take longer for the complete spontaneous restoration of the activity. A decrease in uterine activity caused by epidural analgesia may be easily corrected by administering oxytocin infusion.

The conflicting findings of the different studies may be related to the differences in method used by the different studies. This is hardly surprising because the way in which obstetrics is practiced varies among different countries, institutions, hospitals, and obstetricians. When one considers yet another important factor,

namely patient variability, one has to come to the inescapable conclusion that no hard and fast rules may be laid with respect to anesthetic management of labor and that the management has to be tailored to suit the needs of the patient and her obstetrician. The provision of complete analgesia for second stage labor (T10-S4) is a controversial issue. The anesthesiologist must know ahead of time what the obstetrician's preferences are. The decision to provide complete second stage analgesia must be made on a case-by-case basis. Whereas some women bear down effectivly in the presence of pain, others are unable to cooperate at all.

Conduct of Epidural Block

Epidural blocks are started when the cervix reaches a 3 to 4 cm dilatation in primiparous women, and a 3 cm dilatation in multiparous women. By this time, the process of labor has usually entered the acceleration phase and is therefore not likely to be slowed by the central neural blockade. At least 1 L of Ringer's lactate solution must be administered intravenously before the block is performed. The epidural catheter is inserted through the L2-L3 intervertebral space rather than the L3-L4 space because with the former approach, the catheter tip is more likely to lie close to the segments that conduct first stage labor pains. A true segmental block of the segments between T10-L2 may be obtained with a minimum dose of anesthetic, if the catheter is inserted through the L1-L2 intervertebral space. A test dose of 3 ml of lidocaine 1.5% with 1:200,000 epinephrine is injected to detect accidental intrathecal or intravenous placement of the catheter. Some suggest injecting the test dose though the needle to facilitate easy insertion of the catheter. Modern nylon catheters usually advance through the needle without difficulty thereby obviating the need for the "lubricating dose".

After having determined that the catheter has not inadvertently been placed in the subarachnoid or intrathecal space, the definitive dose must be injected. A further injection of 3 ml of lidocaine 1.5% with epinephrine will usually produce excellent pain relief for approximately 80 minutes. The addition of epinephrine to the local anesthetic solution offers many advantages: (1) it prolongs labor analgesia, (2) it renders the local anesthetic more effective in producing pain relief, (3) it decreases the number of injections required during labor, (4) it decreases the likelihood of development of tachyphylaxis to subsequent injections and (5) it decrease fetal levels.[15–17] The β-mimetic effects of epinephrine are rarely a problem in a healthy parturient. The possible disadvantage of epinephrine added to local anesthetic is the slight decrease in uterine activity following injection. The uterine activity, however, returns to normal within 30 minutes and the duration of first stage is not prolonged when epinephrine containing solutions are used.[18] Subsequent top-up injections will be required once every 90 minutes.

Six ml of bupivacaine in either 0.25% or 0.5% concentrations or 6 ml of 2-chloroprocaine in 2% concentrations also produce excellent analgesia. Regardless of the anesthetic used as the therapeutic agent, lidocaine with epinephrine must be used for the test dose because it produces reliable evidence of spinal anesthesia in a short period of time. Bupivacaine is not reliable for this purpose. The duration of action of a 0.25% bupivacaine solution is approximately 75 minutes and that of a 0.5% bupivacaine solution is close to 2 hours.

The patient must remain on her side and her blood pressure should be measured frequently in the first 20 minutes following the block. For top-up injections, the same volume of local anesthetic is used until the patient is ready for delivery. This dose of local anesthetic is not usually sufficient to abolish the sensations of rectal pressure that are felt by the patient late in the second stage. Patients will therefore be able to bear down. If the patient does not feel the contractions, rectal pressure, or lower pelvic distention because of excessive blockade, the help from a coach or a nurse may be invaluable. The coach or the nurse may ask the patient to start bearing down as soon as a uterine contraction starts. The start of the contraction may be felt by a hand placed on the maternal abdomen or from a tocodynamometer tracing. When the obstetrician feels that the baby may be delivered without difficulty, a perineal dose of the local anesthetic may be injected (10 to 15 ml of 1.5% lidocaine solution with epinephrine, 0.5% bupivacaine solution, or 3% 2-chloroprocaine solution in 5 ml increments in the sitting position). The anesthesiologist must ascertain that the perineum is well anesthetized for performing the episiotomy. Occasionally, it may be impossible to anesthetize the perineum with a lumbar epidural approach, in which case local infiltration of the perineum or a pudendal block may be done before performing the episiotomy.

The successful conduct of epidural analgesia for labor and delivery depends on the cooperation between the anesthesiologist and the obstetrician. When perineal sensations are preserved by careful titration of the local anesthetic dose, the voluntary expulsive forces of the patient will not be severely affected. It is only when intentional blockade of the lower lumbosacral roots is produced that bearing-down efforts may become inefficient. It is a good policy to avoid blockade of perineal segments until the obstetrician feels that the baby may be delivered atraumatically. It is true that pain relief will be incomplete during the second stage when sacral roots are not blocked, however, providing blockade of T10-L1 segments will bring significant pain relief, which will enable the patient to cooperate and bear down more effectively. Should the patient become extremely uncomfortable because of the unblocked segments, there is nothing to be gained from withholding a perineal dose. This should be discussed with the obstetrician and a sacral blockade should then be instituted at the earliest opportunity.

Epidural Narcotics

Substances with opioid activities are being injected into the epidural space to provide labor analgesia (see Chapter 6). The pain relief with this method is not as effective as the one achieved with local anesthetics. To overcome their ineffectiveness, some investigators have used a mixture of local anesthetic and opioid substance. For instance, fentanyl and butorphanol have been used in combination with the local anesthetic solutions.[19,20] Compared to the individual agent, the combination provides longer duration of analgesia. At the present time, the experience with this new approach is limited. One should remember, however, that narcotics are absorbed into the maternal systemic circulation from the epidural space. They will easily cross the placenta and accumulate in the fetus; thus the rationale for this approach does not seem valid to me. Epidural analgesia became the analgesic method of choice during labor because it obviated the need for depressant medications. With the use of a narcotic-local anesthetic mixture, we seem to be reverting back to an era when sedatives and depressant medications were being routinely prescribed, the only difference being that the route of administration of the narcotic is novel (epidural).

Continuous Infusion Techniques

The local anesthetics may be administered continuously into the epidural space with an infusion pump.[21,22] A number of advantages are claimed to result from this method. This method is claimed to provide a steady analgesic state without the need for top-up injections, and by suitably positioning the patient, lower lumbosacral block may be avoided in the early stages of labor. Also, as labor progresses, the patient may be eased into a reclining or sitting position to facilitate blockade of the lower segments. Another advantage attributed to this method is that because only dilute solutions of local anesthetics are used, motor block of the lower extremities is minimal. The block is induced as usual with a loading dose but the infusion of dilute anesthetic solution is started using an infusion pump (Fig. 8–5). The currently available infusion pumps are controlled by a microprocessor. An ideal pump for this use must be easy to program and, be capable of accepting all syringe sizes. It should also be equipped with a security system that allows only the anesthesiologist access to the local anesthetic solution, it must be able to display on command the total volume infused, and it must have dual power (battery and mains). One such device is shown in Fig. 8–5.

In order to maintain a symmetrical block, the patient must be turned from side to side at half-hour intervals. If the patient complains of insufficient analgesia, the infusion rate may be increased. The rate may also be decreased if significant motor block develops in the lower extremities or the sensory level exceeds T8. Occasionally, the block may have to be reinforced with bolus injections.[19] The cephalad ascent must be monitored carefully by a pinprick and if an excessive level is detected, the infusion rate must be decreased. The infusion rate and the type and concentration of the local anesthetic used for infusion is summarized in Table 8–2.

During continuous infusion, the mother and her fetus must receive the same degree of monitoring as they would when intermittent injections are being used. The mother must be clinically evaluated for inadequate analgesia or excessive levels of sensory block and suitable adjustments should be made in the infusion rate. Equipment malfunction is always a potential problem with this technique. In addition, the catheter may migrate into an epidural vein or into the subarachnoid space during the course of labor. Intravascular injection will not produce a significant problem because the rate of injection is slow and the concentration of the local anesthetic used is weak. Epinephrine is usually omitted from local anesthetic solutions during continuous infusion because of possible overdose.

OTHER BLOCKS

Labor analgesia may be produced by caudal injections. To produce a T10 level, approximately 15 to 20 ml of the anesthetic is required. Because caudal block invariably affects the sacral segments, it may not be suitable for producing first stage labor analgesia. However, it produces excellent analgesia for second stage and for performing forceps deliveries. The technique is more fully described in Chapter 7.

Some have advocated the use of double-catheter technique, one in the lumbar epidural space and the other in the caudal epidural space to facilitate selective blockade of the appropriate segments during first and second stage. The double catheter technique has not gained widespread popularity because of the potential risks associated with multiple needle punctures. Lumbar epidural analgesia alone will be adequate for most purposes in obstetric patients. Paracervical block or the lumbar sympathetic block may also be used for producing labor analgesia during the first stage of labor. Paracervical block is associated with a high incidence of fetal bradycardia. The use of paracervical block and lumbar sympathetic block is described in Chapter 7. Paravertebral block of the T11 and T12 mixed spinal nerves may be performed for producing first stage labor analgesia. The method requires four different painful injections and may be associated with inadvertent spinal injection, intravascular injection, and pneumo-

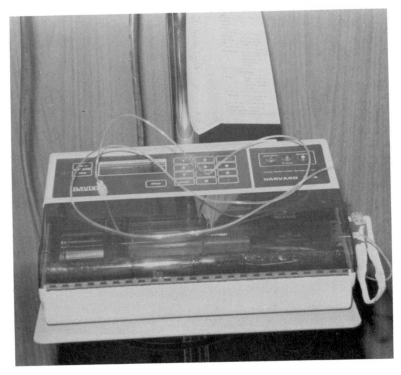

FIG. 8–5. Microprocessor controlled infusion pump for continuous epidural infusion. The unit is also capable of delivering patient controlled analgesia. (Courtesy: Bard Medical System).

thorax. Because of these difficulties, the method is seldom practiced. The use of different regional blocks for producing obstetric pain relief is summarized (Fig. 8–6).

SYSTEMIC MEDICATION

Although not as effective as epidural analgesia in alleviating pain and metabolic and hormonal side effects of labor pains, systemic medication, when judiciously used, is capable of providing satisfactory analgesia in selected patients. Systemic medication may also be used in patients who refuse regional anesthesia. The drugs that are commonly used in obstetrics are discussed in detail in Chapter 4. The most widely used drug is meperidine in 50 to 75 mg doses. The agent may be used alone or in combination with promethazine (25 to 50 mg). The concomitant use of promethazine intensifies analgesia produced by meperidine. The use of intravenous injection produces analgesia within 10 minutes, which lasts up to 2 hours. Two or three injections may be required during the course of labor. All systemic medications cross the placenta and accumulate in the fetus. The fetal neurobehavior is impaired for prolonged periods of time because of accumulation of normeperidine, which is a metabolite of meperidine. Apgar scores may not be significantly affected if the babies were born within an hour of an injection of as much as 100 mg of meperidine; however, even a smaller dose was associated with neonatal depression if the injection-delivery interval exceeded 2 hours. The explanation of this apparent

Table 8–2. Continuous Infusion Technique of Epidural Analgesia

Dose	Suggested technique
Test dose	Lidocaine 1.5% with epinephrine 200,000–3 ml
Loading dose	Lidocaine (1.5%) with 1:200,000 epinephrine–4 ml or Bupivacaine 0.25%–6 ml
Infusion dose	Lidocaine 1%–10 ml/hr (no epinephrine)* or Bupivacaine 0.125%–12 to 15 ml/hr* or Bupivacaine 0.25%–8 to 10 ml/hour.

*See text for further details. The desired dilutions may be prepared using *preservative free* saline.

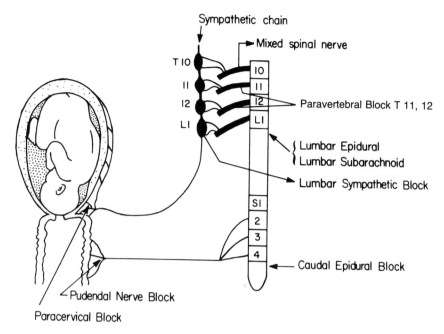

Sympathetic chain

Mixed spinal nerve

T 10

11

12

L1

Paravertebral Block T 11, 12

Lumbar Epidural
Lumbar Subarachnoid
Lumbar Sympathetic Block

S1

2

3

4

Caudal Epidural Block

Pudendal Nerve Block

Paracervical Block

FIG. 8–6. Summary of different blocks available for producing analgesia during labor.

paradox may be related to the significantly higher quantities of meperidine that may be transferred to the fetus when the injection-delivery time is prolonged.[23-25] Butorphanol is gaining increased acceptance for obstetric analgesia.[26,27] The drug resembles meperidine in its ability to produce analgesia and maternal and neonatal side effects. The use of scopolamine, which was once popular has been abandoned because of the high incidence of delirium and amnesia.

Ketamine

Ketamine has been used for producing labor analgesia for second stage. The drug must be injected in 15 mg increments until the patient is pain-free. Its pharmacology is reviewed in Chapter 4.

Inhalation Agents

The relevant pharmacology of inhalation agents is reviewed in Chapter 4. This section will concentrate on the technique of administration of these agents for producing analgesia (not anesthesia) during labor. It must be remembered that when inhalational agents are administered in analgesic concentrations, the patient remains conscious, maintains contact with her environment, and is able to participate actively in the delivery process. Inadvertent overdose may, however, lead to loss of consciousness, vomiting, and/or aspiration of gastric contents. The uterine activity is not affected in analgesic concentrations. Anesthetic concentrations, however, are known to depress myometrial contractility. The neonatal effects are usually negligible when analgesic concentrations are employed. For all agents discussed here, the analgesic concentration is much lower than the anesthetic concentration.

The inhalation agent may be administered intermittently or continuously. During intermittent administration, inhalation is begun at the start of each contraction and is discontinued at the end of the contraction. The start of administration must not be delayed until the patient actually feels the pain. The latency period until onset of analgesia lasts 30 seconds, thus the inhalation must begin as soon as the contraction is sensed. Intrauterine pressure increases of 10 mm Hg may be sensed by abdominal palpation in thin individuals. Pain is not perceived by the patient until the intrauterine pressure has risen to 15 mm Hg. Intrauterine pressure tracings or tocodynamometer tracings (if available) may also be used to aid in commencing inhalation. A review of the previous ten contraction cycles may help in predicting the time of onset of a uterine contraction. Since it is not practical to use an anesthesia machine in the labor room, many portable devices are available for delivering inhalation analgesia during the first stage of labor.

In order to circumvent the difficulties associated with synchronizing the maximal effects of intermittent analgesia with the peak of contraction pain, the continuous inhalation method has been proposed. Continuous inhalation is given usually during the second stage under the supervision of the anesthesiologist. The patient inhales the agent even during the interval between contractions. The concentration of the inhaled agent is slowly increased until the patient is free of pain. The anesthesiologist must make sure that the patient is awake, cooperative, and is able to bear down with each uterine contraction (if needed). Combined with a pudendal block, this method of analgesia can be very satisfactory for vaginal births.

Many of the inhalation agents lend themselves to self-administration by the patient. An apparatus designed for this purpose must be capable of delivering a precise concentration during every breath. The system must permit automatic shut-off should the mother become unduly drowsy. The parturients should be instructed on the proper use of the various devices that are in use for this purpose with special reference to timing of commencement of inhalation. The major draw-back with inhalation analgesia for labor is the environmental pollution by the waste anesthetic gases.

N₂O Analgesia (Entonox). Nitrous oxide is used as Entonox in the United Kingdom (50:50 mixture of N_2O and oxygen). The gas mixture may be delivered by a special apparatus fitted with a pressure reducing demand valve.[28] The valve is connected via a piece of corrugated tubing to the face mask, which has an exhalation valve (Fig. 8–7). A mouth piece may be more acceptable to some patients than the face masks.[29] The entonox cylinders are stored at a temperature not lower than −6°C because of the possible separation of liquid N_2O from the mixture. This will allow oxygen to be delivered first, followed by pure N_2O. Although N_2O has a low blood/gas coefficient (see Table 4–4) maximum analgesia is obtained only after 45 seconds of inhalation. During the first stage, inhalation should commence as soon as the contraction is sensed. Administration must not be delayed until pain appears. Once inhalation ceases, analgesia dissipates rapidly. During the second stage of labor, inhalation must start 30 seconds before the next contraction is expected. During bearing-down efforts, the mother should inhale the gas mixture 3 to 4 times, hold her breath and push. More inhalations may be allowed if analgesia wanes before the contraction is completed. The use of a nasal cannula to deliver a steady supply of N_2O between contractions has been proposed to enhance entonox analgesia.[30] Approximately 30% of patients will fail to experience any analgesia with 50% N_2O, a figure that may be slightly improved by increasing the concentration to 70%. However, with the 70% a significant number of women may become unconscious and/or enter a state of excitement.[31]

Methoxyflurane. The pharmacology of methoxyflurane is discussed in Chapter 4 and its important properties relevant to obstetric anesthesia are summarized in Table 4–4. Methoxyflurane is an ether and possesses excellent analgesic properties at low concentrations (0.2 to 0.3%). The high blood/gas solubility of the agent prevents a rapid decline in blood concentration when inhalation is discontinued at the end of a contraction. Methoxyflurane may be inhaled from a disposable analyzer (Penthrane analgiser) or from a specially designed draw-over type of vaporizer (Cardiff inhaler). The Cardiff inhaler is capable of delivering more concentration than is the disposable analgiser. The disposable analgiser is filled with 15 ml of methoxyflurane. The inhaler is loosely attached to the patient's wrist with a band. The patient is instructed to administer the methoxyflurane to herself by inhaling through the mouth piece. The analgiser delivers 0.3 to 0.9% methoxyflurane in air, the higher concentration being achieved by temporarily blocking the air-intake hole provided at the top. When an excessive amount is inhaled, the patient may become unconscious and her arm may fall to the side preventing any further inhalation. Self-administered methoxyflurane analgesia is safe for the mother and the fetus.[32] Close supervision of the mother is necessary, however, especially during periods of hyperventilation, which may augment uptake of methoxyflurane. Administered in analgesic concentration, methoxyflurane does not usually lead to

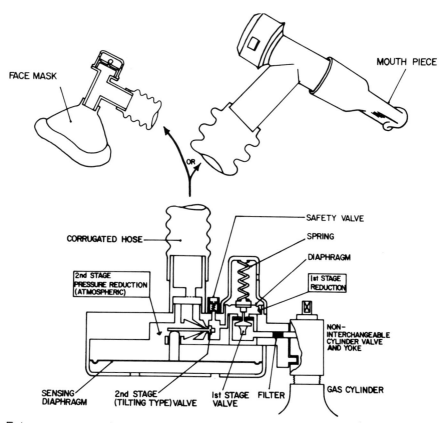

FIG. 8–7. Entonox apparatus for N₂O inhalation analgesia during labor. The patient end can either be a mask or a mouthpiece. The mouthpiece finds more acceptance among parturients. (From Crawford JS: Principles and Practice of Obstetric Anaesthesia. 5th Edition. Blackwell Scientific, 1984.)

fluoride induced nephrotoxicity (see chapters 4 and 22). Nevertheless, it is advisable to limit the total amount of liquid methoxyflurane administered to 15 ml. Methoxyflurane use has been largely abandoned because of the risk of potential nephrotoxicity, although prior to discovery of this risk, it enjoyed widespread popularity in obstetrics because of its analgesic qualities.

Trichlorethylene. This potent agent produces excellent analgesia in 0.3 to 0.4% concentration. It may be inhaled from a draw-over vaporizer. The onset of analgesia is delayed 4 minutes from the start of inhalation, but this is compensated for by the slow rate of elimination, which provides continuous background analgesia during intermittent inhalation. Trichlorethylene may accumulate in significant quantities in the mother and the fetus, thus inhalation must be limited to two hours. It causes nausea and vomiting more frequently than methoxyflurane does.

Enflurane. Enflurane may be used for producing inhalational analgesia in 0.5 to 1.0% in-

spired concentration.[33] It is claimed to achieve an acceptance rate of 90% in obstetric patients. Fluoride induced nephrotoxicity is only slightly a risk in healthy obstetric patients. Isoflurane in 0.2 to 0.7% has also been used in labor.

PSYCHOANALGESIC METHODS

Psychoanalgesic methods became popular after Dick-Read introduced his views on childbirth without fear.[34] Dick-Read felt that the process of childbirth was painless and that the pain of parturition was caused by fear and anxiety. He taught that a properly trained patient could have a natural drug-free delivery. In order to help the parturients relax, he developed some special exercises.

This concept gave rise to many forms of nonpharmacologic methods of labor analgesia. Although these methods do not in any way modify the degree of pain, they may affect the patient's response to pain. Knowledge of what to anticipate, together with support from the delivery room personnel, can reduce anxiety and pain. Many psychoanalgesic methods depend on the extensive mental preparation of the patient for the events to come thus eliminating the fear of the unknown. Courses preparing the woman for childbirth have evolved from the classes that were taught by Dick-Read and Lamaze. The modern preparatory courses not only teach conscious relaxation techniques but also teach anatomy and physiology of child birth. The preparatory courses do not come under the jurisdiction of any governmental regulating agency; therefore it is up to the anesthesia department of each institution to ensure that information on obstetric anesthesia that is given to the participants is accurate and complete. Above all, the main concern of anesthesiologists and the obstetricians in regard to these courses is to ensure that the preparatory courses do not misinform or impart a feeling of guilt to the mother in the event that she requires artificial pain relief during labor.

Lamaze Method

This method of psychoprophylaxis does not deny the existence of labor pain,[35] and use of analgesic is accepted, if pain is intolerable. This method is based on the Pavlovian principle of conditioned response. The parturient is taught to control her pain by using special breathing techniques, whereby she takes a "cleansing" breath at the beginning of a contraction, and exhales gently. Then she begins to breath in a shallow pattern until the pain subsides. In order to divert her attention from the pain, she may also focus her eyes on specific objects or pictures hung on the wall. Many bring pictures of their choice to the labor room.

Although the use of Lamaze methods may reduce the number of parturients requiring chemical analgesia, it will not completely eliminate the need for conventional analgesic drugs.[36] A significant number of patients may still require regional blocks or other types of analgesia. Despite claims that the Lamaze method reduced perinatal mortality,[37] Scott and Rose[36] did not find any major improvement in maternal or fetal outcome in patients who received the Lamaze method of analgesia.

Jacobson Method

This method does not teach the expectant mother either the physiology and anatomy of pregnancy or conscious relaxation techniques. The patient is instead taught to identify her response to tension producing stimulus. This response may be a contraction of a skeletal muscle. She will then be trained to relax groups of muscles. When the stimulus actually occurs she will be able to relax one or many groups of muscles. Training is also given on detecting visual, speech, and emotional tension. The parturient is left undisturbed during labor so that she may continue in her relaxed state.[38]

Bradley Method

This method emphasizes that the labor room be dark and comfortable.[39] Intravenous fluids and medications are usually not prescribed. Breathing patterns are simpler than Lamaze, requiring diaphragmatic breathing (the Lamaze method requires chest breathing). The woman is encouraged to keep her eyes closed in order to achieve a state of relaxation. The partner or coach need not be a trained instructor, but she must have used this method for her own childbirth. The coach is the only person who can communicate with the patient.

Leboyer Delivery

This method, popularized by the French obstetrician Leboyer, concentrates on providing an "ideal environment" into which the neonate is born.[40] The delivery occurs in a dimly lit, dark, quiet room. The baby is placed on the mother's abdomen immediately after birth and the umbilical cord is severed only after the cord pulsations stop. The baby is then given a quiet bath. Leboyer feels that the baby cries at birth because of trauma it suffered during child-birth and these soothing maneuvers are aimed at reducing his suffering.

Both Bradley and Leboyer methods may occasionally endanger maternal and neonatal safety. With the Bradley method, the lack of an intravenous infusion may be hazardous. This may not only lead to maternal exhaustion and dehydration but may also delay immediate access to a vein when urgent fluid therapy or intravenous medication becomes necessary (post-partum hemorrhage). A dark delivery room (used in the Leboyer method) interferes with early detection of cyanosis in the newborn. Placing the infant above the level of the introitus may also lead to neonatal hypovolemia (see Chapter 25). Fortunately, the enthusiasm for these methods has declined considerably in recent years, although they still continue to be practiced by some.

Hypnosis

Subjects with a high degree of susceptibility for hypnosis are good candidates for hypnoanalgesia. Approximately 10 to 20% of all individuals are not susceptible to hypnosis. Those with a low or moderate hypnosusceptibility may require additional pharmacologic analgesia. Under a fully hypnotized state, the patient perceives the uterine contractions as nothing more than a tensing of her abdomen. Several training sessions conducted by a skilled hypnotist are necessary to prepare the subject. The sessions may be given individually or in groups. With each session an increasing degree of trance is induced until arm levitation may be achieved, following which, analagesia is produced in the arm. The patient is then instructed to transfer analgesia from the arm to the abdomen and pubic area by simply rubbing those areas with the "analgesic" arm. The hypnotist need not be present during labor for analgesia transfer. The major disadvantages of this method are that it is time consuming, it is associated with a 15% failure rate, and it may in its own right cause acute anxiety and psychoses.[41]

TRANSCUTANEOUS ELECTRICAL NERVE STIMULATION

Electrical stimulation of the back between T10 to L1 (first stage) via adhesive electrodes is claimed to produce analgesia during labor. Stimulation of S2 to S5 is used for second stage analgesia.[42] The impulse is biphasic (0 to 75 mA, 40 to 150 Hz, 30 to 250 microseconds). Many small hand-held stimulators are available in the market. The stimulus is applied at a steady level and its intensity is increased during each contraction. The level of backgroud stimulation may be increased as labor progresses. The optimum degree of analgesia may be obtained at a level of stimulus, which causes a tingling sensation at the electrode sites. Approximately 50% of all patients will obtain acceptable analgesia with this method. Even when electrical stimulation does not produce complete analgesia, narcotic requirement may considerably decrease during labor.[43] The mechanism of action of electrical stimulation is not known. It may act by stimulating the large A-β fibers leading to blockade of impulse conduction along the A-δ and C fibers (gate closure) or by stimulating the release of β-endorphins. One drawback of the stimulators is that it may cause electrical noise artefact in tracings produced by electronic fetal heart rate monitors.

ACUPUNCTURE

The experience with this method is limited and available data indicates that the method is of questionable efficacy.

ANESTHESIA FOR DELIVERY

If an epidural analgesia was being provided during labor, it is a simple matter to provide analgesia for delivery. The block must be extended to the sacral roots to produce perineal anesthesia for performing episiotomy. The perineal dose must be injected with the patient sitting and sufficient time must be allowed for the onset of anesthesia in the perineum. If adequate anesthesia is not present after 15 minutes, a pudendal block or perineal infiltration may be required for performing episiotomy.

When anesthesia is requested for delivering patients who have not had the benefit of an epidural block during labor, a lumbar epidural block, a caudal block, or a saddle or low spinal block may be performed in the delivery room. A "single-shot" epidural may be particularly suitable under these situations. Following infusion of 1000 ml of Ringer's solution, the epidural space is identified, a test dose of 1.5% lidocaine with 1:200,000 epinephrine is injected through the needle followed by injection of 10 ml of the same agent through the needle (injection rate 0.5 ml/sec). If time permits a catheter may also be inserted. Blood pressure is frequently monitored and hypotension (<100 mm

Hg systolic) is treated with ephedrine. Analgesic effects are noticed within 5 minutes and perineal anesthesia will usually develop in 10 minutes.

A saddle spinal block, or a low spinal block, produces excellent block for delivery. With the patient sitting, the subarachnoid space is entered with a No. 25 or No. 26 gauge needle. Saddle block anesthetizes the sacral roots, whereas low spinal anesthesia extends to the T10 segment. Hyperbaric tetracaine 3 mg or hyperbaric lidocaine 30 mg may be used for this purpose. Low spinal anesthesia requires slightly higher dose. In an average sized female, hyperbaric lidocaine 40 mg, hyperbaric tetracaine 5 mg, or hyperbaric bupivacaine 8 mg may be used for producing low spinal anesthesia. The patient is maintained in a sitting position for 2 minutes and is returned to lithotomy position for delivery. Saddle blocks are suitable for spontaneous deliveries and forceps deliveries require low spinal anesthesia. Complications of spinal anesthesia are described in Chapter 4. Preparations of the anesthetic mixture is described in Table 9–5.

Bilateral pudendal block is used for producing analgesia for second stage, and for performing low forceps deliveries (Chapter 4), and episiotomies. Pudendal block by itself is not adequate for midforceps deliveries, rotations, and extractions; for these procedures, the block must be supplemented by inhalation analgesia (N_2O, enflurane in analgesic concentration) or by ketamine analgesia. Inhalation analgesia is described in detail elsewhere in this chapter. Ketamine analgesia is described in Chapter 4.

Occasionally, general anesthesia may be required for delivering the baby in distress. Endotracheal anesthesia is necesary under these circumstances. Rapid sequence induction must be performed and the trachea must be intubated under succinylcholine induced paralysis. The technique of general anesthesia is more fully described in Chapter 9. General anesthesia may also be needed for manual removal of retained placenta. Endotracheal anesthesia must be used for this purpose. The use of inhalation agents such as halothane, enflurane, or isoflurane in 1 to 1.5 MAC concentration may facilitate myometrial relaxation and easy removal of the placenta. After the delivery of the placenta, the inhalation agent must be discontinued and oxytocin infused to stimulate uterine contraction.

REFERENCES

1. Melzak R, et al: Labour is still painful after prepared childbirth training. Can Med Assoc J 125:357, 1981.
2. Bonica JJ: Pain of parturition. Clin Anaesthesiol 4:1, 1986.
3. Nettelbladt P, Fagerstrom CF, and Uddenberg N: The significance of reported childbirth pain. J Psychosom Res 20:215, 1976
4. Huch A, et al: Continuous transcutaneous monitoring of foetal oxygen tension during labour. Br J Obstet Gynaecol 84S:1, 1977.
5. Pearson JF, and Davis P: the effect of continuous epidural analgesia on maternal acid-base balance and arterial lactate concentration during the second stage of labour. J Obstet Gynaecol of the Br Commonwealth 80:225, 1973.
6. Shnider SM, et al: Maternal catecholamines decrease during labor after lumbar epidural anesthesia. Am J Obstet Gynecol 147:13–15, 1983.
7. Pritchard JA, MacDonald PC, and Gant NF: Williams Obstetrics. 17th Edition. Norwalk, Appleton-Century-Crofts, 1985.
8. Dierker LJ Jr, et al: The midforceps: maternal and neonatal outcomes. Am J Obstet Gynecol 152:176, 1985.
9. Goodfellow CF, et al: Oxytocin deficiency at delivery with epidural analgesia. Br J Obstet Gynaecol 90:214, 1983.
10. Gal D, et al: Segmental epidural analgesia for labor and delivery. Acta Obstet Gynecol Scand 58:429, 1979.
11. Willdeck-Lund G, Lindmark G, and Nilsson BA: Effects of segmental epidural block on the course of labour and the condition of the infant during the neonatal period. Acta Anaesthesiol Scand 23:301, 1979.
12. Hoult IJ, MacLennan AH, and Carrie LES: Lumbar epidural analgesia in labor: relation to fetal malposition and instrumental delivery. Br Med J (Clin Res) 1:14, 1977.
13. Jouppila R, et al: Segmental epidural analgesia in labor: related to the progress of labor, fetal malposition, and instrumental delivery. Acta Obstet Gynecol Scand 58:135, 1979.
14. Phillips KC and Thomas TA: Second stage of labor with and without epidural analgesia. Anaesthesia 38:972, 1983.
15. Ramanathan S, Dursztam M, and Turndorf H: Local anesthetics with freshly added epinephrine produce longer obstetrical analgesia. Anesthesiology 63:3A, 1985.
16. Abboud TK, et al: Maternal, fetal, and neonatal effects of lidocaine with and without epinephrine for epidural anesthesia in obstetrics. Anesth Analg 63:973, 1984.
17. Ramanathan S, Arimendy J, and Turndorf H: The biochemical profile of a well-oxygenated human fetus. Anesthesiology 61:A397, 1984.
18. Catchlove RFH: The influence of CO_2 and pH on local anesthetic action. J Pharmacol Exp Ther 181:298, 1972.
19. Cohen SE, et al: Epidural fentanyl/bupivacaine combinations for labor analgesia. Effects of varying doses. Anesthesiology 65:A368, 1986.
20. Naulty JS, et al: Epidural butorphanol-bupivacaine for

analgesia during labor and delivery. Anesthesiology *65*:A369, 1986.

21. Matouskova A, Hanson B, and Elmen H: Continuous mini-infusion of bupivacaine into the epidural space during labor. Part III: A clinical study of 225 parturients. Acta Obstet Gynaecol Scand Suppl *83*:43, 1979.

22. Abboud TK, et al: Continuous infusion of epidural analgesia in parturients receiving bupivacaine, chloroprocaine, or lidocaine: maternal, fetal, and neonatal effects. Anesth Analg *63*:421, 1983.

23. Kuhnert PR, et al: Meperidine, normeperidine levels following meperidine administration during labor II. Fetus and neonate. Am J Obstet Gynecol *133*:909, 1979.

24. Kuhnert PR, et al: Meperidine and normeperidine levels following meperidine administration during labor. Am J Obstet Gynecol *133*:904, 1979.

25. Shnider SM and Moya F: Effects of meperidine on the newborn infant. Am J Obstet Gynecol *89*:1009, 1964.

26. Hodgkinson R, et al.: Double blind comparison of maternal analgesia and neonatal neurobehavior following intravenous butorphanol and meperidine. J Int Med Res *7*:224, 1979.

27. Maduska AL, and Hajgassemali M: Double blind comparison of butorphanol and meperidine in labor. Maternal pain relief and the effect on the newborn. Can Anaesth Soc J *25*:398, 1978.

28. Cole PV, et al: Specifications and recommendations for nitrous oxide-oxygen apparatus to be used in obstetric analgesia. Anaesthesia *25*:317, 1970.

29. Dolan PF, and Rosen M: Inhalation analgesia in labour. Facemask or mouth piece? Lancet *2*:1030, 1975.

30. Arthurs GJ, and Rosen M: Self-administered intermittent nitrous oxide analgesia for labor. Enhancement of effect with continuous nasal inhalation of 50% nitrous oxide (Entonox). Anaesthesia *34*:301, 1979.

31. Committee on Nitrous Oxide Analgesia in Midwifery, Sir Dugald Bird, chairman. Clinical trials of different concentrations of oxygen and nitrous oxide for obstetric analgesia. Br Med J *1*:709, 1970.

32. Marx GF, Chen LK, and Tabora JA: Experiences with a disposable inhaler for methoxyflurane analgesia during labor: Clinical and biochemical results. Can Anaesth Soc J *16*:66, 1969.

33. McGuinnes C, and Rosen M: Enflurane as an analgesia in labour. Anaesthesia *39*:24, 1984.

34. Dick-Read G: Childbirth Without Fear. 4th edition. (Edited by Wessel H and Ellis H). New York, Harper and Row, 1984.

35. Lamaze F: Painless Childbirth. Psychoprophylactic Method. London, Burke, 1958.

36. Scott JR, and Rose NB: Effect of psychoprophylaxis (Lamaze preparation) on labor and delivery in primiparas. N Engl J Med *294*:1205, 1976.

37. Hughey MJ, McElin TW, and Young T: Maternal and fetal outcome of Lamaze-prepared patients. Obstet Gynecol *51*:643, 1978.

38. Jacobson E: How to relax and have your baby: Scientific relaxation in childbirth. New York, McGraw-Hill, 1959.

39. Bradley RA: Husband-coached Childbirth, revised edition. New York, Harper and Row, 1974.

40. Leboyer F: Birth Without Violence. Westminster, MD, Alfred A Knopf, Inc., 1975.

41. Wahl CW: Contraindications and limitations of hypnosis in obstetric analgesia. Am J Obstet Gynecol *84*:1869, 1962.

42. Augustinsson LE, et al: Pain relief during delivery by transcutaneous electrical nerve stimulation. Pain *4*:59, 1977.

43. Miller Jones CMH: Transcutaneous nerve stimulation in labor (Forum). Anaesthesia *35*:372, 1980.

44. Bonica JJ: Obstetric Analgesia and Anesthesia. 2nd edition. (Edited by Bonica JJ). World Federation of Societies of Anesthesiologists. Amsterdam, 1980.

ANESTHESIA FOR CESAREAN SECTION

The cesarean section (CS) rate has trebled in the last two decades and currently stands at 15% nationally (Fig. 9–1).[1] In some referral hospitals, the rate may actually reach 20%. The indications for cesarean section may be classified into 5 major categories (Table 9–1) with dystocia at the top of the list.[2] Whether the increase in the cesarean section rate is responsible for the declining perinatal mortality rate is open to debate (Fig. 9–1). Some investigators feel that the improvement in neonatal care during this period, rather than the increase in the CS rate, has contributed to the falling perinatal mortality rate.[3] Although the increased CS rate may not affect the perinatal mortality rate under normal circumstances, it may have a salutary effect on the perinatal morbidity rate, especially in babies weighing <2000 g[4] and in breech deliveries. The neonatal mortality rate for infants weighing between 1000 to 2500 g is 2.5 times higher with vaginal breech deliveries than with cesarean breech delivery.[5] One encouraging finding is that under optimum conditions the maternal mortality rate could be reduced to zero.[6] However, the mother faces an increased risk of morbidity from sepsis, urinary tract infection, hemorrhage, and thromboembolism (see Chapter 16) following a CS.[7] Although the use of cesarean section has reduced the birth trauma rate dramatically, it has not eliminated it. For instance, the baby may suffer severe neurologic damage because of head entrapment during cesarean delivery of breech.[7] Respiratory distress is claimed to be higher in babies delivered by cesarean section than in those delivered vaginally. The differences, however, are unlikely to be significant when gestational ages are identical and fetal hypoxia and acidosis are avoided.[7]

Anesthesia has remained a leading cause of maternal mortality. Anesthesia-related factors contribute to between 8 and 10% of maternal

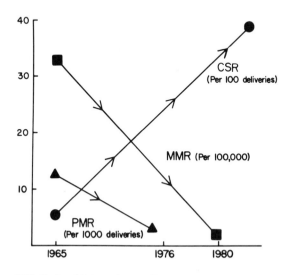

FIG. 9–1. Maternal mortality rate (MMR), perinatal mortality rate (PMR) and cesarean section rate (CSR) in 1965, 1976, and 1980. (From Bottoms SF, Rosen MG, and Sokol RJ: The increase in cesarean birth rate. Reprinted by permission of the New England Journal of Medicine 302:559, 1980.)

Table 9–1. Indications for Cesarean Section in the 80's

Indication	Percentage
Dystocia	33.4
Previous cesarean section	23.1
Breech	18.8
Fetal distress	13.2
Other indications	11.2
Prolapsed cord	
Placenta previa	
Pelvic contraction	
Genital herpes	
Unstable lie	
Unstable maternal condition (preeclampsia)	

(Source: Bottoms SF, Rosen MG, and Sokol RS: The increase in cesarean birth rate. N Engl J Med *302*:559, 1980.)

deaths. A full description of anesthesia-related mortality appears in Chapter 1. Aspiration of gastric contents, failed intubation of the trachea, and intravascular or subarachnoid injection of local anesthetic during attempted epidural anesthesia are the leading causes of anesthetic mortality. Although the reports published by the Confidential Enquiries into Maternal Mortality in England and Wales (CMED, 1973–1975; 1976–1978) indicate that factors related to general anesthesia (aspiration of gastric contents, hypoxia) are the leading cause of maternal mortality, there appears to be a change in the pattern of factors contributing to maternal mortality in this country. Local anesthetic cardiovascular toxicity is becoming a major factor in this country.[8] It is thus seen that both regional and general anesthesia may be associated with serious problems to the mother and the baby. A well planned and cautious approach to anesthesia is of paramount importance in minimizing maternal and neonatal mortality.

COMPLICATIONS OF ANESTHESIA USED FOR CESAREAN SECTION

Although complications may develop even under the most controlled circumstances, the emergency cesarean sections performed for fetal distress are more likely to lead to mortality. In these cases, the anesthesiologist does not have sufficient time to evaluate the patient properly and the patient is not adequately prepared for surgery. The anesthesiologist should therefore evaluate all patients that are admitted to the labor ward, regardless of whether they are going to require anesthetic services later.

Fetal distress is usually diagnosed from an abnormal fetal heart rate tracing and/or from fetal scalp pH values. Many fetal distress situations may be managed with regional anesthesia. The only absolute indications for an immediate delivery is the presence of cord prolapse or persistently slow fetal heart rate that fails to improve. Although a pH of <7.25 is an indication of delivery without delay, it by no means calls for immediate action. One may try to improve the fetal condition by administering oxygen to the mother, maintaining lateral tilt, discontinuing oxytocin infusion, and optimizing the status of the circulating volume. The patient is moved to the operating room with the fetal monitor still in place. An epidural or a spinal anesthesia may be provided if the fetal heart rate shows enough resiliency. The presence of short term variability in the fetal heart tracing is usually an encouraging sign because it means the hypoxic insult has not been prolonged (see Chapter 24). Some have even recommended the use of tocolytic agents to improve uterine blood flow for treating fetal distress (see Chapter 20). The anesthesiologist must take active part in performing intrauterine stabilization of the fetus. These measures may help buy time so that a safer anesthesia can be planned.

PREOPERATIVE EVALUATION

The preoperative evaluation of a patient scheduled for cesarean section is no different from that of a nonobstetric patient, except that the anesthesiologist must also evaluate the fetal condition so that the right type of anesthesia may be chosen. The major difference of obstetric anesthesia from nonobstetric anesthesia is that the anesthesiologist is responsible for two lives, namely the mother and her baby. In evaluating the materal condition, a thorough medical and obstetric history must be obtained. When medical disorders are noted, further evaluation of the condition must be done using guidelines provided for different conditions throughout Section II of this book. Healthy pregnant women do not require any extensive laboratory tests other than routine blood tests, urinalysis, and routine clotting tests (partial thromboplastin time, prothrombin time, platelet count). A baseline clotting study is recommended because pregnancy affects the coagulation system; obstetric hemorrhage may be caused by or result in coagulopathy; and not infrequently, very low platelet counts are detected in routine tests (see Chapter 11).

Every preanesthetic note must contain information about the patient's airway. The presence of loose teeth or any other anatomic abnormality, which may render endotracheal intubation difficult, must be noted. Patients with a short neck, wide mandibles and/or an anterior larynx are difficult to intubate. Patients whose airways appear suspicious may further be evaluated by simple bedside tests. There are two simple ways of predicting difficult intubation. Intubation will be difficult if the distance between the lower incisors and the temporomandibular joint is less than 3.6 times the posterior depth of the mandible (distance between the alveolus immediately behind the last molar and the lower border of the mandible, Fig. 9–2). The difficulty occurs because the wide mandibles prevent displacement of the periglottic soft tissues.[9] These two measurements may be obtained at the bedside using a pair of calipers. The inability to visualize the faucial pillars, and uvula can also be used as a predictor of difficult intubation (Fig. 9–3). The patient is asked to open her mouth widely and protrude her tongue maximally. If the faucial pillars and the uvula are hidden by the base of the tongue, one should anticipate difficult endotracheal intubation. These two predicting systems are summarized in Figures 9–2 and 9–3.

ASPIRATION OF GASTRIC CONTENTS

Aspiration of gastric contents is a major problem of anesthesia for cesarean section. When a single pulmonary lobe is involved, the mortality may reach 20 to 30% and it may reach a staggering 90% if more than one lobe is involved.[11] It may occur in a patient who is receiving an anesthetia with an unprotected airway, or during induction of anesthesia. Difficult or failed intubation is frequently associated with this complication (CEMD reports, 1973–1975; 1976–1978). Aspiration of gastric contents still remains a single major cause of anesthetic death of the mother in the United Kingdom. The fac-

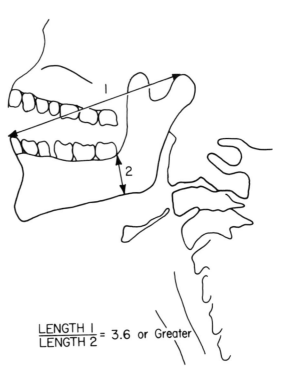

$$\frac{\text{LENGTH I}}{\text{LENGTH 2}} = 3.6 \text{ or Greater}$$

FIG. 9–2. A simple way to predict difficult laryngoscopy. The distance between the lower incisors and the temporomandibular joint (Distance 1) must be at least 3.6 times longer than the posterior depth of the mandible (Distance 2), length of the perpendicular between the alveolus immediately behind the last molar and the lower border of the mandible. When the ratio is <3.6, visualizing the cords may be difficult. (From White A and Kander PL: Anatomical factors in difficult direct laryngoscopy. Br J Anaesth 47:468, 1975.)

tors that predispose to aspiration in pregnant patients, including anatomic and physiologic changes in the gastrointestinal system, have been reviewed in Chapter 2. Patients who are in labor are exposed to added risk because not only is gastric emptying slowed by pain and anxiety but medications such as narcotics, sedatives and tocolytics[12] may further accentuate the problem.

Gastric Fluid Volume and pH

It is generally accepted that when the gastric fluid volume is greater than 25 ml and pH <2.5, the probability of severe aspiration pneumonia increases. These values were based on data derived from unpublished observations made in monkeys[13] and have taken deep roots in anes-

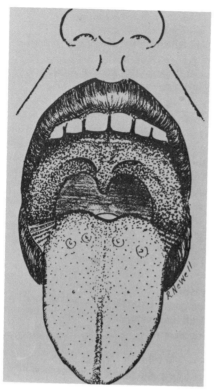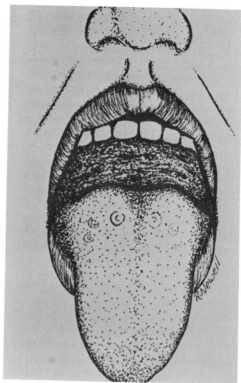

FIG. 9–3. Prediction of difficult intubation. Left: The uvula and faucial pillars are well-seen (easy intubation); Right: The uvula and the faucial pillars are not seen (difficult intubation). (From Mallampati SR, et al: A clinical sign to predict difficult tracheal intubation: A prospective study. Can Anaesth Soc J *32*:429, 1985.)

thesia literature. Several reporters used these criteria not only to define patients at risk, but also to determine the efficacy of various aspiration prophylaxis regimens. These regimens included administration of clear nonparticulate antacids;[14] administration of H_2-histamine blockers, such as cimetidine or ranitidine;[15] and administration of agents that accelerate gastric emptying time (metoclopramide).[16] Even a combination of H_2-blockers with metoclopramide has been investigated.[17] Anesthesia literature was inundated with hundreds of such reports. The problems with these claims are numerous.

No human data exists to show that the criteria from animals (monkeys, rats) can be applied to a pregnant human subject. In addition, a smaller volume (0.2 ml/kg) of gastric fluid has been shown in animal experiments to result in aspiration pneumonia.[18]

It is not known whether the "prophylactic" regimens designed to work against the development of aspiration pneumonia actually prevent this problem. As a matter of fact, the CEMD reports from England and Wales have shown that despite the routine use of antacids, the incidence of aspiration pneumonia has not decreased in England and Wales. According to these reports, four patients who died of aspiration pneumonia had indeed received nonparticulate antacid therapy prior to delivery (CEMD reports: 1979, 1982). Liquid antacids themselves will increase the gastric fluid volume.

The prophylactic agents themselves are not benign. Aspiration of a suspension antacid may lead to severe pneumonia on its own right.[19] The use of cimetidine, especially by the parenteral route, may be associated with severe cardiac arrhythmais, hypotension, reduction in hepatic blood flow, and impaired hepatic metabolism of drugs. The impaired liver function may interfere with elimination of diazepam, propranolol, and lidocaine. Plasma lidocaine levels are reported to be higher with concomitant cimetidine therapy. Ranitidine does not appreciably alter liver function. Both cimetidine and metoclopramide inhibit vascular smooth muscle directly[20] and may therefore result in systemic hypotension, especially when used in combination.

It is also not known which of these regimens will protect the mother at the time of extubation. It is thus seen that there is no fail safe prophylaxis against the possibility of gastric aspiration. Observing the following simple precautions during induction and recovery will minimize the risk of aspiration:

Avoid general anesthesia (GA) whenever possible.

Do not administer mask anesthesia.

Administer sodium citrate 0.3 M, 15 ml, 30 minutes before induction.

For patients with heartburn, ranitidine 150 mg PO at least 90 minutes before induction.

Use rapid sequence induction with cricoid pressure.

The only routine prophylactic regimen that is safe and effective is administration of 15 ml of 0.3 M of sodium citrate solution. Because the duration of the antacid is limited (<20 minutes) it must be administered within 30 minutes before the expected time of anesthesia[14] (Fig. 9–4). Patients who complain of heartburn may benefit from ranitidine therapy because they have diminished esophageal sphincter tone, which re-

sults in easy passage of acidic gastric fluid into the esophagus.

Pathophysiology of Aspiration

Aspiration is of two types, aspiration of acidic gastric juice and aspiration of solid particulate matter. Symptoms of acid aspiration may begin acutely with bronchial spasm or may be delayed for several hours (Table 9–2).[21] Cyanosis unresponsive to oxygen therapy may develop. Pulmonary edema with pink frothy fluid appearing at the mouth or at the endotracheal tube outlet may also be evident. The pulmonary edema is of the "capillary leakage variety" caused by damaged lung capillaries with normal pulmonary capillary wedge pressures.[22] The extravasation of large volumes of fluid into the alveoli and pulmonary interstitium causes systemic hypotension to develop.[21] Severe hypoxemia develops as a result of diffusion abnormality, increased $\dot{Q}s/\dot{Q}t$ ratio, and pulmonary vasconstriction.[21] Metabolic acidosis usually develops as a result of diminished tissue oxygenation and systemic absorption of hydrochloric acid.[21] Chest x-rays may appear normal in the early phases of the syndrome, but soon assume the

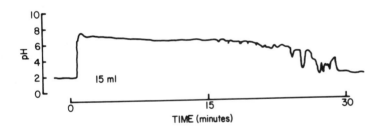

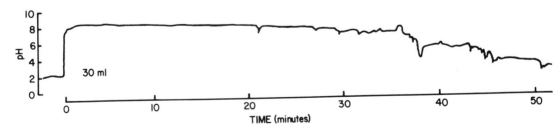

FIG. 9–4.   Intragastric fluid pH with 15 and 30 ml of sodium citrate administered orally. Note the lack of significant difference in the duration of action of these two doses. (Reprinted with permission from the International Anesthesia Research Society from O'Sullivan G and Bullingham RES: Does twice the volume of antacid have twice the effect in pregnant women at term? Anesth Analg 63:752, 1984.)

Table 9–2. Clinical Features of Aspiration

Phase	Characteristics
Phase 1	Profound tachypnea, bronchospasm, and dyspnea Chest x-ray is normal
Phase 2	Latent phase Increasing cyanosis, hypoxemia Minor chest x-ray abnormalities
Phase 3	Respiratory failure Profound hypoxemia Reduced pulmonary compliance Bilateral infiltrates
Phase 4	Hypoxemia unresponsive to oxygen Metabolic and respiratory acidosis

characteristic diffuse mottled apperance (Fig. 9–5). Histopathology of pulmonary aspiration is mainly one of chemical injury with infection being superadded in later phases.[24] The clinical features of acid-aspiration are summarized in Table 9–2. The histopathologic findings are described in the following list:

Impaired mucociliary transport.

Interstitial edema due to transudation of fluid.

Disruption of alveolar-capillary membrane: Destruction of type I and type II pneumocytes.

Bronchitis, bronchiolitis, mucosal necrosis.

Signs of infection (polymorph infiltration).

Hyaline membrane in the alveoli.

Signs of consolidation.

A typical histopathologic picture is presented in Figure 9–6. Resolution starts within 72 hours and it may take up to 3 weeks for complete normalization. The treatment of acid-aspiration syndrome is ineffective.

The immediate treatment consists of the rapid intubation of the trachea and the suctioning of as much gastric fluid as possible from the trachea. Tracheal instillation of saline, alkali, or steroid solution is not recommended as it may further worsen the condition by spreading the aspirate to the distal portions of the lung and such instillation may cause pulmonary damage on their own. In animal experiments, institution of positive pressure ventilation at the earliest opportunity has been shown to decrease mortality caused by aspiration.[22] Thus one may make a case for starting endotracheal intermittent positive pressure ventilation (IPPV) even in

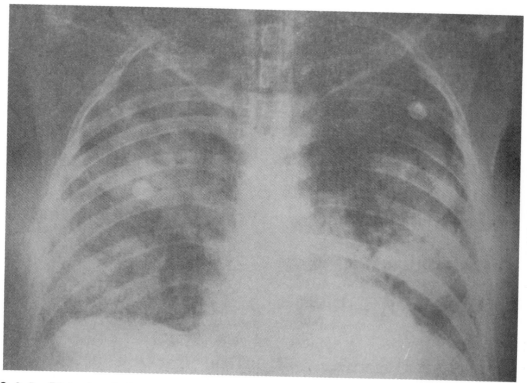

FIG. 9–5. Bilateral aspiration pneumonia. (From Dustins DM: Anaesthesia for obstetrics. *In* A Practice of Anaesthesia. 5th Ed. Edited by Churchill-Davidson HC. Chicago, Year Book Medical Publishers, 1984.)

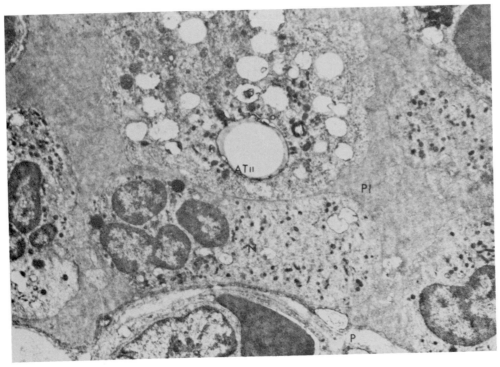

FIG. 9–6. Histology of pulmonary aspiration 48 hours after aspiration. The alveoli are lined by hyaline membrane consisting of plasma (P) debris (Pl), alveolar type II cells (AT II), and alveolar macrophages. The perivascular space (P) is dilated. N = Nucleus (Magnification × 9200). (From Greenfield LJ, Singleton RP, and McCaffree DR: Pulmonary effects of aspiration of hydrochloric acid. Ann Surg 170:74, 1969.).

cases of suspected aspiration. Obviously, severe hypoxia warrants IPPV without delay. Positive end expiratory pressure (PEEP) may be considered in those with severe hypoxemia or evidence of pulmonary edema. The use of steroids for the treatment of acid aspiration syndrome is controversial. Many feel that they offer no specific advantage and in fact may interfere with the natural healing process.[23] Because of the risk of pulmonary edema in these patients, monitoring CVP or pulmonary artery pressure is often helpful.

Aspiration of particulate matter produces more of granulomatous reaction than does acid aspiration.[22] Aspiration of large particles may also obstruct the airway, leading to severe mechanical obstruction of the airway. Rigid bronchoscopy may be needed to remove bigger particles. A saline lavage of the tracheobronchial tree may be used to loosen smaller food particles.

Failed Intubation Protocol

Nothing is perhaps more distressing to the anesthesiologist than failure to intubate the tra-

chea during general anesthesia for cesarean section. Failed intubation may lead to aspiration of gastric contents and/or severe maternal and fetal hypoxemia. Occasionally, ventilation of the mother may become impossible, leading to hypoxic cardiac arrest. The recent CEMD reports show that 15 mothers died because of failed intubation and accompanying complications. Every anesthesiologist must have a well planned protocol ready in case of difficulty in intubating the trachea. In most instances, the external appearance of the patient may not arouse any suspicion.

The most important rule in dealing with difficult intubation is to accept failure and resort to alternate approaches. The anesthesiologist must make one or two attempts. If he fails to intubate the trachea, the failed intubation protocol must be immediately instituted. Repeated attempts at intubation leads to laryngeal edema in pregnant patients, who already have a narrow rima glottidis. When the anesthesiologist is not able to visualize either the epiglottis or the glottis, further attempts at intubation are usually futile and must be quickly abandoned.[25] When only epiglottis is seen, a leader (a flexible stylet) may be introduced into the trachea by sliding it against the epiglottis. The endotracheal tube is then advanced over it. A special angled laryngoscope can also be used in difficult intubation (the Bellehouse laryngoscope, Fig. 9–7).[26] A prism attached to the blade will facilitate visualization of structures behind the epiglottis.

When intubation is determined to be impossible, another course of action should be decided upon immediately. This will depend on why the CS is being performed. If the CS was an elective one, the patient has to be awakened immediately and a regional anesthetic procedure must be performed. If regional anesthesia is not possible, an awake, blind, nasal intubation or bronchofiberscope-facilitated intubation is considered. Topical anesthesia of the nose with cocaine may be used to avoid epistaxis or small doses of intravenous diazepam and/or fentanyl can be used for sedating the patient. The use of these agents for this purpose has been described in Chapter 4.

If the CS is being performed for fetal distress (which precludes awakening the patient) and if the patient can be ventilated easily via a face mask, anesthesia may be administered with N_2O, oxygen, and 0.5% of halothane adminis-

tered with the aid of the mask. Maintaining muscle paralysis with succinylcholine infusion, and carefully ventilating the patient with cricoid pressure, will minimize the hazard of vomiting. Light planes of anesthesia in an inadequately paralyzed patient predisposes to vomiting.

A most difficult situation arises when following the failure to intubate the trachea, it is impossible to ventilate the lungs. The patient rapidly becomes cyanotic and will develop cardiac arrhythmias. The first course of action involves establishing oxygenation. There are several methods available to handle this situation. All these methods require considerable previous experience and extra personnel being available in the operating room. The anesthesiologist chooses any one of the methods outlined below to ensure oxygenation. The choice of the method depends on the equipment available, anesthesiologist's expertise and the type of personnel available in the operating room.

Transglottic Jet Ventilation. A bronchofiberscope may be introduced under direct vision into the glottis. The suction channel of the bronchofiberscope is attached to a Saunders jet ventilation device connected to a 50 PSI source (Fig. 9–8).[27] Each delivery suite must have a bron-

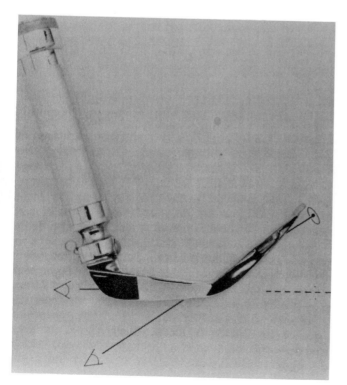

FIG. 9–7. The Bellehouse laryngoscope with detachable prism and an angled blade. (Avulunga Pty Ltd, Elouera Terrace, Murvillumbah 2484, New South Wales, Australia.) (From Tunstall ME and Geddes C: Failed intubation in obstetric anesthesia. Br J Anaesth 56:659, 1984.)

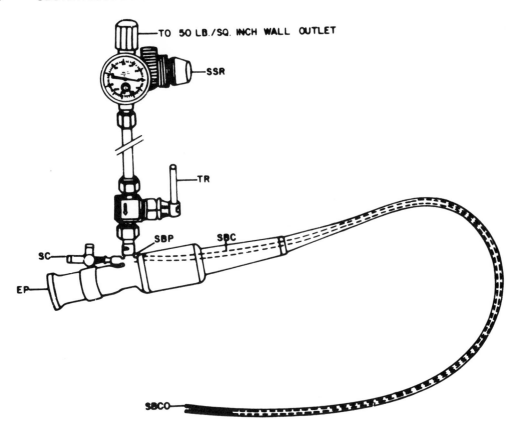

FIG. 9–8.   Saunders jet has been attached to the suction port of a bronchofiberscope. Single stage regulator (SSR); stop-cock (SC); toggle release (TR); suction-biopsy port (SBP); suction-biopsy channel (SBC); eye piece (EP). (Reprinted with permission from The International Anesthesia Research Society from Satyan-arayna T, et al.: Bronchofiberscopic jet ventilation. Anesth Analg 59:350, 1980.)

chofiberscope and a Saunders jet ventilation device (which is an inexpensive item, Fig. 9–8).

Using a No. 16-Gauge Cannula With Jet Ventilation. A No. 16-gauge cannula is inserted into the trachea through the crico-thyroid membrane and its free end is connected to the Saunder's jet system via an i.v. extension tube. Because the only means of gas escape during jet ventilation is the glottis, upper airway obstruction will lead to a tension pneumothorax. Consequently, the anesthesiologist must ascertain after each jet inspiration that the chest is adequately decompressing. It is advisable to start with a low driving pressure of 20 PSI and carefully increase it until adequate chest excursions are noted. Every attempt must be made to maintain patency of the upper airway by jaw elevation and proper head positioning to allow unimpeded exhalation. Anesthesia can be maintained with i.v. methohexital and muscle relaxant. If a jetting device is not available, the oxygen flush from

the anesthesia machine can be used to act as a jet. This, however, is not as effective as the jet.

Emergency Cricithyroidotomy. An emergency cricithyroidotomy cannula (Fig. 9–9) is inserted into the trachea and is attached to the anesthesia circuit using suitable connectors. These cannulae are large and may result in serious trauma to the upper airway and esophagus.

Two Other Positive Pressure Devices. Two other devices have recently been described. These devices enable the anesthesiologist to deliver positive pressure ventilation without the necessity of an endotracheal tube.

The Esophageal Gastric Tube Airway (EGTA).[26] This device is a mask bearing a cuffed endotracheal tube. The endotracheal tube is introduced into the esophagus blindly and the cuff is inflated (Fig. 9–10). The mask end of the endotracheal tube is left open allowing vomitus or secretions to escape. A nasogastric tube is passed through the endotracheal tube to deflate the

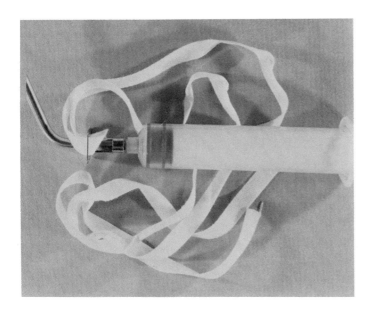

FIG. 9–9. Emergency cricothyroidotomy set.

stomach. The mask also bears an adapter to which the anesthesia circuit is attached. When the mask snugly fits around the nose and mouth of the patient, bag ventilation is possible. The esophageal tube facilitates ventilation by allowing air to pass on its sides and by displacing the glottis forward.

The Laryngeal Mask. This device is a specially designed airway that forms a seal around the glottic opening without actually passing through the vocal cords (Fig. 9–11).[28] A tight fit around the glottis is obtained by inflating the seal with air. A stylet is required to introduce this device into the correct position. This device

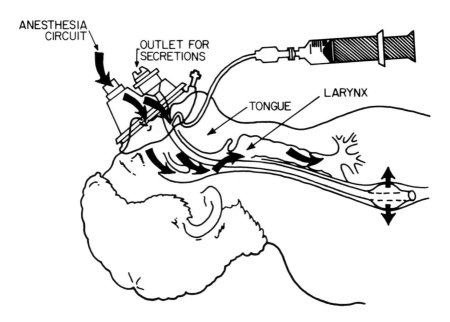

FIG. 9–10. Esophageal gastric tube airway. The tube in the esophagus displaces the tongue forwards, thereby improving air flow to the larynx. The esophageal tube opens to atmosphere to allow escape of gastric contents. The device may be obtained from Eschmann Ltd, Peter Road, Lancing, Sussex, BN58TJ) (Reprinted with permission from the International Anesthesia Research Society from Satyanarayna T, et al.: Bronchofiberscopic jet ventilation. Anesth Analg 59:350, 1980.)

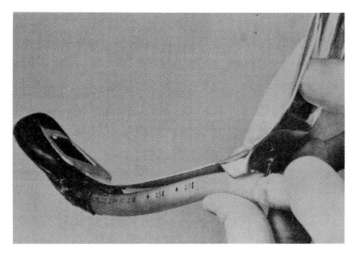

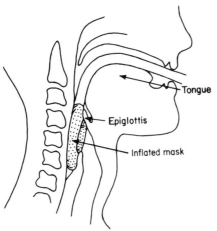

FIG. 9–11.   The laryngeal mask airway containing the stylet (top). The mask in situ during use (bottom). The device is marketed by the Portex Company in UK. (From Brain AIJ, et al.: The laryngeal mask airway. Development and preliminary trials of a new type of airway. Anesthesia *40*:356, 1985.)

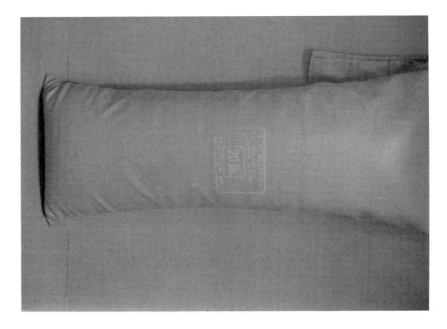

FIG. 9–12.   A 20-lb sandbag for left uterine displacement.

and the EGTA have been used to provide anesthesia to patients whose trachea could not be intubated.[26,29,30] Considerable training is required before these devices can be put to general use. In view of the gravity of the situation, however, investing time in learning the new methods will prove to be worthwhile.

REGIONAL ANESTHESIA

Lumbar epidural or subarachnoid blocks are suitable for anesthesia for cesarean section. The anatomy, pharmacology, and the technique of these blocks have been reviewed in Chapter 7. In this section only the clinical conduct of the procedures will be discussed.

EPIDURAL ANESTHESIA

The patient is given 15 ml of 0.3 M of sodium citrate PO, and is then prophylactically hydrated with at least 1200 ml of crystalloid solution. The infusion of colloid solution offers no particular advantage over crystalloid infusion. The incidence of maternal hypotension and ephedrine requirement are not significantly different with the two prophylactic i.v. solutions.[31] The induction of anesthesia may be done in the operating room or in a well equipped induction area. The induction area must have good lighting, an EKG monitor, an oxygen source, and a suction source. The epidural space is identified at L3-L4, or preferably at L2-L3, and the catheter is inserted 2 to 3 cm cephalad (see Chapter 7). The L2-L3 space is preferred to the L3-L4 space because a more rapid cephalad spread may be achieved with the former approach.

A test dose of lidocaine 2% with a 1:200,000 concentration of epinephrine is injected. Adding the epinephrine solution freshly to lidocaine is recommended because the fresh mixture has a higher pH than the premixed solution. A sand bag is placed under the right hip to produce a 15° left uterine displacement (Fig. 9–12). If the test dose shows no evidence of subarachnoid anesthesia (severe motor weakness in the lower extremities) or intravascular injection (complaints of palpitation), more anesthetic (lidocaine 1.5 or 2% with epinephrine, or bupivacaine 0.5%) is administered in increments of 5 ml. At least 3 to 5 minutes must be allowed to pass

between injections. The sensory level is checked with a pinprick. Blood pressure and pulse rate must be frequently recorded. Any hypotension (systolic blood pressure <100 mm Hg) must be immediately treated with ephedrine injected in 5 mg increments. Severe systemic hypotension that does not respond to ephedrine may require phenylephrine injection in 100 μg increments. Patients must inhale at least a 50% concentration of oxygen before the infant is delivered. Maternal hyperoxia not only increases fetal oxygen stores, but optimizes fetal acid-base status (see Chapter 3). Other methods of optimization of placental gas exchange are described in Chapter 3.

A sensory level of T5-T4 is necessary for satisfactory operating conditions. When the local anesthetic is injected with the patient tilted 15°, the cephalad spread of the anesthetic will be uneven with a lower level (2 to 3 dermatomes) on the right side. However, the dermatomal level will become symmetric with time. If the level on the right side is 5 or more segments lower than the level on the left side, the patient must be turned to her right side and more anesthetic injected. Occasionally, the anesthetic spread will be one-sided. The reason for this is not clear. It is attributed to the presence of a midline septum in the epidural space[32] or the tip of the catheter entering an intervertebral foramen, preventing symmetrical spread of the local anesthetic. The latter situation may be remedied by withdrawing the catheter slightly. With a midline septum, either general or spinal anesthesia may be used. Complications of epidural anesthesia include systemic hypotension, inadvertent intravascular or subarachnoid injection, or an accidental meningeal perforation. Management of these complications are discussed in greater detail in Chapter 7.

SPINAL ANESTHESIA

Spinal anesthesia may be used for CS with good results. Because the total dose of the local anesthetic to be used is small, maternal and fetal drug exposure is small. Pregnancy reduces the dose requirement for local anesthetic needed for spinal anesthesia.[33] The advantages of spinal anesthesia include rapid onset, more profound sensory and motor block, especially a complete blockade of the S1 root.[34] The spread of the anesthetic in the intrathecal space may be quite erratic and unpredictable. In contrast to epidural anesthesia administered via a catheter, the sensory level cannot be reliably controlled with the spinal anesthetic, which is usually administered as a single injection.

Systemic hypotension develops precipitously with spinal anesthesia, which does not allow sufficient time for the physiologic compensatory mechanisms to become fully operational. Several methods may be used for reducing the incidence and severity of hypotension with spinal anesthesia. These methods include using infusions of up to 2000 ml Ringer's lactate solution before spinal anesthesia is induced, or using colloid infusion (5% human albumin) to reduce the incidence of hypotension.[35] Two other methods involve the use of prophylactic administration of ephedrine 25 to 50 mg IM or the rapid administration of ephedrine containing Ringer's lactate solution (50 to 100 mg/500 ml) at the first sign of hypotension.

There are some disadvantages to using spinal anesthesia. Pregnancy reduces the dose requirement for the local anesthetic by approximately 30 to 50%; however, the reduction in dose requirement is not uniform. In order to avoid inadequate blocks, a higher dose than is necessary is used in all patients (Table 9–3), leading to high blocks in certain patients. I have seen total spinal blocks with 8 mg of tetracaine injected into the intrathecal space of a patient in the sitting position. Another major disadvantage of spinal anesthesia is spinal headache. Even with a No. 26-gauge spinal needle, severe spinal headache can develop.

The spinal anesthetic is administered in either the lateral or sitting position. The sitting position is preferred in obese patients. When the anesthetic is administered in the sitting position, the patient is immediately returned to the supine position and a sand bag is wedged under the right hip. The operating table is left horizontal, with the patient's head resting on a single pillow. When the spinal anesthetic is administered in the lateral decubitus, the block must be performed with the patient lying on her right side. This allows for a more even spread of the block when the patient is returned to the position of left tilt.[36]

Lidocaine, tetracaine, tetracaine-procaine mixture,[37] and hyperbaric bupivacaine[38] have all been used for spinal anesthesia for cesarean section. Dextrose is added to these drugs to make them hyperbaric. The use of tetracaine, in both liquid and lyophilized form, has been associated with a high incidence of failure. It appears that it will be replaced with hyperbaric lidocaine or bupivacaine in the near future. The efficacy of epinephrine in prolonging the duration of action of local anesthetics is controversial. This issue is more fully discussed in Chapter 7.

Complications of spinal anesthesia include severe hypotension, high block, total spinal anesthesia, and headache. Occasionally, severe hypotension will lead to ischemia of the brain stem, resulting in apnea. Restoration of perfusion pressure will restore respiratory activity. When a high block occurs, no attempt should be made to arrest the cephalad spread of the anesthetic by raising the patient's head. When the spinal level is at T3 or T4, total sympathectomy may have already occurred. Raising the head end of the operating table is therefore not warranted. Such a maneuver, however, will further decrease the cerebral perfusion pressure that leads to apnea. When total spinal anesthesia is suspected, the patient must be quickly intubated and oxygenated. The systemic perfusion pres-

Table 9–3. Guidelines for Spinal Anesthesia

Drug	How dispensed	Dose	Duration
Lidocaine	5% in 7.5% dextrose (premixed)	70 mg	60 min
Tetracaine	1% solution: Mix with equal volume of 10% dextrose	8 mg	120 min
Tetracaine + Procaine	1% solution + 10% hyperbaric Procaine	8 mg tetracaine + 80 mg of procaine	150 min
Bupivacaine	0.75% with 8.25% dextrose (premixed)	12 mg	100 min

Doses given are for a patient 168 cm tall. With taller patients, add 5 mg of lidocaine, or 1 mg of tetracaine, or 1 mg of bupivacaine for every 7.5 cm difference between the patient's height and 168 cm. When the patient is shorter than 168 cm, reduce the dose by the same amount. For the effect of epinephrine on the duration of spinal anesthesia see Table 7–4.

sure must be restored by administering ephedrine. The treatment of spinal headache is described in Chapter 7.

GENERAL ANESTHESIA

The pharmacology and placental transmission of agents used for general anesthesia have been reviewed in Chapter 4 Perinatal Pharmacology. This section will focus on the technical aspects of administration of general anesthesia in pregnant patients. General anesthesia is needed for cesarean section for fetal distress, in patients who refuse regional anesthesia, or when contraindications exist for regional anesthesia (coagulation disorders, anatomic abnormalities of the spine). Patients must be given antacid prophylaxis as was previously discussed. Left uterine displacement must be maintained with a sand bag wedged under the right hip. Following prophylactic hydration with at least 800 ml of Ringer's lactate solution, anesthesia is induced.

Preoxygenation of the mother before induction is an important precaution. Preoxygenation increases both maternal and fetal oxygen stores and therefore delays arterial desaturation in the event that intubation takes longer than expected. Because of the decreased functional residual capacity (FRC) and increased $\dot{V}O_2$, a pregnant subject will develop arterial desaturation faster than a nonpregnant subject. Some studies have claimed that 4 maximal deep inspirations of 100% oxygen will increase the maternal Pa_{O_2} to 400 mm Hg, the same level achieved by conventional 3 or 5 minute oxygenation.[39] There are two possible problems associated with the shortened preoxygenation. Although four-breath preoxygenation will effectively denitrogenate the lungs, it will not denitrogenate tissue stores,[40] which are more extensive in pregnant patients. In the event of prolonged apnea, nitrogen will build in the alveoli and cause reduction in PA_{O_2}. The other problem is that the fetal blood P_{O_2} lags considerably behind maternal Pa_{O_2}, with the result that fetal P_{O_2} may not rise appreciably with abbreviated preoxygenation. Consequently, if time permits, a full 3 minute preoxygenation must be performed. The shortened preoxygenation must be reserved only for emergency situations.

All agents used for induction and maintenance of general anesthesia cross the placenta easily and achieve detectable levels in fetal circulation. Agents like diazepam and barbiturates are detectable in neonatal circulation for hours (see Chapter 4). When these agents are used in clinical doses, however, the baby may not be depressed. When the injection-delivery interval increases, the maternal/fetal concentration ratio of some agents increases (time-dependent transfer). These agents include volatile agents, pentothal, and pancuronium (see Chapter 4).

Although there is no need to rush unnecessarily to deliver the baby in order to avoid neonatal depression, the delivery must still be performed without delay. Unnecessary delay in delivering the baby creates two problems. It causes the potential neonatal hazard of time-dependent transfer; and when the delivery does not occur, the anesthesiologist is forced to administer depressant medications or increasing concentrations of volatile agents to maintain anesthesia in the mother. Administration of one-third of the initial dose of pentothal will increase the maternal and fetal levels of the drug to the same values caused by the original dose (Fig. 4–3). An induction-delivery interval of more than 8 minutes has been noted to be associated with significantly higher incidence of low, 1 minute Apgar scores and fetal acidosis.[41]

A uterine-incision to delivery time (UD interval) greater than 3 minutes has also been shown to be associated with fetal acidosis and greater incidence of 1 minute Apgar scores,[41] regardless of the type of anesthesia. Prolonged UD intervals must be avoided because intrauterine manipulation may stimulate constriction of the umbilical and placental blood vessels and may also stimulate fetal respiration, leading to meconium or amniotic fluid aspiration by the fetus. In general, irrespective of the type of anesthesia being used, undue delay in delivering the baby must be avoided because anesthetic induction results in many physiologic alterations in the mother, and currently, there is no reliable way of ascertaining fetal welfare from the time of anesthetic induction to delivery.

The administration of a defasciculating dose of a nondepolarizing muscle relaxant has been recommended to avoid succinylcholine induced fasciculations and possibly to avoid rises in intragastric pressure produced by fasciculations. However, fasciculations are usually not intense in pregnant patients. The use of a defasciculating dose may decrease the effectiveness of succinylcholine.[42] Because the onset of facial fasciculations heralds the onset of muscle paralysis, their absence makes it difficult to assess whether or not muscle paralysis has occurred.

Thiopental (3 to 4 mg/kg) is a commonly used inducing agent. Alternate agents are diazepam[43] or ketamine (1 mg/kg). Cricoid pressure is applied by an assistant before induction of anesthesia. If the assistant is not an anesthesiologist, he or she must be coached on how to apply proper cricoid pressure (Fig. 9–13) without distorting the anatomy. The cricoid pressure must be released after the endotracheal tube has passed through the vocal cords. Intravenous administration of succinylcholine (80 to 100 mg) offers unsurpassed intubating conditions in a short period of time. Therefore it is the method of choice for intubating normal obstetric patients. A 7 or 7.5 mm internal diameter (ID) endotracheal tube is suitably sized for most pregnant patients. A 6.5 mm tube must also be available in case it is needed. Only after ascer-

taining that the endotracheal tube has indeed passed through the vocal cords and both hemithoraces are being ventilated equally, surgery must commence because repositioning or reinserting the tube is difficult once surgery is under way. If difficulties are encountered in intubating the trachea, failed intubation protocol must be instituted (vide supra). Anesthesia is maintained with N_2O/oxygen in equal proportions with a volatile agent added to diminish awareness. Enflurane 0.75%, halothane 0.3 to 0.5%, or isoflurane 1% is suitable for this purpose. The use of 50% N_2O alone may be associated with a 10 to 20% intraoperative awareness.[44] Although the incidence of awareness may be decreased to 5% by increasing the N_2O concentration to 75%,[45] the neonatal condition is worsened by this because of the concomitant decrease in FIO_2.[46]

Muscle relaxation is maintained either with nondepolarizing relaxants, such as pancuronium, atracurium, d-tubocurarine, vecuronium, or with succinylcholine infusion. All muscle relaxants cross the placenta and are detectable in the newborn. Used in clinical doses, they do not

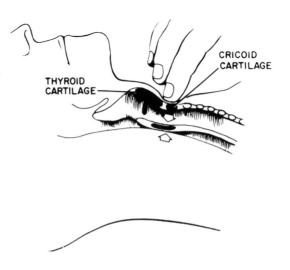

FIG. 9–13. The technique of cricoid pressure.

cause any significant neonatal problems (see Chapter 4). When mechanical ventilation is instituted before the delivery of the infant, hyperventilation must be avoided because maternal hypocarbia is implicated in decreasing fetal oxygenation by shifting the maternal oxyhemoglobin-dissociation curve to the left (see Chapter 3). When babies are delivered expeditiously (within 8 minutes) of induction, general anesthesia is usually not associated with an increased incidence of fetal acidosis or neonatal depression compared to regional anesthesia. Prolonged skin incision to delivery or UD interval will affect neonatal outcome during general anesthesia.

FETAL DISTRESS

An emergency cesarean section may be required for fetal distress. The parturient must receive 15 ml of 0.3 M of sodium citrate PO before induction. The choice of anesthesia depends on the fetal condition. If severe bradycardia develops suddenly and does not respond to intrauterine resuscitation, general anesthesia must be used. If the cesarean section is being performed for late decelerations, which show good recovery, for decreasing scalp pH, or for the presence of meconium, a spinal or an epidural anesthesia may be used.[47] If an epidural catheter is already in place, it is relatively simple to extend the anesthetic level. If an epidural catheter is not available, a "single-shot" epidural may be performed. Lidocaine 2% with 1:200,000 concentration of epinephrine (freshly mixed) 15 ml, provides rapid onset of anesthesia. Spinal anesthesia also provides quick onset. The fetal heart rate must be continuously monitored with a scalp electrode in the operating room when the regional anesthesia is being induced.

REFERENCES

1. Morrison JC, et al.: Cesarean section? What is behind the dramatic rise? Perinatol Neonatol 6:87, 1982.
2. Bottoms SF, Rosen MG, and Sokol RJ: The increase in cesarean birth rate. N Engl J Med, 302:559, 1980.
3. O'Driscoll K, and Foley M: Correlation of decrease in perinatal mortality and increase in cesarean section rates. Obstet Gynecol 61:1, 1983.
4. Williams RL, and Chen PM: Identifying the sources of recent decline in perinatal mortality rates in California. N Engl J Med 306:207, 1982.
5. Sachs BP, et al.: Cesarean section. Risk and benefit for mother and fetus. JAMA 250:2157, 1983.
6. Frigoletto FD Jr, Ryan KJ, and Philippe M: Maternal mortality rate associated with cesarean section: An Appraisal. Am J Obstet Gynecol 136:969, 1980.
7. Pritchard JA, MacDonald PC, and Gant NF: Williams Obstetrics. 17th Edition. Norwalk, Appleton-Century-Crofts, 1985.
8. Ravindran RS, and Ragan WD: Anesthetic causes of maternal mortality in the state of Indiana from 1960–1980. In Abstracts of Scientific Papers, 15th Annual Meeting, Society for Obstetric Anesthesia and Perinatology, 1983.
9. White A, and Kander PL: Anatomical factors in difficult direct laryngoscopy. Br J Anaesth 47:468, 1975.
10. Mallampati SR, et al: A clinical sign to predict difficult tracheal intubation: A prospective study. Can Anaesth Soc J 32:429, 1985.
11. Dustins DM: Anaesthesia for obstetrics. In A Practice of Anaesthesia. 5th edition. (Edited by Churchill-Davidson HC). Chicago, Year Book Medical Publishers, 1984.
12. Creasy RK (ed): Preterm parturition. Seminar Perinatol 3:191, 1981.
13. Roberts RB, and Shirley MA: Reducing the risk of aspiration during cesarean section. Anesth Analg—Current Researches 53:859, 1974.
14. O'Sullivan G, and Bullingham RES: Does twice the volume of antacid have twice the effect in pregnant women at term? Anesth Analg 63:752, 1984.
15. Moore J, et al: H-2 receptor blockade and gastric hyperacidity during labor. Abstract of the Scientifc Paper Presented at the Annual Meeting of the Society for Obstetric Anesthesia and Perinatology, 1984.
16. Brock-Utne JG, et al: The effect of metoclopramide on the lower esophageal sphincter in late pregnancy. Anaesth Intensive Care 6:26, 1978.
17. Rao TLK, et al: Metoclopramide and cimetidine to reduce gastric fluid pH and volume. Anesth Analg 63:1014, 1984.
18. James CF, et al: Pulmonary aspiration—Effects of volume and pH in the rat. Anesth Analg 63:665, 1984.
19. Gibbs CP, et al: Antacid pulmonary aspiration in the dog. Anesthesiology 51:380, 1979..
20. Ramanathan S, Arismendy J, and Turndorf H: Direct inhibitory action of cimetidine and metoclopramide on vascular smooth muscle. Anesthesiology 61:A85, 1984.
21. Santos GD: Acid-aspiration: Pathophysiological aspects, prevention and therapy. Int Anesthesiol Clin 24:31, 1986.
22. Cameron JL, et al: Aspiration pneumonia: Results of treatment with positive-pressure ventilation in dogs. J Surg Res 8:447, 1968.
23. Wynne JW, et al: Steroid therapy for pneumonitis induced in rabbits by aspiration of food stuff. Anesthesiology 51:11, 1979.
24. Greenfield LJ, Singleton RP, McCafree DR: Pulmonary effects of experimental graded aspiration of hydrochloric acid. Ann Surg 170:74, 1969.
25. Cormack RS, and Lehane J: Difficult intubation in obstetrics. Anaesthesia 39:1105, 1984.

26. Tunstall ME, and Geddes C: Failed intubation in obstetric anesthesia. Br J Anaesth 56:659, 1984.

27. Satyanarayana T, et al: Bronchofiberscopic jet ventilation. Anesth Analg 59:350, 1980.

28. Brain AIJ, et al: The laryngeal mask airway. Development and preliminary trials of a new type of airway. Anaesthesia 40:356, 1985.

29. Tunstall ME, and Shiekh A: Failed intubation protocol: Oxygenation without aspiration. Clinics in Anaesthesiology 4:171, 1986.

30. Brain AI: Three cases of difficult intubation overcome by the laryngeal mask airway. Anaesthesia 40:353, 1985.

31. Ramanathan S, et al: Maternal and fetal effects of prophylactic hydration with crystalloids or colloids before epidural anesthesia. Anesth Analg 62:673, 1983.

32. Bose N: Unusual behaviour of extradural analgesia, correspondence. Br J Anaesth 47:806, 1975.

33. Marx GF, and Bassell GM: Physiologic considerations of the mother. In Obstetric Analgesia and Anesthesia. (Edited by Marx GF, and Bassell GM). New York, Elsevier, 1983.

34. Galindo AJ, et al: Quality of spinal extradural anesthesia. The influence of spinal nerve root diameter. Br J Anaesth 47:43, 1975.

35. Matru M, et al: Intravenous albumin administration for prevention of spinal hypotension during cesarean section. Anesth Analg 59:655, 1980.

36. Sprague DH: Effects of position and uterine displacement on spinal anesthesia for cesarean section. Anesthesiology 44:164, 1976.

37. Chantigian RC, Datta S, and Burger GA: Anesthesia for cesarean delivery utilizing spinal anesthesia. Reg Anesth 9:195, 1984.

38. Santos A, et al: Hyperbaric bupivacaine for spinal anesthesia in cesarean section. Anesth Analg 63:1009, 1984.

39. Norris MC, and Dewan DM: Preoxygenation for cesarean section: A comparison of two techniques. Anesthesiology 81:A 400, 1984.

40. Barton F, and Nunn JF: Totally closed circuit nitrous oxide/oxygen anaesthesia. Br J Anaesth 47:350, 1975.

41. Datta S, et al: Neonatal effect of prolonged anesthetic induction for cesarean section. Obstet Gynecol 58:331, 1981.

42. Cullen DJ: The effect of pretreatment with non-depolarizing muscle relaxants on the neuromuscular blocking action of succinylcholine. Anesthesiology 35:572, 1971.

43. Bakke OM, Haram K, Lygre T, and Wallem G: Comparison of the placental transfer of thiopental and diazepam in caesarean section. Eur J Clin Pharmacol 21:221, 1981.

44. Abboud TK, et al: Comparative maternal and neonatal effects of halothane and enflurane for cesarean section. Acta Anaesth Scand 29:663, 1985.

45. Palahniuk RJ, et al: Maternal and neonatal effects of methoxyflurane, nitrous oxide and lumbar epidural anesthesia for cesarean section. Can Anaesth Soc J 24:586, 1977.

46. Marx GF, and Mateo CV: Effects of different oxygen concentrations during general anesthesia for cesarean section. Can Anaesth Soc J 18:587, 1981.

47. Marx GF, Luykx WM, and Cohen S: Fetal-neonatal status following caesarean section for fetal distress. Br J Anaesth 56:1009, 1984.

PART

II

HIGH-RISK PREGNANCY

10

PREECLAMPSIA

Hypertensive disorders of pregnancy are classified into four types: preeclampsia and eclampsia; chronic hypertension caused by various causes; chronic hypertension with superimposed preeclampsia or pregnancy-aggravated hypertension; and late or transient hypertension.[1] This terminology was advocated by the American College of Obstetricians and Gynecologists (ACOG) and is presently the most concise and descriptive classification of the disorders.

PREECLAMPSIA

Unfortunately, a great deal of confusion has surrounded diagnosis of preeclampsia. There is a tendency to diagnose any patient with a slight elevation in blood pressure as having preeclampsia. The diagnosis should instead be based on a set of stringent criteria.[2] Because the condition is relatively rare in multiparous women, a diagnosis of preeclampsia is more likely to be erroneous with them than with nulliparous women.[2] The ACOG has therefore introduced a new category called transient, late, or gestational hypertension. It is defined as a rise in blood pressure during pregnancy, labor, or in the early puerperium with normalization of blood pressure within ten days after delivery. The other condition that may further compound the difficulty of diagnosis is the presence of preexisting renal disease that is latent in midpregnancy but becomes active in late pregnancy. Chealey[2] therefore recommended that the di-

agnosis of preeclampsia be made in a hypertensive patient only when the following criteria are met: nulliparity; abundant proteinuria; a reliable past history with respect to normal renal and cardiovascular systems; age less than 25 years; and hyperuricemia. Proteinuria, however, may present a problem in diagnosing preeclampsia because it can occur very late in the course of the disease. In about 10% of eclamptic women, no proteinuria occurs before the onset of convulsions. Edema is also not a reliable sign.[3] Pedal edema in a pregnant patient may be caused by compression of the inferior vena cava. Up to 64% of pregnant women may have edema in the nondependent portions of the body. Certain conditions, notably diabetes mellitus and multiple gestations, predispose to preeclampsia. The following factors predispose to preeclampsia:

1. Obesity
2. Diabetes
3. Multiple pregnancy
4. Essential hypertension
5. Renal disease
6. Hydramnios
7. Hydatiditiform mole (second trimester)

Hypertension is defined in a pregnant patient as follows: the systolic pressure is 140 mm Hg or greater, the diastolic pressure is 90 mm Hg or greater, and the mean pressure is 105 mm Hg or greater. An increase of 30, 15, and 20 mm Hg, respectively in systolic, diastolic, and mean pressure is considered abnormal. Obviously, more than one blood pressure reading is essential before a diagnosis of hypertension can be made. If no previous readings during pregnancy are available, a reading of 140/90 is considered hypertensive. A proteinuria of at least 0.3 g/L/24 hours (1^+ to 2^+ by the dipstick measurement) is diagnostic. The disease is considered severe if one or more of the following features are present (Table 10–1): severe hypertension; excessive proteinuria; oliguria; and symptoms such as convulsions, headache, seeing halos around bright light (retinal ischemia), or left ventricular failure.

PATHOPHYSIOLOGY OF PREECLAMPSIA

Preeclampsia is a multisystem disease that affects almost every organ in the body. In order to safely administer anesthetic to these patients, the anesthesiologist must possess a working knowledge of the pathophysiologic effects of the disease.

Cardiovascular System

The basic pathophysiologic derangement caused by preeclampsia is the widespread arteriolar constriction occurring throughout the body.[3] This obviously increases the afterload of the heart, which subsequently becomes hyperdynamic to overcome this afterload. The heart rate and cardiac output are increased. The myocardial function is excellent in most patients. A majority of patients with preeclampsia will display a hyperdynamic left ventricular function in relation to the pulmonary capillary wedge pressure[4–7] (Fig. 10–1). Approximately 25% of all patients will show evidence of suboptimal myocardial function (Fig. 10–1). Another interesting finding is the poor correlation between central venous pressure (CVP) and pulmonary artery capillary wedge pressure (PCWP) (Fig. 10–2) in some patients with severe preeclampsia, whether pulmonary edema is present or not.[4–7] It is especially true of patients with a CVP value of 6 mm Hg or greater. The PCWP may indeed be much higher than the CVP.[6] The indications for using a pulmonary artery catheter include the presence of pulmonary edema; failure of the CVP to increase despite adequate volume infusion; failure of improvement in renal function, despite a good CVP and adequate volume replacement; and a large alveolar-arterial oxygen gradient ($AaDo_2$ gradient), which may be caused by interstitial pulmonary edema. A sudden deterioration in left ventricular function has been noted to occur immediately after the delivery of the baby.[6] Autotransfusion, which characteristically occurs at this time, causes a rise in PCWP with only a disproportionate rise in left ventricular function. Thus, the stage is set for the development of pulmonary edema, especially in those who received a large volume of colloid or crystalloid infusion prior to delivery.[7] Intravenous fluid administration is routinely done before administering epidural anesthesia. Intravenous fluids may also be required for replacing blood loss. Judicius monitoring of the PCWP pressure is necessary before large

Table 10–1. Mild and Severe Preeclampsia

	Abnormality	Mild	Severe
	Diastolic pressure	<100 mm Hg	110 mm Hg or higher
	Proteinuria	Trace to 1^+	2^+ or higher
	Headache	Absent	Present
	Visual problems	Absent	Present
	Epigastric pain	Absent	Present
	Oliguria <400 ml/24 H	Absent	Present
	Convulsions	Absent	Present
	Serum creatinine	Normal	Elevated
	Thrombocytopenia	Absent	Present
	Hyperbilirubinemia	Absent	Present
	SGOT* elevation	Minimal	Pronounced
	IUGR†	Absent	Overt

*SGOT = serum glutamate oxaloacetate transaminase
†IUGR = intrauterine growth retardation
Reproduced with kind permission from Pritchard JA, McDonald PC, and Gant NF: Hypertensive disorders in pregnancy. *In* Williams Obstetrics. 17th Edition. Norwalk, Appleton-Century-Crofts, 1985.

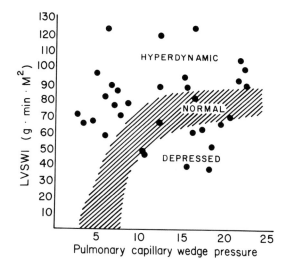

FIG. 10–1. Hyperdynamic circulation in patients with preeclampsia. For every given pulmonary capillary wedge pressure (PCWP), the left ventricle must generate a certain amount of work. The PCWP represents the filling pressure and the left ventricular stroke work index (LVSWI), which is the Y-axis, represents the myocardial function. The shaded area represents the work output of the normal myocardium. Note that in preeclamptic patients the ventricular function lies in the hyperdynamic range. Each circle represents a single patient. Patient data were derived from Newsome LR,[4] Benedetti TJ,[7] and Rafferty TR.[49]

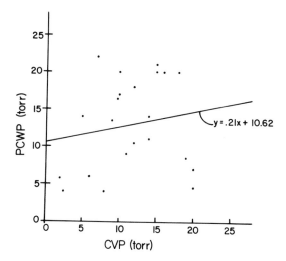

FIG. 10–2. Lack of correlation between central venous pressure (CVP) and pulmonary capillary wedge pressure (PCWP) in patients with preeclampsia. Individual patient data derived from Newsome LR,[4] Benedetti TJ[7], and Phelan JP.[6]

volumes of fluid are administered in severe preeclamptics.

The preeclamptic patient is remarkably sensitive to exogenous and endogenous catecholamines. A pregnant patient does not usually show a pressor response to angiotensin II. In those who are resistant to the vascular effects of this agent, preeclampsia is unlikely to develop later in pregnancy. Of those who show a pressor response to the agent, 92% subsequently became hypertensive.[8] During a 10 week period preceding the onset of preeclampsia, the pregnant patient may become hypertensive on rolling over to the supine position.[9] The reason for this is not clear and is attributed to the increased vascular sensitivity. The basal activity of the angiotensin-converting enzyme is believed to be higher in those who manifest hypertension on "rolling over."[10] The heightened sensitivity to vasopressor was originally attributed to the increased intracellular sodium concentration in the vascular smooth muscle cells. However, recent experimental data do not support this contention.[11]

The circulating fluid volume is diminished 10 to 15% (Table 10–2).[9] The average reduction in blood volume compared to a nonpreeclamptic patient is 10 to 15%. Although many older studies showed that the blood volume was reduced to a greater degree than the 10 to 15%, the results of these older studies may be misleading because the blood volume measurements were not standardized for the weight of the baby. Preeclamptics deliver smaller babies than do normal patients (Fig. 10–3).[11] A smaller baby produces a smaller expansion in blood volume.[9] Therefore, when blood volume comparisons are made between preeclamptics and normal patients, the comparisons must be made only after standardization for fetal weights. One interesting feature of the disease is that the reduction in intravascular volume occurs before any other manifestations appear (Fig. 10–3).

Edema. Preeclamptic patients also have considerable generalized edema. The edema fluid accumulates both in the intracellular and extracellular compartments, favoring slightly the intracellular compartment. Many severe preeclamptics, however, do not have edema and many normal patients, especially those bearing large babies may have considerable edema (Fig. 10–4). Therefore, the presence or absence of

Table 10–2.   Mean Plasma Volume (ml) in Normal and Preeclamptic Pregnancy

Study	Normals	Preeclampsia	Difference
Cope (1961)	3470(29)	2820(14)	650
Honger (1967)	3800(20)	3300(19)	500
Brody (1967)	4245(46)	4010(34)	235
MacGillivray (1967)	4040(18)	3535(35)	505
Blekta (1970)	3133(55)	3524(29)	239
Campell (1980)	3763(55)	3524(29)	239
Hays (1985)*	2345/M²(9)	1763/M²(4)	582/M²
Total means	3742(223)	3297(145)	445

*See Hays PM, Cruikshank DP, and Dunn LJ.[50]

(From MacGillivray I, Pre-Eclampsia; The Hypertensive Disease of Pregnancy. Philadelphia, WB Saunders, 1983.

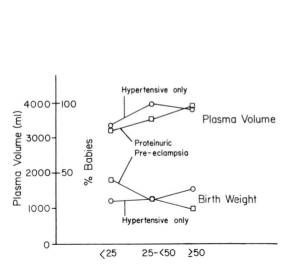

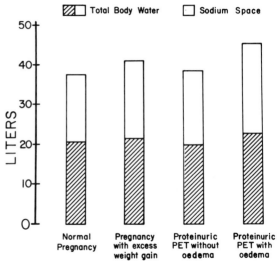

FIG. 10–3.   Newborn birth weight percentile distribution versus plasma volume in patients with hypertension only and in patients with preeclampsia. The plasma volume measurements were made before the onset of preeclampsia. In preeclamptic patients, the birth weight distribution is weighted in favor of small babies. When plasma volumes are compared in patients who delivered babies with similar gestational weights (25 to 50 percentile), the failure of the plasma volume to expand adequately even before the onset of the condition is noticeable in preeclamptic pregnancy. Patients with uncomplicated hypertension are expected to have expansion in plasma volume similar to normal patients. Data derived from MacGillivray.[11]

FIG. 10–4.   Extra- and intracellular spaces (ECF and ICF, respectively) in normal pregnancy with or without excessive weight gain and in preeclamptic pregnancy with or without edema. Darkened area represents ECF and the light area ICF. The ECF to ICF ratio and the total body water (TBW) content are similar in normal pregnancy and preeclamptic pregnancy without edema. Also, the TBW content is increased in normal pregnancy with excessive weight gain and in preeclamptic pregnancy with edema. Thus edema can occur in normal pregnancy and preeclampsia may occur in the absence of edema. The presence or absence of edema is therefore not diagnostic of preeclampsia. (From MacGillivray I: Pre-Eclampsia: The Hypertensive Disease of Pregnancy. Philadelphia, WB Saunders, 1983.)

edema is really not a reliable diagnostic feature. If present, the edema fluid consists of both albumin (0.18 g/100 ml of edema fluid) and globulin (0.16 g/100 ml of edema fluid). The urine also contains albumin and globulin at a ratio similar to the one in the edema fluid. The loss of protein into the interstitium, together with albuminuria, causes a reversal of the plasma's albumin-globulin ratio. The cause of edema is subject to controversy. Reduced plasma oncotic pressure (POP), increased hydrostatic transcapillary filtration pressure, and altered capillary permeability are the possible mechanisms. These factors may also result in increased pulmonary parenchymal water content leading to increased $AaDO_2$ gradient. Because of similar albumin-globulin ratios, the mechanism of edema fluid formation and the mechanism of albuminuria are believed to be the same.[11]

Coagulation. Preeclampsia affects the coagulation system in many ways. Thrombocytopenia is the most common abnormality, followed by HELLP syndrome (hemolysis, elevated liver enzymes and low platelet count syndrome) and disseminated intravascular coagulation (DIC) (Table 10–3).[12] Occasionally burr cells and schistocytes may be seen in peripheral smears suggesting microangiopathic hemolytic anemia.[12] In addition, plasma antithrombin III activity is decreased in patients with preeclampsia.[13] This may predispose to widespread thrombin deposition in many organs, especially in the kidney and the placenta.

Central Nervous System

Whenever the mean arterial pressure exceeds 140 mm Hg, the cerebral circulation loses its autoregulatory capacity, creating an ideal situation for the development of cerebral edema. This situation is usually referred to as the forced dilatation syndrome.[14,15] Although severe hypertension is well-tolerated by those who had been chronically hypertensive, a young preeclamptic patient will not tolerate acute elevations in blood pressure. The cerebral perfusion will increase in response to the increasing perfusion pressure, leading to cerebral edema or hypertensive encephalopathy. Ring hemorrhages (Fig. 10–5) may occur in the brain, which may be a harbinger of a severe cerebrovascular accident. Strokes are a leading cause of maternal mortality in patients with preeclampsia. Severe hypertension may occur especially during endotracheal intubation. The anesthesiologist must try to minimize responses to intubation with prophylactic use of intravenous vasodilators. Hyperreflexia is believed to be caused by cerebral edema, although it may also be present in nonpreeclamptic women.

Kidney

A preeclamptic patient may have a significant plasma volume deficit, an increase in total body exchangeable sodium, and markedly expanded interstitium. The cause of sodium retention is unknown but is believed to be caused by extraadrenal conversion of progesterone to deoxycorticosterone acetate (DOC), a potent antinatriuretic hormone.[16] Diminished glomerular filtration rate may also lead to sodium retention. Oliguria is highly suggestive of a severe disease. Oliguria may be caused by either plasma volume deficit or by actual intrinsic renal disease. Oliguria caused by hypovolemia may respond to intravenous fluid therapy. When this does not happen, one must suspect intrinsic renal involvement by the disease process. A markedly increased blood-urea nitrogen (BUN) and uric acid may give a clue as to the presence of intrinsic renal disease. When renal involvement

Table 10–3. Coagulation Abnormalities in 303 Cases of Preeclampsia

Abnormality	Percentage	Diagnostic criteria
Thrombocytopenia (<150,000)	17	—
HELLP syndrome	9	—
Disseminated intravascular coagulation (DIC)	7	Platelet count <150,000/mm³ Fibrinogen <300 mg% Fibrin split products >400 µg/ml

For explanation of HELLP syndrome, see text.
(Source: Sibai BM, et al: Pregnancy outcome in 303 cases with severe preeclampsia. Obstet Gynecol, 64:319, 1984.)

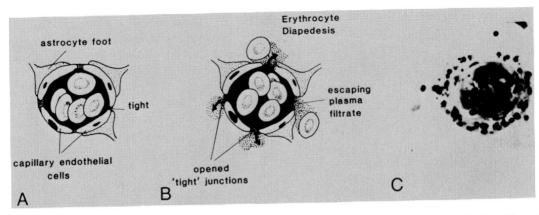

FIG. 10–5. Ring hemorrhage in eclamptic hypertensive encephalopathy. A = intact cerebral capillary: B = ruptured capillary junctions with leakage of red blood cells and plasma; C = a thrombosed cerebral precapillary surrounded by hemorrhage. Clusters of small hemorrhages and infarctions may be found in the occipital lobe of the cerebral cortex, which may lead to blindness. (From Donaldson JO: Neurologic emergencies during pregnancy. *In* Critical Care of the Obstetric Patient. (Edited by Berkowitz RL). New York, Churchill-Livingstone, 1983.)

is present, it usually consists of edema and swelling of the glomerular tuft; pouting of the tuft into the collecting system; narrowing of the glomerular capillary lumen; fragmentation of capillary endothelium; electron dense deposit (probably fibrin derivative) in the capillary basement membrane (Fig. 10–6);[17] and protein casts in the collecting system.

Liver

There are no pathognomonic lesions produced by the disease process in the liver. The nonspecific lesions are mainly caused by fibrin deposition (disseminated intravascular coagulation–DIC). Periportal hemorrhages and midzonal necrosis caused by vasospasm of the hepatic artery branches may also be seen. The epigastric pain is believed to be caused by small subcapsular hemorrhages, which may occasionally culminate in the rupture of the liver. Sudden development of systemic hypotension in a severely ill preeclamptic patient should arouse a high degree of suspicion of spontaneous rupture of the liver (Fig. 10–7). The edema and the hemorrhages are probably responsible for the hepatic dysfunction as evidenced by increased blood SGOT (serum glutamate oxaloacetate transaminase) and SGPT (serum glutamate pyruvate transaminase) (HELLP syndrome).

Placenta

Multiple areas of ischemic necrosis of the villi (placental infarcts) may be found. Massive perivillous fibrin deposition may occur in the periphery of the placenta. Deposition of fibrinoid material is noticed in the intervillous space. Placental abruption occurs with increased freqeuency. There may be narrowing of the intramyometrial portion of the spiral artery. Obliterative endarteritis of the fetal stem arteries may also occur. A true atheroma of maternal decidual artery has also been reported.

In early stages of normal pregnancy, the cytotrophoblastic cells invade the lumen of the dicidual portion of the maternal spiral artery. The elastic tissue of the media is destroyed, and fibrin deposition occurs in the lumen. There is a secondary invasion starting at 16 weeks of gestation into the myometrial segment of the spiral artery. In preeclamptic pregnancies, the early invasion of the spiral artery occurs, but the second wave fails to occur. With the result, the intramyometrial portion of the spiral artery remains narrow (Fig. 10–8).[11,18] The pathologic changes in the placenta are probably responsible for the intrauterine growth retardation of the fetus.

Fetus

Preeclampsia causes intrauterine growth retardation (Fig. 10–3). Perinatal survival is af-

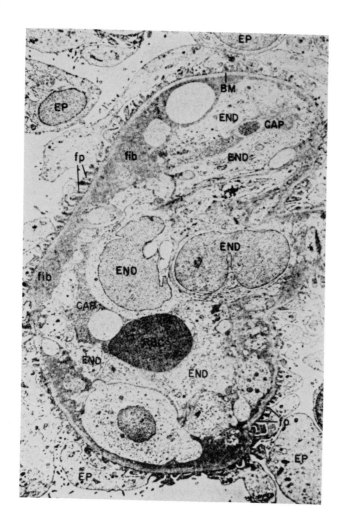

FIG. 10–6. Electron microscopic appearance of the glomerular tuft in a patient with severe preeclampsia. Fibrinoid material deposited on the basement membrane (BM); obliterated capillary lumen (CAP); fragmented endothelium (END); foot processes (fp). The most striking features are the deposition of fibrinoid material on the basement membrane and the obstruction of the capillary lumen with swollen fragmented capillary endothelium (From Dennis EJ and Hester LL: The preeclampsia-eclampsia syndrome. *In* Obstetrics and Gynecology. (Edited by Danforth, DN). New York, Harper and Row, 1982.)

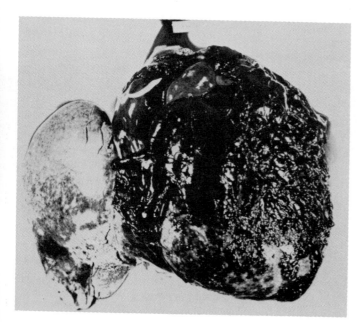

FIG. 10–7. Spontaneous rupture of the liver in patient with severe preeclampsia. (From Dennis EJ and Hester LL: The preeclampsia-eclampsia syndrome. *In* Obstetrics and Gynecology. (Edited by Danforth, DN). New York, Harper and Row, 1982.)

INTERVILLOUS SPACE

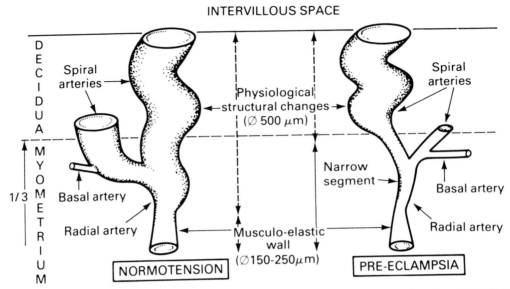

FIG. 10–8. Diagrammatic representation of changes in decidual vessels in normal and preclamptic pregnancy. Note that in preeclamptic pregnancy the intramyometrial portion of the spiral artery fails to undergo dilatation because of the lack of invasion by the cytotrophoblasts. The narrow segment probably accounts for the diminished placental perfusion. Any reduction in perfusion pressure will further reduce blood flow through the segment. For further details see text. (From MacGillivray, I: Pre-Eclampsia: The Hypertensive Disease of Pregnancy. Philadelphia, WB Saunders, 1983.)

fected by maternal hypertension (Collaborative Perinatal Project, Task Force on Toxemia of the National Institute of the Neurologic and Communicative Disorders and Stroke). Hypertension alone without proteinuria was associated with a three-fold increase in the fetal death rate. Large placental infarcts, small placentas, and abruptio placentae constituted the majority of causes for fetal demise[3] (Table 10–4). Because many babies are small at birth, the incidence of respiratory distress is higher than in neonates born of normal mothers.[11] The British Birth Survey (1970) showed that neonatal mortality was higher in preeclamptics who smoked than in those who did not.[11]

TREATMENT OF PREECLAMPSIA

The goals of therapy are (1) adequate control of blood pressure, (2) optimization of circulating fluid volume, (3) prevention of eclampsia (convulsions), (4) delivery of viable baby with the least amount of trauma to the mother and her fetus,[3] and (5) expert postpartum care of the mother. Ambulatory management has no place in the treatment of preeclamptics with severe hypertension and intrauterine growth retardation. Some multipara with moderate elevations in blood pressure without proteinuria may be managed at home.[3] When the patient is at or near term, all these goals can be simultaneously

Table 10–4. Fetal Death Rate per 1000 Births

Diastolic pressure (mm Hg)	Proteinuria					
	None	Trace	1+	2+	3+	4+
65–74	9.3	8.0	5.6	32.9	41.54	—
75–84	6.2	7.44	6.2	19.22	—	—
85–94	8.68	9.3	23.56	—	22.32	—
95–104	19.22	17.36	26.66	55.8	115.32	143.22
105+	20.46	27.9	62.62	68.82	125.24	110.98

(Data modified from Friedman EA and Neff RK: Pregnancy outcome as related to hypertension, edema and proteinuria. *In* Hypertension in Pregnancy. (Edited by Lindheimer MD, Katz AI, and Zuspan FP). New York, Wiley, 1976.)

achieved by proper perinatal management and delivery of the infant. Controversy surrounds the maternal use of steroids for diminishing respiratory neonatal distress. A limited number of studies have claimed that steroid administration is not fraught with any dangers in the hypertensive patients.[19] Many feel, however, that this is an unnecessary risk because respiratory distress occurs less frequently in premature neonates born of preeclamptic mothers than in neonates born of normal mothers at similar gestational age.[3] Surfactant maturation occurs earlier in preeclamptic pregnancy than it does in normal pregnancy.[3,20]

MgSO$_4$

Magnesium sulfate (MgSO$_4$) is used for preventing convulsions, and hydralazine is used for controlling blood pressure. Phenobarbital may be used for sedation. MgSO$_4$ is very popular in North America for the treatment of preeclampsia but this same enthusiasm is not shared by physicians on the other side of the Atlantic Ocean. Mg^{++} is used for its anticonvulsive properties. Its other actions include the inhibition of acetyl choline release from the neuromuscular junction, and the desensitization of the postjunctional membrane of the myoneural junction. Mg^{++} potentiates both depolarizing and nondepolarizing relaxants.

In subhuman primates, Mg^{++} suppresses neuronal burst response and electroencephalogram (EEG) spike activity in experimentally induced epilepsy.[21] Thus it appears that the anticonvulsant action of Mg^{++} is not caused by a nonspecific CNS depression, but by a specific action on the EEG. Mg^{++} is excreted by the kidneys and is partly reabsorbed by the renal tubules. Mg^{++} excretion is impaired in renal disease. An increase in plasma creatinine is a reliable index to monitor kidney function during Mg^{++} therapy. In vitro experiments have shown that Mg^{++} attenuated the contractile responses of umbilical blood vessels to angiotensin II and prostaglandin F$_{2\alpha}$.[22]

The loading dose is usually 4 g i.v. (administered slowly) followed by 10 g i.m. in severe cases. Maintenance administration can be done either by i.m. administration (5 grams every 4 hours) or by i.v. infusion at 1 to 2 grams/hour. In mild cases, the i.v. loading dose is omitted.

Table 10–5. Magnesium Toxicity

Observed condition	Plasma content (mEq/L)
Normal level	1.5–2.0
Therapeutic range	5.0–7.0
ECG changes	
P-Q prolonged, QRS widened	5.0–10.0
Loss of tendon reflexes	10.0
Respiratory arrest, cardiac arrest	12 and higher

Recently, it has been reported that there is no therapeutic advantage to the use of intravenous infusion because adequate therapeutic levels may be maintained by just intermittent intramuscular injections alone.[23,24] The use of a loading dose, however, increases the possibility of an overdose. An infusion pump is used for administering Mg^{++} infusion. Mg^{++} toxicity is an ever-present danger in those who are on treatment. Diminished renal function increases the likelihood of toxicity. The most dangerous toxic effect of Mg^{++} is the possibility of respiratory arrest. The various toxic effects of Mg^{++} and the plasma levels at which they are likely to occur are given in Table 10–5. The therapeutic level of Mg^{++} lies between 5 to 7 mEq/L. When Mg^{++} levels reach 12 mEq/L, respiratory arrest is a real threat.[3] Mg^{++} crosses the placenta. When maternal overdose is avoided and the plasma level of Mg^{++} is kept within a therapeutic range, neonatal hypermagnesemia is unlikely to occur. Neonatal magnesium toxicity causes respiratory inadequacy in the neonate.[25]

Hydralazine for Hypertension

Mg^{++} has only limited action on blood pressure. Hydralazine, a vasodilator is the preferred drug for reducing blood pressure in preeclamptic patients. This drug has stood the test of time and has proved to be safe for the mother and fetus. Any blood pressure higher than 170/110 requires treatment with an antihypertensive drug. Because of the unpredictable response of uteroplacental circulation in severe preeclamptics, the blood pressure should be maintained at a level no lower than 130/90 during therapy. A sudden reduction in blood pressure to levels normal for nonpreeclamptic women may be associated with fetal bradycardia. A severe preeclamptic may also complain of dizziness, suggestive of diminished cerebral perfusion at perfusion pressures normal for nonpreeclamptic patients. For severe hypertension (diastolic pressure >120 mm Hg) a 5 mg injection of hydralazine is given, followed by 5 mg increments at 20 minute intervals. The fullest extent of hydralazine effect will not be evident for 20 minutes. Therefore, if sufficient time is not allowed between injections, severe hypotension may ensue.[26] The patient may complain of headache and flushing of the face during therapy with hydralazine. Hydralazine may not be adequate in some patients with severe hypotension. A small dose of diazoxide may be used to supplement hydralazine under those circumstances.

Drugs Used During Hypertensive Crisis in a Preeclamptic Patient

Hypertensive crisis in a preeclamptic patient requires a more potent and fast acting vasodilator, such as sodium nitroprusside or nitroglycerin. The ganglion blocker, trimethaphan, has also been used for this purpose. An indwelling arterial cannula is necessary for monitoring blood pressure continously when nitroprusside, nitroglycerin, or trimethaphan is being used.

Nitroprusside and Nitroglycerin. The use of nitroprusside is associated with the release of cyanide in the mother and fetus following excessive administration for prolonged periods of time.[27] However, sodium nitroprusside infusion may be used for a short period of time in dire emergencies and discontinued when other modes of therapy become fully effective.[28]

Sodium nitroprusside has been used to produce hypotensive anesthesia in pregnant patients.[29] Both sodium nitroprusside and nitroglycerin have been shown not to reduce uterine blood flow despite a reduction in mean arterial blood pressure in animal experiments.[30] Both these agents counteract uterine vasoconstriction induced by norepinephrine infusion. They do not, however, decrease the uterine blood flow, despite a 20% reduction in perfusion pressure. Both agents may, however, increase the heart rate significantly. The advantages of these two agents are that they act rapidly; that minute to minute control of blood pressure is possible, especially with the use of continuous monitoring and an infusion pump; their action is evanescent,

so that prompt restoration of blood pressure is possible on discontinuation of the drug; and they can be used for controlling hypertensive response to intubation.[31]

Trimethaphan. Trimethaphan is a ganglion blocker with a molecular weight of 600, and therefore its placental passage is limited. It is hydrolyzed rapidly by plasma cholinesterase making it an attractive agent for use in obstetrics. Its use, however, is associated with histamine release, troublesome tachycardia, and tachyphylaxis. Ganglion blockade also causes vasodilatation, which might cause reduced venous return. This may decrease the cardiac output in those with normal cardiac function. Although there is a theoretic possibility that the use of trimethaphan may cause a prolongation of succinylcholine induced paralysis (because it utilizes pseudocholinesterase), this has not been a problem in clinical practice. Many preeclamptics may continue to be hypertensive even after delivery. Therefore, the antihypertensive therapy must be continued in a suitable form until the patient is normotensive. The agent α-methyl dopa is suitable for chronic use during pregnancy and for postpartum use. The use of antihypertensive drugs in pregnancy is summarized in Table 10–6.

Should convulsions occur when the patient is being stabilized, diazepam may be used as an anticonvulsant. The protection of the airway also assumes paramount importance in a convulsing patient. Some recommend intravenous administration of $MgSO_4$ for treating convulsions in a preeclamptic. Although Mg^{++} is effective as an anticonvulsant, a large intravenous dose may result in overdose and respiratory arrest. Occasionally, convulsions may occur with alarming frequency necessitating the use of a muscle relaxant and mechanical ventilation.

ANESTHETIC CONSIDERATIONS

Although mild cases of preeclampsia may be anesthetized without any extensive monitoring, patients with severe disease do require invasive monitoring. In addition to the indwelling arterial cannula, a CVP catheter is usually needed to avoid overhydration and to detect severe hypovolemia. A pulmonary artery catheter may be needed if cardiac decompensation is suspected.

Table 10–6. Acute and Chronic Therapy of Hypertension

	Drug	Action	Administration	Problem	Comments
A C U T E	Hydralazine	Vasodilator resistance vessels	Administer 5 mg increments to a diastolic pressure to 110, maintenance 5–10 mg/hour	Tachycardia	Safe for fetus, widely used
	Labetalol	α and β blocker	Initial dose i.v. or oral 50–100 mg to 300 mg in 30 min or constant infusion 1–2 mg/min	Less side effects than hydralazine	Only limited experience, questionable safety for compromised fetus
	Diazoxide	Vasodilator resistance vessels	30–60 mg i.v. every 5 min, repeat every 5 min as necessary or 10 mg/min infusion	Inhibits labor, hyperglycemia	To supplement hydralazine
	Nitroglycerine	Dilates the capacitance vessels more	Infusion 30 μg/min—increase as needed	Raised ICP (questionable)	To blunt intubation hypertension
	Nitroprusside	Dilates the resistance vessels	25 μg/min and increase as needed	Cyanide release	Hypertension unresponsive to other drugs, to blunt intubation response
	Trimethaphan	Ganglion blocker	Infusion 300 μg/min	Tachycardia, histamine release	MW-600, rapid hydrolysis in the baby
C H R O N I C	α-methyl dopa	α-2 blocker, central sympatholytic	1–3 g daily in divided doses orally		Safe, extensive clinical trial
	Labetalol	α and β blocker	100–300 mg TID or QID orally		Questionable safety for the fetus under stress
	β-blockers: Atenolol Metoprolol Propranolol		50–100 mg daily orally 50–225 mg daily orally 40–240 mg daily orally		Safety questionable for stressed fetus

Indications for the use of a pulmonary artery catheter and the pitfalls of monitoring CVP have been outlined before. The pulmonary capillary wedge pressure is elevated to 20 to 25 mm Hg if there is cardiac decompensation. The CVP is usually a poor index for detecting left ventricular dysfunction.

The plasma oncotic pressure (POP) is reduced in preeclamptic patients because of albuminuria and extravasation of proteins into the interstitium. Although colloids appear to be a tempting choice to raise the POP during the stabilization period, their routine use may not be advisable, because albumin may not remain intravascular in the preeclamptic patient as long as it does in a nonpreeclamptic patient.[11] Even in normal subjects, rapid administration of albumin causes escape of albumin into the interstitium by stretching the capillary pores.[32,33] The increased venous presssure probably causes the stretching

of the pores, increasing the transcapillary diffusion gradient.[34] The normally occurring transcapillary escape accounts for the presence of proteins in the interstitial fluids.[35] In preeclamptics, the protein escape is likely to be faster because of the altered capillary permeability. If the protein escapes into the pulmonary interstitium, pulmonary edema may ensue.

It takes at least 50 g of albumin to raise the POP significantly in pregnant patients.[36] It is not unusual for the POP to decrease to values as low as 12 mm Hg in the postpartum period without evidence of pulmonary edema. The POP-PCWP gradient, which was once thought to be a major determinant of pulmonary edema, is no longer thought to be a reliable predictor of pulmonary edema.[37] The treatment for a decreased or negative POP-PCWP gradient is not raising the POP, but decreasing the PCWP by using nitroglycerin or nitroprusside.[28,38]

LABOR ANALGESIA

In patients with only mild disease, routine anesthetic care during labor analgesia is sufficient. However, in those with severe preeclampsia, a carefully planned approach is necessary. The following important laboratory tests must be done in all preeclamptics:

1. Routine blood work-up
2. Urinalysis (protein casts)
3. 24 hour urine protein
4. BUN, creatinine, uric acid
5. PT, PTT, fibrinogen, fibrin split products
6. Platelet count, peripheral smear (to detect burr cells and schistocytes)
7. Arterial blood gas tensions and pH serum Mg^{++} levels
8. Liver function tests (HELLP syndrome)

In addition to the routine laboratory tests, tests for coagulation abnormalities and renal and hepatic dysfunction are particularly useful. Measurements of POP may help assess the severity of hypoalbuminemia. Measurement of Mg^{++} level may be useful in determining adequacy of therapy and detecting impending toxicity during labor and in the postpartum period. In the absence of a coagulopathy, the preferred anesthetic technique is lumbar epidural anesthesia. Preload optimization with crystalloid infusion is important using either CVP (7 to 8 mm Hg) or PCWP (10 mm Hg) as an index. A Foley catheter must be inserted at the earliest opportunity and the urinary output must be maintained at least at 30 ml/hour. An indwelling arterial cannula is useful for monitoring blood pressure. The epidural catheter is inserted at the L3-L4 or L2-L3 intervertebral space. Bupivacaine 0.25% should be injected in 3 ml increments until the dermatomal level reaches the T10 level. Blood pressure should be maintained at 140/90. If, however, the patient complains of lightheadedness, a higher baseline pressure must be aimed for. Ephedrine in 5 mg increments is recommended for this purpose. A carefully performed lumbar epidural analgesia is not associated with a greater degree of systemic hypotension in preeclamptics than in normotensive subjects.[39] In addition to its other beneficial effects, epidural analgesia for labor reduces the requirements for Mg^{++} and hydralazine. When the block extends from T10 to L3, it may also increase the intervillous blood flow significantly[40] (Fig. 10-9). A

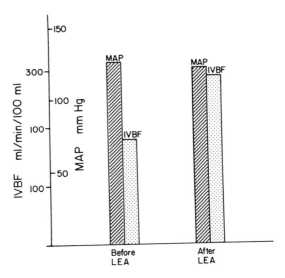

FIG. 10-9. Placental intervillous blood flow (IVBF) and mean arterial pressure (MAP) before and after epidural analgesia in patients with a baseline diastolic blood pressure of at least 100 mm Hg. Data from Jouppila P[40] and Jouppila R.[41]

strictly segmental block extending between T10 and T12 has a less pronounced effect on the intervillous blood flow.[41]

There is some recent evidence to suggest that the clearance rate of lidocaine from maternal circulation may be slower in preeclamptic patients than in normal subjects probably because of hepatic dysfunction.[42] Repeated injections of lidocaine may lead to toxic concentrations in preeclamptics. Because the fetus is compromised somewhat in preeclamptic pregnancy, the paracervical block is not recommended. If epidural analgesia is contraindicated either because of the presence of coagulopathy or because of patient refusal, then a liberal intravenous analgesia is used because pain will increase the dose requirement for Mg^{++} and hydralazine. Intravenous analgesia for labor pains is discussed in Chapters 4 and 8.

CESAREAN SECTION

There is concern among obstetricians that conduction anesthesia for cesarean section in a preeclamptic patient may lead to profound hypotension. The following precautions must be taken to minimize the incidence of this complication: the cardiac filling pressure must be optimized (the use of CVP or pulmonary artery pressure measurement is recommended); epidural anesthesia must be induced slowly by injecting the local anesthetic into the epidural space in increments through an epidural catheter; single shot technique must not be used because it entails injecting a large volume of anesthetic into the epidural space (which may result in precipitous hypotension); left uterine displacement must always be used; spinal anesthesia must be used with great caution (or not al all) because of the possibility of sudden hypotension. Ephedrine in 5 mg increments must be used for treating hypotension. Preeclamptic patients may complain of lightheadedness even with a seemingly innocuous reduction in their blood pressure. A 5 mg dose of ephedrine will usually correct the symptom. The need to monitor the arterial pressure continuously cannot be overemphasized. The greatest advantage of epidural anesthesia in preeclamptics is perhaps that it obviates the need for general anesthesia, which may often be hazardous.

General anesthesia may however be needed if the patient has coagulopathy, or for an emergency intervention for fetal distress. The blood pressure must be stabilized at 140/90 with hydralazine, sodium nitroprusside, or nitroglycerin. This is is absolutely essential to avoid hypertensive responses to intubation.[31,43] Induction is usually done with pentothal (3 to 4 mg/kg) and the trachea is rapidly intubated under succinylcholine induced muscle paralysis. The nondepolarizers are potentiated approximately 20 times more than the depolarizers are. Patients who are on Mg^{++} do not fasciculate with succinylcholine and therefore the usual defasciculating dose of a nondepolarizing relaxant can be omitted in these patients during induction of general anesthesia.[44]

Great caution must be exercised in using nondepolarizing relaxants when the patient is receiving Mg^{++}. A nerve stimulator must be used to monitor the response to the "train-of-four" (T4) stimuli. Inhibition of the first twitch by 95 to 75% is believed to be associated with optimum muscle relaxation in nonpregnant subjects. In pregnant subjects, acceptable relaxation of the abdominal musculature may be obtained at 75% twitch inhibition because abdominal musculature is stretched by the gravid uterus. The third and fourth responses usually disappear at 80% inhibition of the first twitch. At 90% inhi-

bition of the first twitch, the second response is no longer present.[45] Therefore, when a nondepolarizing relaxant is being used, the initial and the maintenance doses of the agent are adjusted so that at least the first two twitches are preserved. Long-acting relaxants are added only after making sure that the residual effects of succinylcholine are worn off. A continuous infusion of succinylcholine may also be used for maintenance of muscle relaxation. The T4 responses must be carefully assessed at the end of the case to detect the presence of fade, which is indicative of a phase-II block caused by excessive succinylcholine administration.

The maintenance of anesthesia is done with an N_2O-oxygen mixture, supplemented with liberal doses of a narcotic or 0.5% halothane, 1.0% enflurane, or 0.75% isoflurane. If, however, severe hepatic dysfunction is suspected, halothane must be used with caution. Ergot preparations must be avoided because they can cause hypertension. Residual effects of the muscle relaxant must be reversed and the patient's trachea must be extubated after ensuring that all the usual extubation criteria are satisfied. If adequate neuromuscular reversal cannot be obtained, the patient must be transferred to the intensive care unit. Artificial ventilation must be provided until she is able to breath adequately. Mg^{++} is excreted by the kidneys and therefore urinary output must be maintained to facilitate rapid elimination of this ion. Contrary to earlier reports, the maternal use of Mg^{++} is not associated with any neonatal problems, provided that the maternal Mg^{++} levels are maintained at a therapeutic range.[46] Even in the presence of severe thrombocytopenia, spontaneous antepartum bleeding is rare.

Correction of coagulation anomaly is not necessary before delivery, unless the platelet count is $<50,000/mm^3$ and there are signs of active bleeding from the skin puncture sites. Under these circumstances measurements of bleeding time may be useful. Fibrinogen replacement with cryoprecipitate is usually not necessary because the fibrinogen levels generally exceed 100 mg/dL.[47] Only very rarely is the DIC associated with preeclampsia also associated with significant intraoperative bleeding. Should this occur, appropriate blood-products must be used to correct the DIC. The nadir platelet count occurs in the first postpartum day and spontaneous resolution of the platelet count occurs within 72 hours.[47] When inserting a Swan-Ganz catheter via the internal jugular vein in a patient with coagulopathy, special care must be taken to avoid accidental perforation of the carotid artery. This may lead to a severe neck hematoma. In such cases, the antecubital or the femoral vein may offer a safer route of insertion.

General anesthesia is hazardous for a number of reasons. Mg^{++} therapy potentiates the action of the neuromuscular agents, and intubation may be difficult because of the possible presence of airway edema. The danger of aspiration of gastric contents always exists, and tracheal intubation, performed under light planes of anesthesia, elicits a severe hypertensive response.

POSTOPERATIVE CARE

Many patients will remain hypertensive in the postpartum period. Therefore, the continued use of antihypertensive therapy is necessary. Magnesium infusion should also be continued. Pulmonary edema may occur in the postpartum period often because of overzealous fluid therapy in the prepartum period[7] and because of the normally occurring mobilization of fluid into the intravascular compartment in postpartum patients.[48] Patients with indwelling monitoring lines must be cared for in an intensive care unit. Occasionally, prolonged postoperative ventilation may be needed for respiratory inadequacy caused by Mg^{++} muscle relaxant interaction. Fluid balance, acid-base status, arterial oxygenation, renal function, and coagulation parameters must be carefully evaluated in the first week. Preeclampsia is not cured (as it is often thought) immediately after the delivery of the baby. Patients may remain severely hypertensive during the first postpartum week.

The leading causes of maternal mortality in preeclamptic patients include convulsions, which lead to hypoxia or aspiration of gastric contents; cerebrovascular accidents caused by uncontrolled hypertension; and cardiac failure. These complications may also develop in the postpartyum period.

CHRONIC HYPERTENSION

All chronic hypertensive disorders regardless of their etiology predispose to superimposed preeclampsia. Coincidental (gestational) hypertension is diagnosed when the history of antecedent hypertension in a previous pregnancy (140/90 or greater) is present; and when hypertension develops before the 20th week of pregnancy (except in cases of molar pregnancy). Pregnancy can cause acceleration of hypertension even in the absence of superimposed preeclampsia. Women with preexisting essential hypertension are prone to develop abruptio placentae. Retardation of intrauterine fetal growth may occur with increased frequency. Treatment with α-methyl dopa is said to minimize the development of preeclampsia. With the development of superimposed preeclampsia, maternal and fetal morbidity increases considerably.[3] The management depends on the degree of hypertension. Patients with severe hypertension (pregnancy-aggravated hypertension) or those who have superimposed preeclampsia should be managed as if they have preeclampsia. Patients with only mild elevations may not require more than routine precautions.

In some women, hypertension develops without proteinuria in the last trimester, but the blood pressure returns to normal by the 10th postpartum day. The outcome for the mother and the fetus is usually good. The condition is called late or transient hypertension and the patients who develop this condition are prone to develop essential hypertension in later life.

REFERENCES

1. Lindheimer MD, and Katz AI: Current Concepts: Hypertension in pregnancy. N Engl J Med *313*:11, 1985.
2. Chealey LC: Diagnosis of Preeclampsia. Obstet Gynecol 65:423, 1985.
3. Pritchard JA, McDonald PC, and Gant NF: Hypertensive disorders in pregnancy. *In* Williams Obstetrics. 17th Edition. Norwalk, Appleton-Century-Crofts, 1985.
4. Newsome LR, Bramwell RS, and Curling PE: Severe preeclampsia: hemodynamic effects of lumbar epidural anesthesia. Anesth Analg 65:31, 1986.
5. Berkowitz RL: The Swan-Ganz catheter and colloid-osmotic pressure determinations. *In* Critical Care of the Obstetric Patient. (Edited by Berkowtiz RL). New York, Churchill Livingstone, 1983.
6. Phelan JP, and Yurth DA: Severe preeclampsia: Peripartum hemodynamic observations. Am J Obstet Gynecol *144*:17, 1982.
7. Benedetti TJ, Kates R, and Williams V: Hemodynamic

observations in severe preeclampsia complicated by pulmonary edema. Am J Obstet Gynecol *152*:330, 1985.

8. Gant NF, Chand S, Whalley PJ, and MacDonald PC: The nature of pressor responsiveness to angiotensin II in human pregnancy. Obstet Gynecol *43*:854, 1974.

9. Spinapolice RX, Feld S, and Harrigan JT: Effective prevention of gestational hypertension in nulliparous women at high risk as identified by the rollover test. Am J Obstet Gynecol *146*:166, 1983.

10. Lee MI, and Todd HM: Plasma catecholamines and angiotensin-converting enzyme activity in hypertensive subjects with positive rollover tests. Obstet Gynecol *63*:511, 1984.

11. MacGillivray I: Pre-Eclampsia: The Hypertensive Disease of Pregnancy. Philadelphia, WB Saunders, 1983.

12. Sibai BM, et al.: Pregnancy outcome in 303 cases with severe preeclampsia. Obstet Gynecol *64*:319, 1984.

13. Weiner CP, and Brandt J: Plasma antithrombin III activity: An aid in the diagnosis of preeclampsia. Am J Obstet Gynecol *142*:275, 1982.

14. Berkowitz RL: The management of hypertensive disease in pregnancy. Critical Care of the Obstetric Patient. (Edited by Berkowitz RL). New York, Churchill-Livingstone, 1983.

15. Redman CWG, Beilin LJ, and Bonnar J: Treatment of hypertension in pregnancy with methyldopa: blood pressure controls and side-effects. Br J Obstet Gynecol *84*:419, 1977.

16. Barron WM, and Lindheimer MD: Renal sodium and water handling in pregnancy. Obstet Gynecol Annu *13*:35, 1984.

17. Dennis EJ, and Hester LL: The preeclampsia-eclampsia syndrome. *In* Obstetrics and Gynecology. 4th Edition. (Edited by Danforth DN). New York, Harper and Row, 1982.

18. Brosens IA, Robertson WB, and Dixon SG: The role of the spiral arteries in the pathogenesis of preeclampsia. Obstet Gynecol Annu *1*:177, 1972.

19. Ruvinsky ED, et al.: Maternal administration of dexamethasone in severe pregnancy induced hypertension. Am J Obstet Gynecol *149*:722, 1984.

20. Pritchard JA, McDonald PC, and Gant NF: Preterm and post-term pregnancies and fetal growth retardation. *In* Williams Obstetrics. 17th Edition. Norwalk, Appleton-Century-Crofts, 1985.

21. Borges LF, and Gucer G: Effect of magnesium on epileptic foci. Epilepsia *19*:81–91, 1978.

22. Altura BM, Altura BT, and Carella A: Magnesium deficiency-induced spasms of umbilical vessels: Relation to preeclampsia, hypertension, growth retardation. Science *221*:376, 1983.

23. Sibai BM, Graham JM, and McCubbin JH: A comparison of intravenous and intramuscular magnesium sulfate regimens in preeclampsia. Am J Obstet Gynecol *150*:728, 1984.

24. Sanders R, and Hayashi R: Intravenous versus intramuscular magnesium sulfate for preeclampsia. Society for gynecologic investigation, 30th annual meeting, Washington DC, March 17–20, 1983, (Abstract No. 25).

25. Pritchard JA: The use of magnesium sulfate in preeclampsia-eclampsia. J Reprod Med *23*:107, 1979.

26. Naden RP, and Redman CWG: Antihypertensive drugs in pregnancy. Clin Perinatol *12*:521, 1985.

27. Naulty J, Cefalo RC, and Lewis PE: Fetal toxicity of nitroprusside in the pregnant ewe. Am J Obstet Gynecol *139*:708, 1981.

28. Stempel JE, O'Grady JP, Morton MJ, and Johnson KA: Use of sodium nitroprusside in complications of gestational hypertension. Obstet Gynecol *60*:533, 1982.

29. Rigg D, and McDonogh A: Use of sodium nitroprusside for deliberate hypotension during pregnancy. Br J Anaesth *53*:985, 1981.

30. Wheeler AS, et al.: Effects of nitroglycerin and nitroprusside on the uterine vasculature of gravid ewes. Anesthesiology *52*:390, 1980.

31. Hood DD, et al.: The use of nitroglycerin in preventing the hypertensive response to tracheal intubation in severe preeclampsia. Anesthesiology *63*:329, 1985.

32. Studer RK, Morgan J, Penkoske M, and Potchen EJ: Regional vascular volume and extravascular accumulation of labeled protein during plasma volume expansion. Am J Physiol *224*:699, 1973.

33. Shirley HH, Jr, Wolfram CG, Wasserman K, and Mayerson HS: Capillary permeability to macromolecules: stretched pore phenomenon. Am J Physiol *190*:189, 1957.

34. Friedman JJ: Transcapillary protein leakage and fluid movement effect of venous pressure. Microvasc Res *12*:275, 1976.

35. Granger DN, Gabel JC, Drake RE, and Taylor AE: Physiologic basis for the clinical use of albumin solutions. Surg Gynecol Obstet *146*:97, 1978.

36. Ramanathan S, et al.: Maternal and fetal effects of prophylactic hydration with crystalloids or colloids before epidural anesthesia. Anesth Analg *62*:673, 1983.

37. Rafferty TD, Keefer JR, and Barash PG: Fluid management in the massively bleeding obstetric patient. *In* Critical Care of the Obstetric Patient. (Edited by Berkowitz RL). New York, Churchill Livingstone, 1983.

38. Cotton DB, et al.: III: Role of intravenous nitroglycerin in the treatment of severe pregnancy-induced hypertension complicated by pulmonary edema. Am J Obstet Gynecol *154*:91, 1986.

39. Moir DD, Victor-Rodriguez L, and Willocks J: Epidural analgesia during labor in patients with pre-eclampsia. J Obstet Gynaecol Br Commonwealth *79*:465, 1972.

40. Joupilla P, Joupilla R, Hollemen A, and Koivula A: Lumbar epidural analgesia to improve intervillous blood flow during labor in severe preeclampsia. Obstet Gynecol *59*:158, 1982.

41. Joupilla R, Joupilla P, Hollemen A, and Koivula A: Epidural analgesia and placental blood flow during labour in pregnancies complicated by hypertension. Br J Obstet Gynaecol *86*:969, 1979.

42. Ramanathan J, et al.: The pharmacokinetics and maternal and neonatal effects of epidural lidocaine in preeclampsia. Anesth Analg *65*:120, 1986.

43. Hodgkinson R, Husain FJ, and Hayashi RH: Systemic and pulmonary blood pressure during caesarean section in parturients with gestational hypertension. Can Anaesth Soc J *27*:389, 1980.

44. DeVore JS, and Asrani R: Magnesium sulfate prevents

succinylcholine-induced fasciculations in toxemic parturients. Anesthesiology *52*:76, 1980.

45. Ali HH: Monitoring of neuromuscular function. *In* Muscle Relaxants. New York, Grune & Stratton, 1985.

46. Green KW, Key TC, Coen R, and Resnik R: The effects of maternally administered magnesium sulfate on the neonate. Am J Obstet Gynecol *146*:29, 1983.

47. Romero R: The management of acquired hemostatic failure during pregnancy. *In* Critical Care of the Obstetric Patient. (Edited by Berkowitz RL). New York, Churchill Livingstone, 1983.

48. Zinaman M, Rubin J, and Lindheimer MD: Serial plasma oncotic pressure levels and echoencephalography during and after delivery in severe pre-eclampsia. Lancet *1*:1245, 1985.

49. Rafferty TD, and Berkowitz RL: Hemodynamics in patients with severe toxemia during labor and delivery. Am J Obstet Gynecol *138*:263, 1980.

50. Hays PM, Cruikshank DP, and Dunn LJ: Plasma volume determination in normal and preeclamptic pregnancies. Am J Obstet Gynecol *151*:958, 1985.

COAGULATION AND HEMOGLOBIN DISORDERS

Although pregnancy is normally associated with augmented coagulation, many severe coagulopathies may occur during pregnancy. Many types of coagulopathies that may preexist in the patient can affect the course of the pregnancy, and conversely, the pregnancy may affect the nature of the coagulopathy. For a thorough understanding of the nature of these coagulopathies, a knowledge of pregnancy-induced changes in coagulation is essential. These changes are discussed in the chapters on thromboembolism and maternal adaptation to pregnancy (Chapters 16 and 2, respectively). Table 11–1 lists the important coagulopathies in pregnancy. Table 11–2 lists the most recent terminology for factors involved in blood clotting.

DISSEMINATED INTRAVASCULAR COAGULATION

Pregnant women are at an increased risk for developing disseminated intravascular coagulation (DIC). For instance, a fulminant DIC may develop during amniotic fluid embolism. The DIC deposits insoluble fibrin in the blood vessels. The formation of fibrin from fibrinogen requires the enzyme thrombin, factor XIII, and Ca^{++}. Soluble intermediates are formed when fibrinogen is converted to fibrin (Fig. 11–1).[1]

Also incorporated into the final clot are fibrinonectin, which is a protein released by the platelet, and α_2 antiplasmin. The fibrinonectin increases surface adhesion of the cells and the antiplasmin increases the resistance of the clot to lysis by plasmin (Fig. 11–1).

It has long been known that the injection of tissue extract into the blood stream of an animal, renders its blood incoagulable. The concentrations of fibrinogen and other coagulation factors decrease and so does the platelet count because they are consumed in blood clots. When the tissue extract is injected slowly, there may be incomplete polymerization of fibrin, resulting in the formation of soluble polymers. Soluble complexes may be formed between the fibrin monomer and fibrinogen, or between the fibrin monomer with fibrin degradation products.[1]

The blood clots are cleared from the small vessels by the plasma fibrinolytic activity, which increases in an attempt to clear the fibrin clots from the blood vessels. Fibrin degradation products (FDP) are thus formed, and they are believed to be responsible for the inhibition of thrombin action in patients with DIC. The immunologic methods used in the detection of FDP also detect soluble fibrin complexes.[1] The term fibrinogen-fibrin related antigens (FRA) is more descriptive of the nature of the FDA. The

Table 11–1. Coagulation Disorders

Type	Disorder
Associated with possible DIC	Abruptio placentae. Dead fetus syndrome. Amniotic fluid embolism. Maternal sepsis. Preeclampsia. Postpartum hemolytic uremic syndrome. Massive transfusion.
Inherited clotting factor deficiency	von Willebrand's disease. Hemophilia A and C. Deficiencies factors I, II, V, VII, VIII, IX, X, XI, XII, XIII. Contact factors deficiency. Antithrombin III deficiency. α_2 antiplasmin deficiency.
Disorders of platelet function	Immune thrombocytopenia. Thrombotic thrombocytopenic purpura.
Obstetric hemorrhage without DIC	Placenta previa. Abnormally adherent placenta (percreta, accreta, and increta).

reticuloendothelial system is also responsible for clearing fibrin related debris from the circulation, thus preventing further deposition. The opsonic protein present in cryoprecipitate is said to enhance the activity of the reticulendothelial system, thus preventing renal complications of DIC.[2]

The DIC process may occur with or without a decrease in fibrinogen level. Hemorrhagic diathesis does not usually occur until the fibrinogen level decreases below 100 mg/dL.[1] A fulminant DIC may develop with amniotic fluid embolism or with abruptio placentae, leading to hemorrhage from exposed wounds and venepuncture sites. When DIC lasts longer, ecchymoses may appear and the patient may bleed into the body cavities.[1] Microthrombi may result in ischemic organ damage. The DIC may occur without hypofibrinogenemia. Under those circumstances, the presence of FRA and fibrinopeptide A or the microangiopathic changes in the RBC will give a clue to the presence of the condition. Fibrinopeptide A is split from fibrinogen by the action of thrombin (Fig. 11–1).

Table 11–2. Blood Clotting Factors

I	Fibrinogen
I′	Fibrin monomer
I″	Fibrin polymer
II	Prothrombin
III	Tissue thromboplastin
IV	Calcium++
V	Labile factor
VII	Proconvertin
VIII	Antihemophilic globulin
IX	Christmas factor
X	Stuart factor
XI	Plasma thromboplastin antecedent
XII	Hageman factor
XIII	Fibrin stabilizing factor
HMW-K	Kininogens (Fitzgerald factor)
Pre-K	PreKallikrein (Fletcher factor)
Ka	Kallikrein
PL	Platelet phospholipid

Reproduced with permission from Krupp MA, Schroeder SA, Tierney LM, Jr (editors).: Current Medical Diagnosis and Treatment 1987. Copyright 1987 by Appleton and Lange. (Norwalk, Connecticut/Los Altos, California).

FIBRINOLYTIC BLEEDING SYNDROMES

The fibrinolysis can be primary or secondary. Primary fibrinolysis occurs without any other coagulation abnormality, whereas secondary fibrinolysis occurs in response to DIC. Plasmin is the protease, which causes fibrinolysis. It is formed from a precursor called the plasminogen. There are several activators of plasminogen, which include urokinase, blood vessel endothelium, and substances present in the myocardium and uterus.[3] These are called extrinsic activators because they are not present in the blood. The intrinsic activators present in the blood are dependent on factor XII, prekallikrein, and high molecular weight kininogens.[3]

Plasmin is not specific for fibrin. It can hydrolyze many plasma proteins including prothrombin and factors V and VIII. The plasmin itself is held in check by α_2-antiplasmin, α_2-an-

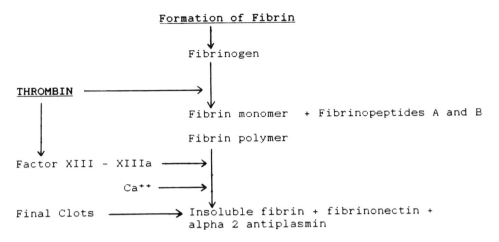

FIG. 11–1. Formation of fibrin from fibrinogen. The final fibrin clot incorporates both fibronectin, which causes further aggregation of platelets, and α_2 antiplasmin, which makes the clot more resistant to fibrinolysis.

titrypsin, and α_2 macroglobulin.[4] The most important inhibitor is the α_2 antiplasmin. The levels of this protein are reduced in patients with DIC. Free plasmin is never present in circulating blood but may appear suddenly when fulminant DIC develops because of amniotic fluid embolism. The presence of fibrinolytic activity may be detected by whole blood clot lysis time (Table 11–3). The euglobulin clot lysis time is measured using the euglobulin fraction of the plasma, which is nothing but an isoelectrically precipitated fraction of the plasma proteins containing plasminogen, fibrinogen, and plasminogen activators. Plasminogen inhibitors are left behind in the euglobulin supernatant. Normal lysis time is 150 minutes, and in severe fibrinolysis, it is less than 30 minutes. Neither clot lysis time or the euglobulin clot lysis time will be able to pinpoint whether the fibrinolysis is caused by the increased presence of activators or to the presence of plasmin. A fibrin-plate as-

say, which uses two types of fibrin is used for this purpose. Lysis of plasminogen-free fibrin indicates the presence of plasmin, whereas lysis of plasminogen-containing fibrin shows the presence of activators. Whole blood clot lysis time may be done without the aid of any elaborate laboratory facility. Euglobulin lysis time and fibrin plate assay are simple enough to be used in routine clinical laboratories. The routinely used tests such as partial thromboplastin time (PTT), thrombin time (TT), and prothrombin time (PT) are moderately prolonged in primary fibrinolysis because of depletion of fibrinogen and/or the effects of FDP on thrombin action. Their prolongation therefore does not exclude the diagnosis of fibrinolysis. If, however, these tests are within normal limits or show only minimum abnormality in a patient with severe hemorrhage, primary fibrinolysis is the likely diagnosis.

Plasmin digests both fibrinogen and fibrin. Lysis of fibrin is harmless but lysis of fibrinogen causes severe hemorrhage. The fibrin monomer is formed by the action of the thrombin on fibrinogen and not by plasmin function. Too much reliance has been placed in the past on the measurement of FDP for the diagnosis of fibrinolysis. Latex particles coated with antibodies to fibrinogen and fibrinogen fragments D and E are used. The test is not specific and may detect fibrin monomer and fibrin monomer-fibrinogen complex. Thus, the detection of FRA does not distinguish between the lysis of fibrin and the lysis of fibrinogen. However, failure to dem-

Table 11–3. Signs and Symptoms of Placental Abruption

Disorder	Percentage
Vaginal bleeding	78
Fetal distress	60
Repeated contractions	17
Hypertonus	17
Idiopathic premature labor	22
Dead fetus	15

(From Hurd, WW: Midovnik M, Hertzberg V, and Lavin JP: Selective management of abruptio placentae: A prospective study 61:467, 1983.)

onstrate any ERA or FDP virtually excludes the possibility of fibrinolysis or fibrinogenolysis. The detection of α_2 antiplasmin/plasmin complex by two dimensional immunoelectrophoresis may circumvent some of the problems.[2] Measurement of plasma plasminogen levels is now possible. Plasminogen levels are reduced in any active fibrinolytic state where plasminogen is being converted to plasmin. The most conclusive proof for the presence of primary fibrinolysis is little or no depletion of clotting factors.

The primary fibrinolytic bleeding syndromes are rare. They may be congenital or acquired. The congenital conditions include α_2 antiplasmin deficiency and excessive presence of plasminogen activator. Acquired conditions include thrombolytic therapy (see Chapter 16 Thromboembolism). Of the disease states producing fibrinolysis, systemic lupus erythematosus is of particular interest because the disease primarily occurs in young women. Primary fibrinolysis may be treated (after establishing the diagnosis) by administration of inhibitors of fibrinolysis. Epsilon aminocaproic acid (EACA) will inhibit the activation of plasminogen completely and at higher doses will inhibit plasmin as well. The loading dose is 3 g followed by 3 g every six hours. Tranexamic acid is more potent than is EACA.[3] The use of these agents is not indicated if whole blood clotting time and euglobulin lysis time are within normal range. Their use is definitely contraindicated in fibrinolysis associated with DIC because of the risk of the formation of widespread microvascular thrombin.[2] The secondary fibrinolysis associated with DIC, although beneficial in removing microvascular thrombi, may cause hemorrhage by digesting fibrinogen and factors V and VII.[1,3]

PREGNANCY CONDITIONS ASSOCIATED WITH DIC

Abruptio Placentae

Abruptio placentae is the premature separation of the normally situated placenta (Fig. 11–2) and is associated with 15 to 25% of all perinatal deaths.[5] Even in neonates who survive the abruption, the incidence of neurologic abnormality may be evident in the first year of life. However, when properly managed, the perinatal mortality remains low. Regardless of the severity of the abruption, some changes in coagulation can always be demonstrated.[1] The condition occurs more frequently in multiparous women. Placental abruption starts with hemorrhage into the decidua basalis. The resulting hematoma slowly enlarges and causes more separation.[6] The rupture of a decidual spiral artery may cause severe bleeding into the decidual bed. The myometrium starts contracting to control local hemorrhage (physiologic ligature), thus explaining the onset of premature labor and the increased resting tension of the uterus. The lack of visible vaginal hemorrhage does not exclude the diagnosis of placental abruption because the hemorrhage may be concealed by the presenting part. Negative sonography does not rule out life-threatening abruption.[7] Retroplacental hematoma is detectable in only 1 out of 59 cases. The signs and symptoms of abruption are summarized in Table 11–3. Vaginal bleeding, tender rigid uterus, and premature labor are common symptoms.[7] There is a 10% recurrence rate in subsequent pregnancies, and therefore, a previous history of abruption makes it necessary to assign the present pregnancy to the high risk category.[8]

The major problems that the anesthesiologist encounters are related to hemorrhagic hypovolemia of the mother, maternal coagulopathy, and poor fetal condition. The hemorrhagic shock may be caused by severe intrauterine and/or vaginal hemorrhage. Local hemorrhage occurring into the myometrium and uterine serosal surface gives the uterus an appearance of cherry fruit. This condition, which is called uteroplacental apoplexy or couvelaire uterus, is associated with shock and fetal death if not promptly treated. Occasionally, fetal to maternal transfusion may happen, which further jeopardizes the fetus.[6]

The DIC results from the release of tissue thromboplastin from the decidual bed into the maternal systemic circulation. The most common cause of hypofibrinogenemia (<150 mg/dL) in pregnancy is placental abruption. The DIC elicits the fibrinolytic response with the result that the serum fibrin-degradation products (FDP) increase. When hypovolemia is not corrected without delay, acute renal failure may ensue because of cortical necrosis or acute tubular necrosis. Postpartum pituitary necrosis, adult respiratory distress syndrome, and overt

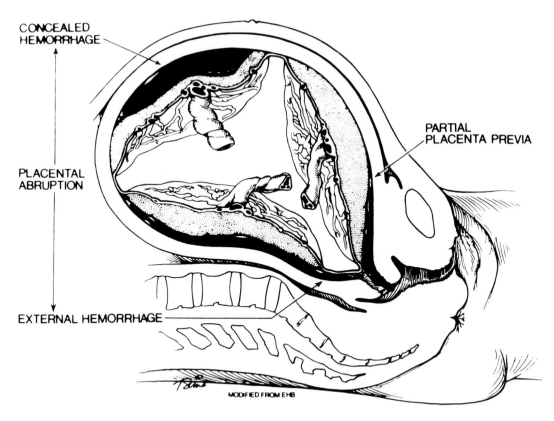

CONCEALED
HEMORRHAGE

PARTIAL
PLACENTA PREVIA

PLACENTAL
ABRUPTION

EXTERNAL HEMORRHAGE

MODIFIED FROM E H B

FIG. 11–2. Placental abruption and placenta previa. Extensive abruption (Top, left) with peripheral placenta still attached to the decidua and with no hemorrhage (also considered to be a "concealed hemorrhage"); placental abruption with external hemorrhage (Bottom, left); and partial placenta previa with abruption and external hemorrhage (Top, right). (From Pritchard JA, McDonald PC, and Gant NF: Obstetric Hemorrhage. *In* Williams Obstetrics. 17th Ed. Norwalk, Appleton-Century-Crofts, 1985.)

hemorrhagic diathesis can also occur.[5] The need for prompt treatment of hypovolemia cannot be overemphasized. Emergency cesarean section is needed if the fetus is in distress. If the fetus is already dead, vaginal delivery is usually preferred. If the fetus does not show signs of distress, a vaginal delivery may be planned.

Assessment of Coagulation

The coagulation status must be assessed at the earliest opportunity. Platelet count, plasma fibrinogen concentration, prothrombin time (PT), plasma thromboplastin time (PTT/APTT), clotting time, and serum FRA must be measured.[8] Within hours of the onset of symptoms, the fibrinogen concentration may decrease to 40 mg/dL or less. Table 11–3 lists useful laboratory and bedside tests for clotting function. A bedside clotting test may be performed by observing the

patient's blood clot in a test tube. Failure to form an adequate clot within 5 to 12 minutes is diagnostic of clotting abnormality. A clot lysis test may be performed by adding patient's plasma to the donor's clot. The lysis of donor clot is usually suggestive of the presence of fibrinolytic activity. Although these tests are crude, they are useful because the results are immediately available.

A severe case of placental abruption requires immediate skillful treatment. An indwelling arterial cannula, a central venous cannula, and two large bore peripheral cannulae must be inserted at once. The immediate goals are to restore circulating fluid volume with crystalloid and/or crystalloid infusion. As soon as blood becomes available, it must be administered to raise the maternal hemoglobin concentration. Severe maternal anemia will hamper fetal oxygenation. If bedside coagulation tests show defective clotting, appropriate component therapy must be instituted. Blood components (Table 11–4) must be requested from the blood bank immediately. Because fibrinogen deficiency frequently develops in the abruption syndrome, cryoprecipitate administration must be considered. Cryoprecipitate also contains the opsonic protein fibronectin, which stimulates the blood and tissue macrophages to clear debris from the blood and tissues, thus minimizing the possibility of renal failure in the postpartum period.[2] Another useful component is fresh frozen plasma, which corrects deficiency of all clotting factors. Platelet transfusions may be necessary to correct low counts (<50,000 to 75,000/mm³). All clotting components must be subgrouped for Rh in women of child-bearing age.[8]

Regional anesthesia may be hazardous in these patients because overt coagulopathy may be present, and considerable hypovolemia may be present at the time of evaluation. Therefore in all but the mildest cases with normal coagulation, regional anesthesia is better avoided. In severely hypovolemic patients, ketamine induction (1 mg/kg) may be considered. The use of pentothal may lead to further deterioration of maternal systemic pressure, consequently affecting the already stressed fetus. The use of ketamine, however, may not be considered a substitute for adequate volume replacement. When severe hypovolemia is present, ketamine may diminish tissue perfusion, and thus may increase blood lactate levels.[9] Therefore, the baby must be delivered as early as possible after the induction of anesthesia. A narcotic may be administered for maintenance of anesthesia. The

Table 11–4. Coagulation Screening in DIC Syndrome

Bedside tests	Results	Lab tests	Results
Thrombin: 0.1 ml thrombin + 23 ml blood.	If solid clot forms immediately, then fibrinogen >150 mg%. If a jelly-like clot forms fibrinogen is 100–150 mg%. If no clot forms, fibrinogen <50 mg%.	Platelet count.	Normal range is 150,000 to 300,000/mm³.
Clotting time: Put some blood in a red-top tube.	If it clots in <6 min., blood fibrinogen 150 mg%.	Ivy bleeding time.	Normal is <6 minutes.
Clot lysis: Patient's plasma plus donor clot.	Lysis suggests fibrinolysis.	Activated partial thromboplastin time (APTT). Requires Kaolin for surface activity.	>5 seconds prolongation is abnormal. Checks the intrinsic pathway.
		Thrombin time: Excess thrombin plus plasma.	Excess thrombin plus plasma >5 sec. prolongation is abnormal.
		Fibrin degradation products: (Fibrin/fibrinogen related antigen).	Tested by immunologic technique (clumping of latex particles coated with antibody to fibrin fragments D and E or by staphylococcal clumping.
		Fibrinogen.	<300 mg% abnormal. (Remember that in pregnancy the fibrinogen concentration is elevated).
		Clot stability test.	Ability of the clot to withstand 5M urea solution of 1% monochloracetic acid.
		Euglobin lysis time.	Ability of the euglobulin precipitate of the plasma to lyse a clot. (The precipitate is devoid of inhibitors of fibrinolysis).
		Whole blood clot lysis time.	A normal clot does not lyse within 8 hours.
		Prothrombin time.	Tests the integrity of extrinsic pathway prolongation >2 sec. abnormal.

use of an inhalation agent is not recommended because a significant number of patients with placental abruption are prone to spontaneous postpartum hemorrhage. Inhalation agents will only worsen the condition. In the postoperative period, the patient must be closely watched for the development of additional clotting abnormalities, renal failure, or adult respiratory distress syndrome.

Dead Fetus Syndrome

Retention of a dead fetus may lead to DIC and hypofibrinogenemia.[3,5,8,10,11] The potential ability of heparin to correct DIC was first discovered when the agent was used for correcting DIC associated with dead fetus syndrome. The syndrome is relatively rare nowadays as fetal demise can be diagnosed accurately with ultrasound and more reliable pharmacologic agents are available to induce labor at any stage of gestation. The longer the dead fetus is retained in utero, the higher is the risk of developing a coagulopathy. When the retention is longer than 5 weeks, one-third of the patients will have hypofibrinogenemia (<150 mg%).[11]

The release of placental thromboplastin into the maternal circulation, activates the extrinsic pathway of coagulation. The fibrinolytic system is activated secondarily, leading to increased bleeding tendency. Excessive fibrinolysis is implicated in the etiology of coagulopathy because hemorrhagic diathesis is known to persist even after correction of hypofibrinogenemia. Dead fetus syndrome may develop in twin gestation after one of the fetuses dies in utero while the other continues to live.

The coagulation system must be evaluated in every woman with a dead fetus because often the only sign of DIC may be a severe postpartum hemorrhage (Table 11–4). If the abnormality includes only elevated FDP with no abnormality either in the platelet count or in the fibrinogen level, the risk of hemorrhage is small. If the platelet count and the fibrinogen level are also low, they must be corrected, especially when the patient is already in labor. For appropriate component therapy see Table 11–5. If the patient is not in labor, heparin therapy may be considered to slow the DIC process. Heparin may be particularly useful in case of twin gestation when one of the fetuses has died in utero and the other one is too small to be delivered.[10] If the twin gestation is monozygotic, placental mingling of the two fetal circulations may occur, leading to coagulopathy in the surviving fetus. When heparin is administered for this purpose, the PTT is usually maintained at 2.5 times the

Table 11–5.   Common Blood Components

Product	Uses	Remarks
Stored blood	Volume replacement.	Lacks factors V, VIII, platelets; may result in dilutional coagulopathy; 2-3 DPG decreased.
Fresh blood	Useful in coagulopathy, must be used within 24 hrs after collection.	Hepatitis screening, AIDS screening may be incomplete.
Fresh frozen plasma	200–250 ml bags, contains all clotting factors, used in factor XI deficiency, coumarin overdose.	Each bag is derived from one unit of blood. Hepatitis risk, ABO-RH cross matching needed.
Cryoprecipitate	One unit = 15–25 ml, prepared by thawing FFP at 1–6°C.	10 units will increase fibrinogen 50 mg/dL; increased fibronectin content, improved renal function.
	Used for fibrinogen, and factors VIII, XI deficiencies and for von Willebrand's disease.	
Platelets	Thrombocytopenia DIC, platelet dysfunction. Prolonged bleeding time.	One unit will increase the count by 5000–10,000/M² body surface.
Factor IX complex	Contains factors II, VII, IX, X. Reconstituted before use. Used when large FFP volumes are harmful.	Significant hepatitis risk, increased thrombosis.

FFP = fresh frozen plasma. Note that fibrinogen concentrate is no longer recommended for correcting fibrinogen deficiency.

control. Heparin administration may cause the fibrinogen concentration and platelet count to rise.[11] The goals of heparin therapy is to achieve a fibrinogen level of at least 200 mg/dL and a platelet count of at least 60,000/mm.[3]

The services of the anesthesiologist may be required for administration of labor analgesia, anesthesia for vaginal or abdominal delivery of the dead fetus, or for the evacuation of the placenta. Regional anesthesia is contraindicated in the presence of coagulopathy. A complete screening of the coagulation system, including an assessment of the fibrinolytic system must be performed. The anesthesiologist must also be prepared for managing postpartum hemorrhage. The safety of regional anesthesia in patients in whom heparin therapy is discontinued at the onset of labor is discussed in Chapter 16.

Amniotic Fluid Embolism

Amniotic fluid embolism is rare and there is no treatment for the condition.[12–14] In early pregnancy, amniotic fluid is a dialysate of maternal plasma, and as pregnancy advances, it gets diluted by fetal urine. Fetal epithelial squames, lanugo hairs, vernix caseosa, and mucin are present in the amniotic fluid. Amniotic fluid embolism usually presents itself suddenly, with respiratory distress, hypoxia, cyanosis, and systemic hypotension. Up to 86% of all cases are fatal. If the patient survives the initial episode, a coagulopathy and renal failure may be evident in a few hours. Occasionally, the condition may present itself starting with a coagulopathy.[12] The presenting symptoms are summarized in Table 11–6.[12]

Amniotic fluid embolism is also known to occur after intrauterine instillation of saline into the uterus for inducing abortion.[6]

The major effects of amniotic fluid embolism include pulmonary vascular obstruction, (Fig. 11–3) which leads to cor pulmonale, severe hypoxia, and reduced cardiac output. Vasoactive substances (mainly prostaglandin $F_{2\alpha}$) that are present in the amniotic fluid during labor, have been implicated in producing the cardiorespiratory symptoms. The presence of meconium in the amniotic fluid causes a more severe syndrome.[6] The amniotic fluid contains a considerable amount of mucus. The human mucus can activate coagulation factor X.[2] Amniotic fluid near term is more capable of activating factor X than the fluid obtained from pregnancy remote from term.[6] This may be responsible for triggering the widespread DIC. The serum fibrinogen level and platelet count decrease and the fibrin degradation products increase rapidly and an overt bleeding tendency from venepuncture sites may be seen. The uterus may be atonic, leading to severe postpartum hemorrhage. Differential diagnosis includes aspiration pneumonia, pulmonary thromboembolism, and other causes of DIC.

A definitive diagnosis may be made in a desperately ill patient by demonstrating the presence of fetal elements in the maternal pulmonary arterial blood or in the central venous blood aspirated through a central cannula. Fetal squames have also been noted in the sputum. Special staining techniques using antibodies against human keratin are much more effective in identifying fetal elements in the maternal blood.[15] Recently, the presence of fetal elements have been reported to persist in pulmonary artery blood for many hours following the initial episode of embolization.[6]

The treatment mainly consists of supportive measures. Endotracheal intubation and positive pressure ventilation may be required. Invasive monitoring of the systemic and pulmonary arterial pressure may be needed. The pulmonary

Table 11–6.   Clinical Features of Amniotic Fluid Embolism

Symptoms	Disorder	Percentage
Presenting symptoms	Respiratory	51
	Cardiovascular	27
	Convulsions	10
	Hemorrhage	12
Associated features	Disseminated intravascular coagulation	12
	Pulmonary edema	24
	Bronchospasm	1

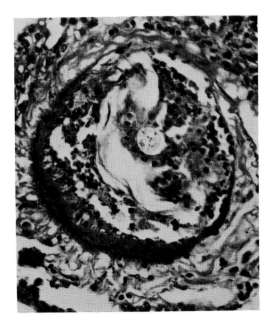
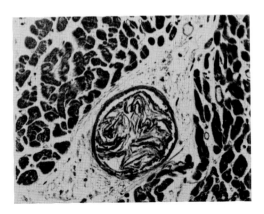

FIG. 11–3.   Fetal squames in the maternal pulmonary artery in a case of amniotic fluid embolism. Left: Note mass of epithelial squames, granular debris, and a lanugo hair (in cross section). Right: Amniotic fluid embolism in the lumen of a myocardial blood vessel. (From Marchesi VT: Disturbances of body water and circulation of blood. *In* Pathology. 7th Ed. (Edited by Anderson WAD and Kissane JM). St. Louis, CV Mosby, 1977.)

artery pressures may be elevated by the obstruction of the pulmonary vascular bed. Dopamine and/or dobutamine infusion may be needed for inotropic support. The DIC must be treated by administration of appropriate blood component therapy (Table 11–5). Postpartum hemorrhage must be treated by appropriate blood replacement. Many other treatment modalities have been suggested, but none with a clear cut advantage. The only hope of survival seems to be related to an unrelenting care by a team of intensive care specialists. Recently, the use of cryoprecipitate has been recommended for the treatment of amniotic fluid embolism. Cryoprecipitate contains significant amounts of opsonic protein which helps the reticuloendothelial system in removing debris from circulation.[15]

Maternal Sepsis

Septic shock in obstetric patients may occur as a result of a complicated abortion or postpartum sepsis, particularly chorioamnionitis. Animal studies have shown that susceptibility to endotoxins increases during pregnancy.[16] Only 5% of septic shock is caused by gram positive bacteria, and the remaining 95% by gram negative bacteria.[17] Escherichia coli (E. Coli) is the offending organism in 50% of these instances. Another 30% is accounted for by the Klebsiella-Enterobacter-Serratia group, the proteus species, and the pseudomonas aeruginosa group. A previously healthy obstetric patient has a favorable prognosis. If, however, she had a debilitating systemic illness such as renal disease or diabetes mellitus, the mortality rate is likely to be very high.

The endotoxins are high molecular weight lipopolysaccharides released from the cell walls of dead bacteria.[17] They cause multiorgan dysfunction, which will ultimately result in death. The major effects of the endotoxins (that are of immediate concern to the anesthesiologist) are DIC and the pulmonary damage leading to adult respiratory syndrome (ARDS)[18] and multiorgan failure. The pathophysiology of septic shock is outlined in Fig. 11–4. The endotoxin damages the pulmonary vascular endothelium. Platelets adhere to the injured vessel wall, resulting in microvascular thrombin. Prostaglandins are released from injured platelets, and the vascular endothelium.[19,20] These substances are potent

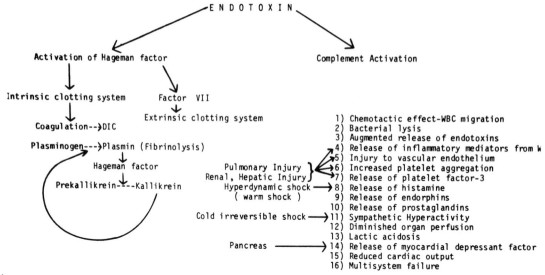

FIG. 11–4. The pathophysiology of septic shock.

pulmonary vasoconstrictors. Cerebral ischemia may also intensify pulmonary vasoconstriction. Complement activation may increase lung damage by causing migration of the WBC into the lung. Proteolytic enzyme elastase has also been implicated in lung injury.[20] Permeability of the pulmonary capillary is increased and the surfactant layer may be disrupted.[21] The increased pulmonary capillary permeability may produce alveolar hyaline membranes.

A myocardial depressant factor has also been identified.[17–20] The concentration of this factor is proportional to the degree of splanchnic ischemia. It causes depression of cardiac output without affecting the heart rate or coronary blood flow. In early phases of septic shock, a hyperdynamic status may be present with increased cardiac output, increasced oxygen consumption, and decreased peripheral resistance (the flushed state). Later in the course of the condition, the enhanced activity of the sympathetic system leads to intense vasoconstriction and diminished tissue perfusion. Pulmonary involvement may produce tachypnea, cyanosis, consolidation, or pulmonary edema. The most common cause of death in septic shock is respiratory failure.

Patients with septic shock must be invasively monitored. Intravascular volume must be adequately restored. Crystalloid solutions or blood (if blood loss has occurred) may be used for this purpose. Dopamine (2 µg/kg/min) may be used

to support circulation. The use of corticosteroids is controversial. If they have to be effective, they must be administered early in the course of the disease. Methyl prednisolone 30 mg/kg is recommended for this purpose.[22] There are several beneficial effects to steroids. They have a positive inotropic action on the heart, and they produce vasodilatation, thereby increasing tissue perfusion. Steroids also depress the myocardial depressant factor released from the pancreas,[21,23] and they inhibit the complement cascade and leukocyte reaction thus preventing cellular autolysis. In addition, they may be helpful in preventing injury to the pulmonary vasculature. Blood component therapy may be required for correcting the coagulopathy (Table 11–5). Appropriate antibiotic therapy must be instituted. Massive doses are usually required. A combination of antibiotics is usually needed. The antibiotics that are commonly used are the following: (1) aqueous penicillin; (2) oxacillin (penicillinase producing staphylococcus), tobramycin (pseudomonas and proteus), clindamycin, and metronidazole.[17] In many patients with septic shock resulting from abortion, suppurative thrombophlebitis develops, which may require heparinization, and ligation of the affected pelvic veins at the earliest opportunity.

Obstetric patients with sepsis may require the services of the anesthesiologist for dilatation and curettage to evacuate the infective material from the uterine cavity; for hysterectomy, if conservative medical treatment fails to improve the septic shock; for a cesearean section if there is evidence of chorioamnionitis; for a cesearean hysterectomy, if a severe endotoxic shock has resulted from sepsis, and for a hysterectomy for a perforated uterus (complication of abortion).[9] Patient's hemodynamic status must be stabilized prior to anesthesia. Invasive monitoring of the systemic and pulmonary arterial pressure must be used. Regional anesthesia is not recommended in these patients because of the possibility of a coagulation abnormality, the presence of severe sepsis, and severe hypovolemia. A high-dose narcotic anesthesia may be suitable for these patients. The use of inhalation agents may be hazardous because the myocardium may have been exposed to the myocardial depressant factor. The use of ketamine may further accentuate the already present lactic acidosis because of its ability to produce peripheral vasconstriction.[9] Postoperative renal failure and ARDS may occur in many patients.

Preeclampsia

Preeclampsia may also produce a coagulopathy including thrombocytopenia, HELLP syndrome, and DIC. The anesthetic considerations in preeclampsia induced coagulopathy is discussed in the chapter on Preeclampsia (Chapter 10). Only recently reported abnormalities in platelet and coagulation functions will be briefly discussed here. Many of the tests of coagulation functions presented here are not generally available for clinical use.

Platelet Studies. The life span of the platelets is shortened. Prostacyclin is a potent vasodilator and thromboxane A_2 is a potent vasoconstrictor. Thromboxane A_2 is released from aggregated platelets. The blood vessels of preeclamptics have been shown to produce less prostacyclin. Thus an imbalance between prostacyclin and thromboxane A_2 is believed to be present in preeclamptic patients. The increased thromboxane A_2 is implicated in the vasoconstriction in preeclamptics.[24]

Coagulation Studies. Thrombin cleaves fibrinopeptides A and B from the fibrinogen molecule (Fig. 11–1). This process is followed by fibrin monomer formation. Fibrin monomers unite with fibrinogen to form a fibrinogen/fibrin complex, which is more soluble. The presence of fibrinopeptide A and the fibrinogen/fibrin complex is detected by immunologic methods.[25] The level of fibrinopeptide A and FRA increase in preeclampsia.[25] The increased thrombin activity may also decrease the half-life of fibrinogen in preeclamptics. Thrombin decreases the procoagulant activity of factor VIII without altering the concentration of factor VIII-related antigen. Thus, the ratio of the antigen/the procoagulant activity ratio is an index of thrombin activity. This ratio is increased in preeclampsia. Under normal circumstances, antithrombin III, which is normally present in the plasma, prevents spontaneous coagulation by inactivaing factor Xa and thrombin. Plasma antithrombin III concentration is decreased in preeclampsia. The extent of decrease may be used as an index of the severity of the disease and as a predictor of fetal morbidity.[26]

Postpartum Hemolytic Uremic Syndrome

The condition is fully discussed in Chapter 22 Renal Disease. Incompletely polymerized fibrin is deposited in the renal glomerular blood vessels, resulting in severe renal failure.

HEREDITARY COAGULATION DISORDERS IN PREGNANCY

The major concerns in the management of hereditary coagulation disorders in pregnant patients are the safety of regional anesthesia, and the severity of intrapartum or postpartum hemorrhage. Also of concern are the fact that some coagulopathies, such as antithrombin III deficiency, may be associated with increased risk of thrombosis in the mother and fetus and not with the hemorrhagic diathesis, and the neonate born with the congenital deficiency of certain coagulation factors is prone to the risk of hemorrhage from the umbilical cord.[27] Platelet deficiency usually causes petechiae. Deficiency of coagulation factors causes hemorrhage into tissues and joint spaces. Under normal circumstances, local bleeding is arrested by the action of the platelet plug, which remains in place for 24 to 48 hours. The platelet plug is unstable in the absence of a firm fibrin plug, thus postoperative hemorrhage may be delayed for 24 to 48 hours in patients with coagulopathy. Many of these conditions occur in women of child-bearing age; therefore knowledge of these conditions is necessary for the proper management of these patients. The degree of deficiency of the clotting factor and the severity of hemorrhage depends on whether the patient is genetically a homozygote or a heterozygote. Table 11–7 summarizes the essential features of some important coagulopathies.

VON WILLEBRAND'S DISEASE

Factor VIII complex consists of at least two protein complexes.[28] The first one is the procoagulant and is referred to as factor VIII:C (antihemophilic factor, AHG). Factor VIII:C Ag is the antigen expressing the activity of the factor during immunologic determinations. The second one is the cofactor involved in causing platelet aggregation in response to a platelet aggregant called the ristocetin. This component is called factor VIII-von Willebrand factor, or the ristocetin cofactor (factor VIIIR:RCo), and the antigen with this activity is the factor VIIIR:Ag). Factor VIII:C is believed to be synthesized by the liver and the larger molecule factor VIIIR:RCo by the megakaryocytes and endothelial cells.[2] Normal pregnancy causes a rise in the serum concentrations of both fractions of the factor VIII complex.

With von Willebrand's disease, the most common hereditary coagulopathy seen in obstetric patients, is caused by the deficiency in VIIIR:RCo. Patients with a mild disease are usually asymptomatic but often bleed excessively during or after incidental disease. Menorrhagia, gastrointestinal bleeding, bruisability, epistaxis, and gingival bleeding are the common symptoms. Bleeding time is prolonged. Factor VIII:C and VIIIR:Rco levels are decreased. Ristocetin induced platelet aggregation is decreased with normal aggregating response to adenosine diphosphate.

Pregnancy causes an increase in both fractions of factor VIII in normal patients, as well as in patients with von Willebrand's disease, which may cause an improvement in bleeding symptoms. If the factor VIII:C level increases to 50% of normal, the bleeding time is considered normal; thus a vaginal delivery is contemplated and no treatment may be required.[27] After delivery,

the concentration of factor VIII:C decreases to pre-pregnancy values in 2 to 3 days and that of the VIII-R:RCo within hours.[27,28] The incidence and severity of postpartum hemorrhage roughly correlates with factor VIII:C level.

Patients with less than 50% of factor VIII:C and/or with an abnormal bleeding time must be treated with cryoprecipitate[28] (15 to 20 units twice daily). Each bag of cryoprecipitate contains approximately 100 U of factor VIII:C. For vaginal delivery, the concentration of factor VIII:C must be raised to at least 50% of normal, and for cesarean section to 80% of normal. Cryoprecipitate therapy must be continued in the postpartum period because risk of hemorrhage continues to be present. The bleeding time must be repeatedly determined during therapy. If the bleeding time has been consistently normal, and the factor VIII:C level is at least 50%, one may consider the use of regional anesthesia. In patients with abnormal bleeding times, general anesthesia must be administered.

HEMOPHILIA

Hemophilia A (factor VIII:C deficiency) may occur in women with a homozygous trait. Heterozygote carriers may also be symptomatic. The carrier state is most reliably diagnosed by the ratio between the concentrations of factors VIII:C and VIIIR:Ag (0.5 or smaller). The prenatal diagnosis of hemophilia A is done by measuring fetal blood concentrations of factors VIII:C Ag and VIIIR:Ag.

The severity of the disease correlates with the level of factor VIII:C in the blood. Severe forms of the disease cause spontaneous hemorrhage, whereas the mild form may cause only surgical bleeding. The PTT is usually prolonged. Carriers rarely become symptomatic during pregnancy. Cryoprecipitate is the accepted mode of therapy. The goal of therapy must be to raise the level of factor VIII:C to at least 30% prior to delivery. Higher levels may be needed in cases of intra- and postoperative bleeding. The level must be maintained for at least 7 days following delivery or surgery to minimize postpartum hemorrhage. The number of units of factor VIII:C needed to raise the activity of factor VIII:C from 10% to 80% in a hemophiliac who weighs 60 kg, and has 70 ml of blood volume per kg is calculated as follows:

$$\begin{array}{ccc} \text{70 ml blood/Kg} & & \text{60 kg} \\ \text{(blood volume)} & \times & \text{(Weight)} \end{array} = \begin{array}{c} \text{4200 ml of blood} \\ \text{(Blood volume in ml)} \end{array}$$

$$\begin{array}{ccc} \text{4200 ml} & & [80 - 10]\% \\ \text{(Blood volume in ml)} & \times & \text{(Change in percentage of} \\ & & \text{factor VIII:C)} \end{array} = \begin{array}{c} \text{2940 Units} \\ \text{(Units of factor VIII:C)} \end{array}$$

Therefore, if one bag of cryoprecipitate has 100 units of factor VIII:C, then approximately 30 bags of cryoprecipitate are needed. One half of the initial replacement therapy will be needed twice daily.[28]

Intravenous infusion of l-d-amino-8-D-arginine vasopressin (DDAVP) has been used to increase the level of factor VIII:C. The hormone increases the level of the clotting factor by eliciting a general stress response. However, there are no well controlled studies available in pregnant patients. The treatment modality may also be used to treat mild forms of von Willebrand's disease. Using a fetal scalp electrode in the fetus with this condition may result in cephalhematomas. Occasionally, the presence of factor VIII antibodies may produce severe hemorrhage in the postpartum period mimicking hemophilia.[29] The condition may develop spontaneously or may occur in combination with systemic lupus erythematosus or rheumatoid arthritis.

Hemophilia B (Christmas disease, factor IX deficiency) is similar to hemophilia A. The homozygote state is associated with severe disease and is rare in women. The clinical picture is quite similar to hemophilia A. The PTT is usually prolonged. Treatment consists of administration of fresh frozen plasma (volume overload) or by administration of factor IX concentrate. Some factor IX concentrates may carry the risk of producing severe thrombotic complications. The risk of hepatitis is also significant. The factor IX level must be raised to 50% of its normal value before surgery.

FIBRINOGEN ANOMALIES

The abnormalities may include decreases in the amount of fibrinogen or a defect in the quality of fibrinogen (dysfibrinogenemia). These conditions are extremely rare. A total of only 200 cases have been reported. In a neonate born with this condition, hemorrhage from the umbilical cord may be severe. Menorrhagia may be a problem later on in life. Repeated miscarriages are said to occur in women with this condition.

In severe fibrinogen deficiency, PT, PTT, and TCT are prolonged, which is corrected by the addition of normal plasma to the patient's plasma. In cases of moderate hypofibrinogenemia, coagulation parameters may actually be normal.

Fibrinogen levels increase during pregnancy, which may cause improvement in symptoms. Dysfibrinogenemia is not usually associated with bleeding tendency, but rather with abnormal thrombotic events and with recurrent first trimester abortions. Cryoprecipitate, which contains 250 mg of fibrinogen per bag is the preferred treatment for hypofibrinogenemic and dysfibrinogenemic states. A fibrinogen level of 100 mg will be associated with adequate hemostasis. Cryoprecipitate administration (3 bags per 10 kg of body weight) is recommended before surgery, followed by a daily maintenance dose of 1 bag per 10 kg every day.[27]

OTHER FACTOR DEFICIENCIES

Factor II Deficiency (Table 11–7)

Prothrombin deficiency is of two types: true hypoprothrombinemia and defective (dys) prothrombinemia. Both conditions are extremely rare. When born with this condition, the neonate may have umbilical cord bleeding. In the adult there may be increased vaginal bleeding during delivery or cesarean section. Both PT and PTT are prolonged with a normal TCT. In severe cases, prothrombin levels may be as low as 10% of normal. The treatment of choice is administration of fresh frozen plasma (FFP). Although commercial prothrombin concentrates are available, their use may be associated with abnormal clotting and increased risk of hepatitis.

Factor V Deficiency (Table 11–7)

Factor V deficiency is rarely associated with increased internal hemorrhage. A relatively large number of congenital anomalies may occur

Table 11–7. Characteristics of Inherited Coagulopathy

Disorder	Bleeding time	Inheritance	Prothrombin time	Partial thromboplastin time	Thrombin clotting time	Clot stability test	Level*	Therapy
Von Willebrand's disease	A	AD/AR	N	N/A	N	N	50–80%	CP
Fibrinogen deficiency	N/A	AR	A	A	A	N/A	100 mg%	CP
Prothrombin deficiency	N	AR	N	A	N	N	50%	FFP/PTC
Factor V deficiency	N/A	AR/AD	A	A	N	N	50%	FFP
Factor VII deficiency	N	AR	A	N	N	N	20%	FFP/PTC
Factor VIII deficiency	N	SLR	N	A	N	N	50%	CP
Factor IX deficiency	N	SLR	N/A	A	N	N	50%	FFP/PTC
Factor X deficiency	N	AR	A	A	N	N	50%	FFP/PTC
Factor XI deficiency	N/A	AR	N	A	N	N	25–50%	FFP/CPS
Factor XII deficiency	N	AR	N	A	N	N	—	—
Contact factors deficiency†	N	AR	N	A	N	N	—	—
Factor XIII deficiency	N	AR	N	N	N	A	10–20%	FFP/CP

*Level: Refers to concentration required for hemostasis.
Abbreviations used: N = normal; A = abnormal; AD = autosomal dominant; AR = autosomal recessive; SLR = sex-linked recessive; PTC = prothrombin concentrate; FFP = fresh frozen plasma; CP = cryoprecipitate.
†Contact factors = Hageman factor, high molecular weight kininogens (Fletcher factor), prekallikrein (Fitzgerald factor).

with this condition, including cardiac septal defects. The PT and PTT are prolonged. Factor V level does not usually rise in pregnancy. The condition is usually associated with postpartum hemorrhage. Fresh frozen plasma (15 ml/kg) is recommeneded to rise the factor V level to 25% of normal. Maintenance therapy with plasma must be continued for at least a week after delivery or after cesarean section.

Factor VII Deficiency (Table 11–7)

Umbilical cord bleeding is usual in the neonate born with this condition. In 15% of adults with this condition, intracranial bleeding may occur. The PT is markedly prolonged, but the PTT is usually normal. Factor VII usually increases in pregnancy. The treatment is with fresh frozen plasma. Commercial prothrombin complex carries the risk of hepatitis. The half-life of infused factor VIII is only hours, and therefore, maintenance therapy is needed every 6 hours.[27]

Factor X Deficiency (Table 11–7)

The presenting symptom in the neonate with this condition is umbilical cord bleeding. Both PT and PTT are markedly prolonged. Hemostasis may be accomplished with a level of 10% of the normal concentration. Fresh frozen plasma administration is the preferred treatment. Maintenance therapy is needed for a week following surgery.

Factor XI Deficiency

This disorder mainly occurs in Ashkenazi Jews. The PTT is prolonged and the PT is normal. Factor XI assay usually shows abnormal levels. The treatment is with plasma or with cryoprecipitate supernatant.

Factor XII and Other Contact Protein Deficiencies

Patients with factor XII deficiency do not have increased bleeding, but they do have increased incidence of thromboembolic disease.[27] Patients with deficiencies of other contact factors (prekallikrein and high molecular weight kininogens) do not have a hemorrhagic diathesis, but they may have serious congenital malformations.

Factor XIII Deficiency

The neonate born with this condition has increased risk of umbilical cord hemorrhage. In adults, postsurgical bleeding, postpartum hemorrhage, and defective wound healing may occur. The incidence of intracranial bleeding is approximately 25%. The clot stabilization test is abnormal, but all other clotting tests may be normal. Factor XIII may be assayed by radioimmunoassay. As little as 10% activity is said to be associated with good clotting, which may be achieved by administering 1 bag of cryoprecipitate at a dose of 1 bag per 10 kg body weight every 3 weeks.

Antithrombin Deficiency

Antithrombin III (ATIII) is a major inhibitor of thrombin and factor Xa. Two to three percent of patients hospitalized for a major thrombotic disorder have ATIII. Many patients with this condition will develop widespread systemic venous thrombosis. The measured ATIII level is only 25 to 50% of normal in these patients. Pregnancy markedly increases the risk of deep vein thrombosis in patients with ATIII deficiency.[27] Recently, it has been shown that patients with preeclampsia have decreased ATIII levels (see Chapter 10.) ATIII deficiency is usually corrected by administration of fresh frozen plasma. Cryoprecipitate should not be used for this purpose. Because of the low levels of ATIII, the anitcoagulant effect of heparin is somewhat diminished in these patients. A 5 to 10 second prolongation of PTT is recommended to diminish thromboembolic complication. A mini-heparin dose schedule may be used for this purpose. Heparin therapy must be continued in the postpartum or in the postabortion period. If thromboembolic events occur in pregnancy, larger doses of heparin may be required. The neonate born with this condition is prone to thrombotic complications as well. When neonatal ATIII levels fall below 10%, fresh frozen plasma administration may be required to correct the problem.

α₂ Antiplasmin Deficiency

Whole blood clotting time and euglobulin lysis time are markedly shortened because of the low resistance of the fibrin clot to plasmin digestion. Patients have been treated with fibrinolytic inhibitors (ε-amino caproic acid).

ABNORMALITIES OF PLATELET FUNCTION

IMMUNULOGIC THROMBOCYTOPENIC PURPURA

Immunologic (idiopathic) thrombocytopenic purpura (ITP), which occurs predominantly in females of child-bearing age is often associated with skin petechiae and ecchymoses, mucous membrane hemorrhages, and menorrhagia. Hemorrhagic diathesis occurs only rarely when the platelet count >100,000/mm³. Excessive bleeding occurs only when the count decreases to 50,000 or less.[30] The mechanism of ITP is related to destruction of the antibody-coated platelets by the macrophages and the spleen. Pregnancy may often induce a relapse.[31]

The diagnosis of ITP is usually confirmed by the demonstration of antiplatelet antibodies. Two types of assays, a direct or an indirect assay, may be performed. In the direct assay, IgG associated with patient's platelets are measured. In the indirect assay, the patient's serum is used to sensitize donor platelets. The amount of IgG adsorbed on the platelet surface is then measured. The indirect assays are simpler to perform but may at times be inaccurate, especially in pregnant women.[30] The treatment usually consists of splenectomy, which causes a significant improvement in the platelet count. Corticosteroids are also effective in increasing the maternal platelet count. Occasionally, immunosuppressive drugs have been used to increase platelet count.

The IgG antibodies, which are formed in the mother, may cross the placenta and produce fetal thrombocytopenia, which puts the infant at increased risk for intracranial hemorrhage, especially after vaginal delivery. No single method currently in use can identify the fetus at risk. A platelet count performed on blood obtained from the fetal scalp may be helpful in this regard. If the scalp blood platelet count is greater than 50,000/mm,³ the risk of neonatal hemorrhage is minimal and labor may be allowed to progress.[32] If the count is less than 50,000, a cesarean section must be performed.[33] Unfortunately, cesarean section does not guarantee that intracranial bleeding will not develop in the neonate.[31] Regional anesthesia may be administered to these patients if their platelet count is above 100,000/mm³ and the bleeding time is within normal limits.

THROMBOTIC THROMBOCYTOPENIC PURPURA

Only a few cases of thrombotic thrombocytopenic purpura (TTP) have been reported in pregnancy. The disease occurs in females between 30 and 40 years of age. The clinical features are fever, bleeding diathesis, and changes in sensorium. Microvascular lesions are found throughout the body. A skin biopsy may reveal the characteristic lesions. Massive plasma infusion with plasmapheresis, total plasma exchange, and blood exchange are the only means of effectively treating this otherwise fatal disease.[31]

HEMOGLOBINOPATHIES

SICKLE CELL HEMOGLOBINOPATHY

Sickle cell anemia (SS disease), sickle cell-hemoglobin C disease (SC disease), sickle cell trait, and β-thalassemia disease (S-thalassemia) are the common sickle cell hemoglobinopathies.[34] The SS disease is usually worsened by pregnancy.[32] Sickle cell crises, pulmonary dysfunction, and infections are ususaly increased in frequency and severity in pregnancy. The maternal mortality and perinatal mortality rates may reach 4.6% and 21%, respectively.[35] The rate of spontaneous abortions may reach 20%. Most patients maintain their hemoglobin at or above 7 g/dL; however, incidental infection may cause a decrease in hemoglobin level. Transfusions are required only if a difficult vaginal delivery or cesarean section is anticipated. The hematocrit under these circumstances must be raised to 35%. An intense sequestration of the red cells may occur, especially late in pregnancy.

Table 11–8. Types of Sickle Cell Crisis

Hemolytic crisis	(May be precipitated by infection).
Infarctive crisis	Sludging in major organs (Local hypoxia and acidosis); Pulmonary infarcts (pleuritic pain); Seizure, stroke, coma (rare).
Aplastic crisis	Viral infection, folate deficiency.
Sequestration crisis	Sequestration of RBC in the liver, spleen, and bone.

Treatment of these crises can include increasing the inspired oxygen concentration, using intravenous hydration, using analgesics, or alkalinization may be necessary.

Table 11–9. Chronic Organ Damage in Sickle Cell Anemia

Organ	Damage
Cardiac	Congestive heart failure (anemia related).
Respiratory	Reduced P_{O_2} (increased intrapulmonary shunting).
Hepatic	Gall stones Jaundice (hemolysis); Infarcted hepatic parenchyma.
Renal	Microinfarcts in renal medulla; (hypertonic environment in the medulla causes sickling); Inability to concentrate urine; Increased water loss and dehydration; Painless hematuria due to papillary infarcts; Renal failure.
Skeletal	Biconcave "fishmouth" vertebrae (bone infarcts); Salmonella osteomyelitis.
Ocular	Retinal infarcts and detachment.
Skin	Leg ulcers.
Neurologic	Cerebral thrombosis, hemiplegia; Subarachnoid hemorrhage.

This is accompanied by bone pain and a sudden decrease in the hematocrit. Patients prone to sequestration anemia may benefit from prophylactic transfusions of normal red cells.[36]

Normal red cells are transfused (hypertransfusion) in quantities sufficient to maintain the hematocrit above 25% and the hemoglobin S at or below 50%.[37] Prophylactic transfusions are said to be associated with decreased maternal and perinatal mortality and morbidity.[32,35,37] Mini-exchanges in which 2 units (500 ml each) of patient's blood are removed and replaced with 500 ml of normal donor blood and 500 ml of normal saline may reduce morbidity, especially from crisis. The hypoxic sickling process increases the viscosity of blood, thus further augmenting the sludging process. When the amount of normal cells are greater than that of the abnormal cells, however, the viscosity of blood may actually decrease, thus optimizing peripheral rheology.[36] Types of crisis in patients with sickle cell crisis are summarized in Table 11–8.

Anesthetic Considerations

The incidence of drug addiction is high in these patients. Because the SS disease involves many systems in the body, a complete evaluation of all organ function must be performed (Table 11–9. The hemoglobin concentration and the ratio of hemoglobin S to normal hemoglobin must be known. Arterial blood gas tensions and hepatic and renal functions must be evaluated. Correction of severe anemia (hematocrit <25%) must be done with fresh cell transfusion. An indwelling arterial line may be necessary for repeated blood P_{O_2} measurement. A central venous catheter may be inserted, if there is a history of congestive heart failure. In addition, a pulse oximeter may be used to monitor oxygen saturation. Because local or systemic hypothermia may predispose to sludging, intravenous fluids must be warmed.

Labor analgesia may be provided in the form of a lumbar epidural anesthetic. Systemic hypotension may lead to a low flow state in the tissues, thus it should be treated promptly with ephedrine. Inferior vena cava compression must be avoided because it may cause sludging in the lower extremity. If cesarean section is required, a lumbar epidural anesthesia is the best technique to use. However, in cases of fetal distress, general anesthesia may be required for cesarean section. A routine general endotracheal anesthesia may be used safely if the patient's circulating fluid volume is adequate. Arterial blood P_{O_2}, pH and P_{CO_2} must be measured during the procedure because of the possibility of increased pulmonary shunting and arterial hypoxemia in these patients.

Sickle-Cell Hemoglobin C Disease

The sickle cell-hemoglobin C (SC disease) occurs approximately in one of every 2000 pregnant black women. It represents a double heterozygous state, the S gene is derived from one parent and the C gene from the other. The hemoglobin concentration is usually normal, unless there is a complication. On electrophoresis the ratio of hemoglobin S to C is almost 1. In nonpregnant women, morbidity from the SC disease is lower than that from sickle cell anemia, and life-expectancy is longer.[32] In pregnant women, however, maternal mortality and morbidity are increased. Painful attacks are frequent. Necrotic bone marrow embolization may cause pulmonary dysfunction. Other systemic manifestations may resemble those in the SS disease (Table 11–9).[39] Maternal mortality reaches 2%, and the perinatal mortality rate reaches nearly 14%. The abortion rate is 14.6%.[36] Prophylactic transfusion regimens, as outlined for the treatment of SS disease, have been generally beneficial in not only minimizing the number of attacks but also maintaining adequate maternal hemoglobin concentration. Anesthetic considerations discussed under the SS disease also apply to the SC disease.

Sickle Cell Trait

The trait (A/S) rarely causes symptoms or signs. Renal concentrating ability may be impaired. Gross hematuria occurs in 3 to 4% of cases. Pulmonary infarcts may also occur occasionally.[38]

β-Thalassemia

The condition is caused by the incomplete formation of the β-globulin chains of hemoglobin. The disease occurs in blacks as well as in patients of Mediterranean extraction. In the latter group, the condition is usually more severe than in the former. Different electrophoretic patterns are recognized. Patients may have Hb S (60%), Hb A_2 (6%) and Hb F (15%). Depending on the amount of Hb A, which may vary from 0 to 40%, the disease may produce clinical pictures of varying severity. When the Hb A levels are very low, the disease is called the Cooley's anemia.[34] These patients develop multiple sites of erythropoiesis. Increased erythropoietic bone marrow in the vertebral bodies may lead to spinal cord compression. Maxillary erythropoiesis causes enlargement of the mandibles, which

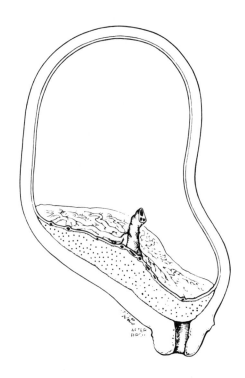

FIG. 11–5.   Placenta previa. (From Pritchard JA, McDonald PC, and Gant NF: Obstetric Hemorrhage. *In* Williams Obstetrics. 17th Ed. Norwalk, Appleton-Century-Crofts, 1985.)

may interfere with laryngoscopy. Congestive heart failure may develop because of either severe anemia or hemosiderosis caused by repeated transfusions.[34]

OBSTETRIC HEMORRHAGE

The leading causes of obstetric hemorrhage in the third trimester are placenta previa and placental abruption. Placental abruption is associated with pain, whereas placenta previa produces painless vaginal hemorrhage. Normally the placenta is attached to the corpus uteri away from the os. When the placenta is implanted close to the os, it is called the placenta previa (Fig. 11–5). The incidence of placenta previa is double in patients who have had a cesarean section in the past.[39] The placenta previa may be total, in which case it covers the os completely, or it may be partial. In the marginal type, only the placental margin reaches the os. The placenta may also lie in the lower uterine segment (low-lying placenta). The advent of sonography has made the diagnosis of placenta previa easy. The placenta is known to migrate towards the fundus as pregnancy advances.[40] Therefore, the diagnosis of a low-lying placenta in early gestation need not cause undue concern.

The low-lying placenta is likely to cause maternal bleeding because it separates from the decidual bed. A complete placenta previa may cause catastrophic hemorrhage (when disturbed during vaginal examination). Unlike placental abruption, placenta previa is not usually associated with DIC. However, DIC may occur if the patient receives a massive replacement therapy. When a patient develops vaginal bleeding in early pregnancy because of placenta previa, she is usually hospitalized and is placed at bed rest. Delivery is delayed, if conditions permit, until the fetus is more mature.

The anesthetic considerations include the need for massive transfusion in a patient who is profusely bleeding, and the possibility of postpartum hemorrhage because the lower uterine segment does not effectively stop hemorrhage from the decidual bed. The anesthesiologist should also be concerned with the premature neonate with a somewhat increased congenital malformation rate, the chance of occasional air embolism, and the possibility of placenta accreta. Air embolism occurs because of the proximity of the open placental sinuses to the outside air.

Abnormally adherent placenta may produce profuse hemorrhage, necessitating hysterectomy.[41] In placenta accreta, the placenta is attached to myometrium. In placenta accreta, the villi actually invade the myometrium. In placenta percreta, the villi may perforate the myometrium. All cotyledons or a single one may be involved in the invasive process.[41] Previous cesarean sections, previous curettage, and multiparity are all associated with increased risks.

REFERENCES

1. Ratnoff OD: Disseminated intravascular coagulation. *In* Disorders of Hemostasis. (Edited by Ratnoff OD, and Forbes CD). New York, Grune and Stratton, 1984.
2. Annest SJ, et al.: Increased creatinine clearance following cryoprecipitate infusion in trauma and surgical patients with decreased renal function. J Trauma 20:726, 1980.
3. Bennett Bruce, and Ogston D: Fibrinolytic bleeding syndromes. *In* Disorders of Hemostasis. (Edited by Ratnoff OD, and Forbes CD). New York, Grune and Stratton, 1984.
4. Walker ID, and Davidson DF: Fibrinolysis. *In* Blood Coagulation and Hemostasis. New York, Churchill Livingstone, 1985.
5. Sher G, and Startland BE: Abruptio placentae with coagulopathy: A rational basis for management. Clin Obstet Gynecol 28:15, 1985.
6. Pritchard JA, McDonald PC, and Gant NF: Obstetric hemorrhage. *In* Williams Obstetrics. 17th Edition. Norwalk, Appleton-Century-Crofts, 1985.
7. Hurd WW, Midovnik M, Hertzberg V, and Lavin JP: Selective management of abruptio placentae: A prospective study 61:467, 1983.
8. Romero R: The management of acquired hemostatic failure during pregnancy. *In* Critical Care of the Obstetric Patient. (Edited by Berkowitz RL). New York, Churchill-Livingstone, 1983.
9. Weiskopf RB, Bogetz MZ, Roizen MF, and Reid IA: Cardiovascular and metabolic sequelae of inducing anesthesia with ketamine or thiopental in hypovolemic swine. Anesthesiology 60:214, 1984.
10. Romero R, Copel JA, and Hobbins JC: Intrauterine fetal demise and failure: The fetal death syndrome. Clin Obstet Gynecol 28:24, 1985.
11. Jiminez JM, and Pritchard JA: Pathogenesis and treatment of coagulation defects resulting from fetal death. Obstet Gynecol 32:449, 1968.
12. Morgan M: Amniotic fluid embolism. Anaesthesia 34:20, 1978.
13. Killam A: Amniotic fluid embolism. Clin Obstet Gynecol 28:32, 1985.
14. Garland IWC, and Thompson WD: Diagnosis of amniotic fluid embolism using an antiserum to human keratin. J Clin Pathol 36:625, 1983.
15. Hall AH, Kulig KW, and Rumack BH: Amniotic fluid embolism. JAMA 256:1892, 1986.
16. Bech-Jansen P, Brinkman CR, Johnson CH, and Assali NS: Circulatory shock in pregnant sheep. I. Effects of endotoxin on uteroplacental and fetal umbilical circulation. Am J Obstet Gynecol 112:1084, 1972.
17. Beller FK: Sepsis and coagulation. Clin Obstet Gynecol 28:46, 1985.
18. Eskridge RA: Septic shock. Crit Care Quarterly 2:55, 1980.
19. Duff P, and Gibbs RS: Bacteremia in Obstetrics. *In* Critical Care of the Obstetric Patient. Edited by Berkowitz RL. New York, Churchill-Livingstone, 1983.
20. Lee CT, et al.: Elastolytic activity in pulmonary lavage from patients with adult respiratory-distress syndrome. N Engl J Med 304:192, 1981.
21. Moss G, Staunton C, and Stein AA: The normal electron histochemistry and the effect of hemorrhagic shock on the pulmonary surfactant system. Surg Gynecol Obstet 140:53, 1975.
22. Schumer W: Steroids in the treatment of clinical septic shock. Ann Surg 184:333, 1976.
23. Glenn TM, and Lefer AM: Antitoxic action of methylprednisolone in hemorrhagic shock. Eur J Pharmacol 13:230, 1971.

24. Weenink JH, ten Cate JW, Treffers PE: Hypertensive disorders. Clin Obstet Gynecol 28:37, 1985.

25. McKillop C, Edgar W, and Prentice RM: In vivo production of soluble complexes containing fibrinogen-fibrin related antigen during ancroid therapy. Thrombosis Res 7:361, 1975.

26. Weenink GH, et al.: Antithrombin III levels in pre-eclampsia correlate with maternal and fetal morbidity. Am J Obstet Gynecol 148:1092, 1984.

27. Caldwell DC, Williamson RA, and Goldsmith JC: Hereditary coagulopathies in pregnancy. Clin Obstet Gynecol 28:53, 1985.

28. Lipton RA, Ayromlooi J, and Coller BS: Severe von Willebrand's disease during labor and delivery. JAMA 248:1355, 1982.

29. Reece EA, Fox HE, and Rapaport F: Factor VIII inhibitor. A cause of severe postpartum hemorrhage. Am J Obstet Gynecol 144:985, 1982.

30. Rote NS, and Lau J: Immunologic thrombocytopenic purpura. Clin Obstet Gynecol 28:84, 1985.

31. Hoffman PC: Idiopathic thrombocytopenic purpura in pregnancy. Clin Perinatol 12:599, 1985.

32. Pritchard JA, McDonald PC, and Gant NF: Medical and surgical illnesses during pregnancy and the puerperium. In Williams Obstetrics. 17th Edition. Norwalk, Appleton-Century-Crofts, 1985.

33. Scott JR, et al.: Fetal platelet counts in the obstetric management of immunologic thrombocytopenic purpura. Am J Obstet Gynecol 145:136, 1980.

34. Bunn HF: Disorders of hemoglobin structure, function and synthesis. In Harrison's Principles of Internal Medicine. (Edited by Petersdorf RG, et al.) New York, McGraw-Hill Book, 1983.

35. Millner PF, Jones PR, and Dobler J: Outcome of pregnancy in sickle cell anemia and sickle cell hemoglobin-C disease. Am J Obstet Gynecol 138:239, 1980.

36. Cunningham FG, Pritchard JA, and Mason R: Pregnancy and sickle hemoglobinopathy. Results with and without prophylactic transfusions. Obstet Gynecol 62:419, 1983.

37. McLaughlin BN, Martin RW, and Morrison JC: Clinical management of sickle cell hemoglobinopathies during pregnancy. Clin Perinatol 12:585, 1985.

38. Wallerstein RO: Blood. In Current Diagnosis and Medical Treatment. (Edited by Krupp MA, Schroeder SA, and Tierney LM, Jr.). Norwalk/Los Altos, Appleton and Lange, 1987.

39. Singh PM, Rodriguez C, and Gupta AN: Placenta previa and previous cesarean section. Acta Obstet Gynecol Scand 60:367, 1981.

40. Comeau J, Shaw L, Marcell CC, and Lavery JP: Early placenta previa and delivery outcome. Obstet Gynecol 61:557, 1983.

41. Pritchard JA, McDonald PC, and Gant NF: Abnormalities of third stage of labor. In Williams Obstetrics. 17th Edition. Norwalk, Appleton-Century-Crofts, 1985.

12

CARDIAC DISEASE

Pregnancy causes an increase in both cardiac work and myocardial oxygen consumption. Severely ill cardiac patients may not be able to tolerate the increased strain on the heart. Additional hemodynamic changes occur during labor, and are especially acute during each uterine contraction. Cardiac output may increase 10 to 20% in the immediate postpartum period because of the sudden increase in venous return caused not only by the relief of inferior vena cava obstruction, but by the contracting uterus, which returns blood from the uterine venous sinuses to the systemic circulation. The pregnant patient with cardiac disease may develop cardiac decompensation any time during the pregnancy, the parturition, or in the puerperium. Table 12–1 summarizes most of the cardiovascular changes that occur in a pregnant patient. For a detailed description of the cardiovascular changes accompanying pregnancy, with special reference to aortocaval compression, refer to Chapter 2 Maternal Adaptation to Pregnancy.

Cardiac disease, which affects 0.5% of all pregnant women, is a leading cause of maternal death even in well developed countries.[1] Rheumatic heart disease constitutes the majority, (83.5%), followed by congenital heart disease (13.4%). Cor pulmonale, cardiomyopathy, and coronary artery disease account for the rest. Table 12–2 lists the types of cardiac disease that are likely to be encountered in pregnancy. The perinatal mortality ranges between 3.3 and 5.7%. For the most part, the maternal mortality is influenced by the type of cardiac decrease (Table 12–3).[2] For instance, Eisenmenger's complex is associated with a very high maternal mortality because of the severe pulmonary hypertension. In many instances, severe cardiac failure contributes to maternal death. The severity of heart disease in pregnancy is graded using the New York Heart Association criteria, which are based on the degree of functional impairment (Table 12–4).[3] Patients in Class I do not have any symptoms nor do they experience any anginal pain. Patients in Classes 2, 3, and 4 may complain of fatigue, palpitations, dyspnea,

Table 12–1. Cardiovascular Changes in Pregnancy

Parameter	Percentage of change with pregnancy	Percentage of change postpartum
Heart rate	+10	−15
Stroke volume	+25	+50
Cardiac output	+40	+50
Plasma volume	+70	−70
RBC volume	+20	−10
V_{O_2}	+20	−10

Table 12–2.   Types of Cardiac Disease in Pregnancy

Form	Disease
Congenital	Aortic valve disease. Hypertrophic obstructive cardiomyopathy. Coarctation of the aorta. Pulmonary stenosis. Left-to-right intracardiac shunts: atrial septal defect, ventricular septal defect, persistent ductus arteriosus. Right-to-left cardiac shunts: Tetralogy of Fallot, Eisenmenger's complex.
Acquired	Mitral stenosis. Mitral insufficiency. Aortic stenosis. Aortic insufficiency. Prosthetic heart valves. Myocardial infarction. Cardiomyopathy. Mitral valve prolapse. Pulmonary hypertension.

or anginal pain to a varying degree. It is important for the anesthesiologist to know the exact symptomatology and the level of physical activity that causes the symptoms.

Excessive weight gain (>10.5 kg), abnormal retention of fluid, and anemia must be avoided because they predispose to congestive heart failure (CHF). Heart failure may occur even with Class I patients.[3] Measurement of vital capacity (VC) at every prenatal visit is recommended to detect heart failure. A decrease in VC is an early warning sign of CHF.[3] The development of preeclampsia worsens prognosis.[3] Pregnant cardiac patients are advised to take rest every day for at least a half hour after each meal. Vaginal delivery is recommended for patients with car-

diac disease and cesarean section is usually reserved for obstetric indication.[3] Many centers use antibiotic prophylaxis to prevent the development of vegetative endocarditis. Sugrue et al[4] have reported that puerperal infective endocarditis very rarely develops and that the antibiotic prophylaxis is unnecessary. However, many authorities are in favor of using prophylaxis because infective endocarditis (if it develops) is a life-threatening condition. Antibiotic administration should begin during labor and be continued for 48 hours. Aqueous penicillin with tobramycin or gentamicin is recommended.[5] Many antiarrhythmic agents have been used safely in pregnancy.[6]

ACQUIRED CARDIAC DISEASE

MITRAL STENOSIS

Pathophysiology

The major derangement in mitral stenosis (MS) is the obstruction to the left atrial outflow.[7-9] Gradually, the left atrial pressure, pulmonary capillary wedge pressure (PCWP), and pulmonary venous pressure rise. Fibrous thickening of the walls of the pulmonary artery capillaries occurs in patients with long-standing pulmonary hypertension. Because of fluid transudation, pulmonary compliance decreases.[9] Intramural thrombi that form in the left atrial appendage may cause cerebrovascular accidents. Major prognostic indices in patients

Table 12–3.   Mortality in Heart Disease

	Disorder	Percentage
Valvular lesions	Class 3–4 mitral stenosis With atrial fibrillation	5 14–17
	Mitral insufficiency Aortic insufficiency Aortic stenosis Prosthetic heart valves	1–5 2–7 6–8 2
Congenital heart disease	Tetralogy of Fallot	4–12
	Eisenmenger's syndrome Primary Pulm. Hypertension Marfan's syndrome Aortic coarctation Peripartal cardiomyopathy	10–30 50 50 3–9 15–60

Table 12–4. Functional Classification of Cardiac Disease*

Class	
1	No limitation on physical activity
2	Ordinary physical activity causes symptoms
3	Less than ordinary activity causes symptoms
4	Marked restriction of activity (may be symptomatic even at rest)

*Based on classification by the New York Heart Association

with MS include the severity of pulmonary hypertension, the presence of atrial fibrillation, and the presence of paroxysmal atrial tachycardia. Because increased left atrial pressure predisposes to tachyarrhythmias, PCWP measurement is recommended. Tachycardia will decrease the time available for left ventricular filling and reduce the cardiac output.

The diastolic filling time is of paramount importance in those with atrial fibrillation because of the absence of atrial "kick", which helps in left ventricular filling. Patients who are in chronic atrial fibrillation may be receiving digoxin. Digoxin levels are lower in pregnant patients for a given dose than they are in nonpregnant subjects.[6] Patients who develop symptoms of pulmonary congestion may benefit from beta blockers such as propranolol. Although there were earlier reports of fetal problems with this drug, recent reports have not been able to corroborate this.[6]

Rapid intravenous infusion of fluids may increase pulmonary congestion and may precipitate atrial fibrillation or congestive heart failure. Pulmonary arterial pressure monitoring may be of benefit under these circumstances. An acute reduction in preload and afterload can ensue after the administration of epidural anesthesia. The preload is reduced because of venous pooling and the afterload is reduced because of arteriolar vasodilatation. This always results in tachycardia, which may be harmful to a patient with MS. An α-mimetic drug such as phenylephrine that is injected in 100 μg boluses may be used to counteract the effects of epidural anesthesia on preload and afterload. The use of ephedrine is associated with a slightly higher heart rate.

Patients with MS have a variety of symptoms, which include palpitations, dyspnea, orthopnea, anginal pain, unexplained cough, and hemoptysis. On auscultation of the chest, a diastolic murmur with a presystolic accentuation, which is usually accompanied by a thrill is present at the apex. The pulmonic component of the second heart sound is accentuated. The two components of the second heart sound are closely split. In addition, the opening snap of the mitral valve may be heard. One may also look for distended neck veins, edema in the lower back, and a palpable liver edge, if heart failure is suspected.[9] A chest x-ray may show signs of increased pulmonary congestion including Kerley B lines. The EKG may show left atrial hypertrophy (P-mitral), and right ventricular hypertrophy (in advanced cases). Cardiac arrhythmias may be also evident in the EKG.

Anesthetic Management During Labor

The majority of Class I patients do not require any invasive monitoring. The EKG, however, must be continuously monitored because the onset of arrhythmias is usually an indication of impending heart failure, or of digitoxicity in patients who are on digoxin.[10] Labor pains cause an increase in cardiac output and heart rate, thereby increasing myocardial oxygen consumption. A segmental lumbar epidural block, by producing effective analgesia, will have a favorable effect on myocardial oxygen consumption. The epidural anesthesia must be induced slowly by injecting small increments of the local anesthetic through a catheter. A combination of epidural fentanyl and local anesthetic may be useful because it helps decrease the requirement for the local anesthetic. Hypotension must be detected and treated promptly. The supine position must be avoided. Perineal anesthesia may be established early in the second stage to minimize the involuntary valsalva maneuver.[2] Some authorities recommend that the second stage of labor be kept short by delivering the baby by low-forceps in order to minimize maternal discomfort.

Patients who are more seriously ill (Class II-IV) must be monitored with an indwelling arterial cannula and a pulmonary artery catheter. Because patients with a tight MS tolerate fluid preload poorly, the customary prophylactic intravenous hydration, (prior to epidural anesthesia) must be done only with PCWP monitoring. Central venous pressure monitoring may be misleading in these patients. In the study by Clark et al., the CVP differed by as much as 10 mm Hg from the PCWP.[11] A carefully performed low-dose epidural anesthesia in combination with fentanyl may be attempted. The addition of fentanyl to local anesthetic may minimize the requirement of the latter. Patients must inhale oxygen throughout the course of labor. A saddle block is suitable for forceps delivery in patients who have not had lumbar epidural analgesia for labor. High spinal blocks can produce severe hypotension because cardiac patients will not be able to increase their cardiac output in response to a decreasing perfusion pressure. General anesthesia is discussed in the section below.

Anesthesia for Cesearan Section

Regardless of the type of anesthesia, PCWP and radial artery pressure must be continuously monitored. The pulmonary artery catheter may be particularly useful in detecting a sudden rise in the pulmonary artery pressure. It also aids in the therapy of pulmonary hypertension with suitable agents. The desirable hemodynamic goals, the recommended anesthetic technique, and the preferred anesthetic agents together with certain special problems are listed in Table 12–5. In a patient with MS, the hemodynamic management must be aimed at maintaining a normal or slightly decreased heart rate and a normal or a slightly decreased preload and afterload throughout the procedure. Excessive fluid administration will quickly result in pulmonary edema.

When anesthesia is required for cesarean section, a well-controlled lumbar epidural anesthesia may be induced by injecting 3 ml increments of the local anesthetic (not the usual 5 ml increments). Should systemic hypotension occur, a 50 to 100 µg injection of phenylephrine may be used to restore blood pressure. Used for correcting systemic hypotension caused by regional anesthesia, phenylephrine, which possesses negligible β-mimetic action, results in a slower heart rate than does the use of ephedrine. Spinal anesthesia is not recommended for cesarean section because it may precipitously reduce systemic pressure. Regional anesthesia is contraindicated in patients who are on antico-

agulant therapy. Postoperative analgesia may be achieved by epidural morphine.

When general anesthesia is required, drugs such as ketamine, atropine, and pancuronium must be avoided because they can increase the heart rate. Patients with mild functional impairment may tolerate the stress of a rapid-sequence induction, whereas those with advanced disease may not do so, necessitating a slow induction. An inhalation induction with a halogenated anesthetic or an intravenous induction with a high-dose narcotic technique (10 to 15 µg/kg) can be used.[9] Patients must have been pretreated with antacids and cricoid pressure must be maintained until the trachea is intubated. Transtracheal lidocaine spray is used to minimize autonomic response to intubation. The pediatric team must be alerted to the possibility of neonatal depression caused by fentanyl or the inhalation agent. Maintenance is carried out with a 50:50 mixture of N_2O-oxygen with or without 0.5% halothane. Succinylcholine infusion can be used for relaxation, which obviates the need for reversal of muscle paralysis at the end of the procedure.

When a long acting muscle relaxant is desired, atracurium or vecuronium are preferred both to pancuronium, which causes tachycardia, and to d-tubocurarine, which causes histamine release. (Please refer to Table 15–5 for a description of the differences among clinically used muscle relaxants with respect to their potential for releasing histamine and causing ganglionic and vagal blockade.) Table 12–6 summarizes the cardiovascular effects of commonly used muscle relaxants. Administration of vecuronium in doses up to 0.28 mg/kg is not usually associated with any deleterious cardiovascular effects (Fig. 12–1).[12,13]

Nitrous oxide has been shown to cause an increase in pulmonary artery pressure in those with preexisting pulmonary artery hypertension.[14] Should tachycardia arise during anesthesia, propranolol may be used to control it. If severe increases are noted in the PCWP with a concomitant reduction in cardiac output, nitroglycerin is infused (0.5 to 1 µ/kg/min) to "unload" the heart. In the postoperative period, the patients must be cared for in the intensive care unit. Prolonged postoperative ventilation may be needed in patients with preexisting pulmonary dysfunction.

Table 12–5. Guidelines for Regulating Preload and Afterload in Pregnant Cardiac Patients

Disease	Desirable heart rate	Desirable preload	Desirable afterload	Anesthesia Labor	Anesthesia C.S.	
Mitral stenosis	N–SD	N–SD	N–SD	L.E.A.	L.E.A.	Avoid ketamine, atropine, pancuronium, atrial fibrillation.
Mitral regurgitation	N–SI	N–SD	N–SD	L.E.A.	L.E.A.	Avoid pentothal, halothane, and inhalation agents; giant v waves in PA tracing.
Aortic stenosis	N–SI	N–SI	N–SI	i.v.	G.A.	Avoid pentothal, halothane; Reduced L.V. compliance; Myocardial ischemia; V5 lead.
Aortic incompetence	N–SI	N–SD	N–SD	L.E.A.	L.E.A.	Avoid pentothal, halothane; Waterhammer pulse; increased end diastolic volume.
Hypertrophic cardiomyopathy	N–SD	N–SI	N	L.E.A.	G.A.	Avoid Digoxin, pancuronium, ketamine, and atropine; Use halothane, beta blockade to improve outflow obstruction.
Peripartal cardiomyopathy	N–SD	N	N	i.v.	G.A.	Avoid pentothal, halothane; Use high dose narcotic anesthesia, S3 gallop, arrhythmias; jugular v waves.
Mitral valve prolapse	N	N	N	L.E.A.	L.E.A.	Tachyarrhythmias increased catecholamines; beta blockade useful.
Marfan syndrome	N	—	SD	L.E.A.	L.E.A.	Aortic dissection; intubation problem.
Ebstein's anomaly	N	N–SD	N–SI	L.E.A.	L.E.A.	Supraventricular tachycardia, Prolonged i.v. induction, pulse oximeter.
Pulmonary hypertension (Eisenmenger syndrome)	N	N–SI	N–SI	L.E.A.	G.A.	Arterial desaturation; Avoid air bubbles, sensitive to blood loss, arrhythmias, pulse oximeter.
Myocardial infarction	N–SD	N	N–SD	L.E.A.	L.E.A.	V5 lead

The table gives guidelines for the maintenance of preload and afterload in pregnant cardiac patients. The desirable goal is shown in each category. It is assumed that invasive monitoring is available. The last column in the table also indicates drugs to avoid or the drugs of choice along with some special problems and recommendations.

It is obviously preferable if all measured hemodynamic variables remain within normal limits. This, however, does not always happen, thus for each hemodynamic variable, the table lists the more desirable situation.

Antibiotic prophylaxis is recommended in most of the categories to prevent vegetative endocarditis. Abbreviations: N = normal, SI = slightly increased, SD = slightly decreased, L.E.A. = lumbar epidural analgesia, G.A. = general anesthesia, C.S. = cesarean section, LV = left ventricle.

Table 12–6. Cardiovascular Effects of Muscle Relaxants

Drug	Ganglion block	Muscarinic vagal block	Histamine release	Under anesthesia			
				SVR	CO	BP	HR
d-tubocurarine	+ +	− −	+ + +	↓	↓	↓	−
Metocurine	+	− −	+ + +	↓	−	↓	−
Pancuronium	− −	+ +	− −	−	↑	↑	↑
Gallamine	− −	+ + +	− −	−	↑	↑	↑
Alcuronium	+	+	− −	↓	↑	↓	↑
Fazadinium	+ +	+ +	− −	↓	↑	↓	↑
Vecuronium	− −	− −	− −	−	−	−	−
Atracurium	− −	− −	− −	−	−	−	−

SVR = systemic vascular resistance; CO = cardiac output; BP = mean arterial blood pressure; HR = heart rate.
(Reproduced with permission by Scott RPF and Savarese JJ: The cardiovascular and autonomic effects of neuromuscular blocking agents. *In* Muscle Relaxants Basic & Clinical Aspects. (Edited by Katz RL). NY, Grune & Stratton, 1985.)

Cardiac arrhythmias can develop during the course of labor, surgery, and the puerperium. Atrial fibrillation is a common problem and is associated with increased maternal morbidity. A case may therefore be made for the need to maintain sinus rhythm in patients with advanced MS. If there is no hemodynamic compromise, atrial fibrillation is treated by intravenous digoxin, followed by quinidine.[6,8] Verapamil may

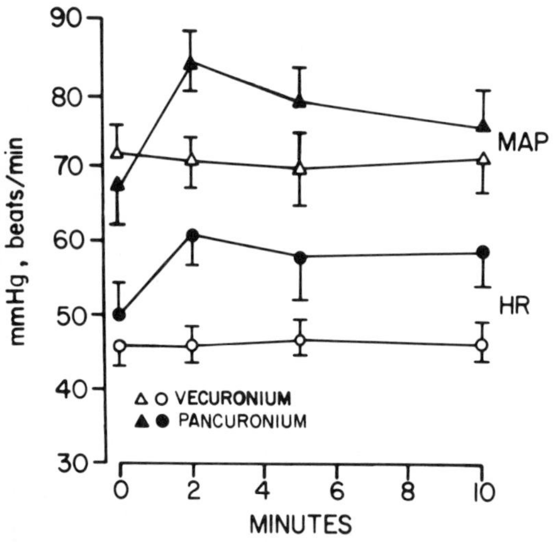

FIG. 12–1. Hemodynamic changes with pancuronium and vecuronium. Note that despite administration of a large dose, vecuronium produces little changes in cardiovascular function. Reproduced with kind permission from Stoelting RK: Choice of muscle relaxants in patients with heart disease. *In* Muscle Relaxants, Basic and Clinical Aspects (Edited by Katz RL). New York, Grune and Stratton, 1985.

be useful in some patients.[6] When rapid ventricular rates cause hemodynamic instability, a DC-cardioversion using 20 watt-second shocks must be performed.[15] Electrical cardioversion in a pregnant patient is not associated with any fetal problems. Paroxysmal atrial tachycardia is usually treated with digoxin. Resistant cases may need propranolol, DC-cardioversion, or temporary overdrive pacing.[8,15] All antiarrhythmic drugs cross the placenta and most of them are secreted in the breast milk.[6] Table 12–7 lists some antiarrhythmic drugs commonly used in pregnancy together with some fetal and maternal problems that may be caused by them.

MITRAL REGURGITATION

Pathophysiology

In more than half of all the patients suffering from mitral regurgitation, the disorder is caused by rheumatic heart disease. The condition also occurs as a result of congenital anomaly of the mitral valve, most commonly a defect of the endocardial cushions. In addition, functional regurgitation occurs as a result of marked left ventricular dilatation.[9] Mitral regurgitation is a self-accentuating condition because the enlarged left atrium puts traction on the posterior mitral leaflet, thereby causing more regurgitation.[8] Mitral regurgitation usually results in volume overload of the left atrium and the left ventricle. The amount of regurgitant flow depends on the systolic pressure gradient between the left atrium and the left ventricle, the duration

Table 12–7. Antiarrhythmic Drugs in Pregnancy

Drug	Indications	Serum level	UV/MV ratio	BM/MP ratio	Use in pregnancy
Digoxin	Paroxysmal SVT, rate control in atrial fibrillation and flutter.	1–2 μg/ml	1	1	Safe, probable intrauterine growth retardation.
Quinidine	Prophylaxis in atrial and ventricular tachyarrhythmias	2–5	1	1	Relatively safe, may cause premature labor
Procainamide	Rx and prevention of atrial and ventricular arrhythmias.	4–8	0.25	?	Relatively safe, lupus-like state.
Disopyramide	Atrial and ventricular tachyarrhythmias.	3–7	0.4	1	Premature labor possible, relatively safe
Propranolol	Rate control, hypertrophic cardiomyopathy, atrial fibrillation.		1	4	Intrauterine growth retardation with chronic administration, relatively safe.
Verapamil	Paroxysmal SVT, rate control in atrial fibrillation.	15–30 ng/ml	0.4	?	Maternal hypotension, relatively safe.
Lidocaine	PVC, digitoxicity.	2–4 μg/ml	0.6	1	Safe

Maternal vein (MV), umbilical vein (UV), breast milk (BM), Supraventricular tachycardia (SVT), maternal plasma (mp). Dilantin causes severe teratogenic effect (fetal hydantoin syndrome). Its chronic use is not recommended in pregnancy. It may be acutely used for the treatment of digitoxicity. Fetal hydantoin syndrome consists of craniofacial anomalies including cleft palate and mental retardation. (From Rotmensch HH, Elkayum U, and Frishman W: Antiarrhythmic drug therapy during pregnancy. Ann Int Med 98:487, 1983.

of the systole and the size of the mitral orifice. The patient will benefit whenever the regurgitant flow fraction decreases. In a patient with mitral regurgitation, the two outlets for blood flow from the left ventricle during systole are the left atrium (from regurgitant fraction), and the aorta (the real cardiac output). The regurgitant fraction produces the giant v-waves in the pulmonary artery pressure tracing[8] (Fig. 12–2). The presence of v-waves may lead to some confusion during wedge pressure measurements. When the regurgitant fraction exceeds 0.6, congestive heart failure develops. Patients with regurgitation usually have less evidence of pulmonary congestion than do patients with MS. In addition, hemoptysis and systemic embolization occurs less frequently.

Mitral regurgitation usually produces a holosytolic murmur at the apex. Compared to a slow heart rate, a normal or slightly increased heart rate will decrease the duration of the systole and therefore reduce the regurgitant flow. A reduced

ECG

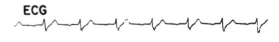

ARTERIAL PRESSURE

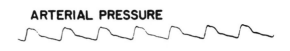

PULMONARY WEDGE PRESSURE

40-

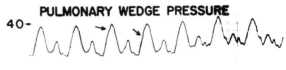

0-

FIG. 12–2. Large v waves in mitral regurgitation (arrow). (From Lake CL: Cardiovascular Anesthesia. New York, Springer-Verlag, 1985.)

preload will decrease the ventricular volume and will therefore decrease the regurgitant flow. Peripheral vasodilatation (reduced afterload) will allow more of the left ventricular output to reach the aorta and therefore decrease the regurgitant fraction. Mitral regurgitation is usually well tolerated in pregnancy. Some patients may actually improve during pregnancy because of the reduced afterload that normally occurs in pregnancy.[7]

Anesthetic Management

Table 12–5 offers some description of anesthetic considerations for mitral regurgitation.

Labor. When the left ventricular filling is increased acutely with volume overload, the compliance of the left ventricle decreases, favoring more regurgitant flow. Volume overload must therefore be avoided. For anesthetic management, a pulmonary artery catheter is useful because it helps to detect the presence of a v-wave. Epidural anesthesia is beneficial because it decreases peripheral vascular resistance, thus favoring a forward flow. By producing venous pooling, it may diminish the end-diastolic dimension of the left ventricle, further favoring forward flow. A lumbar epidural technique is thus useful for relieving labor pains.

Cesarean Section. Invasive monitoring of the pulmonary artery pressure and radial artery pressure must be considered. Lumbar epidural anesthesia is the technique of choice because it obivates the need for general anesthesia, which makes the left ventricle less compliant because of sympathetic stimulation. Lumbar epidural anesthesia may actually improve forward flow from the ventricle.

If general anesthesia is required, a combination of ketamine and fentanyl can be used for induction. Unlike patients with MS, patients with mitral regurgitation will benefit by an increased heart rate. If giant v-waves appear on the pulmonary artery tracing, or if the cardiac output falls, one may elect to improve the forward stroke volume with arterial vasodilators. Arterial vasodilators (such as sodium nitroprusside) are better in this regard than venodilators (such as nitroglycerin).[16] For maintenance, a high dose fentanyl technique is used (refer to the section on MS). Although the use of potent inhalation agents may seem beneficial because of their effect on systemic vascular resistance, their myocardial depressant property makes them less desirable than narcotics. Nitrous oxide increases pulmonary artery pressures in those with preexisting pulmonary artery hypertension. If any increase in pulmonary artery pressure is noted after the addition of N_2O, it should be promptly discontinued.[14]

MITRAL VALVE PROLAPSE

(Systolic click murmur syndrome)

Pathophysiology

With the advent of the echocardiography, the syndrome of mitral valve prolapse (MVP) is being diagnosed with increasing frequency. MVP results from the myxomatous degeneration of the mitral valve and it predominates in females of child-bearing age. The familial tendency suggests a pattern of autosomal dominant inheritance.[9] The condition frequently coexists with Marfan's syndrome or cystic medial necrosis. Occasionally, it may develop as a complication of mitral valvulotomy, ischemic heart disease, or cardiomyopathy. The symptoms usually include atypical chest pain, dyspnea, fatigue, dizziness, and syncope attributable to reduced cardiac output and/or cardiac arrhythmias. Arrhythmias include premature ventricular contractions and supraventricular tachycardia. An isolated midsystolic click with or without a late systolic murmur may be evident at the apex. An EKG shows low or inverted T-waves with or without ST changes. Echocardiography shows a 3 mm pansystolic sagging of one or both leaflets or it shows late systolic dipping of the leaflets (Fig. 12–3). Hypervolemia of pregnancy may modify or abolish the midsystolic click and murmur by mechanical realignment of the mitral valve apparatus.[17]

Anesthetic Considerations

An occasional patient may develop life threatening ventricular arrhythmias when subjected to emotional or physical stress caused by labor pains. Some EKG changes and arrhythmias respond to β-blockade. The degree of leaflet prolapse increases with a smaller ventricular volume. Conversely, an increased left ventricular

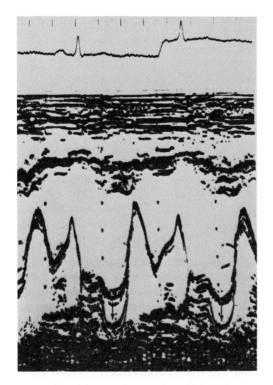

FIG. 12–3. The echocardiogram in mitral valve prolapse. Note the systolic hammocking of the mitral valve leaflet (arrows at the bottom). (From Lake CL: Cardiovascular Anesthesia. New York, Springer-Verlag, 1985.)

end-diastolic volume diminishes the tendency to prolapse.[9] Anesthetic management is aimed at adequate pain control during labor with epidural anesthesia or with intravenous narcotics. These patients also require antibiotic prophylaxis for the prevention of vegetative endocarditis. Epidural anesthesia is suitable for cesarean section. Systemic hypotension caused by epidural anesthesia diminishes end-diastolic volume by diminishing venous return,[18] thus predisposing to an increased tendency to prolapse.

AORTIC STENOSIS

Pathophysiology

Only 20% of patients with symptomatic aortic stenosis are females. Aortic stenosis develops secondary to rheumatic heart disease, a congenital anomaly of the valve, or an idiopathic calcification of the valve.[9] Because of the outflow obstruction, the left ventricle must generate a large pumping pressure. At intraventricular pressures above 250 to 300 mm Hg, myocardial ischemia develops. Over a period of time the left ventricle becomes less compliant and increasingly dependent on atrial contraction for adequate filling. Because a more prolonged systole is needed to eject a given quantity of blood in the presence of significant stenosis, the hypertrophied ventricle becomes vulnerable to ischemia. Any increase in the duration of diastole will reduce the time available for systole. The increased end-diastolic pressure, together with the reduced coronary perfusion pressure (because of the stenotic outflow tract), will reduce the subendocardial blood flow.

The ventricular wall tension, which is a major determinant of myocardial oxygen consumption, is high in patients with aortic stenosis. Patients may thus develop angina pectoris and metabolic evidence of myocardial ischemia (increased lactate production in the myocardium) even in the absence of coronary artery disease.

Exertional dyspnea, angina pectoris, and syncope are the cardinal symptoms of aortic stenosis. Any systemic vasodilatation may result in a reduction in cerebral perfusion pressure because of the inability of the left ventricle to increase its output. Orthopnea, paroxysmal exertional dyspnea, and pulmonary edema occur in advanced disease. The peripheral arterial pulse rises slowly to a sustained peak. The pulse recording shows a marked anacrotic notch, a delayed peak or coarse systolic vibrations. Chest auscultation usually reveals a crescendo-decrescendo murmur during systole at the second right intercostal space. The electrocardiogram reveals left ventricular hypertrophy, and in advanced cases, ST-segment depression, T-wave inversion in leads I and aV_L and in the precordial leads. The echocardiogram shows thickening of the left ventricular wall. Multiple bright echoes are seen when valvular calcification is present.[9] A chest x-ray may show the presence of calcium in the valve leaflets and poststenotic aortic dilatation.

Every attempt must be made to keep these patients in sinus rhythm because atrial systole aids in ventricular filling. Sudden development of atrial fibrillation causes rapid deterioration of patient's condition. A heart rate of 75 to 90 per minute is usually desirable. A heart rate slower than that does not necessarily cause an increase in stroke volume, especially in patients with a noncompliant ventricle. Should atrial fibrillation occur, cardioversion should be done promptly.

Anesthetic Considerations

In symptomatic patients, pulmonary and radial artery pressure must be continously monitored. Monitoring of the V_5 lead of the EKG help detect myocardial ischemia. Since the raised, left ventricular, end-diastolic pressure makes it necessary for the left atrium to produce a stronger than usual systolic contraction, a large a-wave is frequently noticed in the wedge tracing.[9] Under these circumstances, however, the left atrial mean pressure will not increase. It is thus likely that the mean PCWP may underestimate the left ventricular end-diastolic pressure. A true estimate of the end-diastolic pressure is the α-wave height of the wedge tracing.[19]

Labor Analgesia. Epidural anesthesia may not only produce acute vasodilatation but also result in reduction in preload as well. These two situations are poorly tolerated by these patients. Therefore, analgesia is provided by systemic medication. A segmental epidural anesthesia may be considered for producing labor analgesia in patients who do not obtain adequate relief with systemic medication. Should severe hypotension ensue, an infusion of phenylephrine may be considered. The use of epidural narcotics such as fentanyl for producing analgesia is valuable because they do not cause sympathetic denervation.

Cesarean Section. Because of the high sensory levels required for cesarean section, regional anesthesia is not recommended for cesarean section. These patients do well under general anesthesia. Since use of pentothal for induction is associated with severe myocardial depression, a high-dose narcotic technique is preferable (see the section on mitral stenosis). Balanced anesthesia with narcotics is usually preferable to inhalation agents for maintenance because of the possibility of myocardial depression with inhalation agents. Cardioversion is indicated if atrial fibrillation occurs in the periop-erative period.

AORTIC INSUFFICIENCY

Pathophysiology

Almost 75% of all patients with significant isolated regurgitation are males, and in three-fourths of these the valvular deformity is caused by rheumatic disease. However, the ratio of females increases when mitral valve disease co-exists.[9] Cystic medial necrosis of the aorta with or without Marfan's syndrome, or any other condition which causes dilatation of the ventricle (hypertension), may lead to functional regurgitation. In patients with rheumatic causes severe regurgitation may exist without producing any symptoms. The total stroke volume ejected by the heart equals the sum of the forward flow and the regurgitant flow. In contrast to mitral regurgitation, the entire left ventricular stroke volume must be emptied into a high pressure area, namely the aortic root. The increase in end-diastolic dimension of the ventricle constitutes a major hemodynamic compensation. According to La Place's law, the wall tension is the product of intracavity pressure and the radius of the ventricular cavity. A dilated ventricle has a greater radius of curvature, thus leading to increased wall tension required to generate a given ventricular pressure. As left ventricular function deteriorates, the end-diastolic volume further increases and the ejection fraction and forward stroke volume decrease.

Because of the regurgitant flow, the peripheral pulse rises rapidly and collapses suddenly. This occurrence is known as the water-hammer or Corrigan's pulse. The pulse pressure is usually widened. The magnitude of pulse pressure, however, does not correspond to the severity of regurgitation. A diastolic thrill is usually palpable in the left sternal border. A systolic thrill caused by increased flow in the aorta and the carotid arteries may be felt in the jugular notch. The murmur of aortic regurgitation is usually a high-pitched decrescendo variety heard best in the third left intercostal space. In severe regurgitation, a soft, low-pitched rumbling mid-diastolic or presystolic bruit (Austin Flint murmur) is heard at the apex of the heart. An electrocardiogram may indicate left ventricular hypertrophy and signs of ischemia. Aortic insufficiency is usually well-tolerated in pregnant patients because of increased vasodilatation, which improves the forward flow.

Anesthetic Considerations

Invasive monitoring with radial artery cannula and a pulmonary artery catheter is helpful in advanced cases. Bradycardia should be be avoided because it gives the left ventricle a chance to overdistend, thus increasing left atrial distention and pulmonary artery back pressure. A moderate tachycardia will raise diastolic pressure in the aorta, and therefore, will increase coronary perfusion. In addition, slight increases in heart rate will diminish left ventricular end-diastolic pressure and volume, which further improves coronary perfusion. Epidural anesthesia affects both preload and afterload. Preload is decreased as a result of dilatation of the capacitance bed by the loss of sympathetic tone and afterload as a result of dilatation of the capacitance bed by the loss of sympathetic tone and afterload as a result of arteriolar vasodilatation. These patients will therefore benefit from epidural block for both labor analgesia and for cesarean section. Because volume overloading will result in overdistention of the ventricle, fluid infusion must be done with the aid of pulmonary artery pressure measurement. See Table 12–5 for important precautions to be observed during anesthesia.

HYPERTROPHIC CARDIOMYOPATHY

Pathophysiology

In the developing mammalian heart, the interventricular septum is disproportionately thick compared to the posterobasal free left ventricular wall. However, it undergoes regression and reaches normal thickness in the full-term neonate.[20] It has been postulated that failure of the septum to regress results in hypertrophic cardiomyopathy. Adrenergic stimulation of the receptor sites located at the septum by extracardiac catecholamines is believed to result in hypertrophy. The abnormal interaction between the norepinephrine and the receptors causes extensive septal cellular disarray. The basic functional derangement is the dynamic obstruction caused by increased left ventricular contractility.

Increased contractility reduces ventricular systolic volume and increases the flow velocity across the valve. The increased flow draws the anterior mitral valve leaflet close to the septum, thus increasing obstruction. Decreased preload causes narrowing of the outflow tract and decreased afterload will increase flow velocity and at the same time reduce ventricular volume,[8] both of which conditions favor outflow obstruction. The mainstay of diagnosis is echocardiography, which shows left ventricular hypertrophy and disproportionate septal thickness. The two typical hemodynamic features are elevated left ventricular end-diastolic pressure caused by diminished compliance and a pressure gradient between the main chamber and the outflow region of the left ventricle. Digitalis, diuretics, β-agonists, and nitrates usually worsen the condition and therefore are best avoided. Similarly Valsalva maneuvers (bearing-down during second stage) may cause further impairment.

Although the disease progresses slowly over many years, it occasionally may cause sudden death in a person with no previous history. Medical treatment with β-adrenergic blockers or calcium entry blockers has been successful. The symptomatology usually depends on the degree of obstruction. The carotid pulse has a typical spike-dome pattern because the flow in the carotid arteries is brisk at first, followed by diminished pressure as obstruction increases. This is followed by a second peak as ejection proceeds against obstruction (bifid pulse).

Oakley et al.[21] reported their experience in 54 pregnancies in 23 patients with the condition. Ten patients developed dyspnea during pregnancy, but they responded to diuretics. There were no maternal or infant mortality in their series. They advise against the routine use of β-blockers in pregnant patients, and recommend that the decision to use them be made on an individual basis. Cesarean section is reserved only for obstetric indication.

Anesthetic Considerations

Labor. Labor pains cause an increase in circulating catecholamine concentrations thus resulting in increased cardiac contractility. Pain relief can be obtained by producing epidural analgesia with a combination of fentanyl and local anesthetic (see the section on MS). Bearing-down efforts produce maternal fatigue and must therefore be kept to a minimum. Any hypotension is treated with small doses of phenylephrine. Ephedrine is an inotrope and therefore may enhance outflow obstruction. Because both preload and afterload influence the degree of outflow obstruction, monitoring of pulmonary artery pressure is recommended.

Cesarean Section. The anesthetic considerations of aortic stenosis also apply to this condition (vide supra). Regional anesthesia may cause sudden hypotension and diminish the end-diastolic volume, worsening outflow obstruction. Tachycardia also diminishes outflow. Intravenous lidocaine injection is used to blunt some of the autonomic responses to intubation. The use of an inhalation agent, such as halothane 0.5%, is beneficial in decreasing outflow obstruction because of its negative inotropic effect. Oxytocin, when needed, should be administered as a dilute infusion. A bolus injection of oxytocin (10 U) may cause systemic hypotension. Methyl ergometrine (0.2 mg) will increase both systemic and pulmonary artery pressure,[22] thus it must be used with caution.

PROSTHETIC HEART VALVES

Pathophysiology

Successful pregnancy is possible after cardiac valve replacement. Both mechanical (Starr-Edwards prosthesis) and porcine xenografts have been used for valve replacement. The use of the xenograft obviates the need for anticoagulants.[23] In the series reported by Deviri, et al.,[23] patients with bioprosthetic valves were not treated with anticoagulants. Their patients did not have an increased incidence of thromboembolic complication during pregnancy, and the fetal outcome was generally satisfactory. Anticoagulation, however, must be used in those who are in atrial fibrillation or in those who have a history of previous thromboembolism.[24] Fetal wastage is increased in those patients who are chronically anticoagulated.[25] The incidence of congenital malformations is also higher after warfarin therapy. Heparin has also recently been implicated in causing increased fetal wastage.[26] Some workers have used dipyridamole (an antiplatelet drug) for anticoagulation in pregnancy.[27] The safety of this regimen is not well established

because it has received only limited clinical trial. Mitral valve prosthesis is associated with increased incidence of thromboembolic complication. Although fetal problems are increased in patients with prosthetic heart valves, maternal complication caused by either cardiovascular instability or thromboembolic complication seems to be minimal.[25] Closed mitral valvotomy during pregnancy has gained some popularity in the recent years. Closed mitral valvotomy provides safe and effective relief of symptoms in pregnant patients.[28] The prognosis for long-term survival remains excellent. The indication for closed mitral valvotomy in pregnancy is dyspnea at bed rest, which is refractory to medical therapy.

Anesthetic Considerations

Patients who have a normal exercise tolerance after valve replacement may not require any special monitoring. However, those who are symptomatic or show evidence of congestive heart failure must have their radial artery and pulmonary artery pressure continuously monitored. Regional anesthesia is contraindicated in patients who are fully anticoagulated. Chapter 16 Thromboembolism discusses anesthetic considerations in a patient on anticoagulant therapy. Other problems associated with valve prosthesis include paravalvular leaks, and vegetative endocarditis, and some degree of hemolysis. Aortic prosthesis is more often associated with hemolysis than is mitral prosthesis.[9] Thrombocytopenia may also occur occasionally in patients with malfunctioning valves. Red cell survival studies, serum iron, and reticulocyte count may be needed to detect subclinical hemolysis. Platelet count and prothrombin and partial thromboplastin time measurements must be obtained regardless of the presence of anticoagulation.

PERIPARTAL CARDIOMYOPATHY

Pathophysiology

Any cardiomyopathy presenting in the last month of pregnancy or the first six months after delivery without obvious cause is included in this category.[29–31] The incidence is said to be much higher in parts of Africa. The majority of patients in this country are black.[30] The commonest time of onset is the first month of the postpartum period (40%). Approximately 5% will develop the condition in the last month of pregnancy. Multiple gestation places the patient at a slightly increased risk. The maternal mortality ranges between 30 to 60% and the infant mortality is close to 10%.

The cardiac chambers particularly on the left side undergo dilatation with hypertrophy. Myofibrils appear enlarged and disorganized with a great increase in the mitochondrial population. There may be endocardial thickening with mural thrombi. However, none of the histopathologic findings in this condition are specific or pathognomonic. Cardiac involvement in preeclampsia may mimic this condition. In preeclamptic cardiac disease, however, neither arrhythmias nor cardiac enlargement is seen.[31]

The basic functional derangement is the loss of ventricular contractile power and reduction in the ejection fraction. The left ventricular end-diastolic pressure is raised. The pulmonary artery pressure may be raised slightly but severe pulmonary hypertension is an exception rather than the rule. Symptoms include dyspnea, orthopnea, cough, hemoptysis, palpitation, abdominal pain, and chest pain. Physical signs include cardiomegaly, gallop, rales, and severe edema of the legs. In addition, the first heart sound may be decreased in intensity and the pulse pressure may be low because of systolic hypotension. The EKG usually shows low voltage, abnormalities of the T wave and the ST segment, as well as left ventricular hypertrophy and intraventricular conduction defects. Atrial and ventricular arrhythmias are not uncommon. An echocardiogram may show reduced ejection fraction and the presence of mural thrombi. Pulmonary and systemic emboli may occur in 20 to 40% of cases.

Treatment is generally directed toward controlling heart failure with bed rest, digitalis, and diuretics. The use of vasodilators such as prazosin, which dilates both the capacitance and resistance beds has been recommended.[31] Refractory cases may respond to salbutamol a selective β_2 agonist, which increases the ejection fraction.

Occasionally, cardiomyopathy is the result of a recent bout of myocarditis, in which case, steroids are beneficial. Immunosuppression may be considered in cases of inflammatory myocarditis. The diagnosis of myocarditis is usually confirmed by endomyocardial biopsy obtained during cardiac catheterization. In addition, full anticoagulation is necessary to prevent embolic complication. Electrical cardioversion may be necessary to control severe atrial arrhythmias. The mode of delivery is usually vaginal and cesarean section is reserved for obstetric indication. If there is evidence of residual myocardial involvement, future pregnancies are contraindicated.

Anesthetic Considerations

These patients will not be able to tolerate even the slightest reduction in afterload. Therefore, regional anesthesia is suitable for both labor analgesia and for cesarean section. All patients with peripartal cardiomyopathy must be monitored with an indwelling arterial cannula and a pulmonary artery catheter. Labor analgesia may be produced by using intravenous agents. If anesthesia is required for cesarean section, general anesthesia is administered using high-dose fentanyl technique. Ketamine or etomidate may be suitable for induction.[8] The use of pentothal and other potent inhalation agents must be avoided because of the possibility of myocardial depression. The preload must be maintained at normal levels during surgery and in the postoperative period.

CONGENITAL HEART DISEASE

COARCTATION OF THE AORTA

The mortality rate for patients with unoperated aortic coarctation reaches 3.5%. Uncontrolled hypertension leading to cerebrovascular accident and vegetative endocarditis are the common problems. The blood pressure may rise acutely during labor. The use of nitroprusside and/or epidural anesthesia may be needed to blunt the hypertensive response to labor pains. The degree of mechanical aortic compression usually increases during a uterine contraction, causing a further increase in blood pressure.

PULMONARY HYPERTENSION

PRIMARY PULMONARY HYPERTENSION

Pulmonary hypertension (PH) can either be primary or secondary. When no cause can be ascertained the condition is termed the primary PH. It constitutes less than 1% of all cases of PH. The primary PH occurs more frequently in females of childbearing age. Pregnancy may either trigger the condition or aggravate it. PH is thought to be present if the pulmonary artery (PA) pressure exceeds 30/15 mm Hg with a mean pressure of 25 mm Hg or higher. The disease involves smaller branches of pulmonary artery between 40 and 300 μM in diameter. The affected vessels undergo medial hypertrophy and intimal hyperplasia. The use of oral contraceptives has been implicated as an etiologic factor. The right atrial pressure is elevated and giant a-waves are usually detected.[9] In some patients, a favorable outcome has been noted with the use of diazoxide or hydralazine.

Secondary Pulmonary Hypertension (Eisenmenger's Syndrome)

Secondary PH is usually produced by cardiac shunts at aortopulmonary (patent ductus arteriosus), atrial (atrial septal defect), or ventricular level (ventricular septal defect).[32] A bidirectional cardiac shunt and serious pulmonary artery hypertension are hallmarks of the condition. The maternal mortality reaches a staggering 26% (Table 12–8), and fetal mortality is 40 to 45%.[33] The pulmonary hypertension causes severe hypertrophy of the muscular wall of the pulmonary artery branches (Fig. 12–4). The symptoms and signs include central cyanosis, polycythemia, clubbing of the fingers, exertional dyspnea, and syncopal attacks. A sudden fall in systemic vascular resistance will favor the development of a right or left shunt with the result that the arterial desaturation will further worsen. Systemic hypotension will predispose to such a shunt reversal. Valsalva maneuver (bearing-down efforts), hypoxia, acidosis, hypercardia, increased left atrial pressure (volume overload) will further elevate pulmonary artery pressure.[34] The presence of severe pulmonary hypertension precludes any corrective surgery because the increased pulmonary vascular resistance may persist or worsen after surgery.

Anesthetic Considerations. Although there are isolated reports of successful epidural anesthesia[34] in these patients, many authors would seem to agree general anesthesia is the technique of choice for cesarean section because even a small reduction in systemic vascular resistance (as may be caused by epidural anesthesia) may produce shunt reversal.[35] An alternate approach to producing labor pain relief is to use intrathecal or epidural narcotics, which may produce long-lasting pain relief in some patients. It is customary to use a local anesthetic test dose prior to the injection of the epidural narcotic. Because even a test dose may occasionally cause systemic hypotension, a smaller than usual test dose may be used, or the test dose may be completely omitted. In that case, the epidural catheter must be carefully aspirated to rule out the possibility of accidental intrathecal placement. Any form of regional anesthesia is contraindicated if anticoagulation is being used.

An indwelling radial artery cannula is needed for repeated measurements of Pa_{O_2} to detect unexpected arterial desaturation. A pulse oximeter can also be used for this purpose. Although it is tempting to suggest the routine use of a pulmonary artery catheter, the advantages must be carefully weighed against the disadvantages. The possible complications of pulmonary artery catheter in these patients include pulmonary artery rupture, which is always a danger in patients with a high pulmonary artery pressure, paradoxical air-embolus, severe arrhythmias, increased incidence of pulmonary artery thrombosis, and the limited usefulness of the pulmonary artery catheter.[34] Although pulmonary artery pressures are helpful in determining pressure gradients between the left and the right heart in patients with interatrial shunts, it is not helpful for this purpose in patients with interventricular shunts because of the possibility of abnormally high right-heart pressures. In addition, thermodilution cardiac outputs may be misleading because of the varying degree of the diversion of the "coolth" through the shunt.[35] Anticoagulation poses further hazard during cannulation of central veins.

Barbiturates cause a reduction in systemic arterial pressure in addition to myocardial depres-

Table 12–8.   Maternal Mortality in Eisenmenger's Syndrome

Patient	Gestation (weeks)	Procedure	Finding
1	31	Undelivered	Heart failure, pulmonary embolus, pneumonitis.
2	34	NSVD	Died 6 hour postpartum.
3	37	Cesarean	Died 8th postpartum day.
4	39	Cesarean	Died 3rd postpartum day, 400 ml blood in the abdomen.
5		Vaginal hysterectomy	7th postpartum week.
6		NSVD	Died 22nd postpartum day.
7		Ruptured ectopic	Intraoperative death.
8	35	Labor	Toxemia, died intrapartum.
9	37	Low forceps	Toxemia, died 4th day postpartum.
10	36	NSVD	Postpartum hemorrhage, died 4th day.
11	30	Cesarean	Intraoperative cardiac arrest.
12	23	Cesarean	Died 6th postoperative day.

NSVD = normal spontaneous vaginal delivery. (From Gummerus M, and Laasonen H: Eisenmenger complex and pregnancy. Ann Chir Gynecol, 70:339, 1981.)

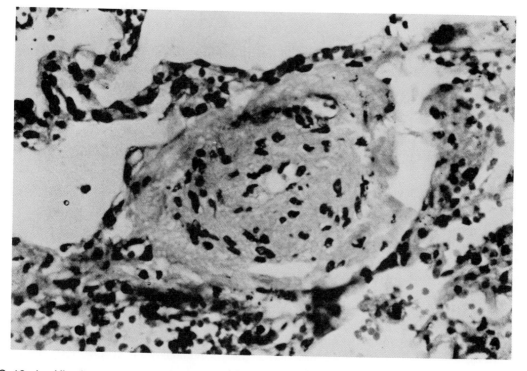

FIG. 12–4.   Histologic section of a small pulmonary artery (center) of a patient with advanced Eisenmenger's syndrome. Note the almost complete obliteration of the lumen caused by medial hypertrophy and intimal hyperplasia. (From Pitts JA, Crosby WM, and Basta LL: Eisenmenger's syndrome in pregnancy. Am Heart J 93:321, 1977.)

sion. Although ketamine may increase the pulmonary artery pressure, it may be less detrimental than pentothal.[9] Diazepam, etomidate, and midazolam do cause a reduction in systemic blood pressure during induction. However, a careful titration of the dose may help minimize some of the deleterious cardiovascular effects. A high-dose narcotic anesthesia with fentanyl is also very suitable (see the section on mitral stenosis). Because of the decreased pulmonary blood flow, the rate of rise of arterial concentration of inhalation anesthetic agents may be slowed, an effect more noticeable with the more soluble agents.[36] An additional problem with inhalation agents such as enflurane, halothane, and isoflurane is their ability to depress the myocardium and diminish the peripheral vascular resistance. The use of N_2O may further increase the pulmonary vascular resistance and therefore its use is not recommended. Air bubbles in intravenous solutions must be avoided because of the fear of paradoxical embolus. Blood loss is not well tolerated; therefore replacement therapy must be quick and adequate.

CARDIAC SHUNTS WITH LEFT-TO-RIGHT SHUNTS

Intra- and extracardiac shunts may occur without a shunt reversal. The left heart pressures are higher than the right heart pressures; therefore the shunt flow occurs from the left-to-right usually. However, this poses an increased workload on the left heart, which will ultimately fail. Over a period of time, pulmonary hypertension develops. The shunts that are commonly seen are the atrial septal defect, the ventricular septal defect and the patent ductus arteriosus. Asymptomatic patients may require no additional precautions; however, patients with congestive heart failure must be adequately treated. A segmental epidural anesthesia is helpful in diminishing systemic vascular resistance and promoting forward flow. The possibility of paradoxical embolus, infective endocarditis, brain abscess, and cardiac arrhythmias must be borne in mind, and the appropriate preventive measures instituted.

FALLOT'S TETRALOGY

Another cause of right-to-left shunt is the tetralogy of Fallot, which consists of infundibular pulmonary artery stenosis, right ventricular hypertrophy, overriding aorta, and a ventricular septal defect. This is the most common cyanotic congenital heart disease. The severity of pulmonic stenosis appears to be the most important determinant of the hemodynamic status of the patient. Systemic hypotension promotes increased right-to-left flow. Similarly, increases in right ventricular outflow obstruction (positive pressure ventilation) increases right-to-left flow. Patients often assume a squatting position to increase the impedance of left ventricular outflow and increase pulmonary artery blood flow, which improves arterial oxygen saturation. Polycythemia, clubbing, increased tendency to fibrinolysis, low platelet count, and thromboembolic complications are often present. Without corrective surgery in childhood, these patients do not usually reach childbearing age. Patients with unrepaired tetralogy usually deteriorate during pregnancy because of the decreasing peripheral vascular resistance, which increases the right-to-left shunt. Poor prognostic signs include a hematocrit above 60%, oxygen saturation less than 60%, and recurrent syncopal attacks.[7] All anesthetic considerations that apply to primary and secondary PH apply to these patients as well. The use of intrathecal narcotics may be considered for labor analgesia. For cesarean section, general anesthesia is recommended. The use of halothane may decrease the outflow obstruction in the pulmonary infundibulum, thus augmenting pulmonary blood flow. The uptake of halothane, however, may be prolonged because of the reduced pulmonary blood flow. Therefore, intravenous anesthetics (a high-dose narcotic technique) may be the agents of choice. Ketamine not only increases pulmonary vascular resistance but also aggravates right ventricular outflow obstruction (see hypertrophic cardiomyopathy). A small dose of phenylephrine may increase systemic vascular resistance and improve pulmonary blood flow. Propranolol 0.05 to 0.1 mg/kg has also been recommended to decrease right ventricular outflow obstruction. A pulse oximeter must be used to monitor arterial saturation continuously.

EBSTEIN'S ANOMALY

In this condition, a portion of the septal and posterior leaflets of the tricuspid valve is attached to the right ventricular wall rather than to the annulus fibrosus. Therefore, a large portion of the right ventricle becomes a part of the right atrium, thus interfering with right ventricular filling. The right atrium is massively enlarged and an atrial septal defect may coexist. A blowing sytolic murmur is heard along the left sternal border. The EKG may show giant peaked P waves, a prolonged PQ interval, right bundle branch block, and occasionally, Wolff-Parkinson-White syndrome.[8] Many patients can reach reproductive age, although their functional status varies widely.[37] Many of these patients may be asymptomatic, wherease others develop cyanosis and dyspnea. Echocardiography, which is useful in delineating the right ventricle, helps obviate the need for cardiac catheterization.

Pulmonary embolization is a constant hazard in these patients. They are particularly prone to the supraventricular arrhythmias, especially during the insertion of a Swan-Ganz catheter. For anesthetic management an indwelling arterial cannula and a pulse oximeter may be helpful. Induction with an intravenous agent may take longer than usual because of the enlarged right atrium. Drugs that produce tachycardia (pancuronium, atropine) are best avoided.[8] A high-dose narcotic technique can be used. Epidural anesthsia has been used safely for cesarean section.[37,38]

MARFAN'S SYNDROME

Marfan's syndrome is a generalized connective tissue disorder. Myxomatous degeneration of the aortic wall occurs that may lead to aortic dilatation, rupture, and dissection of the aortic wall,[7] especially during labor. The increased dissection rate in a pregnant patient has been attributed to increased estrogen levels.[7] Aortic and/or mitral valves may be involved as well. A long narrow face, arachnodactyly, high arched palate, and ectopia lentis are the other features. The high-arched palate may render tracheal intubation difficult. Epidural anesthesia may be of advantage because it obviates the need for tracheal intubation and decreases the hypertensive response to labor pains, thus minimizing the

likelihood of aortic dissection. Awake intubation using a fiber-optic bronchoscope should be considered in patients with an abnormally arched palate (when general anesthesia is needed). All patients with Marfan's syndrome are at risk for developing endocarditis. Severe cases may also have kyphoscoliosis causing respiratory embarrassment and recurrent pneumothoraces.[8]

MYOCARDIAL INFARCTION

The incidence of myocardial infarction (MI) during pregnancy and the postpartum period is 1:10,000. The incidence of coronary artery disease among young women is increasing probably because of the increase of cigarette smoking among this group. More and more women are delaying first pregnancy until they are 35 or older. Myocardial infarction has been reported in patients less than 25 years of age.[39] The maternal mortality rate has reached 35% with most of the deaths occurring either in the third trimester or in the postpartum period (Table 12–9). If the initial infarction occurs in the third trimester, many women will die before delivery can be accomplished. Of these who survive the initial episode, the mortality rate is high (50%), if the patient is delivered within 14 days of the initial infarction.[39] Left anterior descending and left main coronary vessels are the ones commonly involved. Peripartum events, including labor pains and bearing-down efforts, may increase myocardial oxygen consumption. Patients who have suffered an infarct should continue their nitrites and/or β-blockers during pregnancy and labor.

Invasive monitoring is not necessary in all postinfarct patients. However, a patient with a history of a recent infarct or unstable angina, or a patient who is in congestive heart failure may require invasive monitoring. Lead II and a modified V_5 lead must be monitored to detect myocardial ischemia. Ventricular diastolic function deteriorates in patients with myocardial ischemia, leading to restricted diastolic filling. Increase in the amplitudes of the a- or v-waves of the pulmonary artery pressure tracing may occur with the simultaneous development of signs of ischemia (ST-segment changes). A rise in pulmonary artery pressure is therefore an early sign of ischemia. The central venous pressure is usually not reliable under these circumstances. Pa-

Table 12–9. Maternal Mortality with Myocardial Infarction

Outcome	I trimester		II trimester		III trimester		Total percent
	Number	Death	Number	Death	Number	Death	
Died, undelivered	0	0	3	3	11	11	100
Delivered within 14 days of infarction	1	1	0	0	15	7	50
Delivered after 14 days of infarction	8	0	12	0	14	0	0
Recurrent infarction	0	0	2	2	2	1	75
Total	9	1	17	5	42	19	25

(From Hankins GDV, Wendel GD, Leveno KJ and Stoneham J: Myocardial infarction during pregnancy: A review. Obstet Gynecol 65:139, 1985.)

tients with an end-diastolic pressure of >18 mm Hg and an ejection fraction <0.4 and/or patients who have had an infarct in the last 3 months are candidates for pulmonary artery catheter.[9]

Anesthetic Considerations

Lumbar epidural anesthesia is the recommended technique for labor analgesia, because it blunts the hemodynamic responses to labor pains that place additional burden on the myocardium. Epidural anesthesia can also be used for cesarean section. One should, however, look for signs of intraoperative ischemia (EKG, pulmonary artery pressure) and institute therapy immediately. Ketamine and atropine, which produce tachycardia, must be avoided. In patients with normal ventricular function, a slow induction with halothane is used. Patients must have been pretreated with antacids to increase the gastric fluid pH and the cricoid pressure must be continuously applied until the endotracheal tube is safely inserted. Lidocaine may be administered to blunt the hemodynamic responses. Maintenance of anesthesia is performed using 0.5% halothane with vecuronium being added to produce muscle relaxation. In those with poor ventricular function, a high-dose narcotic technique may be used for induction and maintenance. If the patient develops tachycardia in response to intubation or skin incision, it is controlled with propranolol. Sodium nitroprusside may be needed to control arterial pressure. Intraoperative ischemia caused by tachycardia may be treated with propranolol. Ischemia caused by increased preload or afterload (diastolic dysfunction) may respond to nitroglycerin (Fig. 12–5).[9] Invasive monitoring must be maintained for a week in the postpartum period because many deaths are known to have occurred during this period.[39]

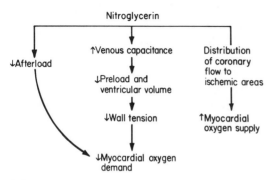

FIG. 12–5. Beneficial effects of nitroglycerin in coronary artery disease. (From Lake CL: Cardiovascular Anesthesia. New York, Springer-Verlag, 1985.)

REFERENCES

1. Sugrue D, Blake S, and McDonald D: Pregnancy complicated by maternal heart disease in National Maternity Hospital, Dublin, Ireland, 1969–1978. Am J Obstet Gynecol 139:1, 1981.
2. Joyce TH: Cardiac disease. In Obstetric Anesthesia: The Complicated Patient. (Edited by James FM, and Wheeler AS). Philadelphia, FA Davis, 1982.
3. Pritchard JA, McDonald PC, and Gant NF: Medical and surgical illness during pregnancy and the puerperium. In Williams Obstetrics. 17th Edition. Norwalk, Appleton-Century-Crofts, 1985.
4. Sugrue D, Blake S, Troy P, and MacDonald D: Antibiotic prophylaxis against infective endocarditis after normal delivery—is it necessary? Br Heart J 44:499, 1980.
5. McNaulty JH, Metcalfe J, and Ueland K: General guidelines in the management of cardiac disease. Clin Obstet Gynecol 24:773, 1981.

6. Rotmensch HH, Elkayam U, and Frishman W: Antiarrhythmic drug therapy during pregnancy. Ann Int Med 98:487, 1983.

7. Lang RM and Borow KM: Pregnancy and heart disease. Clin Perinatol 12:551, 1985.

8. Petersdorf RD, et al. (Eds.): Congenital heart disease. *In* Harrison's Principles of Internal Medicine. New York, McGraw-Hill Book Co., 1983, 1383–1449.

9. Lake CL: Cardiovascular Anesthesia. New York, Springer-Verlag, 1985.

10. Spitzer RC, et al.: Serious arrhythmias during labor and delivery in women with heart disease. JAMA 211:1005, 1970.

11. Clark SL, et al.: Experience with pulmonary artery catheter in obstetrics and gynecology. Am J Obstet Gynecol 152:374, 1985.

12. Stoelting RK: Choice of muscle relaxants in patients with heart disease. *In* Muscle Relaxants: Basic and clinical aspects. (Edited by Katz RL). New York, Grune and Stratton, 1985.

13. Morris RB, et al.: Clinical pharmacology of (ORG NC 45) and pancuronium in patients undergoing coronary artery bypass grafting. Anesthesiology 58:438, 1983.

14. Schulte-Sasse U, Hess W, and Tarnow J: Pulmonary vascular responses to nitrous oxide in patients with normal and high pulmonary vascular resistance. Anesthesiology 57:9, 1982.

15. Cullhead I: Cardioversion during pregnancy. Acta Med Scand 214:169, 1983.

16. Pierpoint GL, and Talley RC: Pathophysiology of valvar heart disease. Arch Int Med 142:998, 1982.

17. Haas JM: The effect of pregnancy on the mid-systolic click and murmur of the prolapsing posterior leaflet of the mitral valve. Am Heart J 92:407, 1976.

18. Ramanathan S, Grant GJ, and Turndorf H: Cardiac preload changes with ephedrine therapy for hypotension in obstetrical patients. Anesth Analg 65:S125, 1986.

19. Lee SJK, et al.: Hemodynamic changes at rest and during exercise in patients with aortic stenosis of varying severity. Am Heart J 79:318, 1970.

20. Perloff JK: Pathogenesis of hypertrophic cardiomyopathy. Am Heart J 101:219, 1981.

21. Oakley GDG, McGarry K, Limb DG, and Oakley CM: Management of pregnancy in patients with hypertrophic cardiomyopathy. Br Med J 1:1749, 1979.

22. Secher NJ, Arnsbo P, and Wallin L: Hemodynamic effects of oxytocin (Syntocinon) and methyl ergometrine on the systemic and pulmonary circulations of pregnant anesthetized women. Acta Obstet Gynecol Scand 57:97, 1978.

23. Deviri E, Levinski L, Yechezkel M, and Levy JM: Pregnancy after valve replacement with porcine xenograft prosthesis. Surg Gynecol Obstet 160:437, 1985.

24. Bodnar AG, and Hutter A: Anticoagulation in valvular heart disease preoperatively and postoperatively. Cardiovasc Clin 14:247, 1984.

25. Lutz DJ, et al.: Pregnancy and its complications following cardiac valve prosthesis. Am J Obstet Gynecol 131:460, 1978.

26. Hall JH, Pauli RM, and Wilson KM: Maternal and fetal sequelae of anticoagulation during pregnancy. Am J Med 68:132, 1980.

27. Ibarra-Perez C, Arevalo-Toledo N, Alvarez-De La Cadena O, Noriega-Guerra L: The course of pregnancy in patients with artificial heart valves. Am J Med 61:504, 1976.

28. Cummerford PJ, Hastie T, and Beck W: Closed mitral valvotomy: Actual analysis of results in 654 patients over 12 years and analysis of preoperative predictors of longterm survival. Ann Thor Surg 33:473, 1982.

29. Homans DC: Current concepts. Peripartum cardiomyopathy. N Engl J Med 312:1432, 1985.

30. Veille JC: Peripartum cardiomyopathies: A review. Am J Obstet Gynecol 148:805, 1984.

31. Julian DG, and Szekely P: Peripartum cardiomyopathy. Prog Cardiovasc Dis 27:223, 1985.

32. Pitts JA, Crosby WM, and Basta LL: Eisenmenger's syndrome in pregnancy. Am Heart J 93:321, 1977.

33. Gummerus M, and Laasonen H: Eisenmenger complex and pregnancy. Ann Chir Gynaecol 70:339, 1981.

34. Midwall J, Jaffin H, Herman MV, and Kupersmith J: Shunt flow and pulmonary hemodynamics during labor and delivery in the Eisenmenger syndrome. Am J Cardiol 42:299, 1978.

35. Foster JMG, and Jones RM: The anesthetic management of the Eisenmenger syndrome. Ann R Coll Surg Engl 66:353, 1984.

36. Stoelting R, and Longnecker D: Effect of right to left shunt on rate of increase of arterial anesthetic concentration. Anesthesiology 36:352, 1972.

37. Waickman LA, et al.: Ebstein's anomaly in pregnancy. Am J Cardiol 53:357, 1984.

38. Linter SPK, and Clarke K: Cesarean section under extradural analgesia in a patient with Ebstein's anomaly. Br J Anaesth 56:203, 984.

39. Hankins GDV, Wendel GD, Leveno KJ, and Stoneham J: Myocardial infarction during pregnancy: A review. Obstet Gynecol 65:139, 1985.

13

ENDOCRINE DISORDERS

THYROID DISEASE

Thyroid dysfunction occurs in 5% of all pregnancies.[1] Because the thyroid secretion is altered in pregnancy, thyroid function tests must be interpreted with caution. In addition, some symptoms of thyroid disease such as fatigue, tachycardia, and a slight enlargement of the thyroid gland are often seen in normal pregnant women. Antithyroid drugs cross the placenta with the result that they may produce hypothyroidism or goiter in the fetus. Severe thyroid dysfunction, such as thyroid storm, may also occur during pregnancy. Please see Chapter 2 Maternal Adaptation to Pregnancy for a discussion on pregnancy induced changes in thyroid function.

THYROID FUNCTION TESTS

About 90% of thyroid secretion consists of thyroxine (T_4) and the other 10% is triiodothyronine (T_3). A considerable portion of the T_4 is converted in the peripheral tissues to T_3. The T_3 hormone is more potent than is the T_4 hormone, but its duration of action is shorter. Both hormones, however, produce similar effects in the body.[2] Both hormones are stored in the acinus of the thyroid gland as thyroglobulin (MW 660.000). The thyroid gland is capable of trapping iodine from blood. The iodine is oxidized by the peroxidase enzyme and the oxidized iodine binds with tyrosine to form mono-, di-, and triiodothyronine (T_3). Two molecules of diiodothyronine unite to form thyroxine (T_4). All these hormones form within the thryoglobulin. The T_3 and T_4 are released into the blood stream by pinocytosis. Upon release from the gland, both hormones are bound by plasma proteins (globulin, prealbumin, and albumin). The T_3 hormone is bound more avidly by proteins than is T_4. When injected systemically, the T_4 has a latency of 1 to 2 days, with a prolonged duration of action. On the other hand, the T_3 effects may be seen in hours, but they do not last longer than 2 to 3 days.[2] The differences in their action are probably a result of their dissimilar protein binding. Some of the T_4 is also converted in the periphery to form "reverse T_3," a metabolically inactive compound, by the removal of one of the iodine atoms from the T_4 molecule. The release of thyroid hormones occurs in response to thyroid stimulating hormone (TSH) of the anterior pituitary. The release of TSH is regulated by the hypothalamic neurohormone, thyrotropin-releasing hormone (TRH).

The concentrations of thyroxine binding globulin (TBG) and of total T_3 and T_4 double between 8 and 12 weeks of gestation. The concentration of free thyroxine may remain unchanged or decrease slightly with the result that the patient is euthyroid.[3] The measurement of free thyroxine is the most accurate test because it is not affected by changes in the concentration of the binding proteins. Measurement of free hormone is usually not available in many laboratories.[4] Radioactive T_3 uptake by resin (RT_3U) is an indirect measure of the thyroxine-binding protein sites in the serum. The free thyroxine index (FT_4I) is an indirect measure of the free hormone activity. It is calculated from the total T_4 and the ratio between RT_3U levels in the patients and in the general population.[3]

Free T_4 index

$$= \text{Total } T_4 \times \frac{\text{Patient's } RT_3U}{\text{Mean normal } RT_3U}$$

Free T_3 index may be calculated by substituting T_3 for T_4 in the above equation. The concentration of TSH can be measured by radioimmunoassay. Normal values of TSH in pregnancy are similar to those in nonpregnant subjects. An elevation of TSH is indicative of hypothyroidism. In normal subjects, administration of TRH produces a prompt increase in TSH level in 30 to 60 minutes. In patients with hyperthyroidism, TRS administration does not produce a similar response. A pronounced and sustained rise in TSH level in response to TRH indicates thyroid failure. Thyroid function tests are summarized in Table 13–1.

HYPERTHYROIDISM

The most common cause of hyperthyroidism in pregnancy in Grave's disease. Toxic thyroid adenoma, multinodular goiter, chronic thyroiditis, viral thyroiditis, hydatidiform mole, and hyperemesis gravidarum, constitute the other causes. Occasionally, hyperthyroidism may manifest for the first time in pregnancy. A hydatidiform mole may be associated with increased FT_4 either because of the TSH released by the trophoblastic tissue or because of the stimulation of the thyroid by the chorionic gonadotropin. Although thyroid function tests are abnormal in 2% of patients presenting with a hydatidiform mole, only rarely are classical manifestations of thyrotoxicosis seen.[5] Hyperemesis gravidarum causes elevations in TT_4 and FT_4I. The TT_3 and FT_3I values may be normal or increased. Thyroid function tests usually return to normal soon after vomiting subsides. The clinical feature, which may help distinguish Graves' disease from hyperemesis is the absence of the severe vomiting in patients with Graves' disease.[1] The other symptoms of thyrotoxicosis are presented in Table 13–2. The diagnosis of thyrotoxicosis is confirmed by FT_4I and/or FT_3I. Thyroid antibodies may be detected in 50% of patients with Graves' disease. Hypercalcemia may be present in 5 to 10% of patients.

The incidence of preeclampsia, premature labor, and congestive heart failure is high in untreated patients. Perinatal mortality and morbidity are also increased. Antithyroid drugs propyl thiouracil (PTU 300 to 600 mg/day) and methimazole (MMI, 30 to 60 mg/day) are administered during pregnancy to control symptoms. Once the patient's symptoms are controlled, and the thyroid function tests begin to normalize, the dose may be decreased. Subtotal thyroidectomy is reserved for those who are allergic or resistant to antithyroid drugs. The drugs may be discontinued if the euthyroid state persists at least 4 to 6 weeks. A recent study showed that the incidence of congenital malformations in neonates born to women who were treated with MMI was only 0.2%, whereas it reached 6% in neonates whose mothers had untreated hyperthyroidism.[6] Both PTU and MMI are secreted in breast milk, but MMI is secreted to a greater degree than is PTU. The use of MMI is not recommended in breast-feeding mothers.

Table 13–1. Thyroid Function Tests in Pregnancy

Test	Normal during pregnancy	Change from nonpregnancy	Thyroid State		
			Normal	Hyper	Hypo
TT_4	5–13 µg/dL	I	15	25	8
RT_3U	25–35 %	D	20	25	18
FT_4I	5–13	N	10	21	4
TT_3	80–220 ng/dL	I	270	480	120
FT_3I	80–220	N	180	400	72
TSH	6–8 miµ/L	I	N	N	I

TT_4 = total thyroxine; TT_3 = total triiodothyronine; RT_3U = radioactive T_3 uptake by resin; FT_4I and FT_3I are free T_4 and T_3 indices; TSH = thyroid stimulating hormone
N = normal; I = increased; D = decreased.

Table 13–2. Symptoms and Signs of Thyrotoxicosis

Symptoms	Signs
Nervousness	Tachycardia
Palpitations	Atrial fibrillation
Tachycardia	Goiter
Fatigability	Bruit over thyroid
Weight loss	Eye signs (stare)
Heat intolerance	Periorbital edema
	Lid lag
	Hyperreflexia
	Tremor
	Pretibial edema
	Wasting
	Osteoporosis

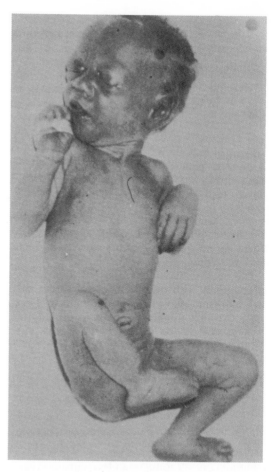

FIG. 13–1. Neonatal Graves' disease. (From Van Der Spuy ZM, and Jacobs HS: Management of endocrine disorders in pregnancy. Part I–thyroid and parathyroid disease. Postgrad Med J 60:245, 1984.

The use of propranolol is reserved only for thyroid emergencies.

The fetus may be affected in patients with hyperthyroidism. Antithyroid medications cross the placenta and consequently may cause fetal goiter and/or hypothyroidism. Fetal goiter is becoming less of a problem because of the availability of more efficient thyroid function tests. When mothers receive properly monitored therapy, postnatal intellectual development of the babies is not affected following in utero exposure to antithyroid drugs.[3] Neonatal thyroid function tests must be performed at the earliest opportunity to exclude neonatal hypothyroidism. Administration of I_{125} may result in severe fetal hypothyroidism and goiter, and therefore its use is contraindicated in pregnancy.

Thyroid stimulating antibodies (TSAb, LATS) are present in 90% of patients with Graves' disease. These antibodies cross the placenta and are believed to cause fetal or neonatal hyperthyroidism. Because of the short half-life of these antibodies, the condition is transient. Thyroid antibodies associated with Hashimoto's disease is not implicated in producing neonatal hyperthyroidism. Even in patients with only a past history of Graves' disease, the risk of neonatal thyrotoxicosis does exist. Neonatal thyrotoxicosis may be present at birth or may develop a few days after birth. A high maternal titer of TSAb in second trimester is said to be associated with neonatal risk for this condition.[7] Fetal tachycardia, growth retardation, and prematurity may occur when fetal thyrotoxicosis occurs. An ultrasonogram of the fetus may show the goiter. When the condition develops in the neonate, the clinical picture may resemble Graves' disease in the adult (Fig. 13–1).

Anesthetic Considerations

Cesarean section is performed in patients with Graves' disease only for obstetric indications. A massive goiter may cause dystocia, necessitating a cesarean section. Occasionally, a cesarean delivery may be necessary for managing fetal tachycardia or distress. The use of β-adrenergic agents for the control of premature labor is contraindicated in these patients. Every attempt must be made to render the patient euthyroid before she goes into labor. Anesthesia in an untreated patient may lead to release of thyroxine hormones and severe cardiovascular problems in the perioperative period. Occasionally, anesthesia may be required for subtotal thyroidectomy in a patient who does not respond to large doses of antithyroid medications. This procedure is usually performed in the second trimester.

During preoperative evaluation, the anesthesiologist must examine the patient's neck carefully to ascertain that the goiter has not distorted the upper airway. If a multinodular goiter is present, the airway must be evaluated with a tomogram or with a nuclear magnetic resonance of the neck. An indirect laryngoscopy is helpful in detecting vocal cord involvement. A fiberoptic bronchoscope can be used for performing tracheal intubations in patients with a distorted upper airway.

Persistent maternal tachycardia is usually suggestive of a hyperthyroid state. Atrial fibrillation often complicates thyrotoxicosis. Facilities must be available for managing a neonatal airway problem (neonatal goiter).

When effective antithryoid therapy has restored the euthyroid state, one need not be unduly concerned about the management of these patients for labor and delivery. When the patient is hyperthyroid because of ineffective treatment, however, special precautions must be exercised. Dehydration caused by vomiting, sweating, and diarrhea must be treated. Epidural anesthesia is the preferred method of pain relief because it diminishes catecholamine release caused by painful uterine contractions. Epinephrine added to a local anesthetic solution may cause tachycardia, therefore its use is better avoided. On occasion, the patient's symptoms worsen because of the stress associated with labor. Propranolol effectively controls tachycardia during labor. Short term administration of β-blockers is not usually associated with any adverse fetal effects.[3]

When cesarean section is required, epidural or spinal anesthesia is preferred to general anesthesia. Should general anesthesia become necessary, however, the following precautions must be observed. Anticholinergic agents must be avoided because they produce tachycardia. Myasthenia gravis occurs with increased frequency in patients with thyrotoxicosis, thus nondepolarizing relaxants must be used with caution in patients with thyrotoxicosis. A nerve stimulator is useful is assessing abnormal response to the muscle relaxants. Generally speaking, use of muscle relaxants that cause tachycardia or histamine release (pancuronium, d-tubocurarine) is not recommended. Inhalation agents do not affect thyroxine release from the thyroid gland.[8] Although halothane has been shown to produce increased hepatotoxicity in mice rendered thyrotoxic by the administration of triiodothyronine,[9] it is doubtful whether the finding is applicable to humans. However, if preoperative testing disclosed abnormal liver function, enflurane or isoflurane is a better choice. During anesthesia, body temperature must be continuously monitored and facilities for cooling must be available. A close watch must be kept for the possible development of thyroid storm in the postoperative period.

Thyroid Storm

Severe infection or stress associated with surgery may lead to excessive liberation of thyroxine leading to a life-threatening thyrotoxic state. If treatment is not instituted promptly, the mortality rate is likely to be very high. The symptoms include toxic psychosis, fever, cardiac tachyarrythmias, and cardiac failure. The treatment is aimed toward stopping thyroxine release from the glands, antagonizing the physiologic actions of the hormone, and providing general supportive care. The treatment is summarized in Table 13–3.[10] Propylthiouracil is preferred to methimazole because it is more effective in blocking the peripheral conversion of T_4 to T_3. Corticosteroids and β-blockers are also believed to block the peripheral formation of T_3.

Postpartum Thyroid Dysfunction

In the last 10 years, the occurrence of postpartum thyroid dysfunction is increasingly being recognized.[1] The cause is uncertain but autoimmune thyroiditis is suspected. The patient develops hyperthyroidism between 6 and 12 weeks after delivery. Spontaneous recovery usually occurs, which is followed by the development of transient hypothyroidism. The disease may recur in future pregnancies.

Autoimmune Thyroiditis

Several forms of autoimmune thyroiditis are known and the commonest is the Hashimoto's

Table 13–3. Treatment of Thyroid Storm

Desired Result	Treatment
To stop thyroxine synthesis	Propyl thiouracil up to a gram loading dose, followed by 200 mg every 4 hours (oral).
To stop thyroxine release	Iodide up to a gram i.v. infusion 300 mg every 4 hours or lithium carbonate.
To stop peripheral T_3 formation	PTU; Glucocorticoids; Propranolol.
To block hormone action	Propranolol i.v. 5–10 mg slowly; oral administration up to 80 mg 4–6 times.
For supportive therapy	Glucocorticoids: hydrocortisone or betamethasone; Treat fever, fluid-electrolyte imbalance and infection: Sedation; Treat cardiac arrhythmias and congestive heart failure.
To remove excess hormone	Plasmapheresis, dialysis.

thyroiditis. The thyroid gland is usually swollen but rarely causes compression symptoms. Very rarely transient myxedema or even thyrotoxicosis (hashitoxicosis) may develop.[5] Antithyroid antibodies are often present. Lymphocytic subacute thyroiditis may present as severe thyrotoxicosis. Propranolol is useful in controlling symptoms. The thyroid dysfunction is related to increased leakage of thyroid hormone rather than increased synthesis. Consequently, PTU is not indicated.

HYPOTHYROIDISM

Up to 95% of the cases of hypothyroidism are caused by primary thyroid disease, which may result from surgical removal of the gland or radioactive iodine therapy for the treatment of hyperthyroidism. Although it is rare to see untreated myxedema in pregnant patients, the chances of seeing one is 10 times greater in females than in males. The replacement therapy during pregnancy is l-thyroxine (synthyroid) 100 to 200 µg/day. Pregnancy modifies the dose requirement for thyroxine.[1] When the condition develops in a pregnant female before the fetal thyroid develops, abortion may ensue.[3]

The untreated condition has protean manifestations.[11] Most important changes occur in the cardiovascular and metabolic status of the patient (Table 13–4). The cardiac output is depressed because of bradycardia, myocardial damage (myxedema heart), and/or pericardial effusion. Blood loss is poorly tolerated for the following reasons: most patients are anemic; plasma volume may be diminished because of persistent vasoconstriction; there is decreased cardiac function; and the metabolism is depressed. Depressed metabolic rate and diminished renal function delay metabolism of opiates. Water intoxication and persistent hyponatremia occasionally develop from inappropriate secretion of ADH and altered renal function.[11] Relevant clinical features of the disorder are summarized in Table 13–4.

Undue concern is not necessary in patients with mild hypothyroidism, but special precautions are necessary in patients with the overt condition. Thyroid swelling, if any, must be carefully evaluated to rule out tracheal compression. Because of the increased incidence of adrenal cortical deficiency in these patients, some suggest supplementation with corticosteroids. General anesthesia is associated with the following problems: increased sensitivity to thiopental, narcotics and inhalation agents; and delayed elimination of many drugs. Regional anesthesia techniques are preferable to intravenous agents for producing labor analgesia. Similarly the use of regional anesthesia is advantageous for anesthesia for cesarean section. The total dose of local anesthetic must be kept to a minimum because of a lowered capacity to eliminate the local anesthetic. The possibility of a diminished plasma volume deserves particular attention before administration of regional anesthesia. The re-

Table 13–4.   Clinical Features of Myxedema

System	Derangement	Effect
Metabolism	Depressed $\dot{V}o_2$	Hypothermia; Delayed drug metabolism.
Cardiovascular	Myocardial damage; Impaired baroceptor response; Diminished cardiac output.	Hypotension; Increased sensitivity to hemorrhage, anesthetics and positive pressure ventilation.
Respiratory	Diminished diffusion capacity. Diminished ventilatory drive.	Respiratory depression.
Fluid-balance	Reduced plasma volume; Edema; Hyponatremia.	Hypotension with regional anesthesia; Water intoxication.
Hematologic	Macro or microcytic anemia.	Inability to tolerate blood loss.
Endocrine	Inappropriate ADH secretion.	Refractory hyponatremia.
Renal	Reduced GFR	Impaired drug excretion.

GFR = glomerular filtration rate

sponse to exogenously administered vasopressors is expected to be normal, therefore hypotension caused by regional anesthesia can be safely treated with incremental doses of ephedrine.

Administration of excessive amounts of noncrystalloid solution may result in water intoxication.[11] Oxytocin has mild water retaining properties; therefore its use must be restricted to small amounts. The balance between intake and output of postoperative fluids and electrolytes must be assessed carefully.[12]

Should general anesthesia become necessary, ketamine may be used in place of pentothal as an inducing agent[11] because it produces less myocardial depression than pentothal. Excessive respiratory minute volumes must be avoided because they not only produce increased intrathoracic pressure but also arterial hypocarbia because of diminished CO_2 production associated with the hypothyroid state. Inhalation agents are better avoided. Anesthesia is maintained using a mixture of N_2O and O_2 and a carefully chosen dose of muscle relaxants and narcotics. Narcotics, including fentanyl, have been implicated in prolonging postoperative recovery. Body temperature must be continuously monitored intra- and postoperatively.[13]

Myxedema Coma. This condition has a reported mortality rate of 80%. The condition must be recognized and treated promptly.[10] Respiratory failure, coma, and hypothermia are the important clinical features of myxedema coma. Occasionally, the condition may present as failure to regain consciousness from anesthesia. The essentials of therapy include (1) protection of the airway; (2) mechanical ventilation; (3) administration of l-thyroxine 7 µg/kg to a maximum of 500 µg; (4) administration of glucocorticoid; (5) treatment of hypothermia; (6) controlling intercurrent infection; and (7) preventing hyponatremia.

PARATHYROID DISEASE

HYPERPARATHYROIDISM

Hyperparathyroidism is caused by the increased secretion of parathyroid hormone by the parathyroid glands. About 70 cases of this condition have been reported.[14] Some cases of maternal hyperparathyroidism have been diagnosed when the infant was found to have tetany at birth.[3] In the majority of cases, the condition is caused by a single adenoma. Occasionally, two adenomas or a cancerous lesion may be responsible. In the United States, irradiation of the neck in the past has been an important etiologic factor in the development of hyperparathyroidism.[3] In untreated patients, the abortion rate reaches 50%.

Hyperparathyroidism is a disease of "renal stones, bones, and abdominal groans." Hypercalcemia leads to nephrocalcinosis and renal damage. Demineralization of the bone produces osteitis fibrosa cystica. Osteoporosis, spontaneous fractures, and vertebral anomalies including kyphoscoliosis may occur.

Occasionally, the syndrome is a part of mul-

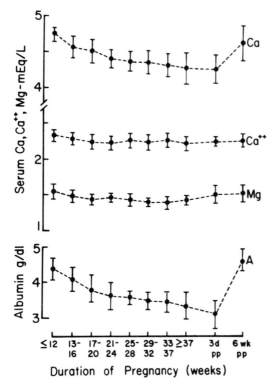

FIG. 13–2. Mean serum Ca, Ca++, Mg, and albumin levels in pregnancy. (From Pitkin RM: Endocrine regulation of calcium homeostasis during pregnancy. Clin Perinatol *10*:575, 1983.

tiple endocrine neoplasia affecting adrenals, pituitary, thyroid, and pancreatic inlets. The clinical features of hyperthyroidism include thirst, anorexia, and vomiting caused by hypercalcemia, hypertension, band keratopathy, peptic ulcers, and acute pancreatitis. The management of life-threatening hypocalcemia is discussed below. Serum total calcium decreases in pregnancy because of reduced albumin concentration but ionized Ca^{++} concentration remains within normal limits[15] (Fig. 13–2, Table 13–5). Parathor-

mone levels also increase 30 to 50% during pregnancy.[15] When only total calcium measurement is available, it may be corrected for hypoalbuminemia by adding 0.8 mg/dL to the measured calcium for every gram of albumin deficiency.[10] Surgical removal of the parathyroid adenoma offers the best prognosis for the mother and infant during pregnancy. If possible, surgery must be deferred until the second trimester.

At term, the serum total calcium level is 0.23 mEq/L lower than in nonpregnant subjects. Serum calcium levels up to 12 mg/dL are considered mild hypercalcemia. Levels of 12 to 14 mg% represent moderate hypercalcemia, and levels in excess of 14 mg/dL call for emergency treatment. Symptoms of hypercalcemia include lethargy, confusion, polyuria, polydypsia, hypertension, cardiac arrhythmias, and coma. Treatment should be instituted immediately. The essentials of treatment include intravenous hydration, extracellular volume expansion, and diuretic administration (furosemide or ethacrynic acid). In severe cases, forced diuresis must be accomplished both by rapid administration of 4 to 6 L of saline, and simultaneous diuretic therapy. Potassium supplementation is necessary to prevent hypokalemia. Oral supplementation of phosphorus is necessary if the serum levels are <3 mg/dL. If these treatments are not successful, mithramycin (plicamycin) a cytotoxic agent specific for the osteoclast may be used to stop bone resorption.

The services of the anesthesiologist may be required either for parathyroidectomy in the second trimester or for anesthesia during labor and delivery. Serum calcium levels must be known and the EKG must be evaluated for the presence of hypercalcemia (a short QT interval and a prolonged PR interval, Fig. 13–3. Renal damage may have occured in patients with long

Table 13–5. Maternal and Neonatal Calcium, Phosphorus, and Albumin Levels

	Maternal vein		Umbilical vein		Umbilical artery	
Calcium++ (mg/dl)	4.46	(2.2)	5.64+	(2.8)	5.62+	(2.8)
Total calcium	8.50	(4.3)	10.60+	(5.3)	10.38+	(5.2)
Phosphate (mg/dL)	4.37		5.96		5.83+	
Magnesium (mg/dL)	1.57	(1.31)	1.69	(1.41)	1.69	(1.39)
Albumin (g/dL)	3.46		4.16+		4.04+	

+ denotes values significantly different from the mother's. Figures within parenthesis are mEq/L. Modified from Pitkin RM: Endocrine regulation of calcium homeostasis during pregnancy. Clin Perinatol *10*:575, 1983.

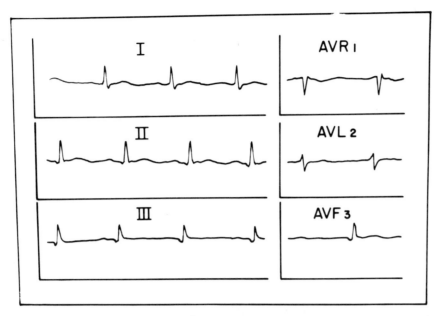

FIG. 13–3.   EKG signs of hypercalcemia. Note the absent ST segment and short QT interval. (From Rolasson WN: Electrocardiography for the anaesthetist. 2nd Edition. Philadelphia, FA Davis, 1969.)

standing hypercalcemia. Anemia resulting from a bleeding peptic ulcer is a possible hazard. Balanced anesthesia with N_2O and a muscle relaxant with narcotic supplementation may be used. Because the patients are prone to fractures, positioning of the patient on the operating table must be carefully done. Anesthesia for nonobstetric surgery during second trimester is considered in Chapter 21.

Spinal or epidural anesthesia can be safely administered to patients who are in labor provided that there is no significant vertebral anomaly, and hypercalcemia induced dehydration has been corrected. General anesthesia may be administered using precautions outlined above. Neonatal calcium levels must be measured at birth and replacement therapy administered if needed. The availability of an ion-specific electrode in many hospitals for the measurement of serum Ca^{++} as a part of auto-analyzers has made it possible to obtain serum Ca^{++} measurement without delay.

HYPOPARATHYROIDISM

Hypoparathyroidism may be caused by parathyroid deficiency, following accidental injury to the parathyroid gland during thyroid surgery; parathyroidectomy for cancer; and previous ir-

radiation of the neck or radioactive iodine administration. Pseudohypoparathyroidsm is a genetic defect associated with a round face, obesity, short metacarpals, hypertension, and ectopic bone formation. In this condition, the parathyroid glands are present but the renal tubules do not respond to the hormone. The lack of 1,25-dihydroxyvitamin D may also play a role.[4] Acute hypoparathyroidism causes tetany, muscle cramps, wheezing, convulsions, stridor, and dyspnea. Chronic disease is associated with cataracts and mental retardation. Chvostek's sign (facial muscle contraction elicited by tapping the facial nerve) and Trousseau's sign (carpopedal spasm on inflating a blood pressure cuff) are the other signs of hypocalcemia. The other major concern for the anesthesiologist is the possible association of the condition with a cleft palate.

Untreated cases develop cardiac dilatation and failure (resistant to digitalis); defective teeth; severe anemia; hypothyroidism; ossification of the intervertebral ligament with nerve root compression; and renal damage from overzealous treatment with calcium salts and vitamin D.[4] Parathyroid hormone preparations are not available for replacement therapy. Treatment is directed at maintaining adequate ionized serum $Ca.^{++}$ Oral calcium salts, a high calcium-low phosphate diet, and calciferol are used for treatment. Aluminum hydroxide gels are used to lower serum phosphate levels. Magnesium deficiency can coexist, which also needs correction.

Acute life-threatening tetany may develop immediately following thyroid or parathyroid surgery or during times of stress. Hyperventilation associated with uterine contractions lowers serum ionized Ca^{++}, and thus may predispose to tetany. Adequate airway must be established in patients who are in respiratory distress. Short acting relaxants may be used to facilitate tracheal intubatin if severe masseter spasms are present. Serum Ca^{++} levels must be raised by the administration of calcium chloride (5 to 10 ml of 10% solution) or calcium gluconate solution (10 to 20 ml). Repeated ionized calcium measurements must be made. Tetany is likely to occur if the Ca^{++} level falls below 3.5 mEq/L. An intravenous infusion containing 25 ml of $CaCl_2$/L in 5% glucose is used for maintenance. Patient must be given oral calcium salts as soon as possible.

ANESTHETIC CONSIDERATIONS

Serum total calcium must be measured repeatedly and maintained above 3.5 mEq/L. Lumbar epidural anesthesia is used for controlling hyperventilation (which lowers serum Ca^{++}) caused by labor pains. If renal impairment exists, adequate precautions are necessary (see Chapter 22 Renal Disease). Administration of spinal or epidural anesthesia may be difficult because of ossification of the vertebral ligaments. Monilial skin infection in the lumbar area (if present) can be an obstacle for performing regional blocks. When general anesthesia is used, the administration of muscle relaxants must be titrated carefully, using a nerve stimulator. Hypocalcemia may theoretically potentiate muscle relaxants. Arterial blood pH, Pa_{CO_2}, and serum Ca^{++} must be repeatedly measured. Respiratory minute volumes must be suitably adjusted to maintain blood pH close to normal values for pregnancy. Rapid blood transfusions (500 ml/10 min.) can lower ionized calcium concentration. Because of the possibility of precipitating laryngeal spasm, tracheal extubation must be delayed until the serum Ca^{++} levels are corrected.

PITUITARY GLAND

ANATOMY AND PHYSIOLOGY

The anterior pituitary is the master endocrine gland regulating metabolism and reproduction. Its hormones are synthesized by hormone-specific cells (thyrotrophs, somatotrophs). Its hormonal releasing function is controlled by neurohormones synthesized by the hypothalamus. The neurohormones reach the median eminence (the lowermost part of the hypothalamus) via neural connections. The neurons then release the neurohormones into the tissue fluid of the median eminence, from where they are absorbed into the capillaries. The neurohormones reach the anterior pituitary via the specialized blood vessels called the portal vessels (Fig. 13–4). The neurohormones regulate synthesis of the six major peptide hormones of the anterior pituitary.[2] Recent evidence has suggested that the neurohormones may also be synthesized in the gastrointestinal tract.[2]

At least a cursory knowledge of the type and function of each one of these anterior pituitary hormones is necessary to be able to predict the specific organ derangement in a given patient. It must be remembered that the placenta has many endocrine functions, which can influence the preexisting endocrine disease in a pregnant patient. A summary of the endocrine function of the placenta may be found in Chapter 2 Maternal Adaption to Pregnancy.

Hypothalamic neurohormones may act on more than one "troph" cell. Not all neurohormones stimulate the secretotrophs. Some of them have an inhibitory action. For instance, somatostatin inhibits the somatotroph and the thyrotroph.[16] All neurohormones are peptides except dopamine, which inhibits prolactroph. In addition, many hormones produced by the end-organ have a negative feed back effect on the secretotroph. For example, even a small excess of thryoxine will inhibit the thyrotroph. The regulatory effect of the hypothalamic neurohormone on the pituitary secretotroph is summarized in Fig. 13–5. In panhypopituitarism, multiple or single hormone deficiency may occur, and in the same patient, the degree of deficiency may vary from one hormone to the other.

The posterior lobe of the pituitary is an out-

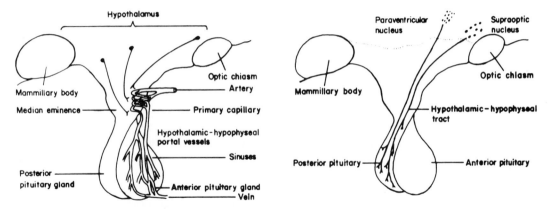

FIG. 13–4.   The relationship between hypothalamus and the two lobes of the pituitary. Note that the different release hormones are liberated from the hypothalamic neurons into the tissue fluid of median eminence from where they are collected by the portal vessels reaching the anterior pituitary. Note the direct neural connections of paraventricular (oxytocin) and supraoptic nuclei (ADH) with the posterior pituitary. (Reproduced from Guyton AC: Endocrinology and reproduction. *In* Textbook of Medical Physiology. 7th Ed. WB Saunders, 1986.

growth of ventral hypothalamus. Neurons originating from the supraoptic and paraventricular nuclei terminate mainly in the posterior pituitary. The two posterior pituitary hormones, namely antidiuretic hormone (ADH, vasopressin) and oxytocin, are synthesized in the hypothalamic nuclei. They are then transported via the specialized neurons along with carrier proteins called the neurophysins to the posterior pituitary (Fig. 13–4).[2] The supraoptic nuclei produce mainly ADH, whereas the paraventricular nuclei produce mainly oxytocin. Thus, the hypothalamus controls the anterior pituitary function through neural and vascular connections and the posterior pituitary function only through neural connection.

Corticotropin releasing hormone (CRH) causes the release of the ACTH precursor, from the anterior pituitary. The ACTH precursor also contains melanocyte stimulating hormone and

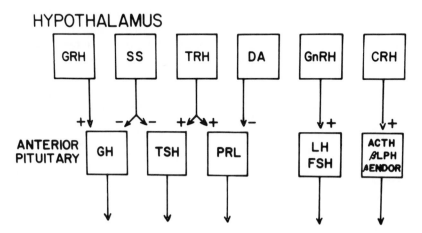

FIG. 13–5.   Regulation of anterior pituitary cell function by the hypothalamic neurohormones. The positive symbol (plus) = stimulatory effect; negative sign (−) inhibitory effect; GRH = growth-hormone releasing hormone; SS = somatostatin; TRH = thyrotropin releasing hormone; DA = dopamine; GnRH = gonadotropin releasing hormone; CRH = corticotropin releasing hormone; PRL = prolactin; Beta LPH = beta lipoprotein; GH = growth hormone; TSH = thyroid stimulating hormone; LH = luteinizing hormone; FSH = follicular stimulating hormone. (From West JB: The hypothalamic-pituitary control system. *In* Best and Taylor's Physiological Bases of Medical Practice. Baltimore, Williams and Wilkins, 1985.)

β-endorphin. (For more information, see Chapter 6 Spinal Opioides). The CRH also activates the sympathetic nervous system. Proper functioning of each of the links in the CRH-ACTH-cortisol axis is vital to the patient's ability to respond to stress, hypovolemia, pain, and other noxious stimuli.[16] The gonadotropin releasing hormone (GnRH) is responsible for releasing luteinizing hormone (LH), and follicular stimulating hormone (FSH). The GRH causes the release of both growth hormone (GH) and thyroid stimulating hormone TSH. Somatostatin inhibits the release of GH. Growth hormone has two major functions: growth regulation and metabolic regulation.[16] The growth response is mediated through insulin-like substances called the somatomedins. The metabolic effects of GH are similar to those of insulin and include increased uptake of glucose by muscle and adipose tissue, increased uptake of amino acid and accelerated protein synthesis in muscle and liver as well as inhibition of lipolysis.

In humans the major function of prolactin is milk production.[2] Prolactin concentrations rise 10-fold during pregnancy. The major regulator of prolactin synthesis is dopamine (Fig. 13–5). Dopamine inhibits prolactin release.[2] Dopamine agonists such as bromoergocryptine are used to inhibit prolactin release. Any drug that interferes with the synthesis of dopamine or antagonizes the effects of dopamine will release prolactin.

The posterior pituitary releases ADH and oxytocin. The plasma osmolarity is sensed by the hypothalamic osmoreceptors, which in turn regulate the synthesis of ADH by the hypothalamic nuclei. The other stimuli for ADH release include changes in circulating fluid volume, pain, stress, and hypoglycemia.[2] Alcohol, α-adrenergic agents, and glucocorticoids inhibit ADH release. Excessive concentrations of ADH may produce vasoconstriction[2] and hypertension. Oxytocin initiates the contraction of myoepithelial cells of the breast and the contraction of the myometrium. The most important disorders of pituitary that are likley to occur in pregnant patients are (1) prolactinomas, (2) acromegaly, (3) panhypopituitarism, and (4) diabetes insipidus.[17]

Prolactinomas

Most prolactinomas are confined to the pituitary fossa but some may extend upward to compress the optic chiasma.[17,18] Treatment with bromocriptine causes prolactinomas to shrink. Patients with prolactinomas are therefore managed conservatively. In some patients prolactinomas may increase in size during pregnancy. Although no known reports of fetal harm exists, bromocriptine is usually discontinued when pregnancy is diagnosed, which may further increase the size of the tumor.[17] The presence of prolactinomas is diagnosed by using provocative tests, which activate prolactin release.[18] Chlorpromazine, metoclopramide, or TRH may be used for this purpose.[18] The blood prolactin levels double in patients with prolactinomas following administration of one of these agents. A CT scan of the pituitary using a fourth generation scanner may reveal the presence of the tumor.[17] Fetal irradiation hazard is minimal if proper pelvic protection is utilized.

If a patient with known prolactinomas develops severe headache or restriction of her visual fields, the infant should be delivered forthwith, if possible. Delivery will usually cause the tumor to shrink. She may require anesthesia for cesarean section. The anesthetic management depends on whether or not she has raised intracranial pressure (ICP). Spinal anesthesia is not safe because it may cause medullary coning in patients with raised ICP. Lumbar epidural anesthesia may be administered, but the threat of accidental spinal tap always exists with this technique. In addition, injecting large volumes of local anesthetic into the epidural space may cause the ICP to rise because of compression of the extracranial dural sac. Not more than 3 ml of local anesthetic must be injected into the epidural space each time, and sufficient time must be allowed for the ICP to stabilize between injections. This issue is more fully discussed in Chapter 17, Neurologic Disease. The technique of general anesthesia for cesarean section in patients with raised ICP is also discussed in that chapter.

When an immature fetus precludes immediate delivery, large doses of bromocriptine may be administered to inhibit prolactin release. If the visual fields continue to deteriorate and headache persists despite therapy with bromocriptine, dexamethasone may be added to the regimen. Dexamethasone not only shrinks brain swelling but lessens fetoplacental production of estrogen, which augments liberation of prolactin. If the patient responds to treatment, the delivery may be deferred until the fetus is more mature. Should the condition deteriorate, emergency neurosurgical decompression may be needed.[17] Furosemide or dexamethasone is used to reduce brain swelling under these circumstances. Occasionally, a ventriculostomy is needed to decrease severe intracranial hypertension before anesthesia is administered.

ACROMEGALY

Up to 25% of patients with acromegaly have hormonally active prolactinomas.[17] Increased prolactin levels reduce fertility.[17] However, when acromegalic patients are treated with bromocriptine, the serum prolactin level falls with the restoration of fertility. Unlike prolactin, the growth hormone level is not affected by pregnancy. In acromegaly, the increased GH secretion is caused by a tumor of the somatrophs of the anterior pituitary. When the tumor develops after puberty, acromegaly usually develops. The clinical manifestations of acromegaly are protean, which depend on the amount of GH released and the size of the pituitary tumor that may produce neurologic symptoms. The encroachment of the tumor on the other trophic cells may lead to multiple hormone deficiency further complicating the course of the disease. The diagnosis is usually established by the following test results: (1) finding an enlarged sella turcica in the skull x-ray, a CT scan, or a pneumoencephalogram; elevated GH or somatomedin C levels; failure of the growth hormone level to decrease after administration of glucose (glucose tolerance test);[18] or demonstration of increased growth hormone levels in response to TRH injection. In normal subjects TRH injection has no effect on the release of growth hormone.[18]

The clinical features, which are of interest to the anesthesiologist are summarized in Table 13–6. Patients with long-standing acromegaly are prone to have diabetes mellitus, hypertension, and cardiac failure. In addition, several upper airway anomalies including recurrent laryngeal nerve palsy is likely to be present. Regional anesthesia may therefore be the best anesthetic method, provided that vertebral anomalies are not severe enough to make the procedure technically difficult. If general anesthesia is planned, airway problems must be anticipated well ahead of time and appropriate equipment, including fiberoptic bronchoscope, should be made available in the delivery room.

Adenomas capable of secreting large amounts of ACTH may cause Cushing's disease. This should not be confused with Cushing's syndrome, which is caused by increased glucocorticoid levels from any source including iatrogenic overdose.[18] Many patients with Cushing's disease do not show suppression of blood or urine glucocorticoid levels after administration of a large dose of dexamethasone.[18] Patients who have undergone bilateral adrenalectomy for the treatment of this condition may develop a rapidly enlarging tumor of the pituitary adenoma, resulting in visual field defects (Nelson's syndrome). Metyrapone, a drug that prevents 11-β-hydroxylation, may be used to diminish adrenal steroid production.

HYPOPITUITARISM

This condition is commonly the result of chromophobe adenomas and craniopharyngiomas of the pituitary, and it may involve one or several tropic hormones. Pituitary tumors may occur in combination with multiple endocrine neoplasia (Wermer's syndrome, type 1). The disease may affect either the pituitary gland itself or the hypothalamic-hypophyseal pathway. Occasionally, severe postpartum hemorrhage may cause ischemic pituitary necrosis (Sheehan's syndrome). It is not necesssary to alter the conventional replacement hormone therapy in view of pregnancy.[17] The diagnosis is usually established by demonstrating decreased tropic hormone level in the presence of diminished target organ secretion.[4] For instance, both TSH and thyroxine levels may be low in patients with hypopituitarism. Provocative tests for growth hormone release have been advocated.[18] Insulin induced hypoglycemia usually results in increased growth hormone release in normal patients. Patients with hypopituitarism have either impaired or no response.[18] Urinary and serum gonadotropins are low and so are the plasma levels of sex steroids. The severity of the clinical picture depends on which tropic hormones are deficient. Pituitary tumors may affect visual fields. Complete replacement therapy with single or multiple end-organ hormones is now pos-

Table 13–6.   Considerations in Acromegaly

System	Abnormality	Anesthesia precaution
Airway	Prognathism; Recurrent laryngeal nerve palsy Large tongue.	Difficult intubation.
Cardiovascular	Cardiac failure; Hypertension.	Sensitivity to inhalational anesthetics.
Skeletal	Vertebral anomaly; Root compression.	Technical difficulty with regional anesthesia.
Metabolic	Diabetes mellitus; glucose intolerance.	Insulin perioperatively.
Neurologic	Raised ICP; Myopathy.	Special precaution; Possible potentiation of muscle relaxants.
Endocrine	Other endocrine adenomas; Failure of other secretotrophs of the pituitary.	Other hormonal hypo or hypersecretion; Pituitary failure.

ICP = intracranial pressure.

sible for the treatment of this condition. Patients thus treated may expect a normal life span. Problems for the anesthesiologist in patients with diminished or absent pituitary function include the possible presence of an intracranial space occupying lesion; the hazard of hyponatremia, hypoglycemia, and increased insulin sensitivity; and decreased stress response. The glucocorticoid dose must be increased during times of stress.

DISEASES OF THE POSTERIOR PITUITARY

Diabetes insipidus is not incompatible with pregnancy.[17] Diabetes insipidus may be caused by abnormality of the posterior pituitary. The condition is familial and is inherited as a dominant trait. Secondary Diabetes insipidus occurs as a result of head trauma or infection (tuberculosis or encephalitis), or metastatic lesions of the posterior pituitary. It also occasionally occurs in the postpartum period.[4] The defect in nephrogenic diabetes insipidus lies in the renal tubules. This may be congenital or acquired. The acquired defect may follow severe pyelonephritis.[4]

Patients with diabetes insipidus drink up to 20 L of water every day to prevent dehydration induced by polyuria.[4] The specific gravity of urine may be 1.006 or less. After administration of 5 units of vasopressin, urine osmolarity promptly rises. Failure to respond to vasopressin usually indicates a nephrogenic condition.[4]

Chlorpropamide (diabenese) an antidiabetic agent is useful in mild cases because it releases ADH and it potentiates the renal action of ADH.[4] More severe cases may need vasopressin tannate, lysine-8 vasopressin (nasal spray), or the new synthetic analogue of arginine vasopressin (DDAVP). Nephrogenic diabetes mellitus is treated with hydrochlorothiazide, which exerts its beneficial action by increasing sodium depletion. This decreases GFR, enhances fluid reabsorption in the proximal tubule,[4] also results in decreased sodium delivery to the ascending limb of the loop of Henle, and consequently reduces tubular capacity to dilute urine.[17]

Accurate fluid balance on total fluid intake and output must be maintained in the perioperative period. Repeated measurements of plasma and urinary osmolarity and urine specific gravity are useful in managing fluid balance. Withholding fluids as a treatment to reduce urine volume can lead to dehydration and shock. Blood sugar measurements are needed when the patient is receiving chlorpropamide therapy. Patients who are receiving diuretics for the treatment of nephrogenic diabetes insipidus may have electrolyte imbalances. Regional anesthesia may be safely administered if the circulating volume is adequate.

Syndrome of Inappropriate ADH Secretion (SIADH)

This disorder is basically one of water intoxication resulting from the presence of inappropriately high concentrations of ADH. Edema is conspicuous by its absence. Plasma arginine vasopressin levels are usually inappropriately high for the plasma osmolarity. Oatcell carcinoma of the lung secretes ADH, thus leading to SIADH. Other etiologic factors include infections (tuberculosis), skull fracture, cerebrovascular accidents, and drugs (general anesthetics, narcotics, chlorpropamide, and oxytocin).[18] Treatment usually consists of water restriction (<1000 ml). Water intoxication must be treated with hypertonic saline. Agents such as butorphanol and naloxone are known to block the release of ADH but their therapeutic efficacy is still to be determined.[18] Demethyl-chlortetracycline blocks the renal action of ADH and therefore may be prescribed in some of the patients. The only known complication of the drug is azotemia.[18]

Anesthesia, surgery, pain, and stress increase the release of ADH and may therefore adversely affect the water balance in patients with SIADH. The concentration of ADH increases 50 to 100 times the postoperative period and may take 5 days to return to normal levels.[19] Severe hyponatremia leading to convulsions and brain damage has occurred in the postoperative period in previously healthy women.[20] In many of these women the diagnosis was not suspected until it was too late. Thus, the maintenance of postoperative osmolarity is critical in women with SIADH. The use of epidural anesthesia to treat labor pains will prevent any further rises in ADH concentration caused by stress. In addition, regional anesthesia also obviates the need for pain relief with narcotics that release ADH on their own right.

Plasma osmolarity and sodium concentration must be measured repeatedly to maintain proper fluid balance. Plasma osmolarity decreases 5 mosm/L in pregnancy because of the resetting of the hypothalamic osmostat to a lower value. (See Chapter 2 Maternal Adaptation to Pregnancy). The use of prophylactic hydration with large volumes of crystalloid (which is customarily done before epidural anesthesia) may pose a hazard. The use of CVP monitoring to gauge adequacy of circulating fluid volume is the rational approach to this problem. It must be remembered that the supine posture has an antidiuretic effect in pregnant patients (see Chapter 22 Renal Disease) and must consequently be

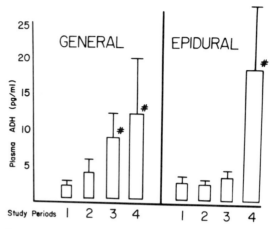

FIG. 13–6.   Plasma ADH concentration changes with general and epidural anesthesia. Study periods: (1) = control; (2) = induction of anesthesia; (3) = skin incision; and (4) = hours after operation. The # symbol identifies those groups significantly different from the control group. There is a lack of change in ADH intraoperatively, whereas postoperatively similar changes are seen with epidural and general anesthesia. (From Bonnet F, Harari A, Thibonnier M, and Viars P: Suppression of antidiuretic hormone hypersection during surgery by extradural anaesthesia. Br J Anaesth, 54:29, 1982.

avoided. Noxious stimuli traveling along the visceral afferents cause the release of ADH. Epidural anesthesia decreases the nociceptive stimuli reaching the brain and may thus diminish ADH response[21,22] (Fig. 13–6). Postoperative pain relief using epidural fentanyl may also at-

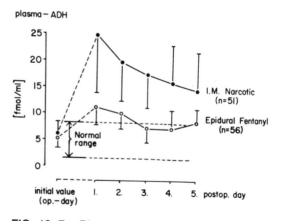

FIG. 13–7.   Plasma levels of ADH in patients receiving parenteral narcotic or epidural fentanyl for postoperative pain relief. (From Bormann BV, et al.: Influence of epidural fentanyl on stress-induced elevation of plasma vasopressin (ADH) after surgery. Anesth Analg 62:727, 1983.

tenuate the ADH response[23] (Fig. 13–7). However, epidural morphine, which is more prone to rostral spread, may cause more release of ADH.[24] Therefore, when epidural narcotics are used for postoperative pain relief, fentanyl is a better choice than morphine for patients with SIADH. Epidural analgesia with a local anesthetic for postoperative pain relief is also known to inhibit ADH release.[24] Thus, a logical approach in managing patients with SIADH is to administer epidural anesthesia for surgery followed by epidural injections of either fentanyl or a local anesthetic for postoperative pain relief.

Although it is small, oxytocin does have some vasopressin-like action. Its use is therefore not without dangers in patients with SIADH. Only small amounts of the drug must be used in the postpartum period. Methyl ergonovine may be used in place of or in combination with oxytocin. In the event that water intoxication develops, it is treated with administration of a diuretic and/or 3% hypertonic saline.

ADRENAL GLAND

The adrenal gland is composed of two different types of tissue of separate embryological derivation.[2,16] The outer cortex is of mesodermal origin and the inner medulla is of neuroectodermal origin. The cortex secretes the steroid hormones: glucocorticoids, mineralocorticoids, and androgenic steroids. The glucocorticoids are cortisol and corticosterone. Aldosterone and deoxycorticosterone are the important mineralocorticoids. The urinary measurements of 17-hydroxysteroids is a measure of the adrenal cortisol production and that of the 17-ketosteroids reflects adrenal adrogen production. The importance of CRH-ACTH-Cortisol axis has already been mentioned. The actions of cortisol are mainly catabolic in the periphery. In the muscle, it causes protein breakdown. It also inhibits peripheral uptake of amino acids and glucose. Cortisol increases lipolysis in the periphery and enhances the other lipolytic stimulants such as catecholamines. Cortisol also produces hepatic anabolic action; it activates gluconeogenesis, and protein synthesis in that organ. The other major effect of cortisol is on immune and inflammatory responses, both of which it blunts.[16]

Aldosterone, the principal mineralocorticoid, increases the reabsorption of sodium in the collecting tubule of the nephron by exchanging Na^+ for K^+ or H^+. Aldosterone production is regulated by the renin-angiotensin system as well as by ACTH and K^+.[16] Whenever the circulating fluid volume decreases, renal perfusion pressure decreases. The juxtaglomerular apparatus releases renin in response to reduced renal perfusion. Renin activates the angiotensin system, which not only causes vasoconstriction but also activates more aldosterone release from the adrenal cortex. Increase in plasma K^+ concentration increases aldosterone synthesis, whereas diminished K^+ concentration has the opposite effect. A more detailed discussion of renal effects of various hormones may be found in Chapter 2 Maternal Adaptation to Pregnancy, and Chapter 22 Renal Disease.

Pregnancy causes a rise in plasma ACTH and cortisol levels. Plasma cortisol levels may rise more than 200% in some patients. One source of increased ACTH in pregnant subjects is the placenta. Thus, diagnostic tests that are used to diagnose adrenal dysfunction must be interpreted with caution in pregnant subjects.[17] Epinephrine is the principal hormone of the adrenal medulla with small amounts of norepinephrine also being produced. The medulla also produces met- and leu-enkephalins (see Chapter 6 Spinal Opioids).

HYPERCORTISOLISM

Hypersecretion of ACTH by a pituitary adenoma is the cause of adrenocortical overactivity in 70% of patients.[4] Hypercortisolism caused by tumor of one adrenal gland may result in atrophy of the contralateral gland. Excessive administration of glucocorticoids causes symptoms of Cushing's syndrome, but at the same time causes adrenals to atrophy. Central obesity, weakness and fatiguability, hypertension, easy bruisability, mental changes, and diabetes mellitus are the relevant clinical features in patients with hypercortisolism. In addition, she might have suffered a cerebrovascular accident or a myocardial infarction in the past. Compression fractures of the spine may be contraindication for regional anesthesia. Routine and special laboratory tests that must be reviewed in the preoperative evaluation are listed in Table 13–7. The treatment

Table 13–7. Laboratory Tests in Disorders of Adrenal Cortex

Tests	Cushing's syndrome	Addison's disease	Conn's syndrome
Routine	Hyperglycemia, glycosuria. Eosinophils <50/uL. Lymphocytes <20%. ↓ Serum Cl-, ↓ K+. ↑ Urine 17–hydroxycorticosteroids. ↑ Plasma cortisol (>20 μg/dL).	Hypoglycemia. Neutropenia, eosinophilia; Lymphocytosis >35%. ↓ Serum Na+. ↑ Serum K, ↑ BUN, ↑ CA++. ↓ Urine 17 OH and keto-steroids. ↓ Plasma cortisol.	↑ Na+. ↓ K+, ↑ HCO3-, ↓ Mg++. ↑ blood pH, ↓ Ca++. ↑ plasma, urine aldosterone. ↓ plasma renin.
EKG	Hypokalemia.	Hyperkalemia. Nonspecific ST-T change.	Hypokalemia. Ischemia.
Radiographic	CT scanning for tumor location. Osteoporosis of the spine.	Adrenal calcification.	CT scan.
Special endo-crine	Failure of urine 17–KS to decrease after dexamethasone.	↑ Plasma ACTH; Corticotropin infusion for 4 days, failure of urine 17–KS to rise.	Failure of i.v. saline to sup-press aldosterone.

KS = ketosteroids

of choice is surgical. If the condition is caused by an ACTH secreting tumor of the pituitary, it is removed through the transphenoidal approach. If the fetus is not mature enough, surgery may be deferred until the baby may be safely delivered. When removal of pituitary adenomas fails to cure symptoms, adrenalectomy must be performed.

Adrenal carcinomas constitute 15% of all conditions producing Cushing's syndrome in pregnant subjects.[17] The remainder is equally divided between pituitary adenomas and adrenal adenomas. Because of the unreliability of routinely used endocrine tests in pregnancy, and a striking incidence of adrenal carcinoma, a CT scan of the adrenals must be performed. The patient must be told of the radiation hazard to the fetus. If carcinoma is diagnosed in the first trimester, pregnancy must be terminated and the lesion must be removed surgically. If the diagnosis is made in the third trimester, the delivery should be done promptly so that adrenal surgery may be performed.[17] Cases that present in the second trimester may be treated with metyrapone until the fetus is more mature.[17] The baby must be delivered at the earliest opportunity so the definitive surgical treatment may be provided. Thus, it may be seen that the services of the anesthesiologist may be required not only during labor and delivery but for adrenalectomy during pregnancy.

Anesthetic Management

Fluid and electrolyte imbalances must be corrected prior to surgery. If bilateral adrenalectomy is contemplated, the patient should receive hydrocortisone, 100 to 300 mg per day, in divided doses, on the day of surgery, and continue to receive similar doses for at least two days. The dose is then tapered to arrive at a proper maintenance dose. Because of the possible presence of myopathy, the dose of muscle relaxants must be carefully titrated with the aid of a nerve stimulator. Hypokalemia may be another factor in inducing muscle weakness. Acute administration of hydrocortisone (>5 mg/kg) may potentiate the action of nondepolarizing relaxants, whereas chronic administration (2 mg/kg, 3 times a week) may potentiate succinylcholine action.[25] Hyperglycemia (if present) must be adequately treated with insulin.

Regional anesthesia may be provided during labor and delivery in patients with untreated Cushing's syndrome or those awaiting treatment. Osteoporosis and compression fractures of the spine, as well as obesity, and skin sepsis may pose problems for regional anesthesia.

ADDISON'S DISEASE

This condition is the result of adrenal cortical failure affecting glucose and mineralocorticoid secretion. Autoimmune involvement of the gland is the most likely etiologic factor, followed by tuberculosis.[16] Anorexia, nausea and vomiting, and striking pigmentation of the skin are the usual presenting symptoms. Multiple electrolyte imbalances and hypoglycemia occur because of the hormone lack (Table 13–7). Contracted blood volume leads to systemic hypotension and reduced GFR. The finding of reduced plasma cortisol with increased ACTH levels is usually diagnostic. Patients with Addison's disease are prone to develop adrenal crisis in times of stress. Severe vomiting seen with Addisonian crisis may be mistaken for hyperemesis during early pregnancy. Labor and delivery place enormous demands on the patient's adrenal reserve and thus can precipitate a crisis. Addison's disease is treated with replacement therapy consisting of 25 mg of hydrocortisone and 0.1 to 0.2 mg of flurocortisone (mineralocorticoid).[18]

During pregnancy, maintenance therapy must be continued. Supplementary hydrocortisone (100 mg, 6 times hourly) is needed during labor. It has been reported recently that a low-dose corticosteroid regimen consisting of 25 mg i.v. hydrocortisone at induction of anesthesia followed by continuous infusion of hydrocortisone (100 mg/1000 ml) is sufficient to achieve adequate cortisol levels in patients who have received long-term corticosteroid replacement therapy.[26] In patients with adrenocortical deficiency, contracted blood volume may be hazardous, especially when regional anesthesia is being considered. Fluid administration must be done with the aid of CVP monitoring. Etomidate interferes with steriod synthesis by affecting 11 β-hydroxylation and side-chain cleavage.[27] Its use is therefore not recommended in patients with limited adrenal reserve. Patients should be watched for the possible development of adrenal crisis during labor and in the postpartum period.

Addisonian or adrenal crisis is precipitated by sepsis or surgery. It is also known to occur following sudden withdrawal of steroids in a steroid dependent patient.[4] Nausea, vomiting, severe abdominal pain, fever, dehydration, lethargy, and finally coma are the classic symptoms of the syndrome. Dehydration must be corrected with the aid of a CVP catheter. Glucocorticoid (hydrocortisone) replacement is life-saving.

HYPERALDOSTERONISM

This rare disorder accounts for 2% of cases of hypertension and is more common in females.[4] Primary hyperaldosteronism is caused by an adenoma (Conn's syndrome) or a localized cortical hyperplasia. Hypertension without edema is the outstanding symptom.[4] The continous exchange of Na^+ for K^+ and H^+ ions in the tubules causes hypernatremia, metabolic alkalosis, and hypokalemia. Alkalosis may cause tetany. Hypokalemia may result in muscular paralysis resembling familial periodic paralysis. Cardiac and renal damage may occur because of hypertension. A CT scan is helpful in visualizing the tumors. Other relevant laboratory findings are listed in Table 13–7. Adrenal adenoma is treated with surgical removal. Adrenal hyperplasia is treated with spiranolactone.[4] Antihypertensive therapy may be needed to correct hypertension.

Because of the possible presence of hypervolemia, hypertension, and renal and myocardial damage, severe cases of Conn's syndrome may benefit from a pulmonary artery catheter. Indwelling arterial cannula is necessary to monitor blood pressure and to obtain arterial blood pH. Epidural anesthesia helps diminish hyperventilation caused by labor pains. Alkalosis may further intensify hypokalemia. Because hypokalemia may potentiate muscle relaxants, a nerve stimulator must be used to monitor the neuromuscular junction during anesthesia. Secondary hyperaldosteronism refers to a state in which aldosterone level is increased in response to increased renin levels. This occurs in edema states (cirrhosis, nephrotic syndrome), renovascular hypertension, or it may be associated with a renin-producing tumor. Hypokalemic alkalosis is a consistent finding in this condition.[18]

PHEOCHROMOCYTOMA

Pheochromocytoma, a tumor of the chromaffin tissue, accounts for fewer than 0.1% of all cases of hypertension.[28] Chromaffin tissue is located not only in the adrenal medulla but in many sympathetic plexus in the body. Most pheochromocytomas secrete both norepinephrine and epinephrine, the former being more abundant than the latter. Several cases of pheochromocytoma have been reported in pregnancy.[29–31] Untreated pheochromocytoma carries maternal and fetal mortality rates over 50%.[17] Pheochromocytoma can be associated with medullary thyroid cancer, neurofibromatosis, and β-cell tumor of the pancreatic islet.

The symptoms include paroxysmal headache, palpitations, and sweating. Severe hypertension and papilledema may also occur. The diagnosis is established by measuring urinary catecholamines (normal up to 130 μg/24 hours) and vanillylmandelic acid (VMA, normal 2 to 7 mg/24 hours) and metanephrines (normal 1.3 mg/24 hours). The direct assay of epinephrine and norepinephrine in urine and blood immediately after a hypertensive attack is reliable.[4] Elevated epinephrine content usually points to adrenal location of the tumor.[4] On the contrary elevated norepinephrine concentration will favor an extra adrenal location. Determination of catecholamine concentration in blood samples obtained via a catheter located at various points in the inferior vena cava helps tumor localization. A CT scan is the most useful test for localizing the tumor. This test exposes the fetus to considerable irradiation. Complications of the untreated condition include hypertensive cerebrovascular accidents, catecholamine cardiomyopathy, and myocardial infarction. Occasionally, postpartum collapse resembling amniotic fluid embolus may occur.[31].

The definitive treatment for pheochromocytoma is surgical removal. In patients who are pregnant, a combined cesarean section and tumor removal may be performed if the pregnancy is not too remote from term. In pregnancies remote from term, medical treatment may buy valuable time until the fetus becomes more mature. The mainstay of medical treatment is producing α-blockade with phenoxybenzamine, and producing β-blockade with propranolol. The institution of β-blockade in the absence of α-blockade may cause severe hypertensive crisis. Phenoxybenzamine diminishes vasoconstriction caused by the catecholamines. This not only reduces blood pressure, but helps blood volume expand. Diminished blood volume caused by prolonged vasoconstriction leads to a decreased plasma volume. Propranolol attenuates the tendency to develop cardiac arrhythmias. Labatelol (a combined α-and β-blocker) has been used, but its α-blocking action is weak. The use of phenoxybenzamine and propranolol for this purpose is usually not associated with any adverse fetal effects.[17]

Patients with pheochromocytomas are usually delivered by cesarean section because of the fear that the stress of labor may release copious amounts of catecholamines. Resection of the tumor may be carried out in early pregnancy, provided that the patient has been adequately investigated. Once the tumor has been successfully removed, pregnancy may be allowed to continue to term. Because of the high recurrence rate, these patients should be followed carefully throughout pregnancy.

When anesthesia is required for removal of the tumor, a pulmonary artery catheter or a CVP catheter together with an indwelling radial artery cannula may be needed. Plasma volume must be expanded prior to anesthesia. An epidural block may be administered for the combined cesarean section and pregnancy. The following drugs must be avoided: ergot preparations because they may cause vasoconstriction; epinephrine with the local anesthetic solution; and excessive amounts of droperidol because it allegedly causes severe hypertension in patients with phaeochromocytoma[32] by causing leakage of catecholamines from the intraneuronal vesicles.[33] Intraoperative hypertension can be treated with sodium nitroprusside infusion.

Epidural anesthesia may not be suitable for resection of multiple tumors or when tumor location is not precisely known. When general anesthesia is being planned, atropine premedication is usually omitted. Tracheal intubation is likely to cause hypertension, which may be attenuated either with sodium nitroprusside or hydralazine. Pentothal or etomidate may be used for induction but ketamine is better avoided. Succinylcholine can be used for facilitating jaw relaxation, d-tubocurarine may release histamine, which is a potent stimulus for liberating catecholamine. Pancuronium has been used in 80 patients with pheochromocytoma without any problems.[28] Halothane may produce cardiac arrhythmias by sensitizing the myocardium to catecholamines. Enflurane or isoflurane are better alternatives for the maintenance of anesthesia. Palpation of the tumor is known to release catecholamine thereby producing hypertension, which is treated with phentolamine (1 to 5 mg) or with sodium nitroprusside. Intraoperative arrhythmias are treated with lidocaine. It is preferred to propanol because it is more effective and has shorter duration of action.[28] Sudden hypotension may follow the removal of the tumor. Volume infusion with careful monitoring of the filling pressures is the treatment of choice.[28] Prophylactic administration of fluids at an increased rate just before the removal of the tumor will minimize this problem. Occasionally, the use of norepinephrine or phenylephrine may be needed to treat persistent hypotension. After surgery 50% of patients will remain hypertensive for a few days. Some will also develop severe hypoglycemia probably related to rebound effects of insulin.[34]

Obesity

The degree of obesity is usually judged by inappropriate body weight for the height (>120%)[35] or by using skin-fold thickness measurements. The obstetric anesthesiologist faces a multitude of problems when managing an obese patient (Table 13–8). These problems may be related either to the mother or the baby. The maternal problems are mainly related to the increased incidence of diabetes mellitus hypertension. Obesity-hypoventilation syndrome (pickwickian syndrome) may occur occasionally. It is characterized by transient upper airway obstruction during sleep because of relaxation of the pharyngeal muscles. The patients are often sleep-deprived, which leads to day time somnolence. Occasionally, life-threatening arrhythmias may occur at night probably related to hypoxia or hypercarbia. Polycythemia, pulmonary hypertension, and cor pulmonale develop as a result of hypoxia.

Fetal macrosomia is common in obese patients. This may be partly responsible for the increased rates of cesarean section and dystocia. The neonate is also prone to develop asymptomatic hypoglycemia. The reason for this is not clear. Even when born with normal blood glucose levels, the fasted neonate of an obese mother may develop hypoglycemia within an hour after birth. Their increased ability to mobilize triglycerides are believed to be responsible for lack of symptoms when hypoglycemia develops.

Anesthetic Considerations

Patients with polycythemia or pulmonary hypertension must have their arterial blood pH and gas tensions measured preoperatively. Carbon dioxide tensions approaching 37 mm Hg are suggestive of respiratory inadequacy in pregnant subjects. A pulmonary arterial catheter is needed in patients with cor pulmonale. The technique of choice is regional anesthesia. However, the increased thickness of the subcutaneous tissue makes it difficult to identify bony landmarks. The distance between skin and the epidural space is increased and needles longer than the ones usually available may be needed.[36,37] Obesity may decrease the dose of local anesthetic required to produce a given dermatomal level[38] following epidural or spinal anesthesia (Fig. 13–8). The increased adipose tissue content of the epidural space together with the increased weight of the abdominal contents may play a role in diminishing the compliance of the epidural and subarachnoid spaces. Because the dose requirement is more unpredictable with spinal anesthesia than with

Table 13–8. Problems in the Obese Patient

Problem area	Disorders
Cardiovascular	Hypertension; Cor pulmonale; Polycythemia; Increased incidence of DVT; Increased supine hypotension.
Respiratory	Hypoventilation; Respiratory failure; Pickwickian syndrome; Upper airway surgery; Restrictive lung disease; Increased closing capacity.
Increased body weight	Increased $\dot{V}O_2$ and $\dot{V}CO_2$; Diabetes mellitus; Technical difficulties; Increased spread of spinal and epidural anesthesia.
Gastrointestinal	Hepatic dysfunction; Increased risk of aspiration.
Neonate	Macrosomia; Hypoglycemia.

DVT = deep vein thrombosis

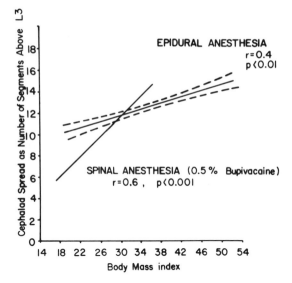

FIG. 13–8. Spread of epidural and spinal anesthesia in relation to Body mass index (BMI). BMI = body weight/height.[2] Graph constructed from the data of Hodgkinson R[38] and McCulloch WJD.[39]

epidural anesthesia, the latter is preferred. The inferior vena cava is subject to more compression in obese patients than in nonobese pregnant patients because of the added weight of the intestines and the abdominal wall. Supine position must at all costs be avoided.

General anesthesia is hazardous because of the increased incidence of hiatus hernia, increased gastric fluid volume, decreased gastric fluid acidity, and increased intragastric pressure. Premedication with a histamine-2 antagonist is beneficial. Endotracheal intubation may be difficult because of increased adipose tissue mass in the neck or in the submandibular area. Massively enlarged breasts make the insertion of the laryngoscope blade difficult. Patients may have had a tracheostomy or pharyngoplasty in the past for the treatment of pickwickian syndrome. An awake fiberoptic tracheal intubation must be considered under these circumstances. The metabolism of volatile agents is altered in obese patients. The increased reduction reaction of halothane releases more fluoride ions. Reductive reaction is implicated in hepatotoxicity of halothane.[40] In addition, the increased levels of bromide may occasionally result in lethargy. This, together with the fact that the incidence of hepatic dysfunction is increased in those who have had jejunoileal bypass, makes halothane a

questionable choice in these patients. Isoflurane is a better alternative. Intraoperative measurement of Pa_{O_2} is necessary because of the potential risk of arterial hypoxemia caused by ventilation-perfusion anomalies or mechanical problems associated with positive pressure ventilation.

The use of epidural opioids for postoperative analgesia allows earlier ambulation of obese patients in the postoperative period.[41] Consequently, their use must be seriously considered for this purpose to minimize postoperative pulmonary morbidity.

REFERENCES

1. Mestman JH: Thyroid disease in pregnancy. Clin in Perinatol *12*:651, 1985.
2. Guyton AC: Endocrinology and reproduction. *In* Medical Physiology. Philadelphia, WB Saunders, 1986.
3. Van Der Spuy ZM, and Jacobs HS.: Management of endocrine disorders in pregnancy Part I—thyroid and parathyroid disease. Postgrad Med J *60*:245, 1984
4. Camargo CA, and Kolb FO: Endocrine disorders. *In* Current Medical Diagnosis & Treatment 1986. (Edited by Krupp MA, and Chatton MJ, and Tierney LM Jr). Los Altos, Lange Medical, 1986
5. Curry SL, et al.: Hydatidiform mole: Diagnosis, management, and long-time follow-up of 347 patients. Obstet Gynecol *45*:1, 1975.
6. Momotani N, et al.: Maternal hyperthyroidism and congenital malformation in the offspring. Clin Endocrinol *20*:695, 1984.
7. Zakarija M, and McKenzie JW: Pregnancy-associated charges in the thyroid-stimulating antibody of Graves' disease and the relationship to neonatal hyperthyroidism. J Clin Endocrinol *57*:1036, 1983.
8. Halevy S, et al.: Serum thyroid hormone changes in patients undergoing caesarean section under general or regional anesthesia. Br J Anaesth *50*:1053, 1978.
9. Wood M, et al.: Halothane-induced hepatic necrosis in triiodothyronine-pretreated rats. Anesthesiology *52*:470, 1980.
10. Robbins J: Thyroid storm. *In* Current Therapy in Endocrinology and Metabolism. Philadelphia, BC Decker, 1985.
11. Murkin JM: Anesthesia and hypothyroidism: A review of thyroxine physiology, pharmacology and anesthetic implications. Anesth Analg *61*:371, 1982.
12. White VA, and Kumagai LF: Preoperative endocrine and metabolic considerations. Med Clin North Am *63*:1321, 1979.
13. Kim JM, and Hackman L: Anesthesia for untreated hypothyroidism: report of three cases. Anesth Analg *56*:299, 1977.
14. Montoro M, and Mestman JH: How to manage parathyroid disease in the pregnant patient and neonate. Contemp Obstet Gynecol *17*:43, 1981a.

15. Pitkin RM: Endocrine regulation of calcium homeostasis during pregnancy. Clin Perinatol *10*:575, 1983.

16. West JB: The hypothalamic-pituitary control system. *In* Best and Taylor's Physiological Basis of Medical Practice. Baltimore, Williams & Wilkins, 1985.

17. Van Der Spuy ZM, and Jacobs HS: Management of endocrine disorders in pregnancy. Part II–pituitary, ovarian, and adrenal disease. Postgrad Med J *60*:312, 1984.

18. Wilson JD: Principles of endocrinology. *In* Harrison's Principles of Internal Medicine (Edited by Petersdorf RG, et al., New York. McGraw-Hill, 1983.

19. Von Bormann B, et al.: Variations in vasopressin (ADH)-levels during NLA combined with epidural fentanyl-analgesia. Reg Anaesth *5*:7, 1982.

20. Arieff AI: Hyponatremia, convulsions, respiratory arrest, and permanent brain damage after elective surgery in healthy women. New Engl J Med *314*:1529, 1986.

21. Bonnet F, Harari A, Thibonnier M, and Viars P: Suppression of antidiuretic hormone hypersecretion during surgery by extradural anaesthesia. Br J Anaesth *54*:29, 1982.

22. Weidler B., et al.: Plasma antidiuretic hormone level as an indicator of perioperative stress (Part I). Anaesth Intensivther Notfallmed *16*:315, 1981.

23. Bormann BV, et al.: Influence of epidural fentanyl on stress-induced elevation of plasma vasopressin (ADH) after surgery. Anesth Analg *62*:727, 1983.

24. Korinek AM, et al.: Effect of postoperative extradural morphine on ADH secretion. Br. J Anaesth *57*:4, 1985.

25. Durant NN, Briscoe, and Katz RL: The effects of acute and chronic hydrocortisone treatment on neuromuscular blockade in the anesthetized cat. Anesthesiology *61*:144, 1984.

26. Symreng T, Karlberg BE, Kagedal B, and Schildt B: Physiological cortisol substitution of long-term steroid treated patients undergoing major surgery. Br. J. Anaesth *53*:949, 1981.

27. Wagner RL, et al.: Inhibition of adrenal steroidogenesis by the anesthetic etomidate. N Engl J Med., *310*:1415, 1984.

28. Desmonts JM, and Marty J: Anaesthetic management of patients with phaeochromocytoma. Br J Anaesth *56*:781, 1984.

29. Davies AE, and Navaratnarajah M: Vaginal delivery in a patient with a phaeochromocytoma. Br J Anaesth *56*:913, 1984.

30. Galletly DC, Yee P, and Maling TJB: Anaesthetic management of combined caesarean section and phaeochromocytoma removal. Anaesth Intens Care *11*:249, 1983.

31. Parsons J, Clunie RWD, Letchworth AT: Phaeochromocytoma in a coeliac ganglion in pregnancy. Postgrad Med J *60*:377, 1984.

32. Bittar DA: Innovar-induced hypertensive crises in patients with pheochromocytoma. Anesthesiology *50*:366, 1979.

33. Hyatt M, Muldoon SM, and Rorie DK: Droperidol, a selective antagonist of postsynaptic alpha adrenoceptors in the canine saphenous vein. Anesthesiology *53*:281, 1980.

34. Chambers S, Espiner EA, Donald RA, and Nicholls MG: Hypoglycaemia following removal of phaeochromocytoma. Postgrad Med J *58*:503, 1982.

35. Kleigman RM, and Gross T: Perinatal problems of the obese mother and her infant. Obstet Gynecol *66*:299, 1985.

36. Palmer SK, Abram SE, Maitra AM, and von Kolditz JH: Distance from the skin to the lumbar epidural space in an obstetric population. Anesth Analg *62*:941, 1983.

37. Brodsky JB: Anesthetic management of the morbidly obese patient. Int Anesthesiol Clin *86*:93, 1986.

38. Hodgkinson R, and Husain FJ: Obesity and cephalad spread of analgesia following epidural administration of bupivacaine for cesarean section. Anesth Analg *59*:89, 1980.

39. McCulloch WJD, and Littlewood DG: Influence of obesity on spinal analgesia with isobaric 0.5% bupivacaine. Br J Anaesth *58*:610, 1986.

40. Bentley JB, Vaughn RW, Gandolfi JA, and Cork RC: Halothan biotransformation in obese and nonobese patients. Anesthesiology *57*:94, 1982.

41. Rawal N, et al.: Comparison of intramuscular and epidural morphine for postoperative analgesia in the grossly obese: Influence on postoperative ambulation and pulmonary function. Anesth Analg *63*:583, 1983.

14

DIABETES MELLITUS

The problem with diabetic pregnancies is four-fold: the diabetes, if severe enough, may cause organ dysfunction; the diabetic state may be worsened by pregnancy; the diabetes predisposes to preeclampsia; and the incidence of metabolic and teratogenic abnormalities is increased in the fetus.[1] The use of insulin has definitely helped to decrease the rates of perinatal morbidity and mortality for diabetics; however, these rates for diabetics still remain slightly elevated compared to those for the general population.

There are two ways of classifying diabetes in pregnancy. The old method, proposed by White (Table 14–1),[2,3] is based on the occurrence of diabetes related complications. The new classification was advocated by the National Diabetes Data Group of the National Institutes of Health (Table 14–2).[3] White has classified diabetes into 8 classes (A, B, C, D, E, F, R, and H) based on

insulin requirement, the duration of the disease and the presence of complications. Patients in classes D to H usually show evidence of vascular disease (see Table 14–1). The classification proposed by the National Diabetes Data Group takes into consideration whether or not the patient is insulin-dependent and whether the diabetes is mainly gestational (see Table 14–2).

DIABETES AND THE MOTHER

The placenta secretes a number of steroid hormones most notably the human chorionic somamammotropin (hCS).[3] This hormone, which is also called the human placental lactogen, is very similar to the human growth hormone. This hormone together with estrogens, progesterones, and free cortisol are responsible for the insulin resistance seen in pregnancy. Because of

Table 14–1.   White Classification of Diabetes in Pregnancy

Class	Age of onset		Duration (year)	Vascular disease	Insulin
A	Any		Pregnancy	No	No
B	>20		<10	No	Yes
C	10–19	or	>10–19	No	Yes
D	<10	or	20	Benign retinopathy	Yes
E	Any		Any	Calcification of pelvic arteries	Yes
F	Any		Any	Nephropathy	Yes
R	Any		Any	Proliferative retinopathy	Yes
H	Any		Any	Heart disease	Yes

(From Friend JR: Diabetes. Clin Obstet Gynecol 8:353, 1981.)

Table 14–2. Classification of Diabetes Mellitus During Pregnancy

New nomenclature	Old names	Clinical characteristics
Type I–(IDDM) Insulin-dependent diabetes.	Juvenile diabetes (JD).	Ketosis prone. Insulin-deficiency caused by islet cell loss. Occurs at any age, common in youth.
Type 2–(NIDDM) Insulin nondependent diabetes.	Adult or maturity onset.	Ketosis resistant. Majority are overweight, requiring insulin during pregnancy.
Gestational diabetes mellitus–(GDM).	Gestational diabetes.	Abnormal glucose tolerance.

(From Hollingsworth DR: Alterations of maternal metabolism in normal and diabetic pregnancies: Differences in insulin d-dependent, non-insulin-dependent, and gestational diabetes. Am J Obstet Gynecol *146*:417, 1983.)

the altered hormonal environment, several changes occur in carbohydrate metabolism.

Starvation that lasts as brief as 12 hours causes lower blood sugar levels in pregnant patients than in nonpregnant subjects. An 18 hour fast leads to ketonemia in an attempt to spare maternal proteins. However, there still occurs a small degree of protein breaking down in response to starvation. The placental steroidal hormones are responsible for the "accelerated starvation" (rapid ketogenesis). The purpose of the ketogenesis is to minimize maternal glucose utilization with the result that the fetus will have a nearly normal supply of this important fuel during maternal starvation.[4]

There is a 2- to 3-fold increase in the secretion of insulin in response to a meal in a pregnant patient compared to a nonpregnant patient. Usually, considerable elevations occur in the blood levels of glucose and other nutrients immediately after a meal. The postprandial increase in blood levels of nutrients as well as that of insulin secretion is also considerably greater in a pregnancy (Fig. 14–1). The purpose of the augmented postprandial hyperglycemia is probably to make available to the fetus a large supply of glucose. Thus, a pregnant patient rapidly achieves a fed state after eating a meal and develops a ketotic or a starved state after even a brief period of starvation (Fig. 14–2).

There are other important interactions between pregnancy and diabetes. The risk of polyhydramnios, preeclampsia, and hypertension is greater in diabetic patients. Pernicious vomiting in early pregnancy may lead to diabetic ketoacidosis. The renal threshold for glycosuria is reduced in pregnancy with the result that glycosuria occurs at normal blood sugar values. Insulin administration should not be based on urine sugar measurments. Lactose, a reducing sugar, may be found in the urine, therefore tests

based on reduction reactions must not be used. Test strips containing glucose oxidase (which is specific for glucose) are available for this purpose. The availability of the test strips has made it possible for the patients to monitor their own blood-glucose levels. Also available are several commercial reflectance colorimeters for reading color changes in the strips. The anesthesiologist must familiarize himself with one of these instruments because they are helpful in deciding the need for insulin therapy in the perioperative

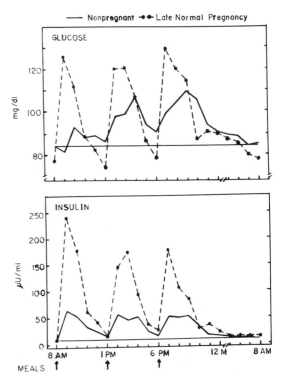

FIG. 14–1. Changes in blood glucose and insulin levels in a pregnant and a nonpregnant subject in reponse to a meal. Note the exaggerated glucose and insulin responses to the meal in the pregnant subject. (From Frienkel N: Of pregnancy and progeny. Diabetes *29*:1023, 1980.)

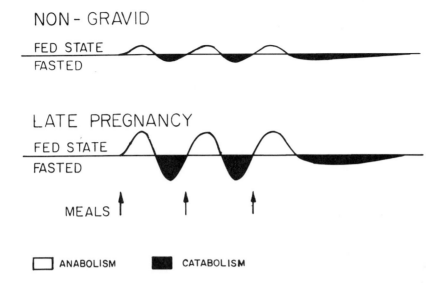

NON - GRAVID

FED STATE
FASTED

LATE PREGNANCY

FED STATE
FASTED

MEALS

☐ ANABOLISM   ■ CATABOLISM

FIG. 14–2.   The accelerated fed (light area) and fasted state (dark area) in a nonpregnant and pregnant subject. Arrows indicate time of meals. Note, in the pregnant patient, the rapid developments of the fed state after eating and the starved state after a short period of starvation. (From Frienkel N: Of pregnancy and progeny. Diabetes 29:1023, 1980.)

period.[5] The accuracy of the units must be verified periodically against measurements made by the hospital laboratory.

DIABETES AND THE FETUS

The incidence of macrosomia, congenital anomalies, and idiopathic respiratory syndrome is higher in the newborn of a diabetic patient (Table 14–3).[6] The fetus secretes increased amounts of insulin in response to the increased placental influx of glucose and other nutrients. Fetal hyperinsulinemia is implicated not only in macrosomia but in the delay in pulmonary sur-

factant maturation. Hyperinsulinemia that occurs at the time of delivery may cause neonatal hypoglycemia. Normalization of maternal metabolic environment by judicious insulin administration is said to minimize many of these complications. The infant may develop hypocalcemia, hyperbilirubinemia, and hypomagnesemia at birth or soon after.

Stillbirths, which occurred frequently a decade ago, have been reduced dramatically by careful monitoring of the mother. The greater the severity of the diabetes, the greater is the perinatal mortality rate (Table 14–4).[7] For instance, the perinatal mortality rate reaches 16 per 1000 live births in Class A patients. The figures for Classes F and R reach a staggering 186 deaths per 1000 births. Congenital anom-

Table 14–3.   Neonatal Morbidity and Mortality in Diabetes

Disorder	Percentage
Deaths	3.2
Hypoglycemia <40 mg%	12.0
Hypocalcemia <7 mg%	26.0
Hypomagnesemia <1.2 mg%	4.0
Polycythemia	11.0
Hyperbilirubinemia	16.0
Respiratory distress syndrome	3.0

Total number of infants is 217 (100%).
(From Lemons JA, Vargas P, and Delaney JJ: Infant of the diabetic mother: Review of 225 cases. Obstet Gynecol 57:187, 1981.

Table 14–4.   Current Perinatal Mortality in Diabetes Mellitus

White's classification	Mortality/1000 live births
A	16
B	48
C	79
D	100
F–R	186

(From Hill DE: Fetal endocrine pancreas. Clin Obstet Gynecol 3:837, 1980.)

alies mainly included neural tube defects and cardiac defects (Table 14–5). Although the perinatal mortality rate has declined over the years, the frequency of congenital anomalies has not shown a similar reduction.[1]

GESTATIONAL DIABETES (GDM)

In 1 to 2% of all women, glucose tolerance decreases enough during pregnancy for the diagnostic criteria of diabetes to be fulfilled. However, these women do not develop overt diabetes. The oral glucose tolerance usually returns to normal after delivery. Patients with GDM have an increased risk of perinatal and neonatal complications. The neonatal complications include macrosomia and hypoglycemia and a slightly increased risk for congenital anomalies. Patients may require only dietary supervision, although some authorities do recommend insulin therapy.[4,8,9] The decision to use insulin will be decided on an individual basis based on fasting blood sugar levels, and the postprandial blood glucose responses.

GLUCOSE TOLERANCE TEST FOR DIAGNOSING GDM

After obtaining a venous sample for fasting blood sugar measurement, 100 grams of glucose is administered orally in the morning. Two or more abnormal measurements are considered diagnostic of GDM. The accepted blood sugar values are 105 mg/dl (fasting), 190 mg (after 1 hour), 165 mg (after 2 hours), and 145 mg (after 3 hours).

Antepartum Surveillance of the Fetus

Tests used for monitoring the antepartum well-being of the fetus are described in Chapter 24. Nonstress testing, contraction stress testing, amniotic fluid lecithin-sphingomyelin ratio (for fetal lung maturity), and fetal α-feto proteins (for diagnosing neural tube defects), fetal biochemical profile, maternal urinary or plasma estriol measurements (for assessing the integrity of the fetoplacental unit) are recommended.[10,11]

Glycosylated Hemoglobin

Ninety percent of adult hemoglobin is hemoglobin A. Glycosylated hemoglobins are normal minor hemoglobins in which a carbohydrate moiety is attached to valine, the N-terminal amino acid of the α-chain.[5,12] The glycosylated hemoglobins are of three different types HbA_{1a}, HbA_{1b}, and HbA_{1c}. HbA_{1c} constitutes the majority of glycosylated hemoglobin. The concentration of glycosylated hemoglobin, which is determined electrophoretically is directly proportional to the fasting blood sugar level and the glucose tolerance. Once formed, the glycosylated hemoglobins are stable for 5 to 8 weeks; therefore they can be used to evaluate whether the treatment regimen has been effective in a given period of time. The current uses of glycosylated hemoglobin measurements in a pregnant patient are: to assess the quality of blood sugar control during critical periods of organogenesis; to assess the effectiveness of antidiabetic therapy; and to help in pregestational counseling. If the levels of glycosylated measurements are high, the patient may be advised to delay conception until the levels are normalized. Inadequately controlled diabetes may be associated with increased fetal teratogenicity.

OBSTETRIC MANAGEMENT

Timing of delivery is no longer based on the severity of the diabetes as indicated by White's

Table 14–5.   Teratogenic Abnormalities in the Infants

Location	Disorder
CNS	Anencephaly, meningomyelocele, spina bifida.
Cardiac	Transposition of vessels, ventricular septal defect, situs inversus, hypoplastic left ventricle.
Renal	Agenesis.
Pulmonary	Hypoplastic lungs.
Gastrointestinal	Anal and rectal atresia, small colon.

(From Cousins L: Congenital anomalies among infants of diabetic mothers. Etiology, prevention and prenatal diagnosis. Am J Obstet Gynecol *147*:333, 1983.)

classification. Several antepartum tests of fetal and maternal well-being are taken into consideration before a decision is made on the timing of delivery. The most important test is probably the one that confirms fetal lung maturity. A combination of an L/S ratio of 2 or greater with the demonstration of the presence of phosphatidyl glycerol in the amniotic fluid provides the most reliable evidence for this.[13] Phosphatidyl glycerol is the final step in the maturation pathway of the fetal surfactant. When antepartum tests are within normal limits and the patient's clinical condition is stable, one can deliver the patient by the 38th week if the tests of fetal pulmonary maturity are satisfactory. In the absence of macrosomia, labor can be induced electively and the infant can be delivered vaginally. Any rapid deterioration in the maternal diabetes or its complications such as nephropathy or retinopathy or sudden deterioration of fetal well-being (as shown by abnormal fetal surveillance tests) calls for delivery as soon as possible.[14]

MEDICAL MANAGEMENT OF DIABETES IN PREGNANCY

Self-measurement of blood glucose with glucose-oxidase-impregnated reagent test-strips are vital to achieving adequate metabolic control in diabetic patients.[4,5,15] Ketone bodies can be tested for in the urine. Insulin administration is timed so that the blood level is not only sustained throughout the day and night but is also adequate to cover postprandial increases in blood glucose levels. The following are several regimens of insulin administration that have been proposed: (1) Two injections of regular and lente insulin (intermediate acting) at breakfast and supper; (2) Injections of regular insulin at breakfast, lunch, supper plus an injection of NPH at night; (3) Three injections of regular insulin (as in regimen no. 2) plus one injection of ultra lente insulin at breakfast. Insulin has also been administered by continuous subcutaneous infusion.

The goal of therapy is to achieve a fasting blood glucose level of 70 to 90 mg/dL and a postprandial blood sugar level of less than 140 mg/dL. Three evenly spaced meals and a bedtime snack are prescribed. Total calorie intake should be 30 kcal/kg in early pregnancy and is increased to 38 kcal/kg per day during the last two trimesters.[4] Forty-five percent of this is given as carbohydrates and 15 to 20% as protein.

Many approaches are available for administration of insulin during labor and delivery. The classical approach is to administer one-third of the total dose in the morning, if the patient has not received her dose. The insulin dose is reduced because of a possible precipitous reduction in the insulin requirement in the post-partum period. A well-controlled diabetic patient who has received a dose of intermediate acting insulin within 12 and 14 hours prior to the onset of labor may not require any more insulin during labor. Some prefer a second approach, which is to give glucose-insulin infusion to minimize ketosis; a glucose load as small as 5 to 10 g is sufficient to suppress the ketogenic response of labor. Glucose is administered at 5 to 10 gram/hour and insulin at 0.02 to 0.04 units of regular insulin/kg/hour.[4] An automatic infusion pump must be used for administering glucose-insulin solution. If glucose-insulin infusion is not used, plasma glucose must be measured every 4 to 6 hours and regular insulin administered accordingly.[16]

Capillary blood sugar must be maintained at 70 to 90 mg/dL. Hypoglycemia can be treated by administration of 5 to 10 g of glucose.[4] Hyperglycemia can be treated by intravenous administration of 2 to 5 units of insulin. One of the commercially available reflectance glucometers may be used for colorimetric reading of the glucose oxidase test strip. The insulin administration rate must be reduced by 50% after delivery to avoid the possibility of postpartum hypoglycemia.[4] Plastic tubing for insulin infusion must be flushed with 40 to 50 ml of insulin-containing solution to prevent adsorption of insulin to the tubing.

Anesthesia for a Pregnant Diabetic

A second intravenous infusion must be started if the patient is already receiving a glucose-insulin infusion. Using the existing infusion line for rapid fluid administration may disrupt the smooth functioning of the glucose-infusion pump. Ringer's lactate (1200 to 1500 ml) must be administered before regional anesthesia is induced to minimize the incidence of systemic hypotension. Administration of glucose in excess of 20 g/hour is associated with neonatal hypo-

Table 14–6.   Signs of Hypoglycemia in the Neonate

Symptom	Percent babies with symptom
Jitteriness	36
Cyanosis	34
Seizure	16
Apnea	11
Hypotonia	7

(From Perelman RH: The infant of the diabetic mother: Pathophysiology and management. Prim Care *10*:751, 1983.)

glycemia and neonatal hyperlactacedemia. Maternal hypoglycemia affects both the mother and the fetus. Maternal hypoglycemia is associated with diminished fetal breathing movement caused by diminished low voltage electric activity in the cerebral cortex. The fetal problems associated with disturbances in maternal glucose homeostasis is discussed in greater detail in Chapter 3. The signs, symptoms, and diagnosis of neonatal hypoglycemia are listed in Table 14–6.[17]

There are studies that suggest that spinal and epidural anesthesia may be associated with increased fetal acidosis.[18,19] The authors of this study attributed this to the increased incidence of hypotension following regional anesthesia. However, the mothers in their studies may have received large volumes of glucose-containing solution prior to delivery. In regard to fetal acidosis, the following precautions must be observed: diabetics must be operated on in the morning to prevent starvation and ketosis; the diabetes must be well controlled; prophylactic hydration must be used; when epidural anesthesia is used, the level must be increased gradually and any hypotension (systolic pressure <100 mm Hg) must be treated promptly with intravenous infusion of ephedrine; inspired air must be enriched with oxygen to ensure adequate oxygenation of the fetus before birth; and aortocaval compression must be avoided. Because of the potential risk for precipitous systemic hypotension associated with spinal anesthesia, one may make a case against the use of this technique.

With diabetics, epidural anesthesia is probably preferable to general anesthesia for cesarean section because general anesthesia may expose the already compromised fetus to the depressant effects of thiopental and other general anesthetics.

The advantages of the use of lumbar epidural analgesia for producing labor analgesia are that it decreases insulin requirements by diminishing catecholamine response to labor pains, and that it minimizes or eliminates the normally occurring lactate accumulation during labor, especially during the second stage of labor.

Neuropathy occasionally complicates diabetes mellitus. Although neuropathy is more common in patients over 50 years of age, it may occasionally occur in pregnant patients. The neuropathy may involve a single nerve or multiple nerves, or it may be an autonomic neuropathy. Regardless of the type of neuropathy, the CSF proteins are usually elevated.[20] Many patients have an unfounded fear that regional anesthesia may further aggravate neuropathy. There is no evidence to suggest that regional anesthesia may either delay recovery from the neuropathy or cause further deterioration of the condition. The anesthesiologist must carefully explain this to the patient before administering regional anesthesia to avoid possible litigation.

DIABETIC KETOACIDOSIS

Occasionally, the anesthesiologist may be required to provide care for a pregnant patient who is in diabetic ketoacidosis (DKA). DKA is caused by lack of insulin and is associated with three types of metabolic derangements.

Carbohydrate Metabolism. Carbohydrate metabolism is affected because of underutilization of glucose and increased hepatic glycogenolysis. Hyperglycemia draws water and sodium out of the cells causing intracellular dehydration. Hyperglycemia also causes osmotic diuresis and renal electrolyte loss causing a shrinkage of extracellular fluid volume. Thus, both intracellular and extracellular water compartments shrink leading to profound shock.

Protein Catabolism. Protein synthesis does not occur in the absence of insulin. Large quantities of amino acids and K^+ are released into the circulation leading to intracellular K^+ depletion.[21] If oliguria ensues, K^+ will not be excreted and this will result in hyperkalemia. The accompanying metabolic acidosis of DKA draws more K^+ out of the cell into the extracellular fluid.

Lipid Metabolism. Fats burn in the hearth of carbohydrates. Defective carbohydrate metabolism interferes with fat metabolism. The lack of carbohydrate fuel makes it necessary for the body to generate energy by intramitochondrial oxidation of fatty acids, consequently releasing keto acids. Keto acids are strong acids and their accumulation will deplete the alkali buffer pool causing a base deficit. Keto acids further compound the acid-base picture by increasing renal sodium excretion.

As mentioned earlier, pregnancy, even in nondiabetic individuals, predisposes to ketonemia. In addition, placental hormones antagonize insulin effect to a certain extent. Any added stress in the form of infection, prolonged starvation, or dehydration is likely to produce ketoacidosis. Severe vomiting, associated with morning sickness, and a stressful labor are the other predisposing factors for DKA in a pregnant patient. Interestingly, failure by the patient to self-administer insulin contributes to only 7% of cases of DKA. Occasionally, malfunction of the continuous subcutaneous insulin infusion pumps may lead to DKA.[22].

Keto acids readily cross the placenta and cause fetal acidosis. The fetal mortality rate may reach 50 to 90% after one episode of DKA. Late decelerations of fetal heart rate are reported to occur with maternal DKA. The fetus is also subject to wide fluctuations in its serum K^+ concentration. Maternal acidosis reportedly decreases uterine blood flow.

The most common symptom of DKA is vomiting, followed by thirst, dehydration, and profound shock. Occasionally, a patient may complain of severe abdominal pains that may be confused with a surgical emergency. Severe acidosis will cause Kussmaul's type of hyperventilation and the patient's breath will have the characteristic fruity odor. It should be remembered that DKA occurs at lower blood sugar levels in pregnant patients.[22] Diagnosis of DKA can be made with certainty when there is marked ketonemia (strong nitroprusside test in undiluted serum), glycosuria or hyperglycemia (serum level 300 to 350 mg/dL), arterial blood pH <7.25 and/or an HCO_3^- concentration <10 mEq/L. Serum Na^+ concentration may be normal or low, and serum K^+ concentration may be elevated. Contracted circulating blood volume often produces prerenal azotemia; therefore blood urea nitrogen (BUN) measurements must also be made.

Treatment of DKA is aimed at correcting the metabolic, electrolyte and acid-base derangements. Central venous pressure measurement is valuable in determining a circulating fluid volume deficit.[20] Two liters of normal saline may be needed in the beginning. The rate of infusion is then decreased to 150 to 200 ml/hour. Half-normal saline must be used, if serum Na^+ exceeds 155 mEq/L. When the plasma glucose level decreases to 200 to 250 mg/dL, a 5% glucose solution may be administered to prevent hypoglycemia. Continuous low-dose insulin infusion not only minimizes the risk of hypoglycemia but also the risk of hypokalemia, which occasionally develops with larger intermittent injections. A loading dose of insulin at 0.3 unit/kg of body weight followed by infusion at a rate of 0.1 unit/kg/hour is recommended. The rate of fall of glucose with the infusion regimen is 75 to 100 mg/dL/hour. The correction of acidosis usually takes longer than with larger intermittent injections.

Plasma K^+ starts falling soon after the initiation of therapy and reaches nadir within 4 hours of therapy. Replacement of K^+ in combination with a neutral phosphate may facilitate treatment of hyperkalemia and hypophosphatemia, which is often seen during therapy of DKA.

Administration of alkali still remains controversial. Excessive $NaHCO_3$ administration may cause hypokalemia. Neutralization of acid with HCO_3^- releases CO_2, which may gain rapid entry into CSF causing worsening of CNS acidosis. Overzealous alkali administration may also shift the maternal oxyhemoglobin dissociation curve to the left, interfering with release of oxygen at the intervillous space. Most authorities administer HCO_3^- only when the arterial blood pH <7.1 and recommend discontinuing HCO_3^- administration when the pH reaches 7.2.

Labor analgesia may be required in a patient who has developed DKA during the course of labor. Because of hypovolemia, lumbar epidural analgesia may produce systemic hypotension. All fluid deficits and acid-base derangement must be corrected before administering lumbar epidural anesthesia. Occasionally, cesarean section may be needed for fetal distress in a patient in DKA. It is then up to the anesthesiologist to treat the DKA intraoperatively. Cardiac arrhythmias caused by hypokalemia or hyperkalemia, and severe systemic hypotension caused by hypovolemia must be considered. Insulin administration must continue intraoperatively. Fluid and electrolyte imbalances must be corrected. Serial serum Na^+, K^+, and glucose measurement, as well as measurements of arterial blood pH, Po_2 and Pco_2 must be made. If the patient is extremely hypovolemic, a combination of ketamine and thiopental may be used for induction. The use of succinylcholine in a hyperkalemic patient with prerenal azotemia may cause further elevations in serum K^+, which can result in life-threatening arrhythmias. Failure to administer insulin intraoperatively may cause plasma levels of glucose to rise rapidly resulting in a hyperosmolar coma. Hyperosmolar state when present at the end of surgery may interfere with regaining consciousness from general anesthesia.

The baby should be evaluated for the presence of hyperglycemia and hypoglycemia and acid-base and electrolyte derangements, which are often more severe than the usual degree of derangements seen in infants born of diabetic mothers without DKA.

REFERENCES

1. Frienkel N: Of pregnancy and progeny. Diabetes 29:1023, 1980.
2. Gabbe SG: Diabetes mellitus in pregnancy: have all the problems been solved? Am J Med 70:613, 1981.
3. Hollingsworth DR: Alterations of maternal metabolism in normal and diabetic pregnancies: Differences in insulin d-dependent, non-insulin-dependent, and gestational diabetes. Am J Obstet Gynecol 146:417, 1983.
4. Buchanan TA, Unterman TC, and Metzger BE: The medical management of diabetes in pregnancy. Clin Perinatol 12:625, 1985.
5. Granados JL: Recent developments in the outpatient management of insulin-dependent diabetes mellitus in pregnancy. Obstet Gynecol Annu 13:83, 1984.
6. Lemons JA, Vargas P, and Delaney JJ: Infant of the diabetic mother: Review of 225 cases. Obstet Gynecol 57:187, 1981.
7. Hill DE: Fetal endocrine pancreas. Clin Obstet Gynecol 3:837, 1980.
8. Kuhl C, Hornes PJ, and Anderson O: Etiology and pathophysiology of gestational diabetes mellitus. Diabetes (suppl 2) 34:66, 1985.
9. Kalkoff RK: Therapeutic results of insulin therapy in gestational diabetes mellitus. Diabetes (Suppl. 2) 34:97, 1985.
10. Diamon MP, et al.: Antepartum fetal monitoring insulin-dependent diabetic pregnancies. Am J Obstet Gynecol 153:528, 1985.
11. Golde SH, et al.: The role of nonstress tests, fetal biophysical profile, and contraction stress tests in the outpatient management of insulin-requiring diabetic pregnancies. Am J Obstet Gynecol 148:269, 1984.
12. Peacock I: Glycosylated haemoglobin: measurement and clinical use. J Clin Pathol 37:841, 1984.
13. Gabbe SG, and Quilligan EJ: General obstetric management of the diabetic pregnancy. Clin Obstet Gynecol 24:91, 1981.
14. Leveno KJ, and Whalley PJ: Dilemmas in the management of pregnancy complicated by diabetes. Med Clin North Amer 66:1325, 1982.
15. Skyler JS: Self-Monitoring of blood glucose. Med Clin North 66:1227, 1982.
16. Friend JR: Diabetes. Clin Obstet Gynecol 8:353, 1981.
17. Perlman RH: The infant of the diabetic mother: Pathophysiology and management. Prim Care 10:751, 1983.
18. Datta S, and Brown WU: Acid-Base status in diabetic mothers and their infants following general or spinal anesthesia for cesarean section. Anesthesiology 47:272, 1977.
19. Datta S, et al.: Epidural anesthesia for cesarean section in diabetic parturients: maternal and neonatal Acid-Base status and bupivacaine concentration. Anesth Analg 60:574, 1981.
20. Adams RD, and Asbury AK: Diseases of the peripheral nervous system. In Harrison's Principles of Internal Medicine, 10th Edition. (Edited by Petersdorf RG, et al.) New York, McGraw-Hill, 1983.
21. Brumfield CG, and Huddleston JF: The management of diabetic ketoacidosis in pregnancy. Clin Obstet Gynecol 27:50, 1984.
22. Peden NR, Braaten JT, and McKendry JBR: Diabetic ketoacidosis during long-term treatment with continuous subcutaneous insulin infusion. Diabetes Care 7:1, 1984.

15

ASTHMA

Asthma affects 1% of all pregnant women.[1] Up to 14% of pregnant asthmatics suffer at least one serious bronchospastic episode during pregnancy.[2] A serious bronchospasm interferes with fetal oxygenation; therefore every attempt must be made to minimize the frequency of bronchospastic attacks during pregnancy and to treat them adequately, if they do occur. Pregnancy causes several alterations in the maternal respiratory system, particularly in arterial blood pH and gas tensions. These changes are described in detail in Chapter 2. Approximately 29% of asthmatics will improve during pregnancy, 49% will remain the same, and the remaining 22% will deteriorate.[3] Women are likely to repeat the same pattern during each pregnancy. Upper respiratory infections are probably the most common precipitating cause of severe asthma during pregnancy.[3]

MATERNAL OUTCOME

In a study of 381 pregnant asthmatic women, Bahna and Bjerkedal[4] reported that hyperemesis, hemorrhage, and preeclampsia were more frequent in this group than in nonasthmatic pregnant patients. Gordon, et al.[5] reported two maternal deaths among 16 asthmatics. However, Shatz, et al.[6] did not report any maternal death among 55 steroid-dependent asthmatics. The decreased complication rate in the study by Shatz, et al. might reflect the closer medical attention given to their patients because of the severity of their disease.

OUTCOME FOR THE INFANT

There are higher rates of prematurity, stillbirth, and perinatal and infant mortality in asthmatic women. The incidence of neonatal hypoxia is slightly higher in asthmatic patients than in the control groups.[4] Gordon, et al.[5] reported a slightly increased incidence of perinatal mortality rate in the asthmatic group as a whole. However, in the sixteen women with severe asthma in their study, the incidence of perinatal mortality and other complications was much higher than in the control groups. Important maternal and fetal complications are summarized in Fig. 15–1.

CLASSIFICATION OF ASTHMA

Asthma is classified according to the causes (Table 15–1).

Extrinsic Asthma. This type is IgE mediated. Inhaling an allergen quickly produces bronchospasm. Whole ragweed pollens or grass pollens present in the atmosphere usually trigger symptoms. Viral infections may precipitate an acute episode. Food preservatives containing metabisulfite release SO_2 in acid solution, which can occasionally stimulate bronchospasm.

Intrinsic Asthma. No specific antigen can be identified.

Mixed Asthma. This type is caused by both IgE and non-IgE related factors. Bronchospasm associated with bronchiolitis in children is a classic example.

Aspirin Intolerant Asthma. Aspirin and other

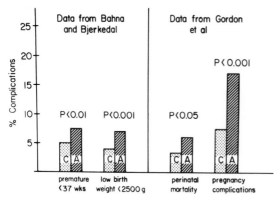

FIG. 15–1. Maternal and neonatal complications in asthma. C = nonasthmatic controls; A = asthmatics. P values given for comparison with controls. Pregnancy complications include hyperemesis, hemorrhage, and preeclampsia. Figures are drawn from the data of Bahna and Bjerkedal[4] and Gordon, et al.[5]

nonsteroidal anti-inflammatory drugs cause worsening of chronic asthma. The incidence of nasal polyps, sinusitis, and parasinusitis is high in this group of patients. Tartrazine, and azo-dye used as a coloring substance in many medications is said to provoke attacks in 5 to 10% of aspirin intolerant asthmatics.

Exercise Induced Asthma. Bronchospasm occurs shortly after discontinuation of the exercise. Cold dry air produces more bronchospasm than does moist warm air in these patients, which suggests that the mechanism of bronchial spasm is related to heat loss from the airways.

Occupational Asthma. Occupation or hobby related allergens, such as bird or chemical antigens may play a role in causing asthma. Symptoms improve when patients are away from the workplace or the hobby causing the asthma.[1]

PATHOPHYSIOLOGY

Contraction of smooth muscle in the large and/or small airways increases airway resistance. Viscid mucus further worsens the obstruction. Hyperinflation of the lungs results in increased residual volume (RV) and functional residual capacity (FRC). The common bronchoconstrictors, such as methacholine, prostaglandin F_2 (PGF_2), and leukotrienes D_4, produce a more intense bronchospasm in asthmatics than they do in nonasthmatics. Although airway spasm is reversible with treatment, these patients may have permanent changes in the lung parenchyma, which include smooth muscle hypertrophy, desquamation of bronchial epithelium, mucosal edema, goblet cell hyperplasma, and basement membrane thickening.

The role of mast cells in the genesis of bronchial spasm is becoming increasingly clear. Mast cells carry a number of reactive sites for IgE antibodies. The attachment of these antibodies to the receptor sites triggers degranulation of the mast cell leading to the release of bronchoactive substances, notably histamine, leukotrienes, PGF_2, and thromboxane A_2. Prostaglandins and thromboxanes are formed from arachidonic acid via the cyclooxygenase pathway whereas leukotrienes are formed via the lypoxygenase pathway. Corticosteroids are believed to exert their beneficial effects in asthma by blocking the formation of arachidonic acid from phospholipid.[7]

Increased resistance to airflow prolongs exhalations and causes airtrapping. The FRC, RV, and total lung capacity increase whereas vital capacity, expiratory reserve volume, and inspiratory capacity decrease. The flow-volume loop

Table 15–1. Types of Asthma

Type	Characteristic
Extrinsic	IgE medicated.
Intrinsic	Not related to IgE.
Mixed	Both IgE and non-IgE related factors (e.g., bronchiolitis in children).
Aspirin intolerant	A small percentage may have IgE-related causes–tartrazine allergy.
Exercise induced	Bronchospasm develops only after discontinuing exercise.
Occupational/hobby related	Symptoms improve on days-off.

(Modified from Greenberger PA: Asthma in pregnancy. Clin in Perinatol *12*:571, 1985.

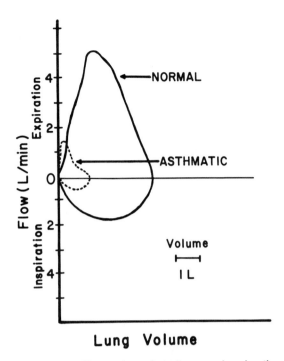

FIG. 15–2.   Flow-volume loop in normal and asthmatic patients. Note the greater residual volume and smaller peak flow in the asthmatic subject. (From Kingston GG and Hirshman CA: Perioperative management of the patient with asthma. Anesth Analg 63:844, 1984.)

becomes abnormal (Fig. 15–2). During moderately severe bronchospasm, FEV_1 may be maintained but the flow in the small airways may be abnormal. Reduction in vital capacity, FEV_1, and peak expiratory flow rates are indications of large airway obstruction but they do not provide any information regarding flows in the small airways. Forced expiratory flow at 25 to 75% of the vital capacity (FEF 25 to 75%) is more indicative of small airway obstruction. An additional advantage of measuring FEF 25 to 75% is that it is, to a large extent, independent of patient effort (Fig. 15–3).[8] Amniotic fluid contains a mixture of prostaglandins. There is a 3-fold increase in urinary metabolites of PGF_2 during pregnancy with further increases occurring during labor and after delivery. It is not known whether the increased levels of these bronchoconstrictors pose any additional risk to the mother.[3]

ANTIASTHMA MEDICATIONS IN PREGNANCY

Theophylline

Theophylline is a methylxanthine derivative. Aminophylline is a preparation of theophylline. Eighty percent of the aminophylline preparation is theophylline. Pharmacokinetic studies have shown that the elimination half-life of theophylline is no different in pregnant subjects from that in nonpregnant patients.[9] Theophylline, which easily crosses the placenta and is excreted in the breast milk has a maternal to fetal blood concentration ratio almost equal to one. Excessive blood concentration of theophylline causes jitteriness, tachycardia, and opisthotonus in the neonate,[10] but fetal side effects are unlikely to occur if the aminophylline levels are less than 13 µg/ml in the mother.[9] There are no other adverse fetal effects or teratogenicity attributed to aminophylline administration in pregnancy.

Although methylxanthine derivatives are believed to produce smooth muscle dilatation by inhibiting phosphodiesterase, recent evidence suggests that there are other mechanisms of action (Table 15–2).[11,12] The additional mechanisms proposed are the liberation of catecholamines from the adrenal medulla, extra adrenal chromaffin tissue, and the myocardium; and the action on intracellular and extracellular Ca^{++}. The cardiac actions of theophylline can be explained on the basis of its effects on excitation-contraction coupling in the myocardium. Aminophylline causes increased Ca^{++} entry into the cell and simultaneously inhibits sequestration of Ca^{++} by the sarcoplasmic reticulum. The concentration of free Ca^{++} in the cytoplasm increases thus augmenting cardiac irritability.

The above-mentioned effects of theophylline may be responsible not only for the cardiac toxicity of theophylline but also for the increased incidence of cardiac arrhythmias when theophylline and inhalation anesthetic agents are used concomitantly. The dosage and mode of administration of theophylline are shown in Figure 15–4. A loading dose of 5.6 mg/kg is sufficient to maintain a therapeutic concentration of 10 µg/ml. When in doubt, selection of dose must be guided by blood concentration measurements. Higher doses may be necessary in smok-

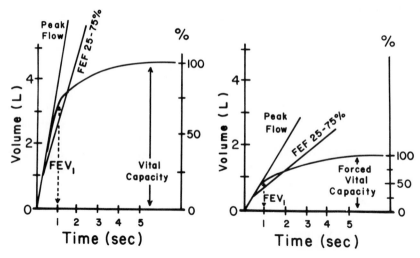

FIG. 15–3. Forced expiratory spirogram tracing the normal patient (left) and the asthmatic patient (right). Note the reduction in peak flow FEF 25 to 75% and FEV₁ in the asthmatic patient. (From Kingston GG, and Hirshman CA: Perioperative management of the patient with asthma. Anesth Analg 63:844, 1984.)

ers because the polyhydrocarbons contained in cigarette smoke are known to cause enzyme induction, thus accelerating the clearance of aminophylline.

β-Mimetic Substances

They produce bronchodilatation by stimulating the bronchial wall β-receptors. Selective β-2 agonists are preferable to mixed agonists, which produce unnecessary tachycardia. The use of epinephrine in the first 4 months of pregnancy has been shown to be associated with slightly increased incidence of congenital malformations in the fetus. A list of β-mimetic substances and their activity is given in Table 15–3.[13] If necessary, one of the beta-mimetic substances such as isoetharine may be administered in the form

Table 15–2. Antiasthma Drugs in Pregnancy

Agents	Mechanism of action	Safety in early pregnancy
Epinephrine (β-mimetic agent)	Stimulates β-receptors.	Congenital malformations.
Other β-mimetic agents	Same as above.	Insufficient data, probably safe.
Theophylline	Posphodiesterase inhibition. Liberation of catecholamines from the adrenal medulla. Affects Ca⁺⁺ turnover in the myocardium.	Safe.
Corticosteroids: Beclomethasone dipropionate aerosol Prednisone Prednisolone Hydrocortisone	Decrease airway edema. Vasoconstriction. Prevents eicosanoid release. Modify β-receptor action.	Safe.
Cromolyn sodium	Prevents mast cell degranulation	Insufficient data.
Iodides	Expectorant.	Fetal goiter. Fetal iodism.
Antihistamines	H₁-blocker.	Safe.

Most of the antiasthma drugs are excreted in the breast milk but do not produce adverse neonatal effects.

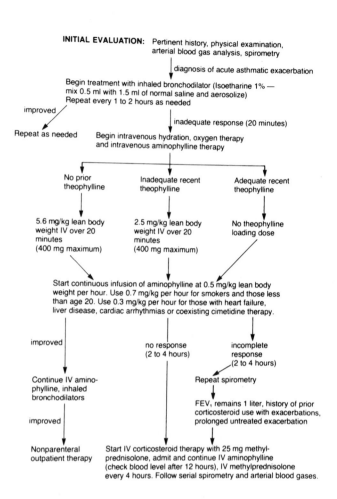

INITIAL EVALUATION: Pertinent history, physical examination, arterial blood gas analysis, spirometry

↓ diagnosis of acute asthmatic exacerbation

Begin treatment with inhaled bronchodilator (Isoetharine 1% — mix 0.5 ml with 1.5 ml of normal saline and aerosolize) Repeat every 1 to 2 hours as needed

improved ↓
Repeat as needed

inadequate response (20 minutes) ↓
Begin intravenous hydration, oxygen therapy and intravenous aminophylline therapy

- No prior theophylline
- Inadequate recent theophylline
- Adequate recent theophylline

5.6 mg/kg lean body weight IV over 20 minutes (400 mg maximum)

2.5 mg/kg lean body weight IV over 20 minutes (400 mg maximum)

No theophylline loading dose

Start continuous infusion of aminophylline at 0.5 mg/kg lean body weight per hour. Use 0.7 mg/kg per hour for smokers and those less than age 20. Use 0.3 mg/kg per hour for those with heart failure, liver disease, cardiac arrhythmias or coexisting cimetidine therapy.

improved

no response (2 to 4 hours)

incomplete response (2 to 4 hours)

Continue IV aminophylline, inhaled bronchodilators

Repeat spirometry

FEV, remains 1 liter, history of prior corticosteroid use with exacerbations, prolonged untreated exacerbation

improved

Nonparenteral outpatient therapy

Start IV corticosteroid therapy with 25 mg methylprednisolone, admit and continue IV aminophylline (check blood level after 12 hours), IV methylprednisolone every 4 hours. Follow serial spirometry and arterial blood gases.

FIG. 15–4. Schematic representation of the step-by-step management of bronchial spasm in asthma. (From Niederman MS, and Matthay R: Asthma and other severe respiratory diseases during pregnancy. *In* Critical Care of the Obstetrical patient. (Edited by Berkowitz RL). New York, Churchill-Livingstone, 1983.)

of an aerosol.[2] The duration of action of isoetharine aerosol is 4 to 6 hours[13] and the drug is not effective if taken orally.

Corticosteroids

The use of corticosteroids in early pregnancy is safe, and although their use has been associated with increased incidence of oral clefts in animals, there are no human data to support this. Corticosteroids are beneficial in asthmatics because they prevent formation of eicosanoids, notably prostaglandin F_2 and E_2 and leukotuences C_4 and D_4, which are potent bronchoconstrictors. Corticosteroids are also beneficial because they abolish T-lymphocyte responses to

Table 15–3. β-Adrenergic Bronchodilators

Agent	α	β_1 activity	β_2 activity	Effective orally	Effective as aerosol	Duration (hours)
Ephedrine	+	+	+	+	−	2
Epinephrine	+	+ +	+ +	0	+ +	2
Isoproterenol	−	+ +	+ +	0	+ +	2
Isoetharine*	−	+ −	+ +	0	+ +	5
Metaproterenol	−	+ −	+ +	+ +	+ +	5
Terbutaline	−	+ −	+ +	+ +	+ +	5
Fenoterol	−	+ −	+ +	+ +	−	5

*Isoetharine (Bronkosol) is particularly suitable for use during acute attacks. A bronchodilator with minimal α and β_1 action must be chosen for use during pregnancy. Excessive α effect may reduce uterine blood flow.

(From Hiller FC and Wilson FJ: Evaluation and management of acute asthma. Med Clin North Am 67:669, 1983.)

specific antigens, and they stabilize lysosomal membranes of both neutrophils and monocytes, thereby preventing the release of proteolytic enzymes. Corticosteroids can restore the sensitivity of the beta-receptor to circulating or exogenous beta agonists,[7] and they may also increase the beta-receptor density on the cell surface.

There are many preparations of corticosteroids available for use. Beclomethasone dipropionate can be administered as an aerosol.[14] The use of corticosteroid in aerosol form has permitted significant reduction in the dose of oral corticosteroid preparations. Prednisone and prednisolone cross the placenta poorly (maternal to fetal concentration is 10:1) and are therefore suitable for long term oral use in pregnancy.[2] Hydrocortisone (2 mg/kg) followed by an infusion 0.5 mg/kg/hour is recommended for the management of status asthmaticus. Guidelines for the use of steroids during an acute attack of asthma are shown in Figure 15–4. Chronic administration of steroids causes adrenal suppression; therefore steroid supplementation may be essential during labor. Maternal administration of steroids is not likely to result in fetal adrenal suppression.[3]

Disodium Cromoglycate

This drug stabilizes the mast cell membrane and prevents its degranulation. About 8% of the drug enters the fetus. Although no fetal malformations have been reported to occur with this agent, the safety of this drug is not fully established in human pregnancy.[3]

Iodide Expectorants

These agents are not recommended because they may cause fetal goiter.

MANAGEMENT OF BRONCHIAL SPASM IN THE PREGNANT PATIENT

Bronchospasm must be relieved promptly to avoid fetal hypoxia. A quick search for the precipitating illness, such as upper respiratory infection, should be made. Questioning the patient about the use of aminophylline or corticosteroids during pregnancy is important. The severity of the attack must then be assessed

Table 15–4. Signs and Symptoms of Severe Asthma

Indicator	Symptom
Pulsus paradoxus	>18 mm Hg
FEV_1	<1 L/min
Pulse	>120 beats/min
Respiration	>30 beats/min
Retractions	Accessory muscle use
Pa_{O_2}	<70 torr
Pa_{CO_2}	>38 torr

(Pneumothorox, pneumomediastinum, or subcutaneous emphysema are also signs of severe asthma.)

(Table 15–4). Increased pulse and respiratory rate, severe dyspnea with audible wheezing, accessory muscle use and pulsus paradoxus are signs of severe asthma. During severe bronchospasm, no wheezes may be heard because of lack of any air movement. Laboratory tests that may help in assessing the severity of the asthma are bedside spirometry (FEV_1) and the measurement of arterial blood pH and gas tensions. An FEV_1 of <1 L/min usually signifies severe asthma. The Pa_{CO_2} is usually lower in a normal pregnant patient (32 to 34 mm Hg) than in a nonpregnant subject. A Pa_{CO_2} of 38 mm Hg or greater is indicative of respiratory failure in a pregnant asthmatic[1,2] (Table 15–4). If the bronchial spasm is not treated promptly, the patient will become progressively hypoxic, hypercarbic, and acidotic.

During mild bronchial spasm, there may be respiratory alkalosis bacause of compensatory tachypnea. Respiratory alkalosis may also interfere with fetal oxygenation, even in the absence of maternal hypoxemia.[1,2] Measurements of arterial blood pH and gas tensions are therefore vital for the proper management of a severe bronchospastic episode.

The guidelines for step-by-step management of a pregnant asthmatic are outlined in Figure 15–4. An aerosolized preparation of a β-mimetic substance such as isoetharine is used first. Excessive use of a β-mimetic substance may be associated with postpartum uterine atony.[2]

If there is no response to isoetharine within 20 minutes, the use of intravenous aminophylline must be considered. If the patient has not taken any aminophylline recently, the recommended dose is 5.6 mg per kg of lean body weight. The drug is administered intravenously over 20 minutes. The dosage must be reduced to half if the patient has taken some oral preparation of aminophylline. The maximum safe loading dose is 400 mg. After the initial therapy, aminophylline must be administered as an infusion.

If aminophylline fails to produce any response in 2 to 4 hours, the use of corticosteroids must be considered. A moribund and cyanotic asthmatic requires endotracheal intubation and mechanical ventilation in addition to the drug therapy outlined above. The use of halothane as a bronchodilator has been recommended to treat life-threatening asthma.[15] Antibiotics are needed if there is evidence of pneumonia. Penicillin, ampicillin, or cephalosporins are safe for this purpose. An occasional patient may develop tension pneumothorax or subcutaneous emphysema, especially on ventilator therapy. The use of muscle relaxants may be necessary if the patient is unduly agitated. Antihistamines, such as pheniramine, chlorpheniramine, and promethazine, are probably safe for use during pregnancy. Promethazine can also be used for sedation in a pregnant patient. The use of diazepam in early pregnancy is suspected of being associated with oral clefts in neonates (see Chapter 18 Tetratology.)

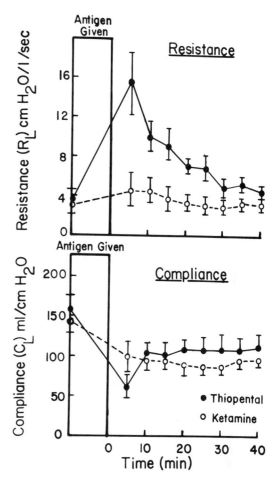

FIG. 15–5. Resistance and compliance changes in an animal model with thiopental and ketamine. The tracheobronchial tree is stimulated with ascaris antigen prior to administration of ketamine or thiopental. (From Kingston GG and Hirshman CA: Perioperative management of the patient with asthma. Anesth Analg *63*:844, 1984.)

ANESTHETIC CARE OF THE PREGNANT ASTHMATIC PATIENT

Whenever possible, regional anesthesia should be used for asthmatic patients because it avoids the need for tracheal intubation, which is probably the worst cause of difficulties in an asthmatic. Bronchial spasms must be adequately controlled prior to an elective cesarean section. Lumbar epidural analgesia either minimizes the stress response to labor and may therefore be beneficial in an asthmatic patient who is in labor. Lumbar epidural anesthesia is also suitable for cesarean section for nonemergency procedures. Epinephrine, used in the local anesthetic mixture, is absorbed systemically. Aminophylline-epinephrine interaction is known to increase the incidence of cardiac arrhythmias. It is therefore advisable to avoid epinephrine in patients who are receiving aminophylline. A low spinal or saddle block may be administered for either spontaneous or forceps deliveries. A high spinal block

must be avoided because it interferes with the motor power in the intercostal muscles and it may cause hyperactivity of the unopposed parasympathetic nervous system, which results in the release of cyclic guanosine monophosphate (cGMP). Increased cGMP concentrations may cause bronchoconstriction.[2]

General anesthesia may be needed for emergency procedures done for fetal distress, or when the patient refuses regional anesthesia. An antacid, such as sodium citrate, must be administered to raise the gastric fluid pH. Administration of histamine-2 antagonists, such as cimetidine, (especially when administered parenterally) can lead to bronchospasm because

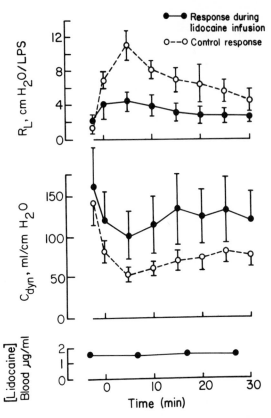

FIG. 15–6. Resistance (top) and compliance (bottom) changes in response to airway stimulation with and without lidocaine administration. Note that the airway is less irritable when the blood level of lidocaine is 1 to 2 μg/ml. (From Kingston GG and Hirshman CA: Perioperative management of the patient with asthma. Anesth Analg 63:844, 1984.)

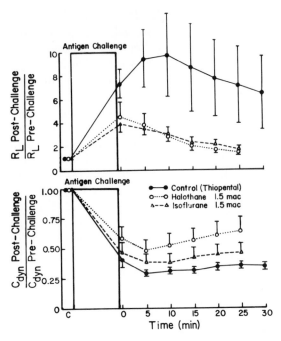

FIG. 15–7. Airway reactivity in the presence and absence of inhalation agents. The airway is stimulated by ascaris antigen in a canine model. Control animals received only thiopental (R_L) resistance of the airway; (C dyn) dynamic compliance. (From Kingston GG and Hirshman CA: Perioperative management of the patient with asthma. Anesth Analg 63:844, 1984.)

of the unopposed histamine-1 receptor activity in the bronchial wall.[16] Although premedication is usually omitted in obstetric patients, the use of atropine may be beneficial because it has been shown to reduce bronchoconstriction caused by antigen reactions.[17] Hydroxyzine is a useful sedative with bronchodilating properties. In addition, it has anticholinergic and antihistaminic properties[18] with no appreciable effect on the fetus.[19]

There is controversy regarding the choice of induction agent for an asthmatic. A 0.7 to 1 mg/kg dose of ketamine may be superior to pentothal for use as an inducing agent. Ketamine produces less pronounced responses in pulmonary resistance and compliance to airway manipulation than does pentothal in animal models (Fig. 15–5). At this dose, the fetus may not be affected

by ketamine. Intravenous lidocaine (75 mg) is useful in decreasing the airway reactivity, especially in patients who are wheezing or who have a history of severe asthma (Fig. 15–6). A serum level between 1 and 2 μg/ml is required for this purpose.[8] Succinylcholine is ideal for facilitating intubation.

The choice of agents for maintenance depends on whether the patient has received aminophylline. Halothane, enflurane, and isoflurane are equally effective bronchodilators (Fig. 15–7).[8] The combination of halothane and aminophylline seems to be more closely associated with greater incidences of cardiac arrhythmia and tachycardia than are either of the combinations of enflurane-aminophylline or isoflurane-aminophylline.[20,21] Arrhythmias are likely to occur during halothane anesthesia, especially when serum aminophylline levels are high (>20 μg/ml). Aminophylline induced changes in Ca^{++} kinetics in the myocardium are believed to be responsible for the cardiac arrhythmias.[12]

Table 15–5. Autonomic Margin of Safety of Nondepolarizing Relaxants in Humans

Drug	Neuromuscular block*	Autonomic margin of safety		
		Ganglion block	Vagal block	Histamine safety†
d-tubocurarine	0.51	2.94	0.59	1
Metocurine	0.28	18.6	2.86	2
Pancuronium	0.07	328.6	2.86	High
Alcuronium	0.25	18.0	1.84	High
Vecuronium	0.056	89.2	40.6	High
Atracurium	0.28	35.7	8.7	3

*ED_{95} in humans (mg/kg)

$$\text{Autonomic margin of safety} = \frac{ED_{50} \text{ for autonomic inhibition in cat}}{ED_{95} \text{ for neuromuscular block in humans}}$$

$$\dagger \text{Margin of safety for histamine release} = \frac{ED_{50} \text{ for histamine release in humans}}{ED_{95} \text{ for neuromuscular block in humans}}$$

(From Scott RPF and Savarese JJ: Cardiovascular and autonomic effects of neuromuscular blocking agents. *In* Muscle Relaxants, Basic and Clinical Aspects. New York, Grune and Stratton, 1984.)

Should arrhythmias occur during anesthesia, lidocaine may be used for treatment.[12] Consequently, before receiving anesthesia, if the patient has not received any aminophylline, halothane may be chosen, whereas if she has received aminophylline, then enflurane or isoflurane may be considered.

d-tubocurarine releases significant amounts of histamine; therefore its use is not recommended in asthmatics. Pancuronium bromide, atracurium, and vecuronium have negligible histamine-releasing potential; therefore one of these three relaxants is used if a long-acting relaxant is required (Table 15–5).[22] The use of a curariform agent requires the reversal of neuromuscular effects with one of the anticholinesterase drugs, which may produce bronchoconstriction. This can be prevented by using atropine.[8] The use of succinylcholine infusion to maintain muscle paralysis obviates the need for an anticholinesterase agent at the end of the procedure. Morphine releases histamine, thus its use is not recommended in asthmatics. Small doses of fentanyl, which lacks histamine-releasing properties, may be used, if a narcotic analgesic is needed for supplementation during anesthesia.[23]

If the patient develops bronchial spasm immediately after induction, the level of anesthesia must be deepened to obtund the airway reflexes.

A β-mimetic agent can be delivered directly into the inspiratory limb of the anesthesia circuit (as close to the endotracheal tube as possible) using a jet nebulizer or a pressurized fluorocarbon canister.[7] If these measures do not control bronchial spasm, aminophylline must be used. As long as serum levels of aminophylline remain below 15 μg/mg, the risk of cardiac arrhythmias resulting from halothane-aminophylline interaction is not significant. The baby must be delivered as quickly as possible because hypoxemia develops rapidly during an episode of severe bronchospasm. Delivering the baby also enables the anesthesiologist to further deepen the anesthetic without the fear of fetal depression. It is likely that volatile anesthetic agents in high concentrations may produce myometrial relaxation. This situation can be improved or overcome by the use of oxytocin. Once other anti-asthma drugs, such as aminophylline, start exerting their protective effect, the inspired concentration of the volatile agent may be reduced to prevent postpartum hemorrhage. Occasionally, the termination of pregnancy may be indicated in order to treat an uncontrollable status asthmaticus. The patient's condition may dramatically improve after delivery of the baby.[24]

Some authors recommend extubation of the trachea before the patient regains airway reflexes. This may be a useful technique to prevent bronchospasm in nonobstetric patients. However, such a practice may lead to aspiration of gastric contents in obstetric patients. Extubation must therefore be performed only after the patient has regained her laryngeal reflex.

REFERENCES

1. Greenberger PA: Asthma in pregnancy. Clin Perinatol 12:571, 1985.
2. Niederman MS, and Matthay R: Asthma and other severe respiratory diseases during pregnancy. In Critical Care of the Obstetric patient. (Edited by Berkowitz RL). New York, Churchill-Livingstone, 1983.
3. Turner ES, Greenberger PA, and Patterson R: Management of the pregnant asthmatic patient. Ann Intern Med 6:905, 1980.
4. Bahna SL, and Bjerkedal T: The course and outcome of pregnancy in women with bronchial asthma. Acta Allergol (Kbh) 27:397, 1972.
5. Gordon M, Niswander KR, Berendes H, and Kantor AG: Fetal morbidity following potentially anoxogenic obstetric conditions. VII. Bronchial asthma. Am J Obstet Gynecol 106:421, 1970.
6. Schatz M, et al.: Corticosteroid therapy for the pregnant asthmatic patient. JAMA 233:804, 1975.
7. Kingston GG, and Hirshman CA: Perioperative management of the patient with asthma. Anesth Analg 63:844, 1984.
8. Dunlap NE, and Fulmer JD: Corticosteroid therapy in asthma. Clin Chest Med 5:669, 1984.
9. Romero R, Kadar N, Govea FG, and Hobbins JC: Pharmacokinetics of intravenous theophylline in pregnant patients at term. Am J Perinatol 1:31, 1983.
10. Labovitz E, and Spector S: Placental theophylline transfer in pregnant asthmatics. JAMA 247:786, 1982.
11. Jenne JW: Theophylline use in asthma: Clin Chest Med 5:645, 1984.
12. Stirt JA, and Sullivan SF: Aminophylline. Anesth Analg 60:587, 1981.
13. Hiller FC, and Wilson FJ: Evaluation and management of acute asthma. Med Clin North Am 67:669, 1983.
14. Greenberger PA, and Patterson R: Beclomethasone diproprionate for severe asthma during pregnancy. Ann Intern Med 98:478, 1983.
15. Rossel P, Lauwers LF, and Baute L: Halothane treatment in life-threatening asthma. Intensive Care Med 11:241, 1985.
16. Manchikanti L, Kraus JW, and Edds SP: Cimetidine and related drugs in anesthesia. Anesth Analg 61:595, 1982.
17. Yu DYC, Galant SP, and Gold WM: Inhibition of antigen-induced bronchoconstriction by atropine in asthmatic patients. J Appl Physiol 32:823, 1972.
18. Smith TC, Cooperman LH, and Wollman H: History and principles of anesthesia. In Goodman and Gilman's The Pharmacological Basis of Therapeutics. 7th Ed. (Edited by Gilman AG, Goodman LS, and Gilman A). New York, Macmillan, 1980.
19. Zsigmond EK, and Patterson RL: Double blind evaluation of hydroxyzine hydrochloride in obstetric anesthesia. Anesth Analg 46:275, 1967.
20. Stirt JA, et al.: Safety of enflurane following administration of aminophylline in experimental animals. Anesth Analg 60:871, 1981.
21. Stirt JA, Berger JM, and Sullivan SF: Lack of arrhythmogenicity of isoflurane following administration of aminophylline in dogs. Anesth Analg 62:568, 1983.
22. Scott RPF, and Savarese JJ: The cardiovascular and autonomic effects of neuromuscular blocking agents. Muscle Relaxants, Basic and Clinical Aspects. New York, Grune and Stratton, 1984.
23. Rosow CE, Moss J, Philbin DM, and Savarese JJ: Histamine release during morphine and fentanyl anesthesia. Anesthesiology 56:93, 1982.
24. Gelber M, et al.: Uncontrollable life-threatening status asthmaticus—an indicator for termination of pregnancy by cesarean section. Respiration 46(3):320, 1984.

16

THROMBOEMBOLISM

Pulmonary embolism (PE), a leading cause of maternal mortality throughout the world, is often preceded by deep venous thrombosis (DVT). The incidence of DVT is higher among pregnant patients because of the hypercoagulability of blood during pregnancy when blood levels of many of the clotting factors increase.[1] Additional evidence for the hypercoagulability of blood comes from elution experiments involving fibrinogen-fibrin antigen.[2] This antigen elutes at an earlier stage in a pregnant patient than in a nonpregnant patient, suggesting increased thrombin activity during pregnancy (Fig. 16–1). This elution is even higher in a preeclamptic pregnant patient than in a normal gravida, which probably explains the greater incidence of thromboembolism in preeclamptic patients.[3] In addition, pregnancy is a state of chronic intravascular coagulation, which occurs mainly in the placenta. Blood fibrinolytic activity is impaired leading to fibrin deposition in the placental intervillous space and in the lumina of the spiral arteries. Increased fibrinolysis causes increased concentration of fibrin-split products.[4] Pregnancy induced changes in coagulation are described in Chapter 2.

CONDITIONS THAT PREDISPOSE TO THROMBOEMBOLISM IN PREGNANCY

In addition to the coagulation changes occurring during pregnancy, there are other factors that also predispose to DVT in pregnancy in-

cluding stagnant venous flow in the lower extremities which results from obstruction of the inferior vena cava by the gravid uterus; the use of estrogen preparations for suppressing lactation; dehydration that may be caused by excessive vomiting (morning sickness) or prolonged labor; and difficult obstetric deliveries. Aaro and Juergens[5] studied the incidence of superficial thrombosis and DVT in over 30,000 deliveries (Table 16–1). They reported that both superficial thrombosis and DVT occurred more frequently in the postpartum period than in the antepartum period. Thus it can be seen that the incidence of DVT is much higher in the postpartum period than during pregnancy.

DIAGNOSIS OF VENOUS THROMBOSIS IN PREGNANCY

Thrombophlebitis is of two types, superficial and deep vein thrombophlebitis. The superficial type usually affects the veins in the leg, whereas the deep vein thrombosis affects the sural, popliteal, femoral, iliofemoral, and pelvic veins in that order. The signs of DVT usually develop on the second postpartum day.[6] The veins commonly affected are listed in Table 16–2.[5] Clinical diagnosis is not conclusive. For instance, Homans' sign is present in only 33% of patients with DVT and in 50% of patients with no DVT at all. Because of the nonspecific nature of the signs and symptoms, treatment cannot be started on clinical grounds alone.[6] The development of clinical signs, however, may draw attention to the possible presence of DVT.[6] The

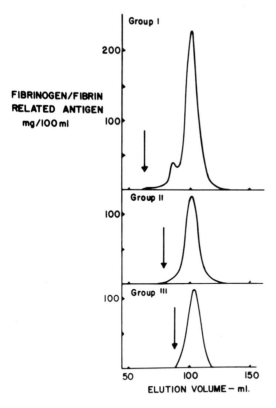

FIBRINOGEN/FIBRIN
RELATED ANTIGEN
mg/100 ml

ELUTION VOLUME — ml.

FIG. 16–1. Elution curves of fibrinogen/fibrin related antigen. Arrow indicates the time at which the antigen was first eluted. (From Weinberger SE, et al.: Pregnancy and the lung. Am Rev Respir Dis *121*:559, 1980.)

clinical and laboratory diagnosis of DVT is outlined in the following list:

1. Pain, swelling, tenderness.
2. Homans' sign–(pain in the calf when the great toe is flexed).
3. Löwenberg test–pain when cuff is inflated to 180 mm Hg.
4. Fever–if septic thrombophlebitis occurs.
5. I_{125} labeled fibrinogen uptake (excreted into the breast milk).

6. Venogram (most definitive).
7. Ultrasound venous flow.
8. Impedance plethysmography (simple and practical).

Cesarean section is associated with a much higher incidence of DVT than is vaginal delivery (Table 16–3).[7]

Noninvasive Tests: Impedance Plethysmography and the Doppler Venous Blood Flow Studies

Both invasive and noninvasive tests are available for diagnosing DVT. Impedance plethysmography and Doppler venous blood flow studies are done noninvasively. The impedance technique measures the rising and falling rates of the electrical impedance of the leg during venous occlusion with an occlusive cuff.[8] The change in the rate of impedence is decreased in patients with DVT. The test detects proximal DVT more reliably than it does distal disease. Although the impedence technique is reported to be the most accurate and simple test in nonpregnant patients, its use in pregnant patients may lead to inaccuracies. The test does not differentiate between thrombotic and nonthrombotic occlusion. The gravid uterus is large enough in the second trimester to cause significant vena caval compression, which may give false positive results. A negative test, however, practically rules out DVT[8] (Fig. 16–2). A positive result must be confirmed with a venogram. The fetal exposure to irradiation from the venogram may be minimized by proper shielding and by limiting the study to the affected limb.[6] The Doppler venous flow studies are extremely subjective. The results depend on the positioning of the patient and on the experience of the investigator. It is also subject to false positive results in pregnancy because of vena caval ob-

Table 16–1. Incidence of Venous Thrombosis

Thrombosis	Type	Number of cases	Incidence
Superficial	Antepartum	52	1:622
	Postpartum	341	1:95
Deep	Antepartum	17	1:1,902
	Postpartum	47	1:688

Total number of deliveries 32,337.
(From Aaro LA, and Juergens JL: Thrombophlebitis associated with pregnancy. Am J Obstet Gynecol *108*:1128, 1971.)

Table 16–2. Sites of Venous Thrombosis

Type	Location	Percent
Superficial venous thrombosis	Leg	61
	Leg and thigh	19
	Thigh	9
	Both lower extremities	11
Deep vein thrombosis	Sural vein	49
	Popliteal vein	6
	Femoral vein	4
	Iliofemoral vein	26
	Pelvic vein	9
	Undetermined vein	6

All incidences for postpartum thrombosis.
(From Aaro LA, and Juergens JL: Thrombophlebitis associated with pregnancy. Am J Obstet Gynecol *108*:1128, 1971.)

struction. Identification of DVT with I_{125} depends on the uptake of the isotope by the developing thrombus. The radioactivity of the calf is assessed using a gamma camera. The isotope crosses the placenta and is excreted into the breast milk; therefore this test is not recommended for use during pregnancy.

Venography

Ascending venography still remains the most accurate test and must be done in all patients with positive plethysmography findings.[2,6] The technique is not reliable for the detection of pelvic thrombi. Proper precautions must be taken to minimize fetal exposure to irradiation. Occasionally, septic thrombophlebitis develops as a complication of puerperal endometritis, a life-threatening condition associated with a 40% incidence of septic pulmonary emboli in untreated patients. Fever that is unresponsive to antibiotic therapy serves as a clue to the presence of this condition.[6]

Table 16–3. Mode of Delivery and Deep Venous Thrombosis

Mode of delivery	Incidence/1000
Spontaneous vertex	1.2
Assisted vaginal breech	3.9
Vaginal, artificial	3.5
Manual removal of placenta	6.5
Cesarean section	25.1

(From Treffers PE, Huidekoper BL, Weeinik GH, and Kloosterman GJ: Epidemiological observations thrombo-embolic disease in the puerpium in 56,002 women. Br J Obstet Gynecol, *21*:327, 1983.)

PULMONARY EMBOLISM

The most dreaded complication of DVT is pulmonary embolism (PE). It remains the second highest cause of maternal mortality, accounting for 30 deaths in every million deliveries.[9] The incidence of fatal PE resulting from untreated (DVT) is about 13%.[10] With prompt treatment, the incidence decreases to less than 1%. Severe PE can occur in patients without any signs of preexisting DVT. It is much more common after

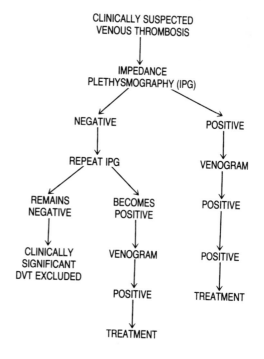

FIG. 16–2. The use of impedance plethysmography for the diagnosis of deep vein thrombosis. (From Hull RD, et al.: The diagnosis of clinically suspected thrombosis. Clin Chest Med 5:439, 1984.)

cesarean section and complicated deliveries than after normal deliveries,[2] a fact which emphasizes the necessity of avoiding cesarean section in patients prone to DVT (Table 16–4).

The most common symptom of PE is dyspnea, and the most common clinical sign is tachypnea. Patients also complain of pleuritic pain, cough, hemoptysis, and nonspecific chest pain. Rales may be heard on auscultation of the chest. Depending on the severity of pulmonary vascular obstruction, varying signs and symptoms may be present[11] (Table 16–5). About 90% of patients with proven PE have a Pao_2 less than 80 mm Hg. Hypoxemia occurs even when the obstruction is less than 25%.[12] The pulmonary artery mean pressure increases after significant embolization has occurred. The increase in mean pressure, however, correlates with the degree of obstruction only in previously healthy patients. In patients with a past history of multiple emboli or those with severe cardiac disease, the correlation is poor (Fig. 16–3).[12]

Laboratory Diagnosis of Pulmonary Embolism

Although diagnostic procedures involving the use of radioactive substances expose the fetus to radiation hazards, the physician should not hesitate to use such procedures when an accurate diagnosis cannot be established otherwise. This becomes necessary in view of the serious complications of anticoagulant therapy needed for treating PE. A chest roentgenogram is of limited value. A method that is widely used in diagnosis of PE is the ventilation/perfusion ($\dot{V}/\dot{Q}$) scintigraphy. Perfusion scan depends on embolization of the pulmonary vasculature with radionuclide particles, which may be either human albumin microspheres or technetium macroaggregates. $Xenon_{133}$ is used for ventilation scanning. Multiple perfusion defects with only minimal changes in ventilation scanning are seen in cases of PE. In the absence of a ventilation study, the diagnostic accuracy of perfusion scan alone decreases.[13] In those cases where the V/Q scans are inconclusive, a pulmonary angiogram must be performed. The angiography is the most definitive of all studies used to diagnose PE. Intraluminal filling defects and/or abrupt cut-off of the intraluminal shadow is considered diagnostic. Useful laboratory findings in patients with pulmonary embolus is summarized in Table 16–6.

TREATMENT OF DEEP VEIN THROMBOSIS AND PULMONARY EMBOLISM

The mainstay of treatment is the use of anticoagulants. Diagnosis of DVT should be promptly established and treatment should be started without delay to prevent PE. Superficial thrombophlebitis occurring during pregnancy usually responds to local heat and bed rest. If conservative measures fail to improve the condition, the use of anticoagulants should be considered. Deep vein thrombosis does require anticoagulation. Anti-inflammatory agents such as phenbutazone and indomethacin are associated with undesirable fetal effects and must therefore be avoided.

Heparin is the anticoagulant of choice during pregnancy. Heparin, a potent thrombin inhibitor, does not cross the placenta because of its high molecular weight (20,000). The therapeutic serum level is 0.3 U/ml and the best coagulation indices for monitoring adequacy of anticoagulation are activated clotting time or activated plasma thromboplastin time (2 to 3 times the control). When used as a continuous infusion, heparin should be mixed in saline solutions rather than in dextrose solutions because it may lose potency in the latter.[14] There is no consensus of opinion with respect to the best mode of

Table 16–4. Maternal Deaths from Pulmonary Embolism

Time of death	1961–1963	1964–1966	1967–1969	1970–1972
After vaginal delivery	0.4	0.2	0.2	0.1
After cesarean section	3.6	2.7	1.8	1.6

Rates per 10,000 deliveries in England and Wales (Reports on Confidential Enquiries into Maternal Deaths in England and Wales). Note that although the number of deaths due to pulmonary embolism is declining, it seems to be 10 to 15 times greater after cesarean section than after vaginal delivery.

Table 16–5. Percent Patients with Signs or Symptoms of Pulmonary Embolus

Form of presentation	Disorder	Percent of patients
Symptoms	Dyspnea	81
	Pleuritic pain	72
	Cough	54
	Hemoptysis	34
	Chest pain	5
Signs	Tachypnea	81
	Rales	54
	Split pulmonic	
	2nd sound	54
	S_3 or S_4 gallop	34
	Arrhythmias	15
	BP <100 systolic	3
	Thrombophlebitis	34

Table 16–6. Lab Methods for Diagnosis of Pulmonary Embolism

Tests	Disorder detected
EKG	Tachycardia
	ST–T changes, P–pulmonale
	S_1–Q_3 pattern, and right axis deviation in severe cases.
Chest x-ray	Inconclusive (atelectasis, occasional effusion).
Arterial blood gases	Arterial hypoxemia.
V/Q scan	Simple and reliable.
Pulmonary angiography	The standard test.

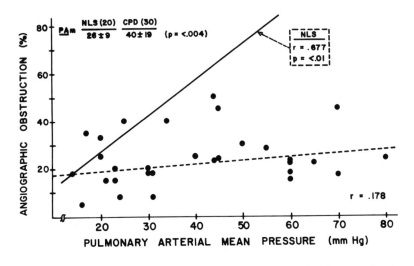

FIG. 16–3. Pulmonary artery mean pressure (PA_M) as it relates to the degree of pulmonary vascular obstruction determined angiographically. Note that in patients with preexisting cardiopulmonary disease (CPD), the pulmonary artery mean pressure does not correlate with the severity of the obstruction (dashed regression line). NLS, no previous history of lung disease: Mean and 1 SD of mean PA_M are shown on upper left. (From Sharma CVRK, McIntyre KM, Sharma S, and Sashahara AA: Clinical and hemodynamic correlates in pulmonary embolism. Clin Chest Med 5:412, 1984.

administration of heparin. Usually, it is started with a loading dose (5000 U) followed by a continuous infusion 15 to 20 U/kg/hr or intermittent intravenous or subcutaneous maintenance administrations. A larger loading dose (10,000 to 15,000 U) is used for the treatment of pulmonary embolus.[11,14] Parenteral administration is required every 6 to 8 hours using coagulation indices as guidelines (activated partial thromboplastin time). Heparin may also be self-administered subcutaneously for long-term management.[15] For treatment of DVT, heparin should be continued for 7 to 10 days. In addition to heparin therapy, other supportive measures are needed in patients with PE. These include the following: oxygen therapy; dopamine infusion (if systemic hypotension is present); and endotrachal intubation and mechanical ventilation (in patients who are severely hypoxic).

Coumarin derivatives are contraindicated in pregnancy because of their teratogenic effects. They may, however, be useful in patients who are allergic to heparin or in those incapable of self-administration.[11] The antithrombotic action of coumarin is caused by the reduction in the concentrations of factors IX and X. Hemorrhagic complications associated with large doses of coumarin are attributed to a reduction in factor VII concentration. The usual therapeutic dose of coumarin is 10 to 15 mg daily to achieve a prolongation in the prothrombin time (1.5 to 2.5 times the control). The use of coumarin derivates is implicated in the production of warfarin embryopathy. For patients who require anticoagulation throughout pregnancy, heparin should be used in the first trimester for the acute episode. She may be taught to self-administer heparin subcutaneously. In those who are not capable of self-administration, coumarin may be substituted in second trimester. Coumarin, when continued well into the third trimester, is associated with increased risk of fetal hemorrhage; therefore some recommend discontinuing coumarin therapy at 37 weeks and restarting heparin.[14] Coumarin derivatives not only cross the placenta, they also are excreted in the breast milk. If premature labor occurs while the patient is receiving coumarin therapy, vitamin K injections and transfusion of fresh frozen plasma may be used. The neonate must be given an injection of vitamin K as well. In spite of such preventive measures, fetal problems may still occur with alarming frequency. Careful dose selection based on repeated prothrombin time measurements and discontinuing the drug well in advance of the expected date of delivery is said to minimize maternal and fetal hemorrhagic problems.[11,16–18]

Heparin must be discontinued as soon as labor starts and be restarted immediately after delivery. In patients with a recent history of pulmonary embolism, patients with prosthetic heart valves, or those with a recent history of iliofemoral vein thrombosis, one may elect to continue heparin infusion throughout labor. A reduced infusion rate (0.1 to 0.2 u/kg/min) is used under these circumstances. The use of estrogen preparations for the suppression of lactation is contraindicated in patients with a history of thromboembolism. A scheme for managing long-term anticoagulation therapy during pregnancy is given in Table 16–7.

Heparin Prophylaxis

In recent years, the minidose heparin therapy has gained considerable popularity for the prevention of DVT. Heparin administered in 5000 unit doses at 8- to 12-hour intervals activates antithrombin III, which is a potent inhibitor of factor X_a. Minidose heparin is believed to decrease the incidence of DVT as well as pulmonary embolism. Patients with a previous history of pulmonary embolism, with previous DVT history, or those with extensive varicosities may be placed on minidose heparin. In pregnancy, the conventional 5000 units may not be adequate because of the hypercoagulability of blood. Some use 7500 units every 12 hours starting at the 13th week of gestation and 10,000 units every 12 hours from the 30th week.[6] The PTT is not usually prolonged with these dosages, when used at the above-mentioned gestational periods.[6]

Other Forms of Therapy

Thrombolitic therapy may be considered in patients with DVT or PE in whom heparin therapy fails to arrest the progression of symptoms. Streptokinase and urokinase, which are used for this purpose, achieve thrombolysis by stimulating the endogenous fibrinolytic system. Streptokinase is used for the treatment of both DVT

Table 16–7. Long-term Anticoagulation During Pregnancy

Trimester	Management
First	1. Treat initial episode with heparin. 2. Discharge patient on subcutaneous heparin. 3. If self administration is not possible, maintain heparin therapy in the hospital or by other means.
Second	1. Maintain subcutaneous heparin. 2. If self administration is not possible, switch to coumarin.

Third	1. Stop coumarin at 34 weeks and switch to heparin.
	2. Stop heparin at the onset of labor.
	3. Restart heparin therapy postpartum in breast-feeding mothers. In others start coumarin.
	    A. *Heparin:* If emergency cesarean section is needed, use protamine.
	    B. *Coumarin:* For premature delivery, use fresh frozen plasma and vitamin K to the mother and neonate.

Prolonged anticoagulation may be required in patients with prosthetic heart valves, with history of multiple attacks of DVT or pulmonary embolism.

Note that patients with history of recent massive DVT or pulmonary embolism, intrapartum heparin therapy is necessary.
Source: Laros RK, Jr.;[14] Spearing;[15] Merrill;[16] Bolan;[17] and Pridmore.[18]

and PE and Urokinase only for treating PE.[19] A loading dose and a maintenance infusion are required for both agents. Coagulation indices that are used for monitoring the adequacey of treatment are euglobulin lysis activity, activated partial thromboplastin time, or thrombin time (2.5 times the control measurement). Patients who are on thrombolytic therapy may ooze blood from indwelling cannula sites.

Patients who are desperately ill because of massive PE that is unresponsive to conventional therapy may require a transvenous catheter embolectomy.[20] The pulmonary artery is entered via the internal jugular vein. If a clot progresses despite adequate anticoagulation or if a serious contraindication exists, such as a previous history of intracranial hemorrhage, a Greenfield filter is placed in the inferior vena cava via the internal jugular vein.[20] Both filter placement and transvenous pulmonary embolectomy can be performed under local anesthesia.

Problems with Anticoagulants

The use of heparin or coumarin is associated with problems for both the mother and the baby. Although the use of heparin is not associated with teratogenicity, it is associated with an increased infant mortality rate and an increase in the occurrence of maternal hemorrhage[21] even in properly monitored nonsurgical patients.[14] Heparin use may also be associated with low

platelet count and osteoporosis (back pain).[6] Despite these problems, heparin is still the anticoagulant of choice in pregnancy because it does not cross the placenta and is not associated with teratogenic effects. Coumarin use is implicated in fetal warfarin embryopathy. The mechanism of embryotoxicity is believed to be caused by the ability of warfarin compounds to prevent the formation of vitamin K epoxide required for fetal bone growth.[21] Warfarin causes both morphologic and behavioral teratogenicity.

1. Nasal hypoplasia.
2. Epiphyseal stippling.
3. Laryngeal calcification, respiratory distress.
4. Optic atrophy.
5. Hypertelorism.
6. Vertebral anomaly.
7. Mental retardation.

Nasal hypoplasia, calcaneal stippling, and mental retardation are the important features of warfarin embryopathy[21] (also see Figure 18–1). Pregnancy outcome in patients treated with heparin or coumarin is listed in Table 16–8.

Anesthetic Considerations

Regional Anesthesia. Regional anesthesia in patients receiving anticoagulation may be associated with serious sequelae, most notably spinal and epidural hematoma.[22–25] Patients who receive anticoagulant therapy are prone to develop even spontaneous spinal hematomas; therefore

Table 16–8. Pregnancy Outcome with Heparin and Warfarin

	Percent pregnancies	
Outcome	Coumarin	Heparin
Liveborn		
Subsequent infant death	2.4	7.4
Persistent sequelae	10.4	0.7
Premature, otherwise normal	1.9	14.1
Spontaneous abortions	8.6	1.5
Stillbirths	7.7	12.5

(From Hall JH, Pauli RM, and Wilson KM: Maternal and fetal sequelae of anticoagulation during pregnancy. Am J Med 68:132, 1980.)

one should avoid regional anesthesia in these patients, especially when other choices are available.

If heparin is discontinued early in labor and all clotting tests have returned to normal, use of regional anesthesia may be considered. Rao et al[26] reported that there were no problems in a large series of patients who were administered anticoagulants approximately an hour after placement of epidural and subarachnoid catheters. Maintenance heparin dose was administered every 6 hours using activated clotting time (ACT) as a guideline. The ACT was maintained at 130 to 150 sec in their study. The epidural catheter was removed the next day an hour before the next maintenance injection was due, when the blood level of heparin would have been low. Allerman, et al.[27] reported a smaller series of patients who received a combination of heparin and dihydroergotamine two hours before surgery and postoperatively for the prevention of postoperative DVT. Both spinal and continuous epidural anesthetics were performed. No patient developed any complications.

Epidural or Spinal Anesthesia. If all anticoagulation has been discontinued at the onset of labor and the clotting indices have returned to normal, one may consider using epidural or spinal anesthesia for labor and delivery. If the patient is on heparin prophylaxis, then 2 hours following the last heparin dose, the epidural catheter may be placed, as long as the clotting indices are within normal limits. Heparin administration is then resumed at least two hours after inserting the catheter. If the patient is receiving intrapartum coagulation, all forms of central neural regional anesthesia are contraindicated. Postpartum anticoagulation is safe

in patients who have received regional anesthesia for labor and delivery.

One should not lose sight of the fact that some patients who require anticoagulation may have severe cardiac disease (mitral stenosis with atrial fibrillation, congenital heart disease). In others, repeated pulmonary embolization may have caused cor pulmonale. The issue in such a patient is not the choice of anesthetic technique (general versus regional anesthesia) but a comprehensive perinatal management (see Chapter 12 Cardiac Disease).

Regional versus General Anesthesia. Regional anesthesia is preferable to general anesthesia in patients with a previous history of DVT. Local anesthetics at low serum levels can prevent adhesion of white blood cells to the vascular endothelium, consequently minimizing endothelial damage.[28] Epidural anesthesia is associated with increased femoral vein blood flow velocity compared to general anesthesia.[29] The use of epidural anesthesia is associated with less incidence of postoperative DVT.[30]

General Anesthesia. When general anesthesia is administered to patients with a recent history of PE, an indwelling arterial cannula is necessary to facilitate repeated arterial PO_2 measurement. Preexisting cardiac disease necessitates the use of a pulmonary artery catheter. In addition, a pulse oximeter and a capnograph (or a mass spectrometer) must be used. Pulse oximeter detects changes in arterial oxygen saturation. End-tidal CO_2 concentration decreases rapidly when pulmonary embolization occurs. Several deaths caused by intraoperative pulmonary embolism have been reported.[31] Systemic hypotension followed by sudden cardiac arrest is the classical feature in all these cases. The immediate post-delivery period may be

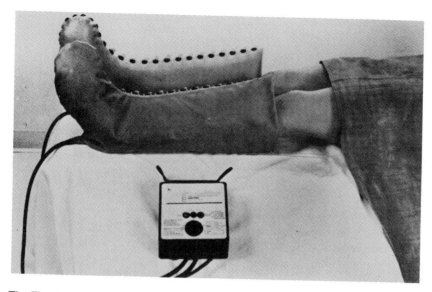

FIG. 16–4.   The Flowtron pump and vinyl boot system. (From Tarnay TJ, et al.: Pneumatic calf compression, fibrinolysis, and the prevention of deep venous thrombosis. Surgery 88:489, 1980.

hazardous because clots are likely to be dislodged from the veins of the lower extremities following sudden release of inferior vena cava compression. Pulmonary thromboembolism is likely to be confused with amniotic fluid embolism. The differential diagnosis is discussed in Chapter 11.

Precautionary Measures. Some simple, practical precautions that one can take to minimize the risk of DVT in those patients at increased risk include using a short acting local anesthetic that permits prompt return of lower limb motor function, avoiding dehydration and aortocaval compression, ambulating the patient at the earliest opportunity in the postoperative period, and using electrical stimulation of the calf muscles (physiotherapy) to augment their pumping action.

The use of epidural narcotics for the relief of postoperative pain permits early ambulation. The use of pneumatic calf-compression is associated with decreased incidence of DVT.[32-34] An air driven motor causes alternating compression and decompression of the calf muscles (Fig. 16–4). Pneumatic compression not only increases venous blood flow in the calf but also releases fibrinolytic substances from the compressed blood vessels. Regardless of the site of compression, the entire systemic fibrinolytic activity is increased.

REFERENCES

1. Weinberger SE, et al: Pregnancy and the lung. Am Rev Respir Dis 121:559, 1980.
2. McKillop C, Edgar W, Prentice RM: In vivo production of soluble complexes containing fibrinogen-fibrin related antigen during ancroid therapy. Thrombosis Res 7:361, 1975.
3. Howie PW: Thromboembolism. Clin Obstet Gynecol 4:397, 1977.
4. Romero R: The management of acquired hemostatic failure during pregnancy. In Critical Care of the Obstetric Patient. (Edited by Berkowitz RL). New York, Churchill-Livingstone, 1983.
5. Aaro LA, and Juergens JL: Thrombophlebitis associated with pregnancy. Am J Obstet Gynecol 108:1128, 1971.
6. Weiner CP: Diagnosis and management of thromboembolic disease during pregnancy. Clin Obstet Gynecol 28:107, 1985.
7. Treffers PE, Huidekoper BL, Weeninik GH, and Kloosterman GJ: Epidemiological observations of thromboembolic disease during pregnancy and in the puerperium in 56,002 women. Br J Obstet Gynaecol 21:327, 1983.
8. Hull RD, et al.: The diagnosis of clinically suspected thrombosis. Clin Chest Med 5:439, 1984.
9. Venous thromboembolism and anticoagulants in pregnancy. Editorial. Br Med J 1:421, 1975.
10. Villasanta U: Thromboembolic disease in pregnancy. Am J Obstet Gynecol 93:142, 1965.
11. Moser KM: Pulmonary embolism. Amer Rev Resp Dis 115:829, 1977.
12. Sharma CVRK, McIntyre KM, Sharma S, and Sashahara AA: Clinical and hemodynamic correlates in pulmonary embolism. Clin Chest Med 5:412, 1984.
13. Polak JF, and McNeil BJ: Pulmonary scintigraphy and

the diagnosis of pulmonary embolism. Clin Chest Med 5:447, 1984.

14. Laros RK, and Alger LS: Thromboembolism and pregnancy. Clin Obstet Gynecol 4:871, 1979.
15. Spearing G, Fraser I, Turner G, and Dixon G: Long term self administered heparin in pregnancy. Br Med J 1:1457, 1973.
16. Merrill LK, ver Burg DJ: The choice of long-term anticoagulants for the pregnant patient. Obstet Gynecol 47:711, 1976.
17. Bolan JC: Thromboembolic complications of pregnancy. Clin Obstet Gynecol 26:913, 1983.
18. Pridmore BR, Murray KH, and McAllen PM: The management of anticoagulant therapy during and after pregnancy. Br J Obstet Gynecol 82:740, 1975.
19. Volgesang GB, and Bell WR: Treatment of pulmonary embolism and deep vein thrombosis with thrombolytic therapy. Clin Chest Med 5:487, 1984.
20. Greenfield LJ: Vena caval interruption and pulmonary embolectomy. Clin Chest Med 5:495, 1984.
21. Hall JH, Pauli RM, and Wilson KM: Maternal and fetal sequelae of anticoagulation during pregnancy. Am J Med 68:132, 1980.
22. Ellison N, and Ominsky AJ: Clinical considerations for the anesthesiologist whose patient is on anticoagulant therapy. Anesthesiology 39:328, 1973.
23. Ginrich TF: Spinal and epidural hematoma following continuous epidural anesthesia. Anesthesiology 29:162, 1968.
24. De Angelis J: Hazards of subdural and epidural anesthesia during anticoagulant therapy. Anesth Analg 51:676, 1972.
25. Varkey GP, and Brindle GR: Peridural anesthesia and anticoagulant therapy. Can Anaesth Soc J 21:106, 1974.
26. Roa TLK, and El Etr AA: Anticoagulation following placement of epidural and subarachnoid catheters. Anesthesiology 55:618, 1981.
27. Allerman BH, and Gruber UF: Ruckenmarksnahe Anaesthesie und subkutan verabriechtes low-dose heparindihydergot zur Thromboembolieprophylaxae. Anaesthetist 32:80, 1983.
28. Cooke ED, Llyd MJ, Bowcock SJ, and Pilcher MF: Intravenous lignocaine in the prevention of deep venous thrombosis after elective hip surgery Lancet II: 797, 1977.
29. Poikolainen E, and Hendolin H: Effects of lumbar epidural analgesia and general analgesia on flow velocity in the femoral vein and postoperative deep vein thrombosis. Acta Chir Scand 149:361, 1983.
30. Modig J, Karlstrom G, Maripuu E, and Sahlstedt B: Thromboembolism after total hip replacement. Anesth Analg 62:174, 1983.
31. Brownne RA, and Catton DV: Massive pulmonary embolism during anesthesia: A report of two cases. Can Anaesth Soc J 14:413, 1967.
32. Knight MTN, and Dawson R: Effects of intermittent compression of the arms on deep venous thrombosis in the legs. Lancet 1:1265, 1976.
33. Tarnay TJ, et al.: Pneumatic calf compression, fibrinolysis, and the prevention of deep venous thrombosis. Surgery 88:489, 1980.
34. Consensus conference: Prevention of venous thrombosis and pulmonary embolus. JAMA 256:744, 1986.

17

NEUROLOGIC DISEASE

Pregnancy may alter the course of neurologic disease that was present before conception.[1] Eclampsia, a serious disorder of the CNS, is considered in the chapter on preeclampsia. This chapter will focus on noneclamptic neurologic disorders. The neurologic conditions to be discussed include the following:

1. Idiopathic epilepsy
2. Multiple sclerosis
3. Myasthenia gravis
4. Cerebrovascular accidents
5. Brain tumors
6. Benign intracranial hypertension
7. Myotonias
8. Autonomic hyperreflexia
9. Familial dysautonomia (Riley-Day syndrome)
10. Guillain-Barre syndrome
11. Genital herpes infection
12. Malignant hyperpyrexia

IDIOPATHIC EPILEPSY

Increased frequency of seizures occurs in one-third of patients during pregnancy. A number of factors are believed to play a role in causing this increase including a decrease in the intake or absorption of the antiseizure drug in early pregnancy, which is a result of nausea and vomiting.[2] An increase in estrogen levels is also implicated in lowering the seizure threshold.[1] Water and sodium retention during pregnancy, the patient's failure to take medication for fear of adverse fetal effects, and decreased serum levels of the anticonvulsant drugs may also increase chances of seizure. The major clinical types of seizures are listed in Table 17–1 and the drug therapy of seizure disorder is described in Table 17–2.

For a given dose, plasma levels of many antiepileptic drugs attain lower levels in pregnant patients than in nonpregnant patients. A 300- to 400-mg dose of phenytoin (hydantoin) results in a therapeutic serum level of 10 to 20 μg/ml in a nonpregnant patient but only achieves 3.6 μg in a pregnant subject. Some pregnant women may require up to 1200 mg of the drug to produce a therapeutic level. The clearance rate of phenytoin and phenobarbitone is increased in pregnancy (Fig. 17–1).[3] Other factors that contribute to decreased levels of phenytoin in pregnancy include increased renal excretion, decreased protein binding, and decreased absorption from the gut. Carbamazepine (Tegretol) and clorazepate metabolism is increased in pregnancy. Because of the unpredictable blood levels of anticonvulsants, the serum concentrations of the drug must be monitored at least once a month during pregnancy. The clearance rate of phenobarbital is not altered in pregnancy, but its absorption rate from the gut is altered. The absorption rate rapidly normalizes after delivery, increasing the likelihood of toxic reactions in the postpartum period.

FETAL EFFECTS OF ANTICONVULSANT DRUGS

All anticonvulsant drugs readily cross the placenta and may cause fetal sequelae. Phenobar-

Table 17–1. Types of Seizures in Adults

Type	Specific types	Main clinical features
Partial or focal	1. Simple with motor, sensory, autonomic, or psychic signs.	No loss of consciousness. Twitching of lips, arms, and face with Jacksonian march to involve contiguous portions of the body.
	2. Complex partial with psychomotor or temporal lobe seizures.	The individual loses contact with the environment; aura, automatism, deja vu (also called temporal lobe or psychomotor epilepsy).
	3. Secondary generalized partial seizures.	Progresses to convulsive activity with loss of consciousness.
Primary generalized	1. Tonic-clonic (grand-mal).	Post-ictal unconsciousness.
	2. Tonic seizures	No clonic phase; head and eyes deviate to one side.
	3. Absence seizures (petit mal)	Brief lapses of awareness occurring many times during the day.
	4. Myoclonic seizures	Sudden, repetitive muscle contractions. No loss of consciousness, may occur in uremia, hepatic failure.
	5. Atonic seizure	Loss of muscle tone, sagging body.
Recurrence patterns		Stimulated by menstruation, reading, special musical composition, tactile or light stimulation.
Status epilectus	1. Tonic-clonic status 2. Epilepsia partialis continua 3. Absence status	Life-threatening continuous partial seizures. May go unrecognized.

Source: Dichter MA.[4]

Table 17–2. Drug Treatment in Epilepsy

Drug	Uses	Daily dose	Serum level/ml	Side-effects, interactions
Phenytoin	Grand mal; focal; complex partial.	300–1200 mg	10–20	Ataxia, altered folate metabolism, skin rash; carbamazepine and phenobarbital therapy decreases level.
Carbamazepine	Grand mal; focal; complex partial.	200–1220 mg	4–12 μg	Ataxia, dizziness, toxicity; level decreased by phenobarbital, phenytoin.
Phenobarbital	Tonic-clonic.	60–200 mg	10–50 μg	Skin rash; level increased by phenytoin.
Ethosuximide	Absence.	500–1500 mg	40–100 μg	Ataxia, bone-marrow suppression.
Clonazepam	Absence; atypical; absence; myoclonic.	1–20 mg	5–70 ng	Ataxia, sedation; may precipitate absence when given with valproic acid.
Sodium valproate	Absence; tonic-clonic	0.75–1 g	50–100 μg	Ataxia, sedation; hepatotoxicity.

Trimethadione and sodium valproate are known teratogens. Their use is restricted to conditions unresponsive to other drugs.

Sources: Noronha A[1] and Dichter MA.[4]

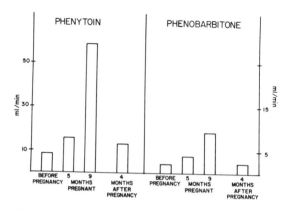

FIG. 17–1. Plasma clearance of phenytoin and phenobarbitone in pregnancy. Note the increase in clearance of both drugs during pregnancy. (From Mygind KI, Dam M, and Christiansen J: Phenytoin and phenobarbitone plasma clearance during pregnancy. Acta Neurol Scand 54:160, 1976.)

bital and valproate are more slowly metabolized in the infant than in the adult, thus neonatal depression may occur. The use of phenobarbital is also associated with fetal withdrawal syndrome.

The use of anticonvulsants in pregnancy has been implicated in the production of fetal teratogenicity. The use of dilantin is associated with the fetal hydantoin syndrome characterized by craniofacial abnormalities, gum hyperplasia, and mental retardation. The anticonvulsants are also implicated in the production of vitamin K deficiency, which may result in neonatal bleeding;[1] thus anticonvulsants are both morphologic and behavioral teratogens. It is recommended that the neonate be given 1 mg of phytonadione intravenously soon after birth[1] to counteract any possible vitamin K deficiency. The teratogenic effects of the anticonvulsant drugs are more fully discussed in the chapter on teratology (Chapter 18).

Most anticonvulsants are secreted into the breast milk. Although most of them do not produce any adverse effects in therapeutic doses, the use of large amounts of diazepam during labor may be contraindicated because of the slow clearance of the drug by the neonate.[1]

STATUS EPILEPTICUS

When the patient does not fully recover between seizures, or a single seizure lasts more than 30 minutes, the maternal mortality may reach 2.5%. The differential diagnosis will obviously include inadvertent intravenous injection of a local anesthetic or unsuspected eclampsia. Another confusing issue is the status hystericus or the psuedoseizures. The hysterical convulsion is differentiated from epileptic convulsion by the presence of pupillary responses to light, which is usually lost during a true seizure.[5] Moreover, the patient rarely loses consciousness during a psuedoseizure. Status epilepticus is accompanied by hypertension, tachycardia, hypoxia, lactic acidosis, and increased cerebral oxygen and glucose utilization.[6] Prolonged muscular contraction may cause rhabdomyolysis, hyperthermia, and myoglobinuric renal failure. In addition, placental separation may occur. Treatment of status epilepticus involves terminating the seizure activity, and maintaining maternal and fetal oxygenation, preventing injury to the mother and the fetus. Diazepam 10 to 20 mg is the drug of choice to obtain immediate control of seizures. This must be followed by a loading dose of phenytoin 14 mg/kg diluted in normal saline and injected at a rate of 50 mg/min. Sufficient brain concentrations of phenytoin does not occur for an hour following injection. Additional diazepam injections may be required in the interim to obtain seizure control. Maternal EKG and fetal heart rate must be continuously monitored. When seizures cannot be controlled by the above-mentioned measures, endotracheal intubation and mechanical ventilation with curarization are required.

ANESTHETIC CONSIDERATIONS

Local anesthetics may be used for producing labor analgesia. Patients with a history of epilepsy are not at increased risk for convulsions caused by local anesthetic toxicity. Adequate lumbar epidural analgesia (LEA) may indeed be beneficial in these patients because it reduces stress, which is often implicated precipitating an epileptic seizure. The anesthesiologist must administer a test dose of local anesthetic to rule out accidental insertion of the epidural catheter into a vein. A local anesthetic seizure may be indistinguishable from a grand-mal seizure. Should seizure occur during epidural anesthesia, blood levels of the anesthetic must be measured to aid in differential diagnosis. The other causes of sudden onset of an actual grand-mal seizure in obstetric patients include malignant hyperpyrexia, water intoxication, amniotic fluid embolism, and cerebrovascular accident.

Antiepileptic drugs (phenytoin, phenobarbital) are potent inducers of hepatic microsomal enzyme. They increase the metabolic rate of many inhalation agents, thereby predisposing to increased toxicity. For instance, the release of fluoride ion (F⁻) from methoxyflurane and enflurane occurs rapidly in enzyme-induced states. Increased serum F⁻ level is associated with nephrotoxicity.

While many drugs used for induction and maintenance of anesthesia are safe in patients with epilepsy, caution must be exercised with the use of some agents.

Enflurane. The use of enflurane is known to induce EEG abnormality (intersuppression bursts) in normal individuals. The burst period may be accompanied by muscular twitching. The activity is generally dose-related and enhanced by hypocapnia. On rare occasions, the use of enflurane has been associated with convulsions in the postoperative period.[7]

Ketamine. The use of ketamine is associated with seizure activity in limbic and thalamic regions (Fig. 17–2) in normal individuals.[8] The drug may also elicit a convulsive response in seizure-prone individuals.[9]

Methohexital. The methyl group attached to the ring of this oxybarbiturate is said to impart convulsive property to this agent. The drug has been shown to induce serious EEG abnormalities in a significant number of epileptics.[10] The use of the drug may occasionally precipitate status epilepticus. The other ultra-short-acting barbiturates, such as pentothal, however, lack this property; therefore they may be safely used in epileptics. Because other excellent alternatives are available, the use of enflurane, ketamine, or methohexital is not recommended in epileptics.

MULTIPLE SCLEROSIS

This is a demyelinating disease of the central nervous system. Depending on the site at which demyelination is occurring at a given time, the symptomatology may be complex. The peripheral nervous system is usually spared. The disease affects individuals between the years of 15 to 40 and the clinical course is punctuated by relapses and remissions.

In 40% of patients, the presenting symptom is related to optic neuritis.[11] Patients may complain of unilateral or bilateral pain in the eye, blindness, and occasionally, disturbances in the color vision. Visually-evoked potentials and somatosensory-evoked potentials are abnormal, and computerized tomography may reveal lesions in the white matter in the brain. Imaging by nuclear magnetic resonance may show multiple defects. The third, fourth, and/or sixth cra-

TRACING FROM ANTERIOR GYRUS

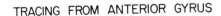

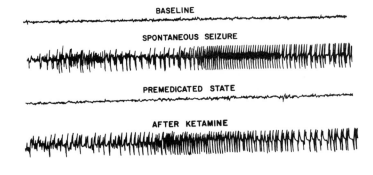

FIG. 17–2. Ketamine (0.5 mg/kg) induced seizure activity recorded by in-depth electrode encephalography in patients with seizure disorders. Preictal tracing from the left anterior gyrus (Baseline tracing). Spontaneous seizure activity in the gyrus (Spontaneous seizure tracing). Tracing from the gyrus in the same patient in the premedicated state (Premedicated tracing). Ketamine induced seizure (After ketamine tracing). Note the resemblance between the spontaneous seizure and the ketamine-induced seizure activities. (From Ferrer-Allado D, et al.: Ketamine induced electroconvulsive phenomena in the human limbic and thalamic regions. Anesthesiology 38:333, 1973.)

nial nerves may also be affected leading to diplopia. Spinal cord involvement includes demyelination of the corticospinal tract (upper motor neuron dysfunction, hyperreflexia), posterior columns (tingling of the extremities), and spinothalamic tracts. Cerebral involvement may result in depression, euphoria, and seizures. Ataxia, nystagmus, and dysarthria may be caused by cerebellar lesions. The inability to adduct one eye on attempted lateral gaze with the other eye in full abduction is virtually diagnostic of multiple sclerosis.[11] The CSF may have raised IgG levels and oligoclonal banding of the IgG.

There is no known treatment for this condition. Glucocorticoids may help during relapses. Azathioprine has been claimed to be successful. Patients may also receive a variety of antiepileptics either for seizures or for facial pain and twitching.[11] Diazepam may be prescribed for spasticity.

Pregnancy itself does not affect the course of the disease, but there is general agreement that the disease worsens in the postpartum period.[1] Relapse may occur after each pregnancy in these patients. The neonate is not adversely affected.[1]

ANESTHETIC CONSIDERATIONS

Even mild elevations of body temperature or electrolyte imbalance may cause exacerbation of the condition by altering the internal milieu of the nerve cell. General anesthesia may be safely administered to these patients without the risk of increased relapse rate.[12] Caution, however, must be exercised, in using succinylcholine in those patients with evidence of massive demyelination in the preceding year because of the possible risk of hyperkalemic response.[12] Atracurium besylate, vecuronium, or pancuronium bromide can be administered for tracheal intubation. Pentothal may be used for intravenous induction of anesthesia. If the patient has extensive muscle weakness, the dose of sedatives and muscle relaxants must be suitably modified.

A great deal of controversy surrounds the use of regional anesthesia mainly because the available information is anecdotal and there are at present no well-controlled studies available on the subject. The anesthesiologist must explain the risk/benefit ratio of regional and general anesthesia to the patient. If the patient prefers

to be awake during the birth of her baby, a regional anesthetic must then be chosen. Epidural anesthesia may be safely administered to patients with multiple sclerosis.[13] A recent report[14] described the development of numbness in the thigh on two different occasions in the same patient following epidural anesthesia. This, however, may be related to postpartum relapse rather than to a specific local anesthetic effect. A short-acting local anesthetic with no known neurotoxicity (lidocaine) can be used.

Although there is no irrevocable evidence that links spinal anesthesia with relapses, this technique is best avoided because the CSF contains a large amount of myelin debris in patients with multiple sclerosis and its protein composition is abnormal. Also the intense losses of sensation and motor power that are produced by spinal anesthesia might be upsetting to the patient. The muscle-relaxant-azathioprine interaction is covered in the chapter on renal disease (Chapter 22).

MYASTHENIA GRAVIS

Myasthenia gravis (MG) is a disorder of neuromuscular transmission believed to be the result of destruction caused by the antibody to acetyl choline (ACh) receptor protein.[1,15] The formation of immune complex is complement mediated and the miniature end-plate potentials vary inversely to the number of immune complexes at the neuromuscular junction. More than 85% of patients with MG will have circulating antibodies to ACh. The storage and the quantal release of acetyl choline remains normal at the neuromuscular junction. The motor end plate becomes elongated and the synaptic cleft is thrown into folds.

The disease mainly affects females (predominantly nonwhite females). The condition is associated with rheumatoid arthritis and other autoimmune diseases, including thyroiditis, systemic lupus erythematosus, and polymyositis. Approximately 65% of patients with MG have thymic hyperplasia, whereas 10% have a thymoma.[16] In 50 to 70% of MG patients symptoms improve after thymectomy. A computerized tomogram scan of the mediastinum is recommended to rule out thymic enlargements in these patients. During pregnancy, the clinical course is generally more favorable in those patients who have had a thymectomy prior to conception.[17]

Diagnosis of Myasthenia Gravis

Typically the patient with MG has an ocular palsy (ptosis, diplopia), facial and pharyngeal muscle weakness (difficult deglutition), laryngeal involvement (choking, aspiration), and respiratory muscle weakness.

The diagnosis of MG is established by using a number of different tests, including intravenous injection of edrophonium, a short acting anticholinesterase, which will restore muscle strength. A six mg dose of edrophonium is divided into three fractions (1, 2, and 3 mg), which are administered two minutes apart. The intramuscular injection of 0.5 to 1 mg neostigmine may also be used; however, the full effects are not seen for 30 minutes. Atropine may be required for treating the cholinergic side effects of these two drugs. A third test that is useful in 50 to 90% of MG patients is the detection of a fade of the twitch response using a 2 to 5 Hz stimulation rate of the motor nerve. A post-tetanic potentiation may also be seen. The abnormal electrophysiologic response is corrected by anticholinesterase (Fig. 17–3). In addition, a single fiber EMG may show variable drop-out of individual muscle fibers. A fourth test is the regional curare test, in which 0.3 mg of d-tubocurarine is injected into the arm vein after application of a tourniquet around the upper arm. Stimulation of the median or the ulnar nerve in such a setting reveals the myasthenic decrement in 95% of patients.

Treatment of Myasthenia Gravis

The currently available treatment modalities include corticosteroids, anticholinesterase, immunosuppressants, and thymectomy. Most myasthenic patients are maintained in a normal functional status by judicious use of anticholinesterase drugs, which include pyridostigmine and neostigmine. The major disadvantage of neostigmine is its short duration of action.[15] A delayed-release form of pyridostigmine is available for nocturnal respiratory muscle weakness. Corticosteroids are used in conjunction with the anticholinesterase in patients in the reproductive age group. Pregnancy can be planned safely when the patient is in a steroid induced remission. Patients who become pregnant while on steroid therapy must be maintained on the lowest possible dose of steroids that is sufficient to prevent exacerbation.[15] In the initial phases of steroid therapy, some patients may complain of increased weakness, which improves spontaneously. Following institution of steroid therapy, about 5 to 8% of patients actually require ventilatory support.[18] Plasmapheresis is recommended for those patients in whom the above-mentioned modalities are inadequate because of a high anti-AChR antibody titer.

PREGNANCY AND MYASTHENIA GRAVIS

During pregnancy, approximately one-third of patients with MG will improve, one-third will

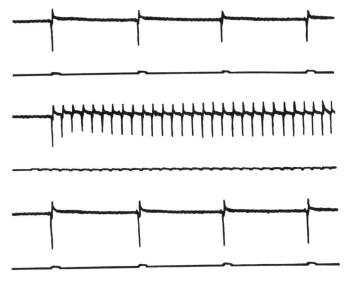

FIG. 17–3. Electromyographic tracing in a myasthenic patient. Note the presence of fade of the twitch response; the fade of the tetanus and; marked post tetanic potentiation. (From Feldman SA: Neurologic conditions and anaesthesia. *In* A Practice of Anaesthesia. 5th Edition. (Edited by Churchill-Davidson HC). Chicago, Year Book Medical Publishers, 1984.

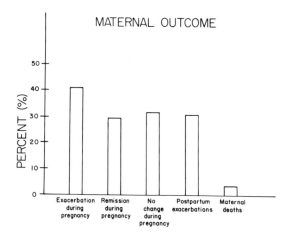

FIG. 17–4. Complication rate in myasthenia gravis in pregnancy. (The maternal deaths were mainly caused by severe myasthenic crisis.)[15]

deteriorate, and the remaining one-third will show no change in their clinical status. A sudden worsening of the condition in the postpartum period has resulted in 9 maternal deaths (Fig. 17–4). The postpartum deaths were caused by a myasthenic state that was unresponsive to treatment, a severe cholinergic crisis, and $MgSO_4$ therapy. It is to be remembered that infections play a key role in the development of a relapse. The live-birth rate reaches 85% in the well treated patients with MG.[15] The perinatal death rate reaches 8%.

One of the most intriguing neonatal problems is the neonatal myasthenia, which may affect up to 20% of the neonates. Symptoms, which include feeble crying, weak suckling, and respiratory distress, appear 12 to 48 hours after birth. The symptoms are not usually apparent at birth because of the persistence of α-fetoproteins in the fetal circulation, which can bind the AChR antibody. Neonatal myasthenia appears when the level of the α-fetoproteins start decreasing in the neonatal circulation. The neonatal myasthenic syndrome may last from 2 to 15 weeks. The higher the titer of the AChR in the mother, the higher is the likelihood of neonatal MG. Most neonates respond to anticholinesterase therapy. Severe cases may require mechanical ventilation and/or plasmapheresis. High titers of anti-AChR antibodies may be present in the breast milk. Therefore breast-feeding is contraindicated.[1]

Labor usually progresses well in myasthenics

and cesarean section is reserved only for obstetric indications; however, the duration of the second stage may be shortened by delivering the baby with forceps. Betamethasone administered for accelerating fetal lung maturity is reported to precipitate life-threatening muscle weakness.[18] Similarly, ritodrine, because of its ability to cause hypokalemia may induce muscle weakness. The use of $MgSO_4$ is contraindicated because of the neuromuscular action of the Mg^{++} ions. Drugs that must be avoided or used cautiously are listed in Table 17–3. Many authorities recommend parenteral administration of the anticholinesterase drugs during labor because of the unpredictable absorption from the gastrointestinal tract. The intramuscular and intravenous dosages for neostigmine are 20 times less than the oral dosage; pyridostigmine i.v. and i.m. dosages are 30 times less than the oral dose.[19] Serial measurement of vital capacity is useful in assessing respiratory muscle strength and the response to anticholinesterase therapy. An EKG is recommended to rule out focal myocardial necrosis that is occasionally seen in these patients.[19]

ANESTHETIC CONSIDERATIONS

For producing labor analgesia, a lumbar epidural technique may be used. Ester-type local anesthetics are best avoided because their metabolism may be slow in patients who are on anticholinesterase therapy. A low spinal block may be used to facilitate delivery. Pontocaine may be used for this purpose (despite the fact that it is an ester) because of the small dose that is used. Methoxyflurane is an ether, and therefore affects neuromuscular transmission. Inhaling devices that use methoxyflurane to produce labor analgesia can increase muscle weakness.

If anesthesia is required for cesarean section, an epidural or a spinal anesthetic may be administered to those who are in remission and to those whose symptoms have adequately responded to anticholinesterase therapy. If, however, the anticholinesterase therapy has been inadequate, and there is evidence of severe respiratory muscle involvement or bulbar muscle weakness, that has affected the laryngeal reflex, a general anesthetic may be preferred.[19]

The use of muscle relaxants is controversial in patients with myasthenia gravis (Table 17–4).

Table 17–3.   Drugs to Avoid in Patients with Myasthenia Gravis

Type	Drug
Antibiotics	Streptomycin
	Kanamycin
	Gentamicin
	Colistin, neomycin, tetracycline, lincomycin, polymyxin
Antiarrhythmics	Quinidine
	Procainamide
Local anesthetics	Ester type local anesthetics for epidural use
Drugs for preeclampsia	$MgSO_4$
Drugs for premature labor	Ritodrine (hypokalemia)
	Betamethasone

Note: All tranquilizers and narcotics may increase muscle weakness, and may cause respiratory embarrassment in patients with bulbar involvement. Therefore the dose must be carefully adjusted.

Patients with MG may initially be resistant to the action of succinylcholine but soon may develop a phase II block. In addition, the duration of succinylcholine may be prolonged. The use of a muscle relaxant is almost inevitable during induction of general anesthesia for cesarean section because the trachea must be rapidly intubated. Some authorities[19,20] advise using 30 to 50 mg of succinylcholine to intubate the trachea. If succinylcholine is administered, a nerve stimulator must be used to ascertain recovery of the neuromuscular junction before more relaxants are administered.

A small dose of d-tubocurarine, pancuronium, or atracurium can also be administered to facilitate intubation (Table 17–4). Atracurium is particularly suitable because it acts rapidly leading to abolition of all twitch responses in most of the cases in 150 seconds.[21] Because the drug is rapidly eliminated, incremental doses are required (0.02 to 0.04 mg/kg) every 10 to 15 minutes (Fig. 17–5). Whatever nondepolarizing relaxant is being used, the dose must be reduced drastically and the administration of the drug must be guided with the use of a nerve stimulator. If a nondepolarizing agent is being used, a single dose will often suffice. The residual effects of muscle relaxants must be reversed with the use of atropine and prostigmine mixture. Pentothal is used for induction. Narcotics, halothane and/

Table 17–4.   The Use of Muscle Relaxants in Myasthenia Gravis

Type	Relaxants	Reaction
Depolarizing	Decamethonium	Initial resistance followed by Phase II block:
	Succinylcholine	Initial resistance.
		Development of phase II block.
		Prolonged duration of action due to anticholinesterase therapy (60–90 min.).
Nondepolarizing	d-tubocurarine	Markedly increased sensitivity, 2–3 mg will produce 90% twitch depression.
		Normal duration of action.
	Pancuronium bromide	0.15 mg will produce 90% twitch suppression.
	Atracurium besylate	Increased sensitivity. 0.1 mg/kg will produce 100% suppression of twitch height.
		Incremental doses may be required (0.02 mg/kg) every 5–10 min.
		Normal duration of action.

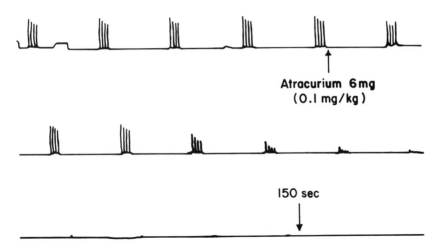

FIG. 17–5. Atracurium besylate in the myasthenic patient. Note the fade to train of four stimuli and the rapid loss of twitch responses following a small dose of atracurium. (From Bell CF, et al.: Atracurium in the myasthenic patient. Anaesthesia 39:961, 1984.)

or nitrous oxide are used for maintenance of anesthesia. If muscle relaxants cannot be reversed adequately or the patient shows signs of bulbar muscle weakness, prolonged endotracheal ventilation must be needed.

Myasthenic crisis may develop in the postpartum period. Mechanical ventilation may be required for respiratory inadequacy. All anticholinesterase drugs must be discontinued and the patients must be mechanically ventilated until the neuromuscluar junction regains its response to anticholinesterase therapy.[15] Some authors recommend plasmapheresis and/or the use of steroids to treat postpartum myasthenic crisis.

CEREBROVASCULAR ACCIDENTS

As in nonobstetric cases, the cerebrovascular accident (CVA) may be caused by cerebral vessel thrombosis or cerebral hemorrhage. Arterial embolic occlusion is the most frequent cause of thrombosis in pregnancy and the puerperium and the middle cerebral artery are more commonly affected than the other vessels.[1] Primary cerebral venous thrombosis may also occur. Cerebral hemorrhage occurs spontaneously as a result of ruptured arteriovenous malformation or an intracranial aneurysm. Cerebral hemorrhage secondary to hypertensive crisis of preeclampsia and other hypertensive disorders are also possible causes. Factors predisposing to CVA in pregnancy are listed in Table 17–5.

Ischemic strokes result in the sudden onset of hemiplegia, aphasia, and hemianopsia. When emboli arise from the heart, immediate anticoagulation must be considered, unless there is evidence of intracerebral hemorrhage. A CT scan must be done to rule out the presence of intracerebral hemorrhage. Paradoxical emboli may arise from pelvic veins. Spontaneous cerebral venous thrombosis, another cause of CVA, may occur up to a month after delivery. The clinical picture includes severe headache and focal seizures. It is also reported to occur in association with the hyperviscosity syndromes and sicklecell crisis. Heparin is used if the CT scan does not show areas of hemorrhagic infarction.

Cerebral hemorrhage is usually accompanied by a very severe headache and neck stiffness. Fifteen percent of patients who recover from the initial episode may have a second attack. A CT scan and cerebral angiography may be required for pinpointing the bleeding vessel. Subarachnoid hemorrhage usually occurs in the third trimester and may precipitate premature labor.[5] Subarachnoid hemorrhage caused by a ruptured arteriovenous malformation or an aneurysm, may indeed start during labor because of hypertension caused by labor pains and because of involuntary valsalva maneuver, which occurs during the second stage. When cerebral hemorrhage occurs during pregnancy or during labor, maternal considerations take priority over fetal considerations. The patient may require a simultaneous cesarean section and a craniotomy

Table 17–5. Causes of Stroke in Pregnancy and Puerperium

Type	Factors
Embolic (Usually middle cerebral artery)	Atrial fibrillation. Rheumatic heart disease. Mitral valve prolapse. Subacute bacterial endocarditis. Fat embolism (Usually encephalopathy): Amniotic fluid embolus; Intrapartum rupture of a dermoid cyst; Hemoglobin S/C disease. Oral contraceptives (Vertebro-basilar artery occlusion). Sickle cell crisis. Thrombotic thrombocytopenic purpura (Transient ischemic strokes). Cerebral venous thrombosis. Cerebral infarction. Sudden, prolonged hypotension. Thrombophlebitis of the legs (paradoxical embolism). Diabetes with vascular disease.
Hemorrhagic	Spontaneous subarachnoid hemorrhage: Arteriovenous malformations (age 20–25 years); Aneurysms (>30 years). Severe hypertension. Preeclampsia. Renal disease. Uncontrolled essential hypertension. Hemorrhage into the metastatic choriocarcinoma.

for clipping of the aneurysm under these circumstances.[22,23]

ANESTHETIC CONSIDERATIONS

Patients with a previous history of subarachnoid hemorrhage will benefit from a lumbar epidural analgesia for labor pains because it blunts both the hypertensive and involuntary valsalva response to strong labor pains. Epidural anesthesia is preferable to a general anesthetic for cesarean section because the latter is associated with a hypertensive response to tracheal intubation. If general anesthesia is required, the hypertensive response to intubation sequelae must be minimized by judicious use of sodium nitroprusside or nitroglycerin (see Chapter 10 Preeclampsia). Ketamine must be avoided in these patients and the use of ergot preparations can cause hypertension.

ANESTHETIC CONSIDERATIONS FOR CLIPPING OF CEREBRAL ANEURYSM

The clipping of a cerebral aneurysm has been successfully performed in pregnant patients.

The major areas of concern are the following: avoiding hypertension during induction; avoiding aortocaval compression; intraoperative fetal well-being; and the effects of hypotensive anesthesia (required for clipping) on fetal well-being.[22,23,24] The hypertensive response may be blunted using the precautions listed above. The fetal heart rate must be monitored continuously and the systemic blood pressure reduced to a level that may be tolerated by the fetus. The intraoperative $PaCO_2$ is maintained at 30 to 34 mm Hg. Severe hypocarbia may diminish fetal oxygenation by interfering with oxygen release by the maternal hemoglobin. Some animal studies have shown that excessive use of mannitol may be associated with fetal hyperosmolarity. When, however, it is used in appropriate clinical doses (up to 1 g/kg), it is not associated with any fetal sequelae.

Several methods have been used for inducing hypotension during clipping of the aneurysm. For a discussion on the hypotensive agents see Chapter 10 on Preeclampsia. Hypothermia has also been used to protect the fetus during induced hypotension. The fetus can tolerate a reduction in uterine blood flow of 40% without showing signs of hypoxia because only 60% of the fetal oxygen demands are utilized for vital cellular functions and the balance for growth needs (see Chapter 3 Respiratory Function of the Placenta). No matter what technique is used for producing hypotension, the period of hypotension should be kept to a minimum because all general anesthetics abolish the fetal responses to hypoxia. Even when fetal oxygen delivery is precariously reduced, the anesthetized fetus will not show any early warning signs such as bradycardia,[25] thus lulling the anesthesiologist into a false sense of security. The safety of halothane is indicated in animal models where maternal halothane anesthesia has been shown not to cause any further deterioration in the metabolic condition of an already stressed fetus (provided that the anesthetic exposure is brief),[26] thus halothane appears to be safe. For a more detailed discussion of the effects of anesthesia on the stressed fetus, see Chapter 9 Cesarean Section.

BRAIN TUMORS

The size of a brain tumor may increase during the second trimester. The neurosurgical treatment is usually postponed until after delivery when the tumor becomes less vascular. Metastatic choriocarcinoma, however, may cause an intracerebral hemorrhage during pregnancy. Pregnancy also causes increased growth of pituitary adenomas. Bromocriptine mesylate is given to patients who have prolactin secreting pituitary adenomas. Bromocriptine may cause resumption of normal menstrual cycle and the patient may become pregnant. Once the diagnosis of pregnancy is established, bromocriptine is usually stopped. Pituitary adenomas may cause sudden loss of vision, in which case an emergency craniotomy may be needed for resecting the tumor. In patients with pituitary adenomas, the visual fields must be assessed once a month.[5]

When a pregnant patient with raised intracranial pressure presents for general anesthesia, the ICP must be reduced with furosemide and/or mannitol. In severe cases, a CSF diversion or a ventriculostomy must be placed before anesthesia is undertaken. Controlled ventilation to decrease the arterial P_{CO_2} to 30 mm Hg is also beneficial. Steroids may be used to reduce the degree of cerebral edema. Thiopental or other barbiturates reduce the ICP. However, ketamine increases the ICP. Fasciculations due to succinylcholine must be avoided. A fentanyl-N_2O anesthesia with or without isoflurane may be used for maintenance. Unlike halothane, isoflurane has little effect on cerebral blood flow and therefore does not increase ICP.[22] d-tubocurarine increases the ICP, and therefore the vecuronium, atracurium, or pancuronium is chosen for producing muscle relaxation.

Spinal anesthesia is hazardous in patients with raised intracranial pressure because of the possibility of herniation after a lumbar puncture. Although epidural anesthesia is superior to spinal anesthesia in this regard, the danger of accidental wet tap is always present with this method. Caudal approach for epidural anesthesia is less likely to be associated with accidental dural punctures. The CSF pressure is likely to increase considerably after a large volume (10 ml) of local anesthetic is injected into the epidural space (Fig. 17–6). The increase is likely to be less severe when 3 ml of the local anesthetic is injected each time and if at least 5 minutes time is allowed between injections. The degree of increase is proportional to the magnitude of baseline intracranial hypertension (Fig. 17–6).[27] The increase is likely to be less pronounced with caudal injection than with lumbar epidural injection.[28]

BENIGN INTRACRANIAL HYPERTENSION

Benign intracranial hypertension (pseudomotor cerebri) occurs predominately in women of child-bearing-age. The lumbar CSF pressure is high, but the CSF itself is acellular with normal protein composition. The CT scan shows no space occupying lesion. Headache and papilledema, however, may be present. Occasionally there may be rapid deterioration of visual fields. The condition often resolves soon after pregnancy. The use of repeated lumbar punctures to drain the CSF, the use of acetazolamide for decreasing the formation of the CSF, and the use of osmotic diuretics or steroids are the common forms of treatment. When visual symptoms do not respond to medical therapy, a CSF shunt and/or a surgical decompression of the optic nerve may be required.[1] Epidural analgesia may be used to blunt the ICP response to uterine

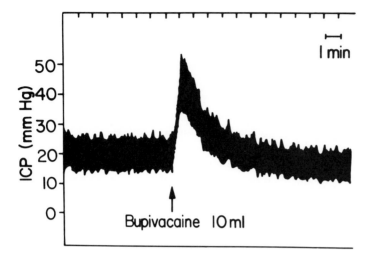

FIG. 17–6. The increase in intracranial pressure following epidural injection of bupivacaine. (From Hilt H, Gramm H-J, and Link J: Changes in intracranial pressure associated with extradural anesthesia. Br J Anaesth, *58*:676, 1986.)

contractions and may also be used for cesarean section.[29] The danger of brain herniation with an accidental dural puncture is minimal (compared to those with raised ICP resulting from brain tumors) because the patients often undergo multiple lumbar punctures for evacuation of excessive CSF. If general anesthesia becomes necessary, the precautions outlined in the section on brain tumors must be observed to prevent further ICP increases during induction of anesthesia. Acetazolamide (carbonic anhydrase inhibitor) may cause metabolic acidosis by causing increased renal excretion of HCO_3^- and diminished H^+ excretion. The CO_2 transport in the plasma may be transiently affected in the early stages of the therapy.

MYOTONIAS

This syndrome consists of a group of diseases inherited by an autosomal dominant mechanism. It is characterized by the inability of the skeletal muscles to relax following contraction.[20] There are two forms of this syndrome, the nondystrophic and the dystrophic types.

Nondystrophic Variety. Myotonia congenita (or Thompsen's disease), which is the classic form, does not not involve either the smooth or the cardiac muscle. The paramyotonia congenita of von Eulenberg is the rarest form of myotonia and the symptoms are produced by exposure to cold. Myotonia congenita of Becker starts at 10 to 20 years of life and is usually mild.

Dystrophic Variety. Myotonic dystrophy (Steinert's disease) is the most severe of the my-

otonias. Cataracts (scintillating subcapsular deposits in the lens) and cardiac involvement (conduction defects) often occurs. The patient's inability to let go after shaking hands may give a clue as to the presence of the disease. Muscular contractures develop late in the disease. The disease is punctuated by several attacks of aspiration pneumonia and pulmonary infection caused by bulbar muscle weakness. Quinidine and procainamide, which block cell-wall ionic channels, help in relieving only myotonic symptoms but not myopathic symptoms.[4] The dystrophic variety often affects the course of pregnancy. When the condition affects the fetus in utero, the inability of the fetus to swallow can result in hydramnios. Lack of fetal body movement results in fetal limb contractures (arthrogryposis). Respiratory difficulty at birth and aspiration pneumonia are not uncommon in the newborn.

The cardiac and respiratory status must be carefully assessed before administering anesthesia. The serum creatine kinase activity is usually moderately elevated.[5] Because of the difficulties associated with the administration of muscle relaxants, epidural or spinal anesthesia is preferred for vaginal delivery and cesarean section. When extensive muscle wasting is present, the patient may be unduly sensitive to pentothal and other sedative drugs. The use of succinylcholine may cause a contracture in the affected muscle (Fig. 17–7). Although the twitch response decreases following succinylcholine, the resting muscle tension will rise, explaining the contracture, the apnea, and the inability to ventilate these patients.[5,30] The succinylcholine

0.1

0.2

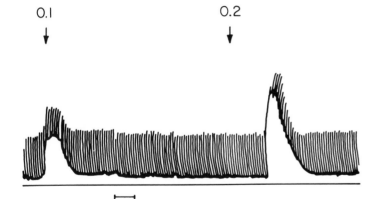

FIG. 17–7. The use of succinylcholine in a patient with myotonia. Note the diminished twitch response with a concomitant increase in the resting tension (contracture). (From Mitchell MM, Ali HH, and Savarese JJ: Myotonia and neuromuscular agents. Anesthesiology, *49*:492, 1978.)

induced contracture is similar to the rigidity seen in malignant hyperpyrexia (MH). Indeed, two cases of MH are reported in patients with myotonias. Because of the unpredictable response to succinylcholine, this drug must be avoided. The response to d-tubocurarine and pancuronium may be prolonged, especially in those with muscle wasting. However, the onset of paralysis is normal. It should, however, be remembered that quinidine, which is prescribed to these patients, usually potentiates the effects of the muscle relaxants. The dose of muscle relaxants must therefore be reduced suitably. Residual curarization must be reversed with neostigmine.[5,30] Atracurium besylate, which undergoes Hoffman hydrolysis, is of benefit to these patients.

A major problem in these patients is the failure to obtain adequate surgical relaxation. Because the defect is in the muscle, muscle relaxants will generally be ineffective. Quinidine, procainamide, local anesthetics, phenytoin, and prednisone have been recommended to overcome contracture caused by handling of the muscles by the surgeon (percussion contracture). When the above measures fail, infiltration of the contracted muscle with a local anesthetic may be tried. Deepening the level of anesthesia with a volatile agent may help but at the risks of causing cardiovascular depression.

AUTONOMIC HYPERREFLEXIA

Sensory stimulation may cause a severe increase in blood pressure, headaches, reflex bradycardia, piloerection, and flushing in patients with spinal cord transection at or above the level T_6. Visceral stimuli, such as pain caused by uterine contractions or distention of the urinary bladder, are potent stimuli for intiating the hyperreflexic response. This condition is belived to be caused by the lack of modulating influences of the inhibitory centers of the brain. Intracranial or retinal hemorrhage may occur as a result of uncontrolled autonomic hyperreflexia. Although a wide variety of vasodilators and alpha blockers have been suggested for controlling the hypertension, epidural anesthesia administered early in the course of labor is the method of choice.[31] Epidural analgesia extending to T_{10} level will block entry of noxious impulses into the spinal cord, thereby interrupting the chain of events that culminate in the hypertensive response. When general anesthesia is needed, a number of precautions must be observed. Hypertensive response to intubation must be prevented with sodium nitroprusside or trimethaphan infusion. Also, succinylcholine must be avoided in patients whose spinal injury is less than six months old because of possible hyperkalemic response. A third precaution is that the upper airway must be properly assessed because these patients may have had a tracheostomy, which causes tracheal narrowing, or they might have had a cervical spinal fusion, which restricts neck motion thus creating difficult conditions for tracheal intubation. A fourth precaution is to determine whether renal function may be impaired because of recurrent urinary infection.

FAMILIAL DYSAUTONOMIA (RILEY-DAY SYNDROME)

This disease which is characterized by severe autonomic instability is limited to Ashkenazi Jews. This multisystem disease is characterized by an extremely labile sympathetic state. The number of sympathetic and autonomic ganglion cells, together with the number of myelinated and unmyelinated cells, is reduced.[32] The clinical features of interest to the anesthesiologist are listed in Table 17–6. Although many patients die at an early age, better medical care has made it possible for these patients to reach child-bearing age. Successful pregnancies have been reported in these patients.[33]

Because of the extremely labile sympathetic system, spinal or epidural anesthesia is not recommended. Indwelling arterial pressure monitoring is required because of the unpredictable changes in blood pressure and CVP monitoring is needed to diagnose and treat preexising dehydration. Adequate crystalloid infusion is necessary to prevent intraoperative hypotensive episodes. Pentothal may be used for induction of anesthesia. The response to succinylcholine and other muscle relaxants is usually normal. Volatile agents must be administered cautiously because they may cause vasodilatation and cardiac depression. A technique of using a high dose of fentanyl (15 ug/kg) is reported to be associated with a greater cardiovascular stability.[31] Should hypertension become a problem during fentanyl anesthesia, halothane may be added in small concentrations. Because these patients lack the ability to sweat, hyperpyrexia may develop perioperatively.

GUILLAIN-BARRÉ SYNDROME

Most cases have occurred in the third trimester. Recurrence during subsequent pregnancy has been reported in two patients.[1] The polyneuropathy is usually motor with little impairment of sensations. There may be, however, cranial nerve involvement, which may affect laryngeal function. Cesarean delivery may be required if the condition develops in late pregnancy. The CSF protein concentration is increased but the cell count is normal. The two important anesthetic considerations are the labile autonomic nervous system (hypotension or hypertension); and the hyperkalemic response to succinylcholine. Arterial pressure and central venous pressure must be continuously monitored. A balanced anesthetic with N_2O, vecuronium, and fentanyl may be administered, if anesthesia is required for cesarean section. Postoperative mechanical ventilation may be needed.

GENITAL HERPES INFECTION

After the membranes rupture, cesarean sections are usually performed on these patients without delay to minimize the neonatal involvement. Neonatal herpes infection usually carries a high mortality. The controversy in this situation revolves around the safety of regional anes-

Table 17–6.   Familial Dysautonomia

Site	Description
Sympathetic system	Increased secretion of catecholamine during crisis, mainly norepinephrine. Loss of temperature control. Loss of vasomotor control. Increased hypersensitivity to exogenous catecholamines. Decreased lacrimation (corneal ulcer).
Somatic nervous system	Decreased sensation with areas of hyperaesthesia.
Cardiovascular system	Labile blood pressure. Orthostatic hypotension. Episodic hypertension.
Gastrointestinal	Dysphagia, prone to aspiration. Vomiting, dehydration, dysautonomic crisis.
Pulmonary	Repeated attacks of pneumonia. Kyphoscoliotic lung disease.
Musculoskeletal	Stunted growth. Scoliosis. Charcot's joints.

thesia because there are some old reports that claim that spinal anesthesia causes reactivation of herpes zoster lesions. Many clinicians consider that spinal or epidural anesthesia is usually contraindicated in these patients.

The genital herpes lesions are caused by two two types of neurotropic viruses: herpes simplex virus 1 (HSV 1) and herpes simplex virus 2 (HSV 2). In some communities, HSV infection is the commonest veneral disease. Both viruses cause a primary infection after which they go into a dormant state. They live in the spinal neural ganglia and cause recurrent local lesions that are known as the secondary infection. The HSV 1 is responsible for 7% of all primary lesions and 2% of all secondary lesions, whereas the HSV 2 causes most of the primary lesions and almost all of the secondary lesions.

The primary infection produces severe generalized symptoms including pyrexia, lymphadenopathy, and signs of meningeal irritation. Viral cultures are often positive. There is always accompanying viremia with transplacental passage of the virus to the fetus. The secondary episodes are not associated with generalized symptoms or neurologic signs and almost always produce only local recurrences. The likelihood of seeing a primary infection for the first time during pregnancy is negligible. The most definitive method of isolating the virus is by tissue culture.[34]

A recent study has shown that epidural anesthesia is safe in patients with active secondary lesions.[35] In many of them, positive culture reports were obtained in the last month of pregnancy (Table 17–7). It is not known whether regional anesthesia is safe in those with primary HSV infection. The safety of spinal anesthesia has not been established.

MALIGNANT HYPERPYREXIA

Malignant hyperpyrexia (MH) is a clinical syndrome of unknown etiology that is characterized by a rapid rise in body temperature. The rate of the rise of temperature may be as great as 1°C per 5 minutes. Even with prompt recognition and treatment of the condition the mortality rate may reach 30%. Almost all inhalation anesthetic agents and depolarizing muscle relaxants (succinylcholine, decamethonium) may trigger the syndrome. Emotional stress or physical stress has also been implicated in awake triggering of MH. Awake triggering is more common in swine than in human beings. The sympathetic nervous system is hyperactive during acute episodes. It is unclear, however, whether the sympathetic response is a primary or a secondary event.

The diagnosis of MH susceptibility is based on family history and a positive skeletal muscle contracture test.[1] A piece of the quadriceps muscle is suspended in a tissue chamber containing Krebs-Ringer biophase. The tissue is stimulated electrically with supramaximal impulses at 0.2 Hz. Three types of tests may be performed; (1) the static caffeine contracture test; (2) the static halothane test; and (3) a dynamic halothane test. With the static test, the muscle preload is held constant at 2 g, whereas with the dynamic test, the muscle is stretched at a rate of 4 mm/minute for 1.5 minutes and held at the new length for 1 minute when halothane is added to the bath (Fig. 17–8). A patient is placed in the MH-susceptible category if a caffeine concentration of 1.5 mmol or less produces a sustained increase of at least 0.2 g in the resting tension in the static test, and if a halothane concentration of

Table 17–7. Anesthesia in Patients with Genital Herpes

Total	Site	General anesthesia	Epidural anesthesia
Number		28	48
Positive cultures		10	25
	Genital (cervical, vulval)	20	29
	Sacral, gluteal	3	3
	Fingers	1	1
	Eye lid	0	1

No patient developed any complication either after general or epidural anesthesia.

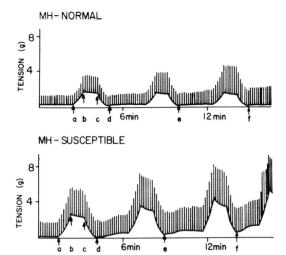

FIG. 17–8. Dynamic halothane contracture test. The muscle is stimulated electrically. The upper tracing is a part of the normal response in an MH-normal patient. The muscle tissue is stretched at 4 mm/ minute (a to b), held constant at the same tension from b to c, and released at the same rate from c to d. After eliciting three such control responses, the test is repeated in the presence of increasing concentrations of halothane at points d, e, and f. In the MH-normal patient the baseline tension does not change. In the MH-susceptible patient, however, the resting tension increases when the muscle is exposed to halothane (lower tracing).

less than 2% produces the same response in the static and dynamic tests.[36]

The basic functional derangement in MH is believed to be related to altered Ca^{++} turnover in skeletal muscles.[37] Under normal circumstances Ca^{++} is stored in the sarcoplasmic reticulum (SR). During a normal contractile response, Ca^{++} ions are released from the SR into the cytoplasm and soon after the contractile response, they are again taken up into the SR. However, when MH develops, there is enormous leakage of Ca^{++} from the SR. The Ca^{++} thus released from the SR is perhaps bound by the mitochondria. The increased mitochondrial Ca^{++} uptake probably causes increased metabolism and heat production. Dantrolene halts Ca^{++} leakage out from the SR, but does not affect the reuptake function. The increased intracellular Ca^{++} content may also explain the tendency toward increased muscle contracture, which causes the masseter spasm.[37]

The syndrome may have an immediate acute onset at the induction of anesthesia or the onset

may be delayed for hours.[37] Hyperthermia, sweating, tachycardia, cardiac arrhythmias, increased CO_2 production, increased oxygen consumption, hyperlactacedemia and hyperkalemia may occur.[37] The clinical manifestations of malignant hyperprexia are the following:

1. Immediate or delayed onset of hyperpyrexia.
2. Masseter spasm with succinylcholine.
3. Increased Pa_{CO_2}, increased blood lactate (respiratory and metabolic acidosis), decreased Pa_{O_2}.
4. Tachycardia, sweating, and hypertension.
5. Edema of the muscles, cerebral edema.
6. Increased serum K^+, Ca^{++}, myoglobin, and creatine phosphokinase.

Blood base excess (BE) values may rapidly increase. Changes in blood pH and BE are detected earlier in central venous blood than in arterial blood.[37] The principles of treatment include removal of the triggering agent (if known); cooling the patient; rapid correction of acid-base and electrolyte abnormalities; correction of volume deficit in order to preserve muscle blood flow; and administration of dantrolene sodium in doses of 2 mg/kg. Dantrolene administration may be repeated if the initial dose fails to produce a response.[37]

The diagnosis of an MH crisis in a pregnant patient is somewhat difficult because the perinatal events are often associated with anxiety, tachycardia, increase in body temperature, and increased plasma catecholamine levels. In addition, prolonged labor causes metabolic acidosis, which is caused by an accumulation of lactate. A BE value of ⁻8 to ⁻10 is not uncommon during strenuous labor. Even in patients undergoing elective cesarean section, a BE value of ⁻6 may be seen.[38] It is uncommon, however, to see a Pa_{CO_2} of >37 mm Hg in an otherwise healthy parturient.[39] The rise in Pa_{CO_2} may therefore be a more reliable diagnostic index of MH than are BE values. It must also be remembered that the serum CPK values rise steadily during labor probably because of uterine activity; however, the rise in CPK levels of an MH-susceptible patient is greater than that in a normal parturient.[40] The administration of a triggering agent such as succinlycholine to the mother may trigger muscle rigidity in an MH-susceptible fetus.[41]

The treatment of MH in a pregnant parturient must take into account the enormous fluid deficit she may have incurred during the course of labor. Dantrolene crosses the placenta.[42] Except for decreased muscle tone, no other adverse neonatal effects have been attributed to dantrolene. Mothers may, however, complain of nausea, muscle weakness, and headache.[43] Extreme caution must be exercised in prescribing prophylactic dantrolene therapy to preeclamptic patients who are on $MgSO_4$ therapy. Dantrolene may also inhibit myometrial contractility, which may result in atonic uterus and severe postpartum hemorrhage.[44] It is therefore recommended that the prophylactic use of dantrolene be restricted to patients who will receive general anesthesia for delivery or for cesarean section.[43] The routine prophylactic use of dantrolene in patients who are in labor, or in patients who will be given an epidural anesthetic for labor analgesia, delivery, or for cesarean section is not recommended.

ANESTHESIA FOR LABOR

Since labor pains are associated with stress, lumbar epidural analgesia may be beneficial. Many have recommended the use of 2-chloroprocaine because it is an ester derivative.[43] Although amide-type local anesthetics have been used without problems for local anesthesia for muscle biopsies,[44] both bupivacaine and lidocaine have precipitated the triggering of MH. If epidural analgesia is not possible analgesia may be safely provided with narcotics. The use of epinephrine-containing local anesthetic solutions are best avoided.[43]

ANESTHESIA FOR CESAREAN SECTION

Epidural anesthesia with 2-chloroprocaine is the preferred method.[43] Intravenous fluids must be administered liberally and aortocaval compression must be avoided at all costs. These general measures are necessary to prevent systemic hypotension which may necessitate the use of sympathomimetic substance such as ephedrine.[43] β-mimetic substances may increase lactate production and α-mimetic substances may lead to diminished heat loss by producing peripheral vasoconstriction.[37] Should use of either of these agents become necessary, they

must be administered in small quantities until the desired end-point is reached.

When general anesthesia is required in an MH-susceptible patient, dantrolene prophylaxis may be considered.[43] The anesthetic must be administered using a system free of anesthetic vapor. Induction may be done with pentothal. Pancuronium bromide may be used for facilitating jaw relaxation.[43] A balanced anesthetic using N_2O, oxygen, narcotic and further doses of pancuronium may be used. Temperature must be monitored at a minimum of two sites. Exhaled CO_2 monitoring is also useful because increased CO_2 production is often an early warning sign.[37] Since measurements of Pa_{CO_2}, BE, and blood lactate levels are useful diagnostic indices, a case may be made for inserting an indwelling arterial cannula. The use of anticholinesterase drugs for reversing neuromuscular block is generally considered safe.[37] Glycopyrrolate may be preferred over atropine as it tends to produce less tachycardia than does atropine. The principles of treatment of MH crisis have been outlined previously in this chapter.

REFERENCES

1. Noronha A: Neurologic disorders during pregnancy and the puerperium. Clin Perinatol 12:695, 1985.
2. Pritchard JA, McDonald PC, and Gant NF: Medical and surgical illnesses during pregnancy and the puerperium. In Williams Obstetrics. 17th Edition. Norwalk, Appleton-Century-Crofts, 1985.
3. Mygind KI, Dam M, and Christiansen J: Phenytoin and phenobarbitone plasma clearance during pregnancy. Acta Neurol Scandinav 54:160, 1976.
4. Dichter MA: The epilepsies and the convulsive disorders. In Harrison's Principles of Internal Medicine. (Edited by Petersdorf RG, et al.). New York, McGraw-Hill, 1983.
5. Donaldson JO: Neurologic emergencies during pregnancy. In Critical Care of the Obstetric Patient. (Edited by Berkowitz RL.) New York, Churchill-Livingstone, 1983.
6. Meldrum BS and Nillson B: Cerebral blood flow early and late prolonged epileptic seizures induced by rats in biculline. Brain 99:523, 1976.
7. Kruczek M, Albin MS, Wolf S, and Bertoni JM: Postoperative seizure activity following enflurane anesthesia. Anesthesiology 53:175, 1977.
8. Ferrer-Allado D, et al.: Ketamine induced electroconvulsive phenomena in the human limbic and thalamic regions. Anesthesiology, 38:333, 1973.
9. Bennett DR, Madsen JA, Jordon WS, and Wiser WC: Ketamine anesthesia in brain-damaged epileptics: elec-

troencephalographic and clinical observations. Neurology 23:449, 1973.

10. Male CG and Allen EM: Methohexitone induced convulsions in epileptics. Anesth Intens Care 5:226, 1970.

11. Antel JP and Aranson BGW: Multiple sclerosis and other demyelinating diseases. *In* Harrison's Principles of Internal Medicine. (Edited by Peterdorf RG, et al.). New York, McGraw-Hill Book Co., 1983.

12. Feldman SA: Neurologic conditions and anaesthesia. *In* A Practice of Anaesthesia. 5th Edition. (Edited by Churchill-Davidson HC). Chicago, Year Book Medical Publishers, 1984.

13. Crawford JS, et al.: Regional anesthesia for patients with chronic neurological disease. Anesth Analg 36:821, 1981.

14. Warren TM, Datta S, and Ostheimer GW: Lumbar epidural anesthesia in a patient with multiple sclerosis. Anesth Analg 61:1022, 1982.

15. Plauche WC: Myasthenia Gravis. Clin Obstet Gynecol 26:593, 1983.

16. Bradley WG, and Adams RD: Myasthenia Gravis, neuromuscular junction disorders, and episodic muscular weakness. *In* Harrison's Principles of Internal Medicine. (Edited by Petersdorf RG, et al.). New York, McGraw-Hill Book Co. 1983.

17. Eden RD and Gall SA: Myasthenia gravis and pregnancy. Obstet Gynecol 328, 1983.

18. Catanzarite V, McHargue A, Sandberg EC, and Dyson DC: Respiratory arrest during therapy for premature labor with myasthenia gravis. Obstet Gynecol 64:819, 1984.

19. Rolbin SH, Levinson G, Shnider SM, and Wright RG: Anesthetic considerations for myasthenia gravis and pregnancy. Anesth Analg 57:441, 1978.

20. Azar I: The response of patients with neuromuscular disorders to muscle relaxants: A review. Anesthesiology 61:173, 1984.

21. Bell CF, et al.: Atracurium in the myasthenic patient. Anaesthesia 39:961, 1984.

22. Newman B, and Lam AM: Induced hypotension for clipping of a cerebral aneurysm during pregnancy. Anesth Analg 65:675, 1986.

23. Lennen RL, Sundt TM, and Gronert GA: Combined cesarean section and clipping of intracerebral aneurysm. Anesthesiology 60:240, 1984.

24. Kofke WA, Wuest HP, and McGinnis LA: Cesarean section following ruptured cerebral aneurysm and neuroresuscitation. Anesthesiology 60:242, 1984.

25. Schwartz J, Cummings M, Pucci W, and Biehl D: The effects of general anesthesia on the asphyxiated fetal lamb in utero. Canad Anaesth Soc J 32:577, 1985.

26. Yarnell R, et al.: The effect of halothane anesthesia on the asphyxiated lamb. Can Anaesth Soc J 30:474, 1983.

27. Hilt H, Gramm H-J, and Link J: Changes in intracranial pressure associated with extradural anesthesia. Br J Anaesth 58:676, 1986.

28. Usubiaga JE, Usubiaga LE, Bea LM, and Goyena R: Effects of saline injections on epidural and subarachnoid space pressures and relation to post-spinal anesthesia headache. Anesth Analg (Cleve) 46:293, 1967.

29. Palop R, Choed-Ampahai E, and Miller R: Epidural anesthesia for delivery complicated by benign intracranial hypertension. Anesthesiology 50:159, 1979.

30. Mitchell MM, Ali HH, and Savarese JJ: Myotonia and neuromuscular agents. Anesthesiology 49:492, 1978.

31. Stirt JA, Marco A, and Conklin KA: Obstetric anesthesia for a quadriplegic patient autonomic hyperreflexia. Anesthesiology 51:560, 1979.

32. Beilin B, et al.: Fentanyl anesthesia in familial dysautonomia. Anesth Analg 64:72, 1985.

33. Porges RF, Axelrod FB, and Richards M: Pregnancy in familial dysautonomia. Am J Obstet Gynecol 132:485, 1978.

34. Corey L and Holmes KK: Genital herpes virus infections: Current concepts in diagnosis, therapy and prevention. Ann Int Med 98:973, 1983.

35. Ramanathan S, Sheth R, and Turndorf H: Anesthesia for cesarean in patients with genital herpes. Anesthesiology 64:807, 1986.

36. A protocol for the investigation of malignant hyperpyrexia (MH) susceptibility. The European Malignant Hyperpyrexia Group Br J Anaesth 56:1267, 1984.

37. Gronert GA: Malignant Hyperthermia. *In* Anesthesia (Edited by Miller RD.) New York, Churchill-Livingstone, 1986.

38. Ramanathan S: The biochemical profile of a well-oxygenated human fetus. Anesthesiology 61:A397, 1984.

39. Greenberger PA: Asthma in pregnancy. Clin Perinatol 12:571, 1985.

40. Sherwood DM, Ridley J, and Wilson J: Creatine phosphokinase (CPK) levels in pregnancy: A case report and discussion of the value of CPK levels in the prediction of possible malignant hyperpyrexia. Obstet Gynaecol 82:346, 1975.

41. Sewall K, Flowerdew RMM, and Bromberger P: Severe muscular rigidity at birth: Malignant hyperthermia syndrome? Can Anaesth Soc J 27:279, 1980.

42. Morison DH: Placental transfer of dantrolene: Anesthesiology 59:265, 1983.

43. Douglas JM, and McMorland GH: The anaesthetic management of the malignant hyperthermia susceptible parturient. Can Anaesth Soc J 33:371, 1986.

43. Weingarten AE, Korsh JI, Neuman GG and Stern SB: Postpartum uterine atony following intravenous dantrolene. Anesth Analg (In Press–1987).

44. Moore DC: Ester or amide local anesthetics in malignant hyperthermia–Who Knows?. Anesthesiology 64:294, 1986.

18

TERATOLOGY

Since the thalidomide tragedy, which occurred in the late 1950s and early 1960s, the teratogenic effects of maternally administered drugs have been the focus of numerous studies.

A pregnant patient may be exposed to several drugs during pregnancy. If nonobstetric surgery is required, the patient is also exposed to several anesthetics. Although the teratogenic effects of many drugs have been studied in animal fetuses, only a limited number of drugs have been studied in human fetuses. Genetic make-up, maternal age, nutritional status, and other underlying coincidental diseases also influence the teratogenic potential of a drug. Both alcohol use and drug abuse, including narcotics and diazepam, are also implicated in teratogenesis.

A federal law requires that the teratogenic potential of a drug must be investigated in animals before it is released for general consumption. Animal experiments can give an indication of a possible teratogenic problem in humans, which may otherwise go unnoticed. Diphenylhydantoin was shown to be a teratogen in animals long before human data were available. The same is true of diethylstilbestrol.

On the contrary, animal experiments have many disadvantages. The metabolic pathways of a particular drug may be species-specific, or dosages used in animal studies are often too high. Drugs that are not teratogenic to animals may be teratogenic to humans. The classic example is streptomycin, which does not produce ototoxicity in animal fetuses but is known to be ototoxic in humans fetuses. Conversely, drugs

that are teratogenic to animal fetuses may not be teratogenic in humans; salicylates and corticosteroids are examples of this problem.

Different types of studies are performed to define the teratogenic risk of a number of different drugs in humans. The different studies include retrospective studies, prospective studies, specially designed clinical trials, data from a centrally maintained register that records all malformations, and isolated clinical reports. Each one of these methods has disadvantages. In each instance, to obtain reliable conclusions a large number of patients must be studied. Retrospective studies may be limited because data are often incomplete, and because information regarding tobacco and alcohol consumption may not be available. Some of these deficiencies are overcome in a prospective study but the results are not immediately available. It may be possible to arrive at conclusions within a reasonable period of time when clinical trials are used. These trials, however, are limited in number and often only well-established drugs are used. In some countries, registrations of malformations is routine; this enables clinicians to reach conclusions regarding a particular type of malformation in a particular geographic area. Case reports may occasionally pin-point the causal relationship between reproductive disturbances and drug-consumption during pregnancy. This approach, however, may be flawed because the author may often make an unwarranted conclusion to prove his hypothesis.

Since 1978, the Swedish catalogue of registered pharmaceutical specialties (FASS) has presented information on some potential problems associated with drug use in pregnancy and breast-feeding. All drugs are assigned to one of the following pregnancy categories: A, B_1, B_2, B_3, C, and D. The letters A to D refer to information based on human data. Drugs are classified into groups I to IV with respect to their potential for being secreted in the breast milk.[1]

PREGNANCY RISKS

CATEGORIZING DRUGS BY TERATOGENIC RISK

Category A. These drugs have been used by a large number of women and are not associated with any increased incidence of malformation or reproductive disturbances.

Category B. These drugs have been used only by a limited number of patients. They are not associated with any harmful effects.

Category C. The pharmacologic effect of these drugs have caused or are suspected of having caused increased reproductive disturbances without directly being teratogenic to the fetus.

Category D. Drugs which are known to have caused increased incidence of malformation.

Comparison of the Categories. The drugs in category A include drugs that have stood the test of time. Local anesthetics, cardiac glycosides, and theophylline are examples of category A drugs. Category B is divided into three subgroups: B_1, B_2, and B_3. In group B_1, animal reproduction studies have not indicated any harmful effects. In Group B_2 drugs, reproduction-toxicology studies are incomplete. In Group B_3, reproduction-toxicology studies have shown an increased incidence of fetal damage or other deleterious effects on the reproductive process.

In clinical practice, drug combinations are often prescribed. For example, trimethoprim (category B_3) and ergotamine (category C) are prescribed in combination for migraine. The combination is usually assigned to the more harmful category C.[1] The intended therapeutic use of the drug may also modify category assignment. For instance, phenobarbital is assigned to category D when used in combination with other drugs for the treatment of epilepsy. It is, however, placed in category A when used

as a sedative. Table 18–1 lists risk classification of certain commonly used compounds.

GROUPING DRUGS ACCORDING TO AFFECTS ON BREAST MILK

Group I. Drugs that do not enter the breast milk.

Group II. Drugs that enter the breast milk, but are not likely to affect the neonate in therapeutic dose-ranges.

Group III. Drugs that enter the breast milk in quantities that may affect the infant even when therapeutic doses are employed.

Group IV. There is no information as to whether or not these drugs enter the breast milk.

PERIODS OF THE PRENATAL STAGE

For the sake of convenience, Hutchings[2] has divided the prenatal stage into three periods: the predifferentiation period; the period of the embryo; and the period of the fetus. A drug that is teratogenic in one period may not be teratogenic when used in the other two periods. The teratogenic effects of the same drug may differ from one period to another.

The predifferentiation period extends from the fertilization of the oocyte to its implantation in the endometrium. This period lasts 6 days in humans. The developing fetus is resistant to teratogenic effects during this period. Except for some reports of altered offspring behavior from phenothiazine exposure in this period,[3] most investigators agree that the fetus is least vulnerable to teratogenicity in the predifferentiation period. The recent advent of in vitro fertilization procedures has made this period critically important for the anesthesiologists. Anesthesia for in vitro fertilization is discussed further in Chapter 21 Anesthesia in Nonobstetric Situations.

The period of the embryo when organogenesis occurs continues up to the 8th week.[2,4] The embryo is highly susceptible to teratogens during this period. The teratogen may damage the actively proliferating cells, resulting in an anatomically defective embryo. The type of defects produced by a given teratogen depends on the gestational period. During this period, with increasing gestational age, the fetus becomes more resistant to teratogenic effects.

Table 18–1.   Pregnancy and Breast-Feeding Risks

Type of drug	Specific drugs	Pregnancy category	Breast milk group
Analgesics:	Codeine, dextropropoxyphene.	A	II
	Methadone, morphine, demerol.	C	II
	Fentanyl, phenoperidine.	C	IV
Anesthetics:	Enflurane.	A	IV
	Halothane, ketamine, thiopental.	A	II
	Methohexital.	B_2	IV
	Propanidid.	B_1	II
	Bupivacaine, lidocaine.	A	II
	Etidocaine.	B_1	IV
Antiaddiction:	Disulfiram.	B_2	IV
	Naloxone.	B_1	IV
Antiasthmatics:	Cromoglicic acid.	A	II
	Theophylline.	A	II
Anticonvulsants:	Phenytoin, valproic acid.	D	II
Antihistamines:	Brompheniramine. Chlorpheniramine.	A	II
Antiemetics:	Diphenhydramine.	A	II
	Promethazine.	A	IV
Antiinfectious:	Aminoglycosides.	D	IV
	Cephalosporins.	A	II
	Penicillins.	A	II
	Sulfonamide.	C	II
	Dapsone.	D	II
	Tetracycline.	D	II
	Para-aminosalicylic acid.	A	IV
	Ethambutol.	A	II
	Rifampicin.	C	II
	Aciclovir.	B_1	IV
	Chloramphenicol.	C	III
	Erythromycin.	A	II
	Metronidazole	B_2	II
	Trimethoprim.	B_3	II
Antimalarials:	Chloroquine.	D	II
	Hydroxychloroquine.	D	IV
Antitussives:	Opium derivatives.	A	IV
Expectorants:	Acetylcysteine.	B_2	IV
	Iodides.	C	III
	Caffeine.	A	IV
Autonomics:	Dobutamine, norepinephrine.	B_2	IV
	Dopamine.	B_3	—
	Ephedrine, (epinephrine).	A	IV
	Pseudoephedrine.	B_2	III
	Terbutaline.	A	II
	Fenoterol, isoprenaline.	A	IV
Anticholinergics:	Atropine.	A	III
	Glycopyrrolate.	B_2	IV
	Scopolamine.	B_2	II
Cardiovascular:	Digoxin.	A	II
	Disopyramide, procainamide.	B_2	IV
	Quinidine.	D	II
Betaadrenoceptor blockers:	All preparations.	C	II

Table 18–1. Continued

Type of drug	Specific drugs	Pregnancy category	Breast milk group
Vasodilators:	Isosorbide.	B_1	IV
	Verapamil.	A	IV
	Nicotinic acid.	B_2	IV
	Nifedipine.	B_3	IV
	Nitroglycerin.	B_2	IV
	Hydralazine, reserpine.	A	II
Antihypertensives:	Clonidine, prazosin.	B_2	IV
	Diazoxide.	C	IV
	Trimethaphan.	C	IV
	α-methyl dopa.	A	III
Diuretics:	Bendroflumethiazide.	C	IV
	Chlorothiazide.	C	III
	Furosemide.	C	I
	Spironolactone.	A	III
Anticoagulants:	Heparin.	B_2	I
	Dicoumarol.	C	III
	Warfarin.	D	II
	Streptokinase.	C	IV
	Protamine.	B_2	IV
Corticosteroids:	Beclomethasone	B_3	IV
Antithyroid drugs:	Carbimazole, Propyl thiouracil.	C	II
Hypnotics:	Phenobarbital	D	III
Sedatives: (anticonvulsant).	Benzodiazepines.	C	III
	Hydroxyzine.	A	IV
	Meprobomate.	B_3	III
	Chlorpromazine.	A	II
Antipsycotics:	Amitryptiline.	A	III
	Imipramine.	A	II
	Lithium salts.	D	III
Oxytocics:	Methylergometrine.	C	II
	Oxytocin	A	IV

See also Chapters 10, 12, 13, 14, 15, 16, 17, 18, 19, 20 and 21 for more information on teratogenicity. For explanation of groups see text.

The period of the fetus extends from the 8th week to the time of delivery. The fetal brain grows very rapidly during this period. In humans, the myelination of the nervous system occurs actively from the seventh month of intrauterine life to the first few months of extrauterine life.[4,5] The fetus and neonate, although refractory to gross structural defect, remain vulnerable to more subtle brain damage, particularly in those areas of the brain that are actively proliferating. This can produce brain dysfunction in the neonatal period or in early childhood.[2]

TERATOGENS

The teratogenic effects can therefore be generally divided into two major categories: morphologic teratogenicity, which involves structural alteration of an organ; and behavioral teratogenicity, which involves subtle brain dysfunction such as learning disability.[2] Behavioral teratogenesis can occur with or without gross CNS structural abnormality. Two other factors, which may play a role in teratogenicity in fetuses born of mothers hospitalized for an incidental illness, are the stress of being confined to a hospital bed (which may lead to increased congenital malformations and mental retardation),[5,6,7] and hypoglycemia (which is implicated in causing defective ossification of axial skeleton and defective morphogenesis of embryonic neural tube.[8] Frequent blood sugar determinations are therefore necessary in hospitalized pregnant patients receiving prolonged parenteral fluid therapy, especially when they have diabetes.

It is beyond the scope of this discussion to describe exhaustively the effects of all teratogens. Therefore this discussion will be limited to the teratogenic effects of the most commonly used drugs and anesthetics (Table 18–2).

Morphologic Teratogens

Anticoagulants. Oral anticoagulants such as warfarin are contraindicated in pregnancy. Exposure during the first trimester is associated with fetal nasal hypoplasia (Fig. 18–1) and chondrodysplasia punctata. Exposure during the second and third trimester may result in optic atrophy, microcephaly, mental retardation, and other central nervous system disorders (warfarin embryopathy). If anticoagulants are required during pregnancy, heparin is preferred to oral anticoagulants. However, the use of heparin is associated with other fetal problems such as prematurity.[9] These problems are more fully discussed in Chapter 16 Thromboembolism.

Table 18–2.   Human and Animal Teratogenicity

Drug	Morphologic teratogenicity	Behavioral teratogenicity
(1) Anticoagulants (humans)	Optic atrophy; microcephaly.	Mental retardation.
(2) Diazepam (humans)	Oral clefts.	
(3) Salicylates (humans)	Neonatal platelet dysfunction, neural tube defects.	
(4) Dilantin (humans)	Facial anomalies; neonatal vitamin K deficiency.	Mental retardation.
(5) Narcotics: (humans) heroin; morphine; methadone	Cranial defects reduced DNA and RNA in the brain.	Hyperactivity; insomnia; learning problems; motor incoordination; neonatal withdrawal; syndrome; neonatal tolerance.
(6) Anesthetics (Human low level exposure)	Fetal loss; ? congenital anomalies.	
(7) Anesthetics (Acute exposure)	Fetal resorption; skeletal defects.	Learning difficulties.
(8) Barbiturates (humans)	Vitamin K deficiency.	Withdrawal symptoms; decreased attention span.
(9) Alcohol (humans)	Craniofacial-limb defects.	Withdrawal syndrome hyperactivity in preschool period Lower I.Q.
(10) Amphetamine	Altered brain catecholamine content.	Hyperactivity; impaired locomotion.
(11) Phencyclidine (humans)	Cranial anomaly.	Hyperactivity.
(12) Antenatal stress (humans)		? Mental retardation; defective motor development.
(13) Tranquilizers: meprobamate; chlordiazepoxide (humans)	Congenital heart disease, microcephaly.	Mental retardation.
(14) Hypoglycemia	Skeletal defects.	
(15) Diabetes with acidosis (humans)*		Lower I.Q.
(16) Antibotics:		
Aminoglycosides (humans)	Cranial nerve defects.	None known.
Cephalosporins	None known.	None known.
Erythromycin	None known	None known
Metronidazole	None known	None known
Penicillin	None known.	None known.
Sulfonamides (humans)	Hemolytic anemia, thrombocytopenia.	None known.
Tetracyclines (humans)	Impaired bone growth, stained teeth.	None known.

*Teratogenic effects reported in humans are indicated in table by the following: (humans). All others are based upon data from animal fetuses. (From Churchill WA, Berendes, and Nemore J: Neuropsychological deficits in children of diabetic mothers. A report from the collaborative study of cerebral palsy. Am J Obstet Gynecol *105*:257, 1969.)

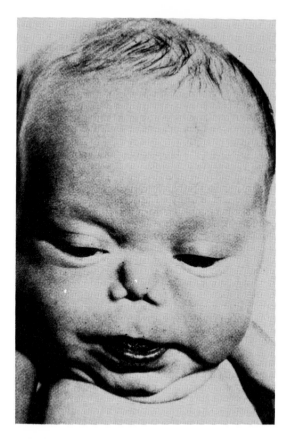

FIG. 18–1.   A baby with nasal hypoplasia resulting from maternal administration of warfarin. (From Pettifor JM, and Benson R: Congenital malformations associated with the administration of oral anticoagulants during pregnancy. J Pediatr 86:459, 1975.)

Lithium. Lithium is implicated in congenital heart disease (Ebstein's anomaly).[1]

Diethylstilbestrol. Intrauterine exposure to this drug causes malformation of the genitourinary tract, and sometimes adenocarcinoma of the vagina in late childhood.

Tranquilizers. Diazepam taken in early pregnancy is associated with oral clefts.[10,11] It is, however, unlikely that one or two doses of the drug used for sedation will result in such a defect. There may be a small risk of congenital heart disease with the use of meprobamate and chlordiazepoxide.[12]

Phenothiazines. Despite a suspicion that antenatal exposure may be associated with cardiovascular malformations these drugs are considered generally safe.[13]

Salicylates. Intrauterine exposure causes neural tube defects, ophthalmic malformations,

and visceral eventerations in the rat. Neonatal platelet dysfunction has also been reported in humans. Acetaminophen may be used as a safe analgesic and antipyretic in the pregnant patient.[14]

Anticonvulsants. Children born to epileptic women have a malformation rate of two or three times higher than do controls.[15,16] The defects include oral clefts and cardiac anomalies. The fetal dilantin syndrome (hydantoin) is the name given to a combination of severe facial anomalies and mental retardation. Both barbiturates and dilantin are also implicated in causing a fetal coagulopathy resembling vitamin K deficiency (see also Chapter 17 Neurologic Disease).

Narcotics. Methadone produces CNS and skeletal abnormalities in laboratory animals.[2] Morphine causes reduced fetal brain size with reduced amounts of DNA, RNA, and total protein content in the brain.[17] Cranioschisis and exencephaly are also reported with morphine use. Heroin is also implicated in CNS malformations. In animals, pretreatment of the mother with a narcotic antagonist (such as nalorphine or naloxone) blocks the teratogenic effects of both single and multiple doses of the narcotic.[18]

Anesthetics. All available data on teratogenicity of anesthetics are based on animal experimentation. There are no reliable well-controlled prospective studies available from human beings. N_2O (0.5% ambient air concentration) is associated with increased fetal resorption, reduced fetal size, and skeletal abnormalities.[19] N_2O may also interfere with folate metabolism by affecting vitamin B_{12} turnover.[20–22] Chronic exposure to trace anesthetics in the operating room is also implicated in increased incidence of miscarriage and congenital abnormalities.[23,24] Using a microbial assay system, Baden et al.[25] noted that fluroxene was more mutagenic than the other halogenated ether anesthetics. Mice exposed to 0.4 minimum alveolar concentration (MAC) per day had an increased incidence of pregnancy resorptions, fetal death, and decreased birth weight.[26] Acute exposure to halothane (0.8% for 12 hours) was associated with increased fetal skeletal abnormalities.[27] Mazze, et al. have recently reported that halothane, isoflurane, and enflurane are not associated with any increased teratogenicity in rats.[28] The same authors, however, reported increased incidence of cleft palate in mice when they were exposed in utero to isoflurane.[28] This shows that the animal teratogenicity is species-specific, emphasizing the need for caution in extrapolating these data to predict human teratogenicity.

There are no known reports implicating local anesthetics in teratogenicity.

High inspired concentrations of halothane has been associated with metabolic disturbances in the rat brain that are suggestive of cerebral hypoxia. Low to moderate inspired concentrations (0.4%) were not associated with any significant change in the metabolic status of the brain.[29] Pentobarbital administered in high doses to the mother (200 mg/kg) has also been shown to protect the fetal rat brain against hypoxia.[29] Based on the nature of the evidence available, we cannot say with certainty that short exposure of the mother to an inhalation anesthetic is associated with any short or long-term harmful effects to her fetus. Enflurane and halothane are assigned to pregnancy category A (Table 18–1).

Behavioral Teratology (Table 18–2).

Fetal Alcohol Syndrome. Infants born to alcoholic women exhibit prenatal and postnatal growth retardation and craniofacial anomalies known as fetal alcohol syndrome. During the neonatal period, tremulousness, hyperactivity, and irritability are seen, suggesting a state of withdrawal. The abnormality may persist for months. Hyperactivity in the preschool age with evidence of mental retardation has also been noted.

The Fetal Hydantoin Syndrome. Low IQ scores with mild to moderate mental retardation has been reported as characteristics of this syndrome.[2]

The Fetal Trimethadione Syndrome. Facial anomalies with developmental delay and speech difficulty have been reported with this syndrome.

Amphetamine. An estimated 570,000 American women of child-bearing age are using amphetamine-containing diet pills. Amphetamine intake may increase the catecholamine contents of the fetal brain. The offsprings have increased nondirected locomotion.[2]

Barbiturates. Following maternal treatment, infants may exhibit withdrawal syndrome characterized by overactivity, restlessness, disturbed sleep, excessive crying, diarrhea, and vomiting.[31] High doses of barbiturates administered to the mother may cause decreased neonatal responses to enviromental stimuli.

Opiates. Approximately 34,000 women of childbearing age, including 10,000 to 12,000 on methadone maintenance programs, are among the 150,000 opiate-dependent persons in the New York metropolitan area alone. Passively addicted neonates show signs of acute narcotic withdrawal (hyperreflexia, tremors, and irritability). Infants may not become symptomatic for 2 to 4 weeks after birth because of fetal storage and prolonged metabolic clearance of the narcotic agents from the fetal tissues. Neonates exposed to narcotics in utero (morphine, methadone, or heroin) experience less tranquil sleep and more active REM sleep. Morphine exposure may be associated with neonatal tolerance to the drug.[32] In early childhood, they demonstrate poor intellectual and cognitive abilities. Heroin exposure is linked with uncontrollable temper and impulsiveness in early childhood. After prenatal exposure to methadone, the compound persists in the brain and liver of the offspring for at least 20 days. This suggests that the hyperactivity, increased state of lability and disturbance of sleep may be the result of the slow clearance of methadone. In summary, both clinical and animal studies suggest that prenatal exposure to opiates produces biphasic effects, the acute phase consisting of an abstinence syndrome with increased CNA arousal, followed by changes in behavior such as hyperactivity, disturbed sleep, and increased lability of behavior. For more information on neonatal withdrawal syndrome see Chapter 22 Drug Abuse.

Anesthetics. The fetal brain is more sensitive to inhalation agents than the adult brain.[33] Intrauterine exposure to halothane and enflurane for short periods of time has been shown to impair learning of the murine progeny (reduced MAC).[34] The learning defects were shown to be present even in the second generation offspring. Intrauterine exposure to halothane also increases murine postnatal autotolerance to the anesthetic. In addition, halothane exposure reduces the offspring brain weight.[35]

Subtle neurologic testing of infants in the early neonatal period has shown that intrauterine exposure to general anesthetics, local anesthetics, or analgesics may impair the neurobehavior of the infant.[36] The neurobehavior testing system elicits the following three aspects of infant behavior: the adaptive capacity of the neonate to his environmental stimuli; skeletal muscle tone; and the presence of some primary reflexes (for further discussion on neurobehavioral testing see Chapter 4). Most of the abnormal neurobehavior resulting from depressant medications is confined to the first 24 hours. Central Nervous System (CNS) depressants have a more pronounced effect on neonatal neurobehavior than do local anesthetic agents. A prospective study of 570 infants, who were tested at regular intervals for four years, showed no significant differences in the developmental status of the children at 4 years of age, regardless of the type of obstetric analgesia or anesthesia used.[37] Thus the transient neurobehavioral change observed in the early neonatal period do not appear to produce any long-term developmental sequelae.

DIAGNOSTIC IRRADIATION

Exposure to diagnostic irradiation may also cause teratogenicity.[38,39] Diagnostic x-rays are often required in the pregnant patient for the evaluation of trauma sustained in an automobile accident. The most frequent abnormalities caused by irradiation were stunted intrauterine growth, microcephaly, mental retardation, microphthalmos, pigmentary degeneration of the retina, genital and skeletal malformations, and cataracts. As little as 5 to 15 rads of irradiation is known to cause fetal death in early murine pregnancy. The majority of organogenesis is complete at 16 weeks of gestations in humans. The CNS, however, may be damaged even after 16 weeks. Neuroblasts are found in human embryo from the 16th day after conception until about two weeks after birth. Neuroblasts can be destroyed by a 25 rad exposure.

Most human data are collected from patients who were exposed to therapeutic irradiation and not to diagnostic irradiation. Studies in mice show that when the radiation dose does not exceed 10 rads, the anomaly rate is not distinguishable from the background rate. At 20 rads, the incidence of malformations are significantly increased. Diagnostic x-ray studies that do not have the pregnant uterus in the direct path of their beam do not expose the fetus to appreciable irradiation (if appropriate beam columnation and pelvic shielding are used). When studies that may cause direct exposure of the uterus are required, the number of views and exposures must be limited. These studies include x-rays of pelvis, hips, lumbar spine, sacrum, and abdomen. Intravenous pyelogram, cystogram, and pelvic angiography may also be needed occasionally. During angiography, fluoroscopy must be kept to a minimum. The use of video-playback equipment allows more viewing time and thus minimizes exposure time. Using the above mentioned measures, the radiation exposure can be decreased to 2 rads per examination.

When computerized tomography scan (CT scan) is needed, a dosimeter can be placed directly on the maternal abdomen to measure skin dose. During CT scan exposures, the dose is approximately 3 rads per slice at any volume of tissue directly irradiated. During CT scan the patient should be moved in programmed increments in such a way that there is no overlap of adjacent slices. Some recommend even small gaps between tissue slices during exposure. A myelogram can be avoided by the use of a CT scan. A small dose of intrathecal metrizimide may be used to provide contrast during CT scan. Emergency pelvic x-ray studies may be performed with doses below 5 rads with the possible exception of pelvic angiography for pelvic hemorrhage, where the dose may exceed 5 rads. In view of the seriousness of pelvic hemorrhage, the study must be performed and the patient must be informed of the possible risk to the fetus. An accurate record of all the x-ray doses must be kept for future references. The National Council on Radiation Protection (NCRP-Report 39) has published guidelines for the maximum permissible dose (MPD) in pregnant patients. The fetal MPD is 0.5 rem. The rem unit takes into account the qualities of different radiations. The MPD for adults is 5 rem per year. Radiation from protons, neutrons, or alpha particles is more damaging than the same degree of irradiation from gamma rays or x-rays.

REFERENCES

1. Bergland F, et al.: Drug use during pregnancy and breast-feeding: A classification system for drug information. Acta Obstet Gynecol Scand (Suppl 126), 5–51 1984.

2. Hutchings DE: Behavioral teratology: A new frontier in neurobehavioral research. *In* Johnson EM, Kochar DM, (eds): Teratogenesis and Reproductive toxicology. (Handbook of Experimental Pharmacology. Ser.: Vol 65). (Chapter 11). New York, Springer Verlag, 1983.

3. Werhoff J, and Havelna J: Postnatal behavioral effects of tranquilizers administered to the gravid rat. Exp Neurol 6:263, 1962.

4. Pedersen H, and Finster M: Anesthetic risk in pregnant surgical patient. Anesthesiology 51:439, 1979.

5. Adamson SK, and Joelsson I: The effects of pharmacologic agents upon fetus and the newborn. Am J Obstet Gynecol 96:437, 1966.

6. Goldman AS, and Yakovac WC: The enhancement of salicylate teratogenicity by maternal immobilization in the rat. J Pharmacol Exp Ther 142:351, 1963.

7. Stott, DH: Physical and mental handicaps following a disturbed pregnancy. Lancet 1:1006, 1957.

8. Hannah RS, and Moore KL: Effects of fasting insulin on skeletal development in rats. Teratology 4:135, 1971.

9. Hall J, Pauli RM, and Wilson KM: Maternal and fetal sequelae of anticoagulation during pregnancy. Am J Med 68:122, 1980.

10. Safra MJ, and Oakley GP: Association between cleft lip with or without cleft palate and prenatal exposure to diazepam. Lancet II: 478, 1975.

11. Saxen I, and Saxen L: Association between maternal intake of diazepam and oral clefts. Lancet 2:498, 1975.

12. Milcovich L, and Van den Berg BJ: Effects of perinatal meprobomate and chlordiazepoxide on human embryonic and fetal development. N Engl J Med 291:1268, 1974.

13. Slone D, et al.: Antenatal exposure to the phenothiazines in relation to congenital malformations, perinatal mortality rate, birth weight, and intelligence quotient score. Am J Obstet Gynecol 128:486, 1977.

14. Niederhoff H, and Zahradnik HP: Analgesics during pregnancy. Am J Med 83:117, 1984.

15. Beeley L: Adverse effects of drugs in the first trimester of pregnancy. Clin Obstet Gynaecol 8:261, 1981.

16. Bodendorfer TW: Fetal effects of anticonvulsant drugs. Drug Intell Clin Pharm 12:14, 1978.

17. Steele WJ, and Johannesson T: Effects of prenatally-administered morphine on brain development and resultant tolerance to the analgesic effect of morphine in offspring of morphine treated rats. Acta Pharmacol et Toxicol 36:243, 1975.

18. Geber W, and Schramm LC: Congenital malformations of the central nervous system produced by narcotic analgesics in the hamster. Am J Obstet Gynecol 123:705, 1975.

19. Vieira E: Effect of the chronic administration of nitrous oxide 0.5% to gravid rats. Br J Anaesth 51:283, 1979.

20. Beeley L: Adverse effects of drugs in later pregnancy. Clin Obstet Gynaecol 8:275, 1981.

21. Chanarin I, et al.: Vitamin B_{12} regulates folate by the supply of formate. Lancet 2:505, 1980.

22. Nunn JF: Faulty cell replication; abortion, congenital abnormalities. Int Anesthesiol Clin 19:77, 1981.

23. Cohen EN, Belleville JW, and Brown BW: Anesthesia, pregnancy and miscarriage. A study of operating room nurses and anesthetists. Anesthesiology 35:343, 1979.

24. Spence AA, et al.: Occupational hazards for the operating room-based physican. JAMA 238:955, 1977.

25. Baden JM, et al.: Mutagenicity of halogenated ether anesthetics. Anesthesiology 46:346, 1977.

26. Wharton RS, et al.: Fertility, reproduction and postnatal survival in mice chronically exposed to halothane. Anesthesiology 48:167, 1978.

27. Basford AB, and Fink BR: The teratogenicity of halothane in the rat. Anesthesiology 29:1167, 1968.

28. Mazze RI, et al.: Reproductive and teratogenic effects of nitrous oxide, halothane, isoflurane and enflurane in Sprague-Dawley rats. Anesthesiology 64:339, 1986.

29. Vanucci RC, and Wolf JW: Oxidative metabolism in the fetal rat brain during maternal anesthesia. Anesthesiology 48:238, 1978.

30. Streissguth AP, Herman CS, and Smith DW: Intelligence behavior and dysmorphogenesis in fetal alcohol syndrome: a report on 20 patients. J Pediatr 92:363, 1978.

31. Desmon MM, Schwanekke RP, and Wilson GS: Maternal barbiturate utilization and neonatal withdrawal symptomatology. J Pediatr 80:190, 1972.

32. Zimmerberg B, Charap AD, and Glick SD: Behavioral effects of in utero administration of morphine. Nature 257:376, 1974.

33. Gregory GA, et al.: Fetal anesthetic requirement (MAC) for halothane. Anesth Analg 62:9, 1983.

34. Chalon J, et al.: Exposure to halothane and enflurane affects learning function of murine progeny. Anesth Anal 60:794, 1981.

35. Chalon J, et al.: Intrauterine exposure to halothane increases murine postnatal autotolerance to halothane and reduces brain weight. Anesth Analg 62:565, 1983.

36. Dailey PA, Baysinger CL, Levinson G, and Shnider SM: Neurobehavioral testing of the newborn infant. Clin Perinatol 9:191, 1982.

37. Ounsted M: Pain relief during childbirth and development at 4 years. J R Soc Med 74:629, 1981.

38. Elliot G, and Rao T: Pregnancy and radiographic examination. *In* Trauma and Pregnancy. (Edited by Haycock CE). Littleton, Mass, PSG Publishing, 1985.

39. Mossman KL: Medical radiodiagnosis and pregnancy: Evaluations of options when pregnancy status is uncertain. Health Physics 48:297, 1985.

19

DIFFICULT OBSTETRIC SITUATIONS

The services of the anesthesiologist are invaluable in the management of difficult obstetric situations such as breech presentation, multiple gestation, or severe shoulder dystocia. The anesthesiologist must act quickly and the ultimate maternal and fetal outcome depends on his skill.

BREECH PRESENTATION

In 10% of all pregnancies the presenting part is breech in the second trimester. The fetus usually corrects itself to the vertex position near term, with the result that only 2% of full-term fetuses present by breech.[1] Spontaneous correction may occur even in the case of dead fetuses.[1] The obstetric terminology used in connection with breech presentation and delivery varies from institution to institution. Table 19–1 provides a brief description of these terms. The breech presentation is associated with increased fetal morbidity and mortality because of prematurity. The congenital malformation rate is 2.5 times higher for breech than for vertex presentation[1-4] (Fig. 19–1). The anomalies include congenital hip dislocation, neural tube defects, anencephaly, familial dysautonomia, myotonic dystrophy, and many other genetic abnormalities.[2] In addition, the prolapse of the umbilical cord may result in severe hypoxia. Umbilical cord prolapse may occur more commonly with footling breech (up to 18%), than

with frank or complete breech.[2] Because the umbilical cord often gets compressed, variable decelerations of the fetal heart rate are likely to occur.[5] When a late component is also present in the fetal heart tracing, neonatal depression and deaths occur more frequently.[5]

The greatest problem of breech delivery for the obstetrician and the anesthesiologist is the possible arrest of the after-coming head during a vaginal delivery. The breech is a poor dilator of the cervix. Although the breech may be born through the incompletely dilated cervix, the shoulders and the head may not fit through the passage. Delivery of the breech draws the fetal umbilicus and the cord into the maternal pelvis. The cord may either be stretched or compressed. If the rest of the body is not delivered promptly, hypoxia and acidosis ensue rapidly. The obstetrician may then make desperate attempts at delivery that not only worsen the cord compression but result in fetal trauma. Intracranial hemorrhage, brachial plexus palsy, spinal cord damage, and damage to the adrenal gland are some common injuries that the neonate is likely to sustain. Adrenal glands, which are often enlarged in fetal life, might be injured during manipulation of the fetal trunk. Head entrapment is a real hazard in premature neonates (26 weeks or more) because the head is disproportionaly larger than the body. Patients are not considered suitable candidates for vaginal delivery when the fetal weight is >3500 g; the fetal

Table 19–1.   Obstetrical Terms Used in Connection with Breech Delivery

Type	Description
Frank breech	Fetal hips flexed, knees extended (50–70%).
Complete breech	Both knees and hips flexed.
Single or double footling breech	One or both feet descend through cervix.
External cephalic version	Manual rotation of the fetus to vertex position at or after 34 weeks.
Partial breech extraction	Spontaneous delivery up to the umbilicus, the rest of the body extracted manually.
Complete breech extraction	The entire body extracted manually.*

*Carries significant mortality.

head is hyperextended; the gestation is longer than 26 weeks (in the case of a premature neonate remote from term); or when the fetus is severely growth retarded. Very small and very large fetuses are likely to benefit from a cesarean section. The umbilical cord cortisol and catecholamine levels are higher in fetuses born vaginally by breech than in those born normally.[6]

The use of cesarean section for the management of breech presentations has tripled in the last decade. While there is general agreement regarding the benefit of cesarean births of large fetuses (>3500 g), there is a considerable dispute regarding the efficacy of the procedure in reducing morbidity and mortality in preterm neonates (<2000 g). The opponents of cesarean section contend that the seemingly improved neonatal morbidity and mortality under these circumstances are really the result of improved neonatal care rather than cesarean delivery.[7] Because the head may be trapped even during a cesarean section, others have expressed concern that cesarean section may not necessarily reduce the incidence of birth asphyxia even in fetuses weighing >2500 g.[3] In many teaching centers, however, cesarean section is being accepted as the delivery mode of choice for fetuses presenting by breech.

ANESTHETIC CONSIDERATIONS

Many obstetricians do not recommend use of epidural analgesia for labor because it may interfere with the voluntary bearing-down efforts of the mother. This interference, however, is not likely to occur unless a high concentration or a large volume of the local anesthetic is used. Injecting 6–8 ml of 0.125% bupivacaine into the epidural catheter when the patient is flat (the patient should not be semirecumbent) will usually preserve not only perineal sensations but also the patient's expulsive efforts.

Many researchers have attested to the safety and benefits of the use of epidural anesthesia for breech presentations. The use of epidural anesthesia will not increase the frequency of breech extraction.[8] If an epidural catheter has been used to produce labor analgesia, perineal relaxation may be provided easily for the application of Piper forceps, which are believed to protect the fetal skull from the trauma caused by the pelvic bones during delivery. Epidural analgesia for labor also improves the fetal acid-base status (possibly because of its beneficial effect on maternal stress response to pain).[9,10] Patients usually bear down strongly when the fetal foot has entered the vagina in the case of footling presentation. This may result in the prolapse of the umbilical cord. Judicious administration of epidural anesthesia will minimize the patient's urge to bear down, thus preventing the potentially disastrous complication.

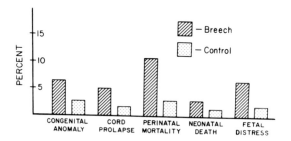

FIG. 19–1.   Increased incidence of neonatal complications associated with breech delivery. Source Pritchard JA, et al.,[1] Collea JV,[2] Green J, et al.,[3] Gimovsky ML, et al.,[4] and Mazor M, et al.[19]

There does exist, however, a potential problem with the use of epidural anesthesia for breech deliveries. The duration of the second stage may be prolonged by this procedure, especially when the fetus is large. Prolongation of the second stage may result in 1 minute Apgar scores that are lower than those of fetuses born to mothers who do not receive conduction anesthesia.[11] The anesthesiologist may circumvent this problem by ensuring that the sacral segments are not blocked at the onset of second stage. This should not only preserve the patient's urge to bear down, but should also maintain her expulsive forces. The block may be reestablished just prior to delivery.

No other obstetric emergency, with the possible exception of shoulder dystocia, is more horrifying than the entrapped aftercoming head during breech delivery. The entrapment is caused by the incompletely dilated cervix and/or by the unrelaxed maternal pelvic muscles. While epidural anesthesia will relax the pelvic musculature, it does very little to diminish the snaring action of the cervix. The role of the anesthesiologist assumes paramount importance in this situation. The obstetrician must discuss with the anesthesiologist how the breech delivery will be conducted well in advance of the actual delivery. An anesthesiologist must always be in attendance during all breech deliveries, regardless of the parity of the patient. The patient must receive a dose of nonparticulate antacid before delivery and must be made to inhale oxygen continuously from a disposable mask. All necessary preparations for administration of general anesthesia must be made even when an epidural catheter is in place. Should entrapment occur, the obstetrician must notify the anesthesiologist immediately. The patient must be induced with pentothal and the trachea intubated rapidly under succinylcholine-induced muscle paralysis. Myometrial relaxation must be obtained with brief administration of 2% (inspired concentration) halothane or 3% enflurane. Muscle relaxation may be maintained with succinylcholine infusion. Using high concentrations of a volatile agent may result in postpartum hemorrhage. Halothane may be discontinued immediately after the baby is born. Anesthesia may be subsequently maintained with N_2O supplemented with a narcotic.

Anesthesia for cesarean section for breech presents less problems. When an emergency cesarean section is required for footling presentation, a spinal or epidural anesthetic may be administered. The presence of variable decelerations alone should not deter the anesthesiologist from administering a regional anesthetic. The fetus must be continuously monitored while the anesthetic procedure is being performed. Because the threat of cord prolapse always exists under these circumstances, the regional procedure must be performed swiftly and skillfully. Spinal anesthesia which uses pontocaine or bupivacaine or epidural anesthesia, which uses either 3% 2-chloroprocaine or 2% lidocaine with epinephrine, both provide rapid onset of action. If, however, there is a rapid deterioration of the fetal condition, general anesthesia with endotracheal intubation is indicated. Although head entrapment is still likely to occur during cesarean sections, the situation is not as desperate as it is during vaginal delivery because the obstetrician can deliver the baby by extending the uterine incision.

Breech presentations are often associated with premature labor; consequently many patients may be placed on tocolytic therapy. Tocolytics may also be prescribed after an attempted external cephalic version. External cephalic version may be associated with fetal death, injury, and fetal maternal transfusion.[1] Tocolytics, such as ritodrine, present additional problems to the anesthesiologist (see Chapter 21 Preterm Delivery).

MULTIPLE PREGNANCY

Multiple pregnancy, which occurs approximately in one of ninety deliveries, is associated with increased maternal and fetal morbidity. The maternal problems that are likely to be encountered by the anesthesiologist are summarized in the following list:

1. Overdistended uterus
2. Increased aortocaval compression
3. Preeclampsia
4. Placental abruption
5. Premature labor
6. Tocolytics (ritodrine)
7. Prolonged bed rest (back edema)
8. Compression of the lung bases by the distended uterus

9. Possible coagulopathy (death of one fetus)
10. Postpartum hemorrhage (uterine atony)

The fetal complications with multiple pregnancy are as follows:[12]

1. Prematurity (RDS, intracranial hemorrhage)
2. Twin-twin transfusion
3. Vasa previa
4. Vilamentous cord insertion
5. Growth retardation
6. Cord entwinement
7. Locked twins
8. Perinatal mortality (10%)
9. Congenital malformations

The advent of sonography has facilitated early and accurate twin pregnancies. The twin gestation may either be mono- or dizygotic. The number of placentas alone is not diagnostic of zygosity. The outer blastocyst layer of the zygote is fully prepared to form the chorion within 72 hours. If the zygote divides before that time, two embryos with two amnions and two chorions will develop (see Chapter 3 Respiratory Function of the Placenta). There may be either two separate placentas or one single, fused placenta (Fig. 19–2,A, B). A single placenta with one chorion and two amnions may result from a single zygote if the embryonic division occurs between the 4th and 8th day (Fig. 19–2,C).[12] Embryonic division occurring after the 8th day, when the amnion is already established, will result in a monoamniotic and monochorionic, monozygote twin pregnancy. Thus both mono- and dizygotic twins may produce a single placenta or two placentas. Vascular complications, such as twin-twin vascular anastomosis, occur more frequently with monochorionic placenta.

Interfetal vascular anastomosis between arterial circulation of one fetus with the venous circulation of the other may develop at the placental bed.[12] The blood is pumped from the artery to the vein. The recipient becomes polycythemic and plethoric and the donor becomes anemic and malnourished. Polyhydramnios and oligohydramnios develop in the recipient and the donor sacs, respectively. The donor may die and induce a coagulopathy in the surviving fetus and in the mother.[12]

ANESTHETIC CONSIDERATIONS

All maternal cardiovascular changes that accompany pregnancy are further augmented in twin pregnancy. Expansion in blood volume is 500 ml greater than that seen in singleton gestation. The average blood loss is also higher by approximately the same amount. In addition,

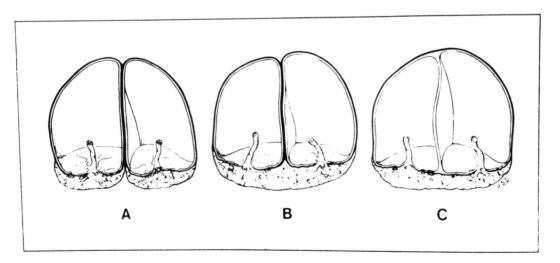

FIG. 19–2.   Placentas and membranes in twin pregnancies. Two placentas, two amnions (dark line), and two chorions (light line) from either dizygotic or monozygotic twins (A). Single placenta, two amnions and two chorions from mono- or dizygotic twins (B). One placenta, one chorion, and two amnions from monozygotic twins (C). (From Pritchard JA, MacDonald PC, and Gant NF: Dystocia caused by abnormalities in presentation, position or development of the fetus. *In* Williams Obstetrics. Norwalk, Appleton-Century-Crofts, 1985.)

the incidence of hypertension is higher. Hypertension may occur early and may be more severe. If preeclampsia coexists, adequate monitoring of the patient is necessary (see Chapter 10 Preeclampsia). Patients may have received tocolytics for arresting premature labor (see Chapter 20 Preterm Labor for more discussion on tocolytics). Because of possible prolongation of labor, many obstetricians do not use epidural analgesia during labor.[12] Both first and second stages of labor may be prolonged by epidural analgesia.[13–14] The prolonged second stage may lead to increased incidence of instrumental deliveries and breech extractions. As in the case of breech deliveries, the analgesia may be permitted to wear off at the onset of second stage and reestablished just prior to delivery of the second twin. This will preserve the patient's perineal sensation with the result that the bearing-down efforts are likely to be more efficient.

However, the use of epidural analgesia for labor is associated with many advantages. It provides complete analgesia and prevents maternal acidosis. It also obviates the need of general anesthesia for the delivery of the second twin by cesarean section or for internal podalic version and breech extraction. The condition of the second fetus is better when epidural analgesia is used than when no analgesia is used.[15] This is particularly true when the delivery of the second twin is delayed. The current obstetric recommendation is to wait for the spontaneous delivery of the second twin (when it presents by vertex and shows no signs of distress).[16] A scalp electrode may be applied to monitor fetal EKG during the waiting period. Because many twin fetuses are premature, avoiding general anesthesia is likely to benefit them.

All vaginal twin deliveries must also be attended by an anesthesiologist. Although in a majority of instances the delivery of the first twin is accomplished without much difficulty, the second twin may require intrauterine manipulation. When the second twin is in oblique lie, an internal podalic version may be performed to deliver it as breech. General anesthesia may be required to deliver the second twin. While internal podalic version may be performed under epidural anesthesia, general anesthesia may be required in uncooperative patients. General endotracheal anesthesia with halothane (or with enflurane or isoflurane) will produce myometrial

relaxation thus providing excellent conditions for performing external podalic versions. The myometrial relaxation will also minimize the chances of head entrapment during the delivery of the second twin. An inhaled halothane concentration of 1 to 1.5%, or an equivalent concentration of enflurane or isoflurane, will produce good results. The inhalation agent must be discontinued as soon as the baby is born and oxytocin administered to contract the myometrium. The remainder of the procedure may be carried out with N_2O supplemented with a narcotic.

While many obstetricians permit vaginal delivery of uncomplicated twin gestation, the majority will resort to cesarean section when there are three or more fetuses. In view of the small size of the fetuses, regional anesthesia is preferred to general anesthesia. Supine hypotension is likely to be more severe because of the increased compression of the inferior vena cava. Consequently, adequate lateral tilt and proper fluid preloading are important. All measures required for optimizing transplacental oxygenation must be carried out (see Chapter 3 Respiratory Function of the Placenta).

SHOULDER DYSTOCIA

Inability to deliver the shoulder of the neonate after its head is born is one of the worst obstetric problems. Maternal obesity, fetal macrosomia, contracted pelvis, and prolonged second stage are some of the predisposing factors.[17] Occasionally, an attempted midforceps delivery of a large baby is likely to result in shoulder dystocia because the forceps help deliver only the head. In shoulder dystocia, the anterior shoulder of the neonate is impacted under the pubic symphysis (Fig. 19–3). The baby becomes asphyxiated rapidly. Consequently, the condition has a 15% intrapartum neonatal mortality rate. In those infants who survive, many will have evidence of severe hypoxic brain damage and birth trauma to brachial plexus and other bodily organs. The longer the delivery is delayed, the greater is the likelihood of neonatal asphyxia. The following maneuvers have been advocated to disengage the shoulder: suprapubic pressure; posterior traction of the head; bringing the anterior shoulder forward (Wood maneuver);

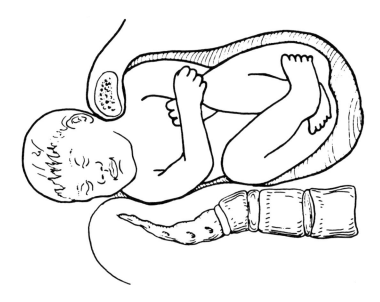

FIG. 19–3. Shoulder dystocia. Note that the anterior shoulder is wedged under the maternal symphysis pubis. (From Harris BA, Jr.: Shoulder dystocia. Clin Obstet Gynecol, 27:106, 1984.)

and flexing the patient's lower extremities sharply against her abdomen (McRobert's maneuver). Symphysiotomy has also been recommended. All these procedures may cause uterine rupture and severe intrapartum hemorrhage. A new solution to the problem of shoulder dystocia has recently been suggested. The procedure, called the Zavanelli maneuver, is based upon reversing the birth process. Instead of attempting to deliver the baby vaginally, the head is pushed back into the vagina and delivery is completed abdominally.[18]

Obviously, shoulder dystocia places tremendous emotional strain on the patient. Regardless of the type of analgesia that was being provided for labor, the patient must be given an immediate general anesthetic. Complete muscle relaxation must be provided with succinylcholine infusion. Uterine relaxation may be provided with one of the halogenated inhalation agents. The use of inhalation agents also permits administration of 100% oxygen. The newborn may sustain a fracture of the ribs or clavicle, which may result in a pneumothorax during resuscitation. Should this happen, appropriate measures must be instituted immediately.

REFERENCES

1. Pritchard JA, MacDonald PC, and Gant NF: Dystocia caused by abnormalities in presentation, position or development of the fetus. *In* Williams Obstetrics. Norwalk, Appleton-Century-Crofts, 1985.
2. Collea JV: The intrapartum management of breech presentation. Clin Perinatol 8:173, 1981.
3. Green JE, McLean F, Smith LP, and User R: Has an increased cesarean section rate for term breech delivery reduced the incidence of birth asphyxia, trauma and death? Am J Obstet Gynecol *142*:643, 1982.
4. Gimovsky ML, and Paul RM: Singleton breech presentation in labor: Experience in 1980. Am J Obstet Gynecol *143*:733, 1982.
5. White PC, and Cibils LA: Clinical significance of fetal heart patterns. VIII. Breech presentations. J Reprod Med *29*:45, 1984.
6. Tomazevic T, Kovacic J, and Vrhovec I: Umbilical cord cortisol in breech delivery. J Reprod Med *30*:53, 1985.
7. Cox C, Kendall AC, and Hommers M: Changed prognosis of breech presenting low birth weight infants. Br J Obstet Gynaecol *89*:881, 1982.
8. Darby S, and Hunter DJ: Extradural analgesia when the breech presents. Br J Obstet Gynaecol *83*:35, 1976.
9. Breeson AJ, Kovacs GT, Pickles BG, and Hill JG: Extradural analgesia—the preferred method of analgesia for vaginal breech delivery. Br J Anaesth. *50*:1227, 1978.
10. Hill JG, Eiolot BW, Campbell AJ, and Pickett-Heaps AA: Intensive care of the fetus in breech labour. Br J Obstet Gynaecol *83*:271, 1976.
11. Confino E, Ismajovich B, Rudick V, and David MP: Extradural analgesia in the management of singleton breech delivery. Br J Anaesth *57*:892, 1985.
12. Pritchard JA, MacDonald PC, and Gant NF: Multifetal Pregnancy. *In* Williams Obstetrics. Norwalk, Appleton-Century-Crofts, 1985.
13. Crawford JS: An appraisal of lumbar epidural blockade in labour in patients with multiple pregnancy. Br J Obstet Gynaecol *82*:929, 1975.
14. Gullestad S, and Sagen N: Epidural block in twin labour and delivery. Acta Anaesthesiol Scand *21*:504, 1977.

15. Jarvis GJ, and Whitfield MF: Epidural analgesia and the delivery of twins. J Obstet Gynaecol 2:90, 1981.
16. Olofsson P, and Rydhstrom H: Twin delivery: How should the second twin be delivered? Am J Obstet Gynecol *153*:479, 1985.
17. Harris BA, Jr.: Shoulder dystocia. Clin Obstet Gynecol *27*:106, 1984.
18. Sandberg EC: The Zavanelli maneuver: A potentially revolutionary method for the resolution of shoulder dystocia. Am J Obstet Gynecol *152*:479, 1985.
19. Mazor M, et al.: Fetal malformations associated with breech delivery. J Reprod Med *30*:884, 1985.

20

PRETERM LABOR

In a majority of cases the cause of premature birth is not known. The following conditions may predispose to preterm labor: premature rupture of the membranes; incompetent cervix, uterine septa, and other anatomic abnormalities of the uterus; overdistended uterus (twins, hydramnios); fetal malformations; placental abnormalities (placenta previa and abruption); fetal death; and serious maternal systemic disease that is complicated by maternal hypoxia.[1] Uterine contractions that occur at least once every 10 minutes and last 30 seconds are suggestive of preterm labor, and dilating cervix is, of course, indicative of the condition. The mortality and morbidity rate among the preterm neonate is disturbingly high, thus there has been over the decades a search for an ideal agent to arrest premature labor. To date no such drug is known. Available studies present only conflicting data. The problems of the premature neonate are discussed in Chapter 25. Anesthesia may be needed under the following circumstances in patients who have received tocolytic therapy: for cesarean section, which is often performed to improve fetal survival; for removal of the retained products of conception; or for relieving labor pains. Many agents currently in use for arresting premature labor produce serious side effects.

ETHANOL

Ethanol is no longer a popular agent for the prevention of premature birth. However, it is used in patients in whom serious contraindications exist for the use of β-mimetic agents. Ethanol is believed to inhibit oxytocin release from the neurohypophysis. The release of anterior pituitary hormones is, however, not affected.

Another possible mechanism of ethanol action is the increased liberation of catecholamine (mainly norepinephrine) from the adrenal medulla. Ethanol administration is associated with a better success rate when the membranes are still intact. The dose and mode of administration of ethanol are given in Table 20–1. The incidence of perinatal mortality and respiratory distress syndrome is higher in babies born to mothers who received ethanol for the arrest of premature labor than in those whose mothers received ritodrine for this purpose.[2] The reason for this is not clear. It may be related to the failure of ethanol to arrest premature labor effectively. Neonatal CNS depression is likely to occur especially when the delivery occurs within 12 hours of ethanol administration. Except for the drunkenness, maternal cardiovascular changes appear to be minimal. Anesthetic requirement will be less in those who receive intravenous alcohol. Because alcohol increases gastric acid secretion, a nonparticulate antacid must be administered before anesthesia. Also endotracheal anesthesia must be performed whenever necessary.

β-MIMETIC SUBSTANCES

The β-mimetic agents, isoxuprine, ritodrine, terbutaline, salbutamol, and fenoterol, have

Table 20–1. Tocolytic Therapy

Drug	Administration	Maternal side effects	Fetal side effects
Ethanol	9.5% solution. 7.5 ml/kg/hour.[L] 1.5 ml/kg/hour.[M]	Drunkenness; Increased gastric fluid acidity.	Hypoglycemia. Mild CNS depression.
Ritodrine	0.05–0.1 mg/min infusion;[L] Increase 0.05 mg/min every 10 min; Oral tablets.[M]	Tachyarrhythmia. Pulmonary edema. Hyperglycemia. Hypokalemia. Hyperlactacidemia.	Tachycardia. Hyperglycemia. Hyperlactacidemia.
Terbutaline	10 µg/min infusion.[L] Maximum 23 µg/min. Tablets 5 mg TID.[M]	As above.	As above.
$MgSO_4$	4 g i.v.[L] 2 g/hour.[M]	Hypocalcemia. Respiratory paralysis.	Muscular hypotonia.
Indomethacin	50 mg orally.[L] 25 mg QID.[M]	Maternal bleeding. Gastrointestinal.	Premature ductal closure. Pulmonary hypertension. Platelet dysfunction. ? Renal dysfunction.
Nifedipine	10 mg PO TID.	Hypotension, edema.	No data.

L–Loading dose; M–Maintenance.

been extensively used for the treatment of premature labor. The beta agonists bind with the receptor on the cell surface activating the adenylcyclase complex. This causes conversion of adenosine triphosphate to cyclic adenosine monophospate (cyclic AMP). Cyclic AMP interferes with Na^+-K^+ pump. The altered activity of Na^+-K^+ pump interferes with Ca^{++} concentration in the cytoplasm. Reduced Ca^{++} level interferes with myosin light-chain phosphorylation, which subsequently results in smooth muscle relaxation.[2] The exchange of intracellular Na^+ for K^+ also causes reduced plasma K^+ concentration. Isoxuprine was the first agent of this type introduced for clinical use. Because the drug produced many cardiovascular side effects, other agents with selective β-2 activity were introduced. Ritodrine, terbutaline, fenoterol, salbutamol, and hexoprenaline are the drugs currently available as β-2 agonists. However, they are also associated with a number of cardiovascular side-effects. Ritodrine is the most widely used agent in the United States.

RITODRINE

Compared to the patients treated with ethanol or placebos, the gestation of ritodrine-treated patients was prolonged by a week (p <0.05).[3] The incidence of neonatal deaths and respiratory syndrome were half of that in either the control group or the placebo group. The infants reached a gestational age of 36 weeks and a birth weight of 2500 g more frequently than did infants whose mothers were not treated. There has been a rash of publications on the use of the drug. The results of these studies are often conflicting, probably because of the lack of uniform criteria for defining premature labor and for patient selection. The ritodrine is administered as an intravenous infusion (Table 20–1). The starting dose is 0.05 to 0.1 mg/minute, which is increased to 0.05 mg/minute until uterine contractions either stop or decrease in frequency to less than 1 in a 15 minute period. If the maternal heart rate increases to 140 beats per minute or the patient complains of chest pain, the dose must be decreased. The onset of maternal tachycardia coincides with the onset of uterine effects.[4] The maternal heart rate follows the blood levels of ritodrine (Fig. 20–1). The recommended maximum dose is 0.35 mg/min. If the therapy is successful, oral therapy with ritodrine tablets is prescribed. The use of different tocolytics in combination (i.e., ritodrine and $MgSO_4$) is not associated with any beneficial effects;[5] in fact, the frequency of serious side-effects, including chest pain and EKG changes suggestive of myocardial ischemia, increases.[4]

The use of β-agonists may improve uteroplacental perfusion either by producing vasodilatation[4] or by decreasing myometrial con-

Table 20–2.   Metabolic Effects of Beta Stimulants

Increased	Unchanged	Decreased
cAMP	Pituitary hormones	Serum iron
Glucose	Calcium	Transferrin
C-Peptide	Phosphorus	Potassium
Glucagon	Cortisol	Cholesterol
Free Fatty Acids	Bilirubin	Alanine
Triglycerides	Haptoglobin	Estriol
Lactate	Creatinine	HCO_3^-
Pyruvate	Sodium	
Glycerol	Chloride	
Beta-Hydroxybutyric acid	Placental lactogen	
Acetoacetic acid		
Renin		

(Reproduced with kind permission from Lipshitz J: Beta-adrenergic agents. Seminars in Perinatology 5:253, 1981.)

tractility. Ritodrine crosses the placenta and produces the same side effects in the fetus as it does in the mother. The side effects, however, are less severe in the fetus than in the mother. There are no known adverse long-term effects on the baby from in utero exposure to ritodrine.

Ritodrine and the other β-mimetic agents produce a number of serious cardiovascular and metabolic side effects. The maternal heart increases and patients may complain of shortness of breath, palpitations, and chest pain probably caused by stimulation of the β-1 receptors. Even EKG changes suggestive of myocardial ischemia have been reported.[6] Occasionally, life-threatening supraventricular arrhythmias requiring electrical cardioversion may occur.[7] The systolic

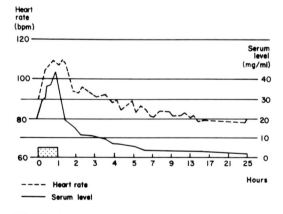

FIG. 20–1.   Heart rate changes in relation to serum ritodrine level. Infusion rate-O.15mg/min. (From Post LC: Pharmacokinetics of β-adrenergic agonists. In: Anderson A, et al. Preterm Labour. Proceedings of the Fifth Study Group of the Royal College of Obstetricians and Gynaecologists, 1977. pp. 134–148.)

blood pressure remains unchanged but the diastolic pressure decreases. Other disturbing side effects include nausea, vomiting, and anxiety. Patients with preexisting heart disease are more likely to develop serious cardiovascular side effects.

A rare but serious complication of β-agonist therapy is pulmonary edema. The mechanism of pulmonary edema is poorly understood. Ritodrine is a cardiac ionotrope. It decreases the end-systolic and end-diastolic dimensions of the ventricle and increases the cardiac output.[8] The mechanism of pulmonary edema is therefore probably not related to cardiogenic causes. Another possible mechanism proposed is that ritodrine causes increased aldosterone levels resulting in sodium and water retention.[9] Increased fluid overload causes a reduction in plasma oncotic pressure, thus further predisposing to pulmonary edema. When pulmonary edema develops the pulmonary capillary wedge pressure is usually high[10] and the arterial blood P_{O_2} is reduced. It is interesting to note that ritodrine administered in clinical doses also causes a 66% decrease in hypoxic pulmonary vasoconstriction, further compounding the problem of arterial hypoxemia (Fig. 20–2).[11] The decrease in cyclic AMP is believed to affect the vasoconstrictive response. Other β-2 agonists also share this effect on the pulmonary vasculature. A common problem identified in many patients who developed pulmonary edema is the iatrogenic fluid overload. The use of excessive volumes of crystalloid solution is particularly hazardous in view of the effects of ritodrine on circulating renin and aldosterone levels. When pulmonary edema is clinically suspected, rito-

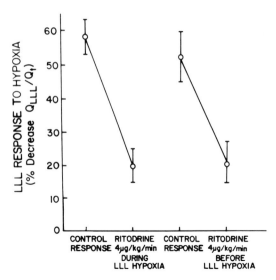

FIG. 20–2. Reduced hypoxic pulmonary vasoconstriction (HPV) during left lower lobe (LLL) hypoxia. The ratio between pulmonary blood flow to the lower lobe and the total pulmonary blood flow was derived before and after hypoxia in the absence and presence of ritodrine. Ritodrine infusion caused a similar reduction in the HPV response whether its administration began during or before hypoxia. (From Conover WB, Benumof JL, and Key TC: Ritodrine inhibition of hypoxic pulmonary vasoconstriction. Am J Obstet Gynecol, *146*:652, 1983.)

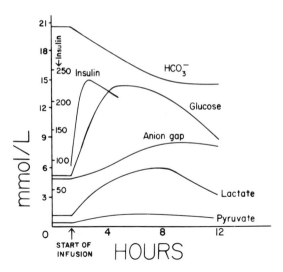

FIG. 20–3. Metabolic effects of ritodrine infusion. Changes in blood of glucose, insulin, lactate, pyruvate, HCO_3^- and anion gap caused by ritodrine infusion. Graphs constructed from the data of Kirkpatrick C, et al.[14] and Schreyer P, et al.[13] Blood anion gap = [$Na^+ + K^+ + Ca^{++}$] − [$Cl^- + HCO_3^- +$ protein].

drine administration must be discontinued. Administration of furosemide will help eliminate the excess fluid overload. Refractory cases may need a pulmonary artery catheter, mechanical ventilation with positive end-expiratory pressure (PEEP). When an epidural anesthetic block is being planned in a patient who is receiving ritodrine therapy, the customary prophylactic hydration must be done cautiously. The chest should be auscultated to detect the possible presence of congestion. Patients with preexisting cardiac disease especially mitral stenosis are at an increased risk for developing pulmonary edema.[12]

Ritodrine and the other β-mimetic agents also produce several metabolic side effects.[2] They increase blood glucose levels and the concentration of insulin.[4] Hypokalemia is a frequent complication. Hypokalemia is a result of the increased entry of glucose into the red blood cell[13] and inhibition of the Na^+-K^+ pump.[2] The serum lactate and pyruvate levels increase and the blood HCO_3^- and anion gap are decreased[14] (Fig.

20–3). Combined therapy with betamethasone is likely to exaggerate the hyperglycemic response but not the hypokalemic response.[14] Ritodrine increases the rate of lipolysis with the result that the serum concentrations of free fatty acids (FFA) and triglycerides rise.[2] Tolerance may develop to the metabolic and cardiovascular effects with prolonged use. However, tolerance may develop to the therapeutic actions also. The metabolic side effects of beta-mimetic agents are summarized in Table 20–2. The use of ritodrine is contraindicated in patients with preeclampsia, diabetes, hypertension, and hyperthyroidism. Rarely, because of the action of ritodrine on the Na^+-K^+ pump, exacerbation of myotonic symptoms can occur.[15] Similarly, symptoms of myasthenia gravis may be worsened by ritodrine administration.[16]

Tocolytic agents may be useful in situations other than preterm labor.[2,4] They can be used to produce myometrial relaxation when the uterine tone is increased, either spontaneously or by oxytocin infusion (Bandle's ring). They may be used to relieve fetal distress caused by increased uterine tone. They may also be used for facilitating delivery of a very small infant during cesarean section, or for producing uterine relaxation during external version.[2] Premature labor often develops in pregnant patients who have undergone cerclage procedures or major surgery and in pregnant victims who have sustained trauma or burns. Tocolytics may be useful in selected patients under these circumstances.

Several precautions must be taken when anesthetizing these patients. Blood levels of sugar and K^+ must be known. Potassium supplementation is usually not necessary if there are no EKG signs of hypokalemia. The anesthesiologist must not only evaluate the fluid balance but must also look for evidence of pulmonary edema. Invasive monitoring may be needed if signs of pulmonary edema are detected. If time permits, pulmonary edema must be treated before administering anesthesia. Ritodrine infusion must be discontinued at the earliest opportunity to prevent tachyarrhythmias at the time of induction. If, however, tachyarrhythmias do not occur, they can be treated with a small dose of propranolol.

Regional anesthesia is preferable to general anesthesia in patients who have received a β-mimetic agent for tocolysis because cardiac arrhythmias may be precipitated by adrenergic activity related to laryngoscopy, and general anesthesia exposes the preterm fetus to the CNS depressants. The ability of epidural anesthesia to effectively decrease preload is beneficial in patients with pulmonary edema. Since significant aortocaval compression occurs from the 20th week of gestation, left uterine displacement must be instituted. Excessive fluid administration may result in pulmonary edema in patients receiving ritodrine tocolysis. When general anesthesia is needed, sympathetic stimulants such as ketamine are best avoided. Atropine must be used with great caution. When volatile agents are needed, isoflurane or enflurane is preferable to halothane because they are less likely to sensitize the myocardium to catecholamines.

OTHER β-MIMETIC AGENTS

Ritodrine is the only β-agent officially approved for tocolysis in the USA, although worldwide, terbutaline is being used. No definite advantages have been demonstrated for the use of terbutaline over ritodrine.[1] The drug is used extensively in Scandinavian countries. A single injection of 125 to 250 μg may be used to terminate

uterine tetany. The mode of administration of terbutaline is given in Table 20–1. Salbutamol and fenoterol have also been used as tocolytic agents.

MAGNESIUM SULFATE

The mechanism by which Mg^{++} decreases uterine activity is probably related to its action on Ca^{++}. Diminished Ca^{++} causes a reduction in ATP levels and decreases interaction between actin and myosin. Serum Mg^{++} deficiency is known to be associated with premature labor.[2] Correcting the deficiency with oral administration of Mg^{++} will sometimes stop premature labor. The success rate of arresting premature labor with Mg^{++} is claimed to 75% when therapy is started before the cervix dilates to 5 cm and when the membranes are still intact. This enthusiasm, however, is not shared by other workers. The drug is usually effective when started very early in the course of labor, a feature associated with most tocolytics.[1] When the membranes rupture, or if the dilatation has proceeded beyond 5 cm, the drug is usually discontinued. The maternal side effects of Mg^{++} are described in Chapter 10 Hypertensive Disorders of Pregnancy. Pulmonary edema-like syndrome has been reported in two patients who received Mg^{++} with betamethasone. In animal experiments, Mg^{++} has been shown to increase uterine blood flow. No major changes have been reported in the fetal heart rate variability. Mg^{++} crosses the placenta freely, occasionally causing neonatal muscular hypotonia. Neonatal magnesium toxicity and anesthetic considerations for patients who have received Mg^{++} therapy are discussed in Chapter 10.

PROSTAGLANDIN INHIBITORS

Prostaglandin (PGE_2, PGF_2) are believed to play a key role in initiating labor in mammals. Prostaglandin levels increase in the amniotic fluid and in the blood during labor. The conversion of the precursor arachidonic acid to prostaglandins is facilitated by the enzyme prostaglandin synthetase. Indomethacin is a potent inhibitor of this enzyme and has been used for the inhibition of premature labor. Indomethacin administration causes a decrease in the level of the circulating prostaglandin metabolite. In 82% of patients, uterine contractions may be stopped for a week, and in others, a transient effect may be noted. The treatment usually fails in 7% of patients.

The major concern with the use of indomethacin is the potential risk for premature closure of the fetal ductus arteriosus in utero, which results in thrombosis of the pulmonary artery. In fetal life, the ductal patency is maintained by prostaglandins. The ductus arteriosus becomes increasingly less sensitive to prostaglandins as gestational age increases, thus diminishing the risk of this serious complication. Indomethacin also interferes with platelet function and hemostasis, which may have lethal consequences in a premature neonate who is already at an increased risk for developing intracranial hemorrhage. The mode of administration and side effects are listed in Table 20–1.

CALCIUM CHANNEL BLOCKERS

The Ca^{++} channel blockers block the influx of extracellular Ca^{++} into the cell, thus interfering with uterine contractility. The antianginal drug nifedipine inhibits uterine contractility both in vivo and in vitro. However, the drug has undergone only limited clinical trial for this purpose. The potential maternal side effects are related to the ability of the drug to cause peripheral vasodilatation. Mode of administration and the side effects are listed in Table 20–1.

MISCELLANEOUS

Diazoxide, a smooth muscle relaxant, has been used to arrest premature labor, but maternal side effects such as hypotension and hyperglycemia have limited the usefulness of this drug. Aminophylline, a phosphodiesterase inhibitor, can produce uterine relaxation. The blood concentration required for producing tocolysis may be associated with serious side effects (see Chapter 15 Asthma).

PREMATURE RUPTURE OF MEMBRANES

Premature rupture of the amniochorionic membrane complicates 5 to 7% of all deliveries.

In the majority of instances, the pregnancy is usually at or near term. In a smaller number of patients, it may occur remote from term. The major problem is the development of chorioamnionitis, which is associated with an increase in the perinatal mortality rate. Some investigators have suggested that premature rupture causes an increased surfactant synthesis, thereby decreasing the incidence of respiratory distress syndrome in infants delivered 24 hours after rupture had occurred. However, there is no agreement on this issue.[17] Amniotic fluid obtained from the mother's vagina has been used for the measurement of the lecithin/sphingomyelin ratio.[17] The use of corticosteroids to hasten surfactant production in patients with ruptured membranes is controversial because of the increased risk of maternal and/or neonatal infection[17,18] and the lack of consensus on efficacy.

CORTICOSTEROIDS IN PRETERM LABOR

Howie and Liggins' study, which was based upon favorable data obtained from animal experiments, used betamethasone injections in the mother to accelerate surfactant maturation in the fetal lungs.[19] Two injections of betamethasone with 24 hours between injections were used. A mixture containing 6 mg each of betamethasone acetate and phosphate was used for each injection. They showed that, if delivery can be delayed for 24 hours by administration of a tocolytic agent, the incidence of neonatal RDS may be lowered.[1] The protective action was diminished if the delivery was delayed more than a week after the administration of the drug. Steroids are widely used for this purpose in many centers. Some investigators, however, have cast doubt on the efficacy of the therapy. They have not found any improvement either in the incidence of RDS or in the perinatal outcome in preterm infants exposed to corticosteroids in utero compared to those infants who were not exposed to this drug.[20] The use of corticosteroids may intensify the metabolic effects of β-2 agonists. Because of their water and salt retaining property, they may also increase the risk of pulmonary edema in those who receive tocolytic therapy with ritodrine.

REFERENCES

1. Pritchard JA, MacDonald PC, and Gant NF: Medical and surgical illnesses during pregnancy and the puerperium. *In* Williams Obstetrics. Norwalk, Appleton-Century-Crofts, 1985.
2. Symposium. (Various authors.) Preterm parturition. (Edited by Creasy, RK). Semin Perinatol 5:191, 1981.
3. Barden TP, Peter JB, and Merkatz IR: Ritodrine hydrochloride: A Betamimetic agent for use in preterm labor. Obstet Gynecol 56:1, 1980.
4. Symposium. (Various authors.) Beta-receptor agonists in obstetrics. (Edited by Ingemarsson, I). Acta Obstet Gynecol Scand Suppl. 1, 108:13, 1982.
5. Ferguson JE, Hensleigh PA, and Kredenster D: Adjunctive use of magnesium sulfate with ritodrine for preterm labor tocolysis. Obstet Gynecol 148:166, 1984.
6. Michalak D, Klein V, and Marquette GP: Myocardial ischemia: A complication of ritodrine tocolysis. Am J Obstet Gynecol 146:861, 1983.
7. Fink BJ, and Weber T: Direct current conversion of maternal supraventricular tachycardia developed during the treatment of a pregnant heroin addict with ritodrine. Acta Obstet Gynecol Scand, 60:501, 1981.
8. Finley J, et al.: Cardiovascular consequences of beta-agonist tocolysis: an echocardiographic study. Obstet Gynecol 64:787, 1984.
9. Philipsen T, Eriksen PS, and Lynggard F: Pulmonary edema following ritodrine-saline infusion in premature labor. Obstet Gynecol 58:304, 1981.
10. Nimrod CA, et al.: Hemodynamic observation on pulmonary edema associated with a β-mimetic agent. J Reprod Med 29:341, 1984.
11. Conover WB, Benumof JL, and Key TC: Ritodrine inhibition of hypoxic pulmonary vasoconstriction. Am J Obstet Gynecol 146:652, 1983.
12. Reichman J, and Goldman JA: Pulmonary edema after ritodrine infusion for premature labor in a patient with mitral valve disease. Acta Obstet Gynecol Scand 60:87, 1981.
13. Schreyer P, et al.: Metabolic effects of intravenous ritodrine infusion in pregnancy. Acta Obstet Gynecol Scand 59:197, 1980.
14. Kirkpatrick C, Quenon M, and Desir D: Blood anions and electrolytes during ritodrine infusion in preterm labor. Am J Obstet Gynecol 138:523, 1980.
15. Scholl JS, Hughey MJ, and Hirschmann RA: Myotonic muscular dystrophy associated with ritodrine tocolysis. Am J Obstet Gynecol 151:83, 1985.
16. Catanzarite V, McHargue A, Sandberg EC, and Dyson DC: Respiratory arrest during therapy for premature labor with myasthenia gravis. Obstet Gynecol 64:819, 1984.
17. Gibbs RS, and Blanco JD: Premature rupture of the membranes. Obstet Gynecol 60:671, 1982.
18. Simpson GF, and Harvert GM, Jr.: Use of beta-methasone in management of preterm gestation with premature rupture of membranes. Obstet Gynecol 66:168, 1985.
19. Howie RN, and Liggins GC: Clinical trial of antepartum betamethasone therapy for prevention of respiratory distress in preterm infants. Proceedings of Fifth Study Group, Royal College of Obstetricians and Gynecologists, Oct. 1977, p. 281.
20. Quirk JG, Jr, Raker RK, Petrie RH, and Williams AM: The role of glucocorticoids, unstressful labor, and atraumatic delivery in the prevention of respiratory distress syndrome. Am J Obstet Gynecol 134:768, 1979.

21

ANESTHESIA IN NONOBSTETRIC SITUATIONS

Anesthesia may be required in any trimester of pregnancy. Approximately 2% of pregnant patients may have to be anesthetized for nonobstetric surgical procedures.[1,2] Cervical cerclage is probably the most common nondelivery procedure for which anesthesia may be required. Anesthesia may also be required for trauma surgery or for the treatment of many other surgical conditions, such as a twisted ovarian cyst or acute appendicitis. Neurosurgery and cardiovascular surgery have also been performed upon pregnant patients. A partial list of surgical conditions that require anesthesia is given in Table 21–1.

The major concerns in anesthetizing pregnant patients are the altered maternal physiology; fullfilling the metabolic needs of the growing fetus throughout the perioperative period; avoiding the use of potential teratogens, especially in early gestation; and preventing premature labor.

MEDICAL EVALUATION OF THE PREGNANT PATIENT

This topic has been extensively dealt with in Chapter 2 Maternal Adaptation to Pregnancy. Because of diminished functional residual capacity (FRC), the uptake rate of inhalation

agents is likely to be faster in pregnant patients. Blood endorphin levels increase in pregnancy, which might reduce the minimum alveolar concentration (MAC). The combination of diminished FRC and decreased MAC will permit achieving surgical anesthesia more rapidly in pregnant patients than in nonpregnant subjects. The triad of diminished FRC, increased ventilation-perfusion anomaly, and increased $\dot{V}_{O_2}$ predispose to rapid development of hypoxia when respiratory obstruction develops. Even at an FI_{O_2} of 1, the Pa_{O_2} reaches only 450 mm Hg in pregnant subjects. Repiratory passages develop increased vascularity; consequently, nasal intubation (if needed) must be done with caution. The glottic opening may be narrowed due to edema, necessitating a smaller endotracheal tube (7 or 7.5 mm OD). Arterial blood pH is slightly alkaline and the Pa_{CO_2} is lowered. A Pa_{CO_2} of 37 mm Hg is highly suggestive of respiratory failure in a pregnant patient (see Chapter 15 Asthma). The fetus is dependent on the mother for its oxygen supply. The maternal cardiac output must be maintained to ensure adequate uteroplacental blood flow. Simple precautions, such as using lateral tilt and administering intravenous fluids prior to induction of regional or general anesthesia, will minimize changes in maternal cardiac output. Systemic hypotension

Table 21–1.   Surgical Conditions in Pregnancy

Condition	Characteristics
Trauma	Blunt trauma: Motor vehicle accident, falls. Penetrating trauma: Gunshot wound. Burns.
Surgical conditions (abdominal)	Twisted or ruptured ovarian cyst (1:2500). Acute appendicitis (1:1000). Intestinal obstruction (1:10,000). Cholecystitis (1:10,000).
Surgical conditions (extra-abdominal)	Breast tumors. Thyroidectomy for intractable Grave's disease. Parathyroidectomy. Adrenalectomy (Adrenal cancer). Open heart surgery. Intracranial surgery for aneurysms, tumor.
Conditions related to pregnancy	Cervical cerclage. Fetal surgery. In vitro fertilization.

resulting from regional anesthesia must be treated with ephedrine rather than with pure α-agents, which constrict uteroplacental vasculature.

Starting early in the second trimester, mask anesthesia must be avoided in pregnant patients. Anatomic and physiologic changes in the gastrointestinal tract put the patient at an increased risk for aspiration of gastric contents. A rapid sequence induction followed by endotracheal intubation is recommended. Measures to diminish gastric acidity must be used judiciously. Cimetidine crosses the placenta freely. The physiologic or the teratogenic effects of blocking the fetal histamine-2 (H-2) receptors are not fully known. Therefore a nonparticulate antacid such as sodium citrate is preferable, especially in the first trimester. The use of H-2 blockers should be reserved for patients who complain of severe heartburn or for those who have developed a stress ulcer during their hospital stay. For more discussion of the use of antacids in pregnant patients see Chapter 9 Cesarean Section.

Distribution, metabolism, and excretion of many drugs are altered in pregnancy because of decreased plasma albumin levels and increased excretion (increased glomerular filtration rate). The ratio between the free and bound fractions of diazepam are increased. For a given dose, the blood levels of drugs, such as digoxin and antiepileptics, are lower than those seen in nonpregnant subjects. Consequently, blood levels of these drugs must often be measured during pregnancy to ensure therapeutic concentrations.

A strict adherence to amount, frequency and time of dosage of these important drugs is necessary in the perioperative period. For instance, omission of a routine dose of phenytoin is more likely to result in a seizure in a pregnant patient than in a nonpregnant subject.

Metabolism of many fuel substrates are altered in pregnancy such as the fuel supply to the fetus is maximized. Pregnant patients are prone to develop an accelerated state of starvation characterized by ketosis. Surgery must be performed in the morning. If surgery has to be delayed, and intravenous infusion containing glucose must be started in the morning. Administration of even 5 to 10 g of glucose is known to halt ketosis in pregnant subjects. Maternal hypoglycemia may interfere with fetal cerebral activity and is implicated in causing congenital malformations. On the other hand, overzealous administration of glucose (>20 g/hour) will be associated with fetal hyperglycemia and lactic acidosis. (For a more detailed discussion of the harmful effects of hyperglycemia, hypoglycemia, and starvation, the reader is referred to Chapters 2 and 14.) It must be borne in mind that glycosuria may occur at blood glucose levels considerably less than the usual critical threshold level of 180 mg/dL. Consequently, urine sugar determinations should not be used as an index of the amount of insulin needed by pregnant diabetic patients.

Blood is hypercoagulable in pregnancy. Fibrinogen levels increase almost 150%. A fibrinogen concentration that is normal for a nonpregnant subject suggests hypofibrinogenemia in a pregnant patient. In addition, normal values for many coagulation indices are different in pregnancy. One clinical situation where the anesthesiologist may have to critically evaluate the coagulation system of a pregnant patient is placental abruption associated with trauma.

Because pregnancy alters several organ functions, interpretation of many routine laboratory results must be done with caution. For instance, a blood urea nitrogen (BUN) level of 15 mg and a serum creatinine level of 1.5 mg/dL are acceptable in nonpregnant subjects but they are highly suspect in pregnant patients. Anemia (hematocrit 34%), decreased plasma protein concentrations, decreased plasma oncotic pressure are normal in pregnancy. Similarly, pregnancy modifies thyroid function tests (see Chapter 13 Endocrine Disease). Table 21–2 lists normal values for some routine laboratory tests of pregnant subjects that might be erroneously interpreted as abnormal when judged by values obtained from nonpregnant subjects.

Teratogenicity. Anesthetics interfere with mitosis.[3] Numerous animal studies have shown that the anesthetic agents may be teratogenic. Anesthetics inhaled in trace concentrations are said to predispose to an increased congenital malformation rate.[4] The problems associated with applying animal data to human beings are discussed in Chapter 22. When a pregnant patient undergoes surgery, she may be exposed to several nonanesthetic drugs that have a much more teratogenic potential than do anesthetics. Aminoglycoside antibiotics, Coumadin anticoagulants, and antiepileptic drugs are implicated in severe teratogenicity. In addition, drug abuse during pregnancy may also lead to teratogenicity.

The Swedish Catalogue of Registered Pharmaceutical Specialists have placed the anesthetic drugs in Category A (no known teratogenicity). (For further description of categorization see Chapter 18 Teratology.) Two recent studies[1,5] have shown that the incidence of congenital malformations is not increased following exposure of the fetus to general anesthetics in utero. The hospitalized pregnant patient is exposed to a variety of chemical and environmental teratogenic stimuli. Diagnostic irradiation, hypoglycemia, emotional stress, and confinement to a hospital bed have all been associated with teratogenicity.[6–8] The preoperative and/or the postoperative note must therefore include a succinct summary of all these confounding variables. Should a baby be born deformed such documentation will no doubt protect the anesthesiologist against possible litigation.

Of equal importance is the gestational period. The fetal growth period may be divided into the predifferentiation period (the first 6 days following fertilization), the period of the embryo (up to 8 weeks) when most of the fetal organs develop, and the period of the fetus, when the fetal brain grows. The fetus is resistant to teratogenicity during the predifferentiation period.

Table 21–2.   Laboratory Evaluation in Pregnancy

Site	Normal Test Values
Cardiovascular system	EKG: PVC, Left axis deviation, ST-T changes.
Blood	Hematocrit 34%. Osmolality 8–10 mosms/L lower. Sedimentation rate increased. Leukocytosis (12,000/mm^3).
Respiratory system	Chest x-ray–Increased lung markings. Pa_{CO_2} = 34 mm Hg.
Blood chemistry	BUN 8 mg/dL. Creatinine 0.6 mg%. HCO_3^- 18–20 mmol/L. Total calcium 8.5 mg/dL. Cholesterol +40%. Triglycerides +80%.
Special studies	Total thyroxine and triiodothyronine increased; SGOT, SGPT (mild elevation). GFR increased.

Morphologic teratogens are likely to produce maximum harm during the period of the embryo. Behavioral teratogens produce maximum harmful effects during the period of accelerated fetal brain growth. Coumadin is a classic example of an agent that produces morphologic and behavioral teratogenicity. For a complete description of morphologic and behavioral teratogenicity see Chapter 18 Teratology.

Preterm Labor. Preterm labor and loss of the fetus may follow anesthesia and major surgery. General anesthesia may be more closely associated with an increased incidence of abortion than is regional anesthesia.[5] The reason for this is not clear. The risk of premature labor is high when surgery is performed on an organ close to the conceptus. For instance, cervical cerclage and pelvic surgery is associated with increased abortions.[5] Similarly intraabdominal sepsis is associated with a disturbingly high rate of perinatal fetal loss. Acute appendicitis complicated by rupture leads to perinatal loss in 28% of cases, whereas only 4% loss is reported in uncomplicated cases.[9] The high incidence of premature labor dictates that uterine activity be monitored intra- and postoperatively so that when spontaneous uterine activity is detected tocolytic therapy can prompty be instituted. Ritodrine is the commonly used tocolytic. For an immediate effect, a single injection of 125–200 μg of terbutaline may be administered. The uses and complications of tocolytic therapy are discussed in Chapter 21 Preterm Labor. Premature labor complicating severe burns is discussed below.

SURGICAL CONDITIONS

ACUTE APPENDICITIS

Sixty-four percent of all abdominal surgical conditions in pregnant women are caused by appendicitis.[9] Intraabdominal trauma (13%), and biliary tract problems (11%), constitute the other major surgical conditions. Diagnosis of appendicitis is difficult in pregnancy because, as the uterus grows, the position of the appendix changes. Right quandrant pain is a consistent finding in the first trimester but is found in only 14% of patients in the third trimester. In addition, the relative leukocytosis (12,000–15,000/mm³) of pregnancy further confuses the issue.

The majority of pregnant patients with appendicitis will have a leukocyte count between 10,000 and 15,000. However, 75% of patients will show a shift-to-the-left in the differential count. The diagnostic error rate may be as high as 40%.[9] The incidence of appendiceal perforation reaches 35%. When it occurs in late pregnancy, it has grave consequences because the appendix becomes an abdominal rather than a pelvic organ during this period.

The site of surgical incision is important. Because of the uncertainty that surrounds the diagnosis, a paramedian incision is preferred to the classic McBurney's incision, especially in the first trimester. In late pregnancy, the appendix is approached via a muscle splitting incision that is placed on the site of maximum tenderness. Unless the surgeon is extremely confident of the diagnosis, general anesthesia is recommended because the patient is likely to be uncomfortable if the appendix cannot be located or the diagnosis is wrong. During surgery, the uterus must be displaced 30° to the left. This not only exposes the appendix but helps avoid inferior vena caval compression. If peritonitis had developed, the patient may develop severe hypovolemia and gram negative shock. Fluid therapy must be guided by central venous pressure monitoring. Aminoglycoside antibiotics and tetracyclines are teratogenic. If the use of aminoglycoside antibiotics is vital to the control of gram negative sepsis, it must be clearly stated in the patient's records. The problems associated with antibiotic use in pregnancy is covered in Chapter 18 Teratology.

CARDIAC SURGERY

Many pregnant patients have been subjected to open heart surgery during pregnancy. Mitral valvotomy, replacement of cardiac valves, emergency repair or replacement of thrombosed or infected prosthetic valves, and coronary artery bypass grafts have been performed. The pathophysiologic characteristics of many of these cardiac conditions are presented in Chapter 12 Cardiac Disease. Only general principles will be discussed here. The majority of cardiac operations have resulted in favorable outcomes for both the mother and the fetus.[11]

Maternal extracorporeal circulation is remarkably well tolerated by the fetus provided that the following conditions are met: (1) bypass time is less than 4 hours; (2) the extracorporeal flow rate must be 2.8 to 3 L/min/M² (rather than the customary 2.4 to 2.6 L/min used in nonpregnant subjects); (3) the mean perfusion pressure is maintained at least at 80 mm Hg; (4) the degree and duration of hypothermia are kept to a minimum; (5) maternal oxygenation is adequate; and (6) aortocaval compression is avoided during surgery.[11-13] The fetal heart rate may decrease immediately after the institution of bypass (Fig. 21–1). Increasing the extracorporeal pump flow rate may remedy the problem. If perfusion pressure is not adequate, adrenalin infusion may be used to restore perfusion pressure.[12] Pure α-agents, such as phenylephrine, are not used for this purpose for fear that they may reduce uteroplacental flow.

Although it is advisable to postpone cardiac surgery until the second trimester, corrective surgery must be done promptly in those who are otherwise doomed to die. Occasionally, emergency cardiac valve replacement is needed in patients who are in labor. Cesarean section and open heart surgery may be performed simultaneously under these circumstances.[14] Bioprosthetic valves are preferable to mechanical valves because they obviate the need for long term anticoagulation.[15] The use of coumarin derivatives is associated with many congenital abnormalities in the fetus. Because the mother is in grave danger under these circumstances, the choice of anesthetic agents must be based on ensuring maternal safety. Fetal teratogenic considerations are of secondary importance. Ritodrine may be required in the postoperative period to prevent premature labor.

OTHER SURGICAL CONDITIONS

Intestinal obstruction occurs more frequently in the third trimester than in the other two.

Because of the delay in diagnosis, the fetal loss and maternal morbidity and mortality rates are high.[10] The most frequent cause is adhesions resulting from previous surgery. Cholecystitis, with or without pancreatitis, occurs in pregnant subjects. When it is complicated by pancreatitis, the maternal mortality may approach 15%, with fetal loss occurring in 60% of these cases. Surgery for uncomplicated cholecystitis is not associated with increased maternal mortality. Only 7% of pregnancy-related jaundice is caused by common duct stones. Hepatitis (42%) and cholestasis (20%) are the other more prevalent causes.[10] Other rare conditions that may require operative intervention during pregnancy include phaeochromocytoma, intractable Graves' disease, hyperparathyroidism, and adrenal cancer with associated Cushing's syndrome. These conditions are covered in Chapter 13 Endocrine Disease.

TRAUMA

Because of the forward shift of the center of gravity of the body, accidental falls are common during pregnancy. Motor vehicle accidents are a leading cause of trauma in pregnant patients. Trauma caused by burns, firearms, and noxious fumes may also occur.[16] In the first trimester, the uterus is well-protected by the bony pelvis, and is therefore is not likely to be injured; but in the second and third trimesters uterine injuries are more frequent. The changes in blood volume and hemoglobin are relatively small in the first trimester and the heart rate increases only 10 to 15 beats per minute. Consequently, in the first trimester, the adequacy of circulating volume may be evaluated and managed based on criteria used in nonpregnant patients.[17] If

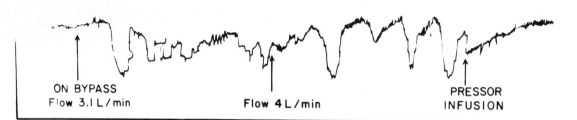

ON BYPASS
Flow 3.1 L/min

Flow 4 L/min

PRESSOR
INFUSION

FIG. 21–1. Fetal heart rate pattern during extracorporeal circulation. The increased pump flow rate produces only temporary improvement in the fetal heart rate. Improving perfusion pressure produces sustained recovery. (From Lamb MP, Manners JM: Fetal heart monitoring during open heart surgery. Br J Obstet Gynaecol 88:669, 1981.)

time permits, all blood products must be cross-matched for ABO and Rh groups to prevent fetal isoimmunization. In dire emergencies O-negative blood may be used.

In the second and third trimesters, the blood volume is considerably higher than in nonpregnant subjects. The pregnant patient may lose a considerable amount of blood without showing signs of shock. The usual clinical indicators of shock such as "cold and clammmy skin" are delayed because of pregnancy induced peripheral vasodilatation. If one depends on blood pressure alone, serious hypovolemia (and the resultant placental vasoconstriction) is liable to be missed.[17] Central venous pressure (CVP) measurement may be used as a reliable index of contracted circulating volume. Left uterine displacement must be maintained continuously during trauma care.

The EKG changes of pregnancy (ST-T changes) are liable to be confused with traumatic myocardial contusion.[17] Any injury to the maternal abdomen may result in fetal death. Fetal death is more likely to occur with penetrating injury than with blunt trauma because of the buoyancy afforded by the amniotic fluid. The fetal heart rate must be evaluated either with a Doppler device or with real time ultrasonography. Ultrasonography is also useful in diagnosing placental tears. When evaluating traumatized pregnant patients, three additional factors must be taken into consideration.

1. Was the trauma sustained in a fall caused by an eclamptic seizure?
2. Is there any evidence of coagulation anomaly caused by traumatic placental abruption?
3. Is there a history of drug abuse?

Further obstetric management depends on the extent of maternal injury and gestational age. If the gestational age is beyond 36 weeks, a cesarean section may be performed at the time of abdominal exploration for trauma.

General anesthesia is preferable for major abdominal trauma. Fractures and superficial trauma, however, can be managed satisfactorily with regional anesthesia. Postmortem cesarean sections have been performed to save the fetus. The success of this procedure depends on the gestational age of the fetus and the timeliness of the procedure.[18] Delivery of a healthy fetus from a woman who had been in a persistent vegetative state for 18 weeks following head trauma has been reported.[19] The use of ritodrine may be considered if preterm labor develops in traumatized pregnant patients.

BURNS

Mortality in burns depends on the extent of the burns. Most burns occur at house fires.[20] Burns involving 30% or more of the body surface usually result in premature delivery of the fetus. Phospholipase A an enzyme that converts arachidonic acid to prostaglandin is liberated by bacteria that frequently cause sepsis in burn victims. Prostaglandins are known to stimulate uterine contractions. Maternal burns may interfere with fetal oxygenation. A severe respiratory burn may cause maternal hypoxia. Carbon monoxide inhalation may interfere with the oxygen carrying capacity of both maternal and fetal hemoglobin, and severe maternal shock and sepsis will seriously curtail uterine blood flow. Fetal hemoglobin has a greater affinity of CO than does maternal hemoglobin. The concentration of carboxyhemoglobin may be measured with a cooximeter. Prolonged artificial ventilation with 100% oxygen and/or hyperbaric oxygenation may be needed until the CO-Hb level decreases to 10%. Ritodrine may be indicated in those who develop premature uterine contractions.

CERVICAL CERCLAGE

Cerclage procedures are usually done in women with repeated second trimester abortions. The procedures are done at 14 to 18 weeks of gestation.[21] They are not performed in the first trimester because most first trimester abortions are associated with some fetal congenital malformations. An ultrasound examination of the uterus is usually done to ascertain that there is a viable fetus, that there is no hydatidiform mole, and that the fetus is not grossly malformed. The McDonald procedure, in which a purse string suture is placed around the cervix, is technically easier to perform than the original Shirodkar procedure.[21] In the Shirodkar procedure, the vaginal mucosa is dissected and the bladder is advanced cephalad before the stitch is placed. Both procedures yield similar success rates. Cerclage procedures are usually not effective after the 26th week of gestation.

Cervical cerclage is associated with many complications: (1) traumatic rupture of the membranes; (2) chorioamnionitis; (3) uterine rupture during subsequent labor when the suture is in situ; (4) subsequent cervical dystocia requiring cesarean section even after the stitch has been removed; (5) premature uterine contractions developing immediately after the procedure; and (6) premature rupture of membranes, which may be caused by premature uterine contractions.[21] Some obstetricians use tocolytic therapy to stop premature contractions. However, there is no consensus of opinion as to their efficacy.

It is generally believed that the fetal salvage improves two- to three-fold after the stitch is placed.[21] However, there is no agreement on this. Recent randomized clinical trials have failed to disclose any improved fetal salvage with this procedure.[22] For cerclage procedures, regional anesthesia is preferred to general anesthesia because it limits the number of drugs that the developing fetus is exposed to. Both spinal and epidural anesthesia may be suitable. A T_{10} level will usually suffice. If general anesthesia is required, balanced anesthesia supplemented with meperidine may be used (vide infra). Endotracheal intubation is recommended because the muscle relaxants may be needed to relax the pelvic musculature and the lithotomy position may increase the intragastric pressure. Some recommend using halothane for its myometrial relaxing properties.[2] Occasionally, the obstetrician may decide to perform an emergency cerclage procedure if he discovers bulging membranes during a routine office visit. The time at which the patient last ate or drank fluids must be known when an emergency procedure is planned.

FETAL SURGERY

Several fetal malformations may now be detected in utero because of advances made in ultrasound and amniocentesis. Fetal cell cultures may be used to diagnose inborn errors of metabolism. Elevation in the amniotic fluid concentrations of fetal α-fetoprotein or acetylcholinesterase is indicative of fetal neural tube de-

fect (see Chapter 14 Diabetes.) Some congenital malformations that may interfere with fetal development may have to be corrected in utero. Many lesions are not amenable to corrections before the baby is born. Anomalies that lend themselves to possible corrections prior to birth include congenital hydronephrosis, hydrocephalus, and diaphragmatic hernia (CDH).[23]

Fetal hydronephrosis may be treated with repeated decompression of the hydronephrotic sac, by placing an indwelling shunt between the fetal bladder and the amniotic sac, or by the decompression of the hydronephrotic sac by exteriorizing the fetus through a hysterotomy. A fetus with malformations of the genitourinary tract is likely to have hypoplastic lungs. Hydrocephalus may be treated by performing serial cephalocentesis or a ventriculoamniotic shunt. Correction of artificially created CDH has been shown in lamb fetuses to minimize damage to the lungs.[23] The correction of fetal CDH has not been done in human beings.

Anesthesia for fetal surgery may be provided in two ways. If the fetal surgery does not involve hysterotomy, local anesthesia of the maternal abdomen will suffice to enter the amniotic sac. Intravenous sedation with diazepam, promethazine, meperidine, or morphine is used for producing maternal sedation as well as fetal sedation. An unsedated fetus will move in response to surgical stimulation and disrupt delicate surgical maneuvers.[24] When a hysterotomy is required, general anesthesia must be administered. The use of halothane for this procedure will ensure a quiescent uterus. Tocolytics may be required postoperatively.[25]

IN VITRO FERTILIZATION

In vitro fertilization (IVF) is a new technique that offers some hope to infertile marriages. The contents of the ovarian follicle are aspirated and the egg is isolated from the aspirate. The egg is suspended in a cell culture medium.[26] Fertilization is done in vitro with a sample of seminal fluid obtained by masturbation. Enough time is allowed for the blastocyst to attain the two-cell stage, following which the blastocyst is transferred transcervically into the uterus. A variety of agents, including clomiphene citrate and human menopausal gonadotropin, are used for stimulating ovulation with a view to obtain multiple ova during aspiration. The chances of a successful pregnancy increase significantly when several fertilized ova are deposited into the uterine cavity.[26]

The two methods of aspirating the follicle are either by a laparoscope or by an ultrasonically guided percutaneous needle aspiration. Whereas percutaneous aspiration may be performed under local anesthesia,[27] laparoscopic aspiration requires either regional or general anesthesia. Although local anesthesia has been used for laparoscopy, it is not recommended for this purpose because the CO_2 pneumoperitoneum may produce extreme discomfort. General anesthesia, epidural anesthesia, and spinal anesthesia[28] have been used for obtaining the follicular aspirate. Because the patient is usually kept in the operating room until the laboratory confirms the presence of eggs in the aspirate, the use of regional anesthesia will obviate the need for prolonged general anesthesia. Some centers do allow husbands in the operating room during aspiration of the follicle. Regional anesthesia is preferable under these circumstances.

The use of general anesthesia may expose the potential embryo to a variety of chemical teratogens. Although there are no human or animal data suggesting that the blastocyst is vulnerable to teratogens in the first week after fertilization, caution is advised. Many volatile anesthetics produce dose-dependent inhibition of cell-multiplication.[29] Nitrous oxide interferes with vitamin B_{12} action by oxidizing it. This decreases the formation of thymidine, which is one of the bases in DNA. The diminished DNA systesis is believed to be responsible for the depressant effects of N_2O on the bone marrow.[30] The use of N_2O either as an anesthetic agent or as a gas for producing pneumoperitoneum before laparoscopy is perhaps not advisable. Thus, one may make a case for the use of regional anesthesia for follicle collection. When general anesthesia is needed, time-honored medications (with the possible exception of N_2O) must be chosen (vide infra).

Carbon dioxide pneumoperitoneum is associated with many hazards, notably gas embolism, increased CVP, decreased cardiac output, hypotension, and increased incidence of cardiac arrhythmias, increased arterial P_{CO_2}[31] and tension pneumothorax. The above-mentioned complications together with the deep Trendeleburg position required for this procedure make endotracheal intubation and controlled ventilation mandatory when general anesthesia is used. Because CO_2 enters the systemic circulation and is excreted by the lungs, continuous measurement of end-tidal CO_2 concentration is recommended.

PRACTICAL CONSIDERATIONS FOR ANESTHESIA DURING PREGNANCY

Nonurgent Surgery. Nonurgent surgery must not be performed in the first trimester. If, however, surgery is needed for malignant tumors (adrenal cancer), it must be performed regardless of the gestational age.

Preoperative Preparation and Medication. The preoperative note must list all medications that the patient has been taking during the pregnancy. Drugs such as antiepileptics and oral anticoagulants are teratogens. History of drug or alcohol abuse must be known.

Preoperative pain caused by trauma or other surgical conditions must be adequately treated with narcotics. Meperidine is safe for this purpose. Promethazine is not teratogenic to humans[32] and may be used either as a sedative or for treating nausea. Diazepam is claimed to produce oral clefts in the neonates; however, it is unlikely that one or two doses of this agent may result in teratogenicity (See Chapter 18).

Patients must receive a nonparticulate antacid 30 to 45 minutes before induction of anesthesia.

The supine position must be avoided in the perioperative period from the 20th week of gestation.

Monitoring the Fetal Heart Rate and Uterine Activity. The fetal heart rate and uterine activity must be monitored throughout surgery and in the postoperative period.[33-34] During general anesthesia the fetal heart rate variability usually diminishes (Fig. 21–2) and it may remain suppressed for 60 to 90 minutes following anesthesia. This, however, does not seem to be associated with harmful long-term sequelae to the fetus. A fetal heart rate of 110-120 beats per minute is not unusual during fetal sleep cycles and therefore does not signify fetal hypoxia. Sudden development of tachycardia (>160 beats per minute) or bradycardia is nevertheless highly suggestive of fetal hypoxia. When confronted

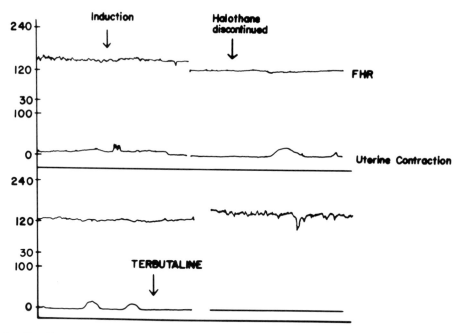

FIG. 21–2. Fetal heart rate (FHR) pattern during general anesthesia. Note: (1) the loss of baseline variability during halothan administration, (2) the onset of premature uterine contractions, which are abolished by terbutaline 0.25 mg s.c. (From Liu PL, et al.: Foetal monitoring in parturients undergoing surgery unrelated to pregnancy. Can Anaesth Soc J, 32:525, 1985.)

with such a situation, the anesthesiologist must ascertain that there is no maternal hypoxia, hypovolemia, or any other factor that may interfere with transplacental gas exchange (see Chapter 3 Respiratory Function of the Placenta). The use of a tocotransducer may indicate the onset of uterine contractions (Fig. 21–2), which can be terminated by appropriate tocolytic therapy using either terbutaline or ritodrine (see Chapter 21 Preterm Labor).

Regional Anesthesia. Regional anesthesia is preferable to general anesthesia for the following reasons: the fetus is subjected to less drug exposure, local anesthetics have no known teratogenic effects;[2] the use of spinal opiate analgesia is possible when epidural or subarachnoid block is performed; the risk of aspiration is minimal; local anesthetics do not interfere with reflex bradycardia, a sensitive index of fetal hypoxia; general anesthetics are known to blunt this response;[35] and the risk of abortion is slightly greater with general anesthesia than with regional or local anesthesia (Fig. 21–3).[5]

Routine precautions such as prophylactic hydration, correction of systemic hypotension (<100 mm Hg systolic, or a 10% decrease from preanesthesia values) with 5 mg increments of ephedrine and maintaining left uterine tilt should not be ignored. Even in early pregnancy, the rate of the spread of local anesthetic is faster in the epidural space than in nonpregnant subjects (Fig. 21–4). As a result of this, induction of epidural anesthesia must be done by incremental injections of the local anesthetic.

General Anesthesia. When general anethesia is needed time-proven anesthetic agents and adjuvants must be used. Atropine (glycopyrrolate), thiopental, succinylcholine, N_2O, d-tubocurarine (or pancuronium) and halothane may be used for anesthesia. Because maternal oxygenation is vital to fetal well-being, an endotracheal tube must be used whenever possible. Maternal hyperventilation must be avoided because respiratory alkalosis decreases oxygen delivery by maternal hemoglobin. The maternal Pa_{CO_2} must be maintained between 30–34 mm Hg. End-tidal CO_2 (ET_{CO_2}) may be continuously monitored with a capnograph. An ET_{CO_2} concentration of 4 to 5% is in the desirable range. Ketamine (2 mg/kg) may increase the uterine tone to a greater degree in early pregnancy than in near-term pregnancy.[37] Unless very specific in-

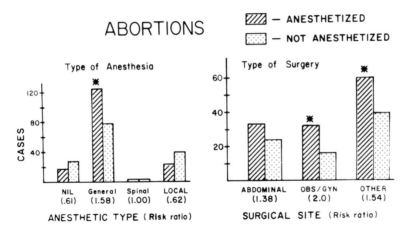

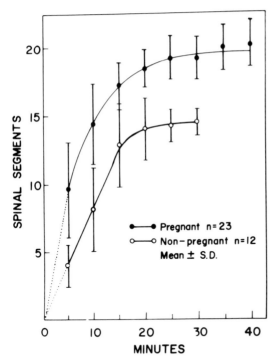

FIG. 21–3.   Number of abortions in patients who received an anesthetic and in patients who did not. Note the increased number of abortions in patients who received general anesthesia. Obstetric and gynecologic procedures are associated with a greater risk than other procedures. (From Duncan PG, Pope WDB, Cohen MM, and Greer N: Fetal risk of anesthesia and surgery during pregnancy. Anesthesiology 64:790, 1986.)

FIG. 21–4.   Increased rate of spread of epidural analgesia in pregnant subjects. (From Fagraeus L, Urban BJ, and Bromage PR: Spread of epidural analgesia in early pregnancy. Anesthesiology 58:184, 1983.)

dications, such as serious hypovolemia, exist for the use of ketamine, its use is better avoided in early pregnancy. At the dosage specified above it is as effective as ergometrine in increasing uterine tone.

Atropine crosses the placenta readily but transplacental transfer of glycopyrrolate is limited with a fetal/maternal ratio of 0.13.[38] Atropine causes a rapid increase in the maternal heart rate, but its effects on the fetal heart rate are delayed.[39] Neostigmine, being a quarternary ammonium compound, is fully dissociated at body pH and consequently undergoes only minimal placental transfer. For reversal of muscle relaxants, a mixture of glycopyrrolate and neostigmine may be used because both agents cross the placenta poorly. Atropine-neostigmine combination may cause transient fetal tachycardia. Placental transfer of muscle relaxants and reversal agents are fully discussed in Chapter 4 Perinatal Pharmacology.

Postoperative Pain. Postoperative pain must be adequately relieved with meperidine or morphine because maternal stress may decrease uterine blood flow because of the catecholamine release.

REFERENCES

1. Brodsky JB, et al.: Surgery during pregnancy and fetal outcome. Am J Obstet Gynecol 138:1165, 1980.
2. Pedersen H, and Finster M: Anesthetic risk in the pregnant surgical patient. Anesthesiology, 51:439, 1979.

3. Davis AG, and Moir DD: Anesthesia during pregnancy. Clin. Anaesthesiol, 4:233, 1986.

4. Cohen EN, Belleville JW, and Brown BW: Anesthesia, pregnancy and miscarriage. A study of operating room nurses and anesthetists. Anesthesiology 35:343, 1979.

5. Duncan PG, Pope WDB, Cohen MM, and Greer N: Fetal risk of anesthesia and surgery during pregnancy. Anesthesiology 64:790, 1986.

6. Goldman AS, and Yakovac WC: The enhancement of salicylate teratogenicity by maternal immobilization in the rat. J Pharmacol Exp Ther 142:351, 1963.

7. Stott DK: Physical and mental handicaps following a disturbed pregnancy. Lancet 1:1006, 1957.

8. Hannah RS, and Moore KL: Effects of fasting and insulin on skeletal development in rats. Teratology 4:135, 1971.

9. Weingold AB: Appendicitis in pregnancy. Clin Obstet Gynecol 26:801, 1983.

10. Kammerer WS: Nonobstetric surgery during pregnancy. Med Clin N Am 63:1157, 1979.

11. Becker RM: Cardiac surgery in pregnant women. In Critical Care of the Obstetric Patient. (Edited by Berkowitz RL). New York, Churchill-Livingstone, 1983.

12. Lamb MP, and Manners JM: Fetal heart monitoring during open heart surgery. Br. J Obstet Gynaecol 88:669, 1981.

13. Koh KS, Friesen RM, Livingstone RA, and Peddle LJ: Fetal monitoring during maternal cardiac surgery with cardiopulmonary bypass. Can Med Assoc J 112:1102, 1975.

14. Martin MC, et al.: Cesarean section while on cardiac bypass. Obstet Gynecol 57:419, 1981.

15. Larrea JL, et al.: Pregnancy and mechanical valve prostheses: a high risk situation to the mother and the fetus. Ann Thorac Surg 36:459, 1983.

16. Jackson FC: Accidental injury–The problem and the initiatives. In Trauma in Pregnancy. (Edited by Buchsbaum HJ). Philadelphia, WB Saunders, 1979.

17. Haycock CE: Emergency care of the pregnant traumatized patient. Emergency Med Clin North Amer 2:843, 1984.

18. Patterson RM: Trauma in pregnancy. Clin Obstet Gynecol 27:32, 1984.

19. Aderet NB, Cohen I, and Abramowicz JS: Traumatic coma during pregnancy with persistent vegetative state. Case report. Br J Obstet Gynaecol 91:939, 1984.

20. Rayburn W, et al.: Major burns during pregnancy: effects on fetal well-being. Obstet Gynecol, 3:392, 1984.

21. Harger JH: Cervical cerclage: patient selection, morbidity, and success rates. Clin Perinatol 10:321, 1983.

22. Rush RW: A randomized controlled trial of cervical cerclage in women at high risk of spontaneous preterm delivery. Br J Obstet Gynaecol 91:724, 1984.

23. Neal R, and Andrassay R: Fetal surgery in utero. Tex Med 80:40, 1984.

24. Spielman FJ, Seeds JW, and Corke BC: Anesthesia for fetal surgery. Anaesthesia 39:756, 1984.

25. Harrison MR, et al.: Fetal surgery in the primate. I. Anesthetic, surgical and tocolytic management to maximize fetal-neonatal survival. J Pediatr Surg 17:115, 1982.

26. Dodson MG, et al.: A detailed program review of in vitro fertilization with a discussion and comparison of alternative approaches. Surg Gynec Obstet 162:89, 1986.

27. Lewin A, Margalioth EJ, Rabinowitz R, and Schenker JG: Comparative study of ultrasonically guided percutaneous aspiration with local anesthesia and laparaoscopic aspiration of follicles in an in vitro fertilization program. Am J Obstet Gynecol 151:621, 1985.

28. Endler GC, Magyar DM, Hayes MF, and Moghissi KS: Use of spinal anesthesia in laparoscopy for in vitro fertilization. Fert Ster 43:809, 1985.

29. Sturrock JE, and Nunn JF: Mitosis in mammalian cells during exposure to anesthetics. Anesthesiology 43:21, 1975.

30. Nunn JF: Faulty cell replication; abortion, congenital abnormalities. Int Anesthesiol Clin 19:77, 1981.

31. Versichelen L, Serreyn R, Rolly G, and Vanderkerchove D: Physiopathologic changes during anesthesia administration for gynecologic laparoscopy. J Reprod Med 29:697, 1984.

32. Slone D, et al.: Antenatal exposure to the phenothiazines in relation to congenital malformations, perinatal mortality rate, birth weight, and intelligence quotient score. Am J Obstet Gynecol 128:486, 1977.

33. Liu PL, et al.: Foetal monitoring in parturients undergoing surgery unrelated to pregnancy. Can Anaesth Soc J 32:525, 1985.

34. Biehl DR: Foetal monitoring during surgery unrelated to pregnancy. Can Anaesth Soc J 32:455, 1985.

35. Swartz J, Cummings M, Pucci W, and Biehl D: The effects of general anaesthesia on the asphyxiated foetal lamb in utero. Can Anaesth Soc J 32:577, 1985.

36. Fagraeus L, Urban BJ, and Bromage PR: Spread of epidural analgesia in early pregnancy. Anesthesiology 58:184, 1983.

37. Oats JN, Vasey DP, and Waldron BA: Effects of ketamine on the pregnant uterus. Br J Anaesth 51:1163, 1979.

38. Murad SH, et al.: Atropine and glycopyrrolate: Hemodynamic effects and placental transfer in the pregnant ewe. Anesth Analg 60:710, 1981.

39. Kanto J, et al.: Placental transfer and pharmacokinetics of atropine after a single maternal intravenous and intramuscular administration. Acta Anaesth Scand 25:85, 1981.

22

RENAL DISEASE

The major concerns in pregnant patients with kidney disease are the increased incidence of hypertension, the possible further deterioration of renal function during pregnancy and the compromised fetus. The kidney is the target organ for several systemic diseases such as systemic lupus erythematosus (SLE) and diabetes mellitus. Anesthesia and surgery also affect kidney function directly or indirectly.

APPLIED PHYSIOLOGY

Pregnancy causes major changes in renal function, the most important one being the ability of the nephron to maintain a positive sodium balance. Most of the changes in renal function during pregnancy have been discussed in Chapter 2. The tubular mechanisms will be briefly reviewed here because the anesthetics may affect the tubular transport process.

Most of the filtered sodium and water are reabsorbed in the tubules (Fig. 22–1).[1] In the proximal convoluted tubule (PCT), the reabsorption is *isosmotic*. The Na^+ reabsorption is a passive process in the proximal convoluted tubule. There is also some active transport of Na^+ in the Pars recta of the proximal tubule. Because of the removal of several solutes in the proximal tube (including HCO_3, amino acids, and glucose), the fluid entering the descending limb of the loop of Henle is hyposmotic. Under normal conditions, only one-third of the glomerular filtrate enters the descending limb of the loop of Henle, which does not reabsorb Na^+ but does

reabsorb H_2O. Because of preferential removal of water, the tubular fluid becomes *hyperosmotic* (rich in NaCl but poor in urea concentration) in the loop of Henle. The ascending limb, however, is permeable to Na^+ but impermeable to water. Active electrogenic Cl^- transport occurs in the ascending limb, with Na^+ following passively. The tubule fluid becomes dilute but the medullary interstitium becomes hypertonic. The fluid reaching the distal convoluted tubule (DCT) thus becomes *hyposmotic*. The active sodium ion reabsorption in this segment of the nephron and in the collecting system is aldosterone-sensitive. K^+ and H^+ are exchanged for Na^+. Most of the distal convoluted tubule is impermeable to water. The antidiuretic hormone (ADH) exerts its effects mainly at the cortical and papillary portions of the collecting duct. In the presence of ADH, water is avidly reabsorbed resulting in hypertonic urine. The antinatriuretic effect of the supine posture in pregnant subjects has been discussed in Chapter 2.

Another important concept involves how the mechanism for renal elimination of a substance will affect the rate at which the substance's plasma concentration will rise in a patient with renal failure (Fig. 22–2).[1] Substances such as urea and creatinine depend entirely on glomerular filtration for their elimination (Fig. 22–2A). When glomerular function deteriorates by 50%, the plasma concentrations of these two substances will rise rapidly.

Substances that depend on tubular excretion (PO_4^-, urate, K^+, and H^+) will not be affected

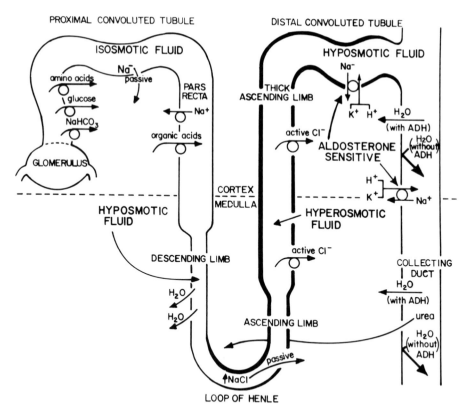

FIG. 22–1. Transport function of the various segments of the nephron. (From Brenner BM, and Hofstetter TH: Disturbances of renal function. *In* Harrison's Principles of Internal Medicine. Edited by Petersdorf RG, et al. New York, McGraw-Hill, 1983.)

to the same degree, unless there is a substantial reduction in kidney function (Fig. 22–2B). A third class of substances (such as Na^+) undergoes glomerular filtration as well as extensive tubular reabsorption. When filtration fails, the nephron can compensate by decreasing reabsorption with the result that a constant quantity of the substance can be eliminated. In other words, a Na^+ balance may be maintained by slow modification of the reabsorptive process in the remaining nephrons. (For nephron sites at which Na^+ reabsorption takes place please see Fig. 22–1.) Thus, whereas plasma Na^+ concentration is not affected until renal disease reaches a terminal stage, blood urea nitrogen (BUN) and creatinine are affected earlier in the course of the disease. Therefore BUN and creatinine levels are more sensitive indices of renal function than are serum Na^+ levels.

RENAL FUNCTION TESTS[2]

In the majority of instances, BUN and serum creatinine measurements are adequate for as-

sessing renal function tests. The clearance tests are popular because they assess the glomerular filtration rate (GFR). The creatinine clearance is simple to perform and requires only urine collection and a plasma creatinine measurement. The amount of creatinine secreted by the tubule is only 10 to 15% of the amount filtered by the glomerulus. Clearance tests indicate the overall elimination of a substance by the kidney. They are not useful for evaluating the individual segment of the nephron. A summary of renal function tests is given in Table 22–1. The concentrations of BUN and serum creatinine are reduced and creatinine clearance is increased in pregnancy because of the increased renal blood flow (RBF). Although a BUN value of 15 mg/dL and a serum creatinine value of 0.85 mg/DL are acceptable in nonpregnant subjects, they are suspect in pregnancy patients.[3]

Insulin clearance and para-aminohippuric acid (PAH) clearance are used to measure GFR and renal plasma flow (RPF), respectively. The Fick equation provides the basis for measuring

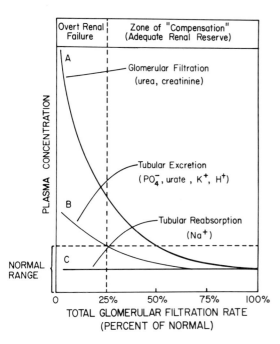

FIG. 22–2. The rate of rise of plasma concentrations of three classes of substances in renal failure due to decreased GFR. (From Brenner BM, and Hofstetter TH: Disturbances of renal function. *In* Harrison's Principles of Internal Medicine. (Edited by Petersdorf RG, et al.) New York, McGraw-Hill, 1983.)

renal plasma flow. Insulin is neither reabsorbed nor excreted and is therefore an ideal substance for measuring GFR. The major problem with PAH is that 10 to 15% of the RPF supplies portions of kidneys that cannot remove the drug. Therefore the renal vein concentration of PAH is not zero. The PAH clearance does not measure the total RPF, but the effective RPF to those portions of the kidney that can remove PAH. Iodohippurate is handled similarly by the kidney.

Two types of tests commonly used to assess the glomerular function are the fractional excretion test and the fractional reabsorption test of a substance. These two tests help distinguish prerenal azotemia from acute tubular necrosis (ATN).

Fractional excretion
of a substance X

$$= \frac{\text{Concentration of X in urine/concentration in plasma}}{\text{Concentration of inulin in urine/inulin concentration in plasma}}$$

For an approximate calculation, the corresponding creatinine concentration may be substituted for insulin concentration.

$$\text{Fractional reabsorption} = 1 - \text{fractional excretion}$$

Free water clearance is an index of the ability of the tubule to concentrate or dilate the urine. When the amount of water excreted exceeds osmolar clearance, the quantity of water excreted is inappropriate for the amount of solute present in the urine, signifying defective tubular function. For instance, a patient with polyuric renal failure will have a positive free water clearance because the volume of water excreted is higher than that needed for excreting isosmotic urine. In prerenal azotemia, the free water clearance will be negative.

PREGNANCY AND RENAL DISEASE

During pregnancy, the severity of renal disease is classified based upon the serum creatinine level.[3] In mild disease, the serum creatinine level is less than 1.4 mg/dL. In moderate impairment, the level is increased to >1.5 mg/dL but <3 mg/dL, and in severe impairment, the serum creatinine levels exceed 3 mg and BUN levels exceed 30 mg/dL. Although many women with severe impairment are usually infertile, an occasional pregnancy can occur.

Davison, et al.[3] has summarized the results of several studies on the effects of renal disease on 584 pregnancies (Fig. 22–3). The antenatal course may be complicated by the development of hypertension, proteinuria, and/or decreased renal function often mimicking severe preeclampsia. The diagnosis of preeclampsia is often difficult in patients with renal disease.[4] The frequency of preterm deliveries, intrauterine growth retardation, still births, and neonatal deaths is higher. Long-term follow-up shows that a significant percentage of patients may develop hypertension and permanent deterioration of renal function. Because of the possible deterioration of renal function caused by pregnancy, patients with severe renal impairment are advised against pregnancy.

The single most important factor that determines pregnancy outcome is probably the development of hypertension. In the absence of

Table 22–1.   Renal Function Tests

Test type	Specific tests	Normal values
Clinical test of glomerular function	Blood urea nitrogen.	10–20 mg/dL (normal), 5–8 mg/dL in pregnancy.
	Serum creatinine.	0.6–1 mg/dL (nonpregnant); 0.58 mg/dL (pregnant).
	Creatinine clearance.	85–125 ml/min (nonpregnant); 120–180 ml/min (pregnant).
Investigational tests of glomerular function	Inulin clearance (C_{in}) [GFR].	110 ml/min (nonpregnant)/1.73M².
	PAH clearance (Effective RPF).	660 ml/min/1.73 m² body surface.
	Effective RBF [= RPF/(1-hematocrit)].	1200 ml/min/1.73m².
	Filtration fraction GFR/RPF or C_{in}/C_{PAH}.	0.2
Tests for tubular function	Fractional sodium excretion.	<1% in prerenal azotemia, >1% in acute tubular necrosis.
	Free water clearance.	Negative in prerenal azotemia zero or positive in acute renal failure.

(RPF)–renal plasma flow, (RBF)–renal blood flow; (PAH)–para-aminohippuric acid; (see text for inaccuracies associated with PAH clearance).

$$\text{Fractional excretion} = \frac{\text{Urine sodium concentration}}{\text{Urine creatinine concentration}} \times \frac{\text{Plasma creatinine concentration}}{\text{Plasma sodium concentration}} \times 100\%.$$

$$\text{Free water clearance} = \text{Urine volume} - \text{osmolar clearance}.$$

$$\text{Osmolar clearance} = \text{Urine osmolarity} \times \frac{\text{Urine volume (min.)}}{\text{Plasma osmolarity}}.$$

hypertension, many patients with only mild renal disease can expect a normal outcome. When hypertension complicates pregnancy, renal function may further deteriorate in 15% of patients. Renal deterioration occurs only in 5% of patients without hypertension. Patients with hypertension often deliver small-for-date babies and develop premature labor (Fig. 22–4).[4] The highest degree of renal impairment is likely to occur in patients with membranoproliferative glomerulonephritis and IgA nephropathy.[3]

TYPES OF RENAL DISEASE IN PREGNANCY

Chronic Pyelonephritis

This disease involves the tubulointerstitial renal tissue. Exacerbations are common during pregnancy because of the increased bacteriuria at this time. Generally, the patients tend to have a more benign antenatal course than those with glomerular condition. Dehydration may lead to excerbations.

Chronic Glomerulonephritis

Histopathologically, the process can be focal, diffuse, proliferative, or of the lupus type. Preeclampsia is more likely to occur in these patients. Chronic glomerulonephritis may lead to nephrotic syndrome. The perinatal mortality can reach 18%.[5] There is a rare form of this condition called the hereditary nephritis, that may be associated with platelet abnormality, which in turn, may lead to hemorrhagic complications.[3]

Systemic Lupus Erythematosus

In addition to renal involvement, this disease has protean manifestations. Endocarditis (Libman-Sacks) and coronary artery narrowing may occur in some individuals. The renal involvement may be one of four histopathologic types: focal proliferative glomerulonephritis, mesangial nephritis, diffuse glomerulonephritis, or membranous glomerulonephritis.[5] The disease will worsen in 50% of those patients who have had an exacerbation in the preceding six months prior to conception.[6] In those who are in remission, a smaller percentage of patients will

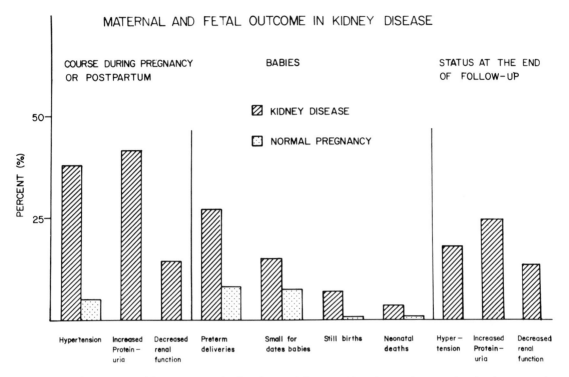

FIG. 22–3.   Maternal and fetal outcome in chronic renal disease. Note the tendency to develop hypertension and proteinuria and the short and long-term deterioration in renal function. Wherever possible data from normal pregnancies are shown for comparison. Histograms constructed from the data of several authors as summarized by Davison JM.[3]

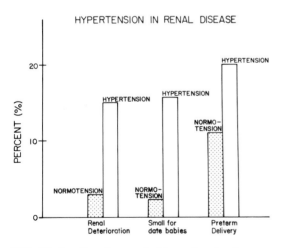

FIG. 22–4.   Development of hypertension in a patient with renal disease causes further deterioration of maternal renal function, increased incidence of preterm deliveries, and small (for their gestational age) infants. Histograms constructed using data of Surian M, Imbasciuti E, and Cosci P: Glomerular disease and pregnancy: A study of 123 pregnancies in patients with primary and secondary glomerular diseases. Nephron 36:101, 1984.)

have a relapse. The results of six studies on pregnancy outcome is summarized in Fig. 22–5.[6] Abortion, perinatal mortality, and premature delivery all occur with increased frequency in lupus nephropathy patients. In addition to clinical exacerbations, some will experience a transient or permanent deterioration of renal function. Proteinuria and reduced creatinine clearance are indicators of a poor prognosis.

Many serologic tests are performed to define the severity and to diagnosis exacerbations. The serum factors include complements (total complements and CH50, C4, and C3 fractions), antibody to nuclear antigens (ANA) and the lupus anticoagulant. Reduction in the concentrations of CH50 and C4 are said to be early indicators of renal exacerbations. The antibody to the soluble DNA [anti-RO(SS-A)] is believed to cross the placenta and cause a neonatal lupus that resembles the adult condition. The incidence of congenital anomalies, particularly heart block, and endocardial fibroelastosis is higher in babies born of patients with SLE than in the general population. Antibody deposition in the devel-

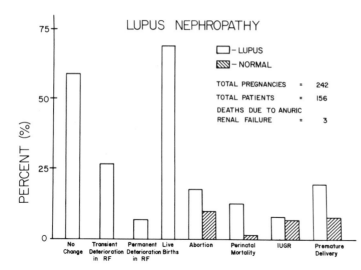

FIG. 22–5. Pregnancy outcome in lupus nephropathy. Maternal renal function tends to worsen somewhat after pregnancy. The rates for abortion, premature delivery, and perinatal mortality are higher compared to normal pregnancies. Histograms constructed using data from several authors.[6]

oping fetal heart is said to play a role in the pathogenesis of the heart block. The lupus anticoagulant is believed to bind with platelet membranes, thus causing platelet aggregation and increased incidence of spontaneous arterial and venous thrombosis. In addition, they are thought to produce extensive thrombotic changes in the placenta resulting in an increased abortion rate. The antibody is only rarely associated with bleeding diathesis. Treatment with low-dose aspirin and/or corticosteroids are said to be beneficial when thrombotic complications occur.[7]

Patients with lupus may be treated with corticosteroids and/or immunosuppressants. There is a fear that the use of these two drugs may be associated with fetal malformations. The risk, however, appears to be small, therefore the drugs should be used, especially if the maternal disease is severe. Renal exacerbations may be diagnosed by examination of urinary sediment for the presence of hematuria.[6]

Diabetic Nephropathy

Diabetic nephropathy is often the cause of death in juvenile diabetics. Life-expectancy after the onset of proteinuria is usually less than 5 years. Diabetes primarily affects the glomeruli. Two types of lesions are seen. The nodular glomerulosclerosis (Kimmelstiel-Wilson syndrome) being more common than the diffuse type. Although there is little evidence to suggest that it is pregnancy that causes severe deterioration of the renal status of the patient, moderate to heavy proteinuria occurs in 50% of women and the incidence of preeclampsia is high. The perinatal mortality reaches 25% is severe cases. It is felt that patients with severe nephropathy must avoid pregnancy. Diabetic retinopathy must always be suspected in these patients. Patients with diabetic nephropathy are often candidates for renal transplantation.[5]

Urinary Calculi

Urinary calculi often produce alarming symptoms during pregnancy. They occur in 0.05 to 0.5% of all pregnancies. Fifty percent of pregnant women with calculi may require surgical removal of the calculus during pregnancy. An intravenous pyelogram (IVP) may be needed for the diagnosis. Lumbar epidural analgesia extending between T11 and L2 segments may be used to relieve ureteric colic. Because of its antispasmodic effect, epidural analgesia may even cause spontaneous passage of the stone.[8]

Transplanted Kidney

Despite earlier encouraging reports, patients with transplanted kidneys have an increased incidence of complications during pregnancy. When therapeutic abortions are excluded, 71% may expect a normal pregnancy outcome. In 9% of women, however, serious rejection episodes may be encountered. Dystocia may occur as a result of the pelvic position of the transplanted kidney. The gravid uterus may also obstruct the ureter. Proteinuria and hypertension are often accompanying features.[9]

Fetal problems include prematurity and intrauterine growth retardation. Urinary estriol measurement may not be reliable in those receiving corticosteroids because they inhibit the formation of estriol precursors in the fetal adrenals. Although azathioprine use is associated with numerous fetal anomalies in animal studies, they do not appear to be risky in human pregnancy. Both azathioprine and its active metabolite 6-mercaptopurine, undergo only limited transfer. Both corticosteroids and azathioprine must be continued throughout pregnancy.

Azathioprine is structurally similar to aminophylline, which is a phosphodiesterase inhibitor. Injected intraarterially, azathioprine increases the excitability of the skeletal musculature, thus producing a dose-related increase in the force of muscular contraction. Because of this property, it reverses the effects of nondepolarizing relaxants and potentiates those of succinylcholine. Monitoring of the neuromuscular transmission is recommended when the patient is receiving this drug.[10]

Permanent Urinary Diversion

Surgical urinary diversion is necessary in women with congenital anomalies of the lower urinary tract. Urinary tract infection and acute pyelonephritis may occur and renal function may decrease transiently during pregnancy. The gravid uterus may obstruct the ileal conduit or the ureterocolic anastamosis. The cesarean section rate may be higher because of the coincidental lower genitourinary tract abnormality. Vaginal delivery is safe in patients with urinary diversion. The presence of an intact anal sphincter, however, is necessary for urinary continence in patients with ureterosigmoid anastomosis. Therefore it may be necessary to avoid damage to the perineum. Blocking sacral 2, 3, and 4 segments with a lumbar epidural anesthetic may help avoid precipitate delivery, thus preventing damage to the anal sphincter. Ureterosigmoidoscopy is only rarely performed nowadays because it may often lead to hyperchloremic acidosis caused by intestinal exchange of Cl^- ion for HCO_3^-.[1]

Nephrotic Syndrome

This condition is characterized by albuminuria (>3.5 g/24 hours), hypoalbuminemia, hyperlipidemia, and edema. The edema occurs as a result of reduced plasma oncotic pressure (POP). The reduced POP is also said to stimulate hepatic lipoprotein synthesis. Serum concentrations of low-density lipoproteins and cholesterol are often elevated. Urinary loss of thyroglobulin and immunoglobulin may produce a hypothyroid state, and IgG deficiency, respectively.

Nephrotic syndrome is more common in the final trimester than in the other two; at this time, the most common cause of the syndrome is preeclampsia. Other causes of nephrotic syndrome are similar to those operative in nonpregnant subjects: diabetic nephropathy, lupus kidney disease, membranous nephropathy, proliferative or membranoproliferative glomerulonephritis, minimal change disease (lipoid nephrosis), and amyloidosis. Patients with nephrotic syndrome are predisposed to bilateral and unilateral renal vein thrombosis. The clinical picture of renal vein thrombosis include fever, severe flank pain, and rapid deterioration of renal function. Some patients may require anticoagulation, especially in the presence of pulmonary embolism. Diuretics are not recommended for the treatment of nephrotic edema, because they may result in hypovolemic renal failure. Salt-poor albumin therapy is not recommended for the treatment of anasarca (except in cases of severe hypoalbuminemia) because most of the albumin will be lost in the urine. The serum albumin decreases approximately 1 g/dL in pregnancy; therefore a reduction of this magnitude in serum albumin must not be mistaken for a deteriorating renal condition.

Chronic Hemodialysis

Patients who are on chronic hemodialysis are usually infertile. When the serum creatinine and BUN level remain consistently elevated above 3 mg and 30 mg/dL, respectively, conception is rare. Pregnancy, however, occurs in one out of every 200 women on dialysis. Spontaneous abortions frequently occur. Therapeutic abortions are often performed in view of the maternal condition. The fetal problems are low birth weight and prematurity. Onset of premature labor, vaginal bleeding, and systemic hypotension are some problems reported to occur in pregnancy during or immediately after hemodialysis. Patients may occasionally require an anesthetic immediately after receiving hemodialysis therapy. Hemodialysis may be associated with a low platelet count, the possibility of rebound or residual heparinization, and hypovolemia (Table 22–2). The reduction in platelet count appears to be caused by retention of platelets on the dialysis membranes. Heparin does not decrease the surface activity of platelets and in fact it is believed to augment ADP induced platelet aggregation.[11] Although a reduction in pseudocholinesterase was reported to occur with the use of older dialysis membranes, the newer ones are devoid of this problem.[12]

Polycystic Kidney Disease

When the other kidney is functionally normal, the outcome is generally favorable. The incidence of hypertension and preeclampsia, however, is higher in this group of patients. In one series, the incidence of hypertension was 40%, but half of those patients were hypertensive prior to conception.[3] The condition has a strong tendency to be inherited.

Solitary Kidney

These patients may have had a nephrectomy in the past for unilateral pyelonephritis. If infection occurs in the solitary kidney and does not respond to antibiotics, pregnancy termination may be indicated. The solitary kidney may be ectopic, which makes it more susceptible to infection.

Polyarteritis Nodosa

Renal involvement occurs in 80% of patients with this condition. Medium and small arteries are usually involved. An immunologic etiology has been proposed and many studies have implicated hepatitis B virus as the antigen. A syndrome indistinguishable from polyarteritis nodosa may also occur in drug addicts. Malignant hypertension is common, which makes the prognosis grave. Therapeutic termination of pregnancy is often performed to protect the mother.

Scleroderma

Diffuse fibrosis of the skin and of internal organs (including the lung, gastrointestinal tract, heart, and kidney) occurs. Cardiac fibrosis may involve both the myocardium and the conduction system leading to heart blocks and arrhythmias. Dilatation of the lower two-thirds of the esophagus caused by destruction of the muscular wall may result in regurgitation of gastric contents and aspiration pneumonia. In the kidney, fibrinoid necrosis of the wall of the afferent glomerular arteriole and the glomerular tuft may occur. Renal involvement may start acutely with malignant hypertension resulting in uremic death. A more benign variant without hypertension but with proteinuria is also reported to occur.[1] An interesting feature of the disease is that renal blood flow may decrease when patients are exposed to cold. Deaths from renal failure usually occur in the fall and winter. It is advisable to warm all the intravenous fluids before infusion.

Table 22–2.   Problems Due to Dialysis

Complication	Manifestation-mechanism
Hypoxia	Excessive HCO_3^- removal.
Hypoventilation	Same as above.
Hypovolemia	Hypotension, excessive fluid removal.
Acetate toxicity	Hypotension, acetate in dialysate.
Thrombocytopenia	Bleeding, surface adhesion.
Rebound heparinization	Bleeding (vaginal bleeding).
Disequilibrium syndrome	Head ache, nausea, raised CVP.
Dialysis encephalopathy.	Slurred speech, death, aluminum toxicity.
Digitoxicity	Cardiac arrhythmias, lowering of K^+.

ACUTE RENAL FAILURE

Acute renal failure (ARF) in pregnancy accounts for 50% of all ARF in young women.[13] The ARF may be caused by prerenal, renal, or postrenal causes. In early pregnancy, the ARF is usually associated with illegal abortion and in late pregnancy with abruptio placentae, obstetric hemorrhage, and/or preeclampsia. The causes of ARF in pregnancy are summarized in Table 22–3.

In obstetric patients, the most common cause of oliguria is systemic hypotension caused by hemorrhage or hyperemesis. During hypovolemia, renal perfusion and GFR decrease. Persistent hypovolemia results in reduced cortical blood flow and acute tubular necrosis (ATN). The differentiation between prerenal oliguria and ATN may be done by infusing 500 ml of saline rapidly, followed by administration of furosemide (100 to 120 mg). If urinary output fails to improve in two hours, a CVP catheter must be inserted, a further 500 ml of saline must be administered, and additional doses of furosemide must be tried. If no improvement occurs in urinary output (despite a normal CVP) the oliguria is most likely due to ATN. The other methods of differentiating between prerenal azotemia and ATN are summarized in Table 22–4.

ATN is the most common cause of ARF in pregnancy. Among the other causes of ARF, preeclampsia deserves special mention. The pathogenesis is related to increased renal vascular resistance in these patients. The complication is more common in multiparous women than in primiparous women. ATN may also be caused by major transfusion reactions. Mannitol administration administered early in the course of the condition may be beneficial.

Renal cortical necrosis (RCN) is another cause of ARF in pregnancy. Although only a limited number of cases of RCN have been reported in the literature, most of the cases have occurred in association with some pregnancy-related condition, such as abruptio placentae or preeclampsia. Renal cortical necrosis produces permanent deterioration in renal function. Whereas total anuria is rare in ATN, anuria lasting for several days is seen in RCN. For the most part, RCN is irreversible. When necrosis is confluent, the mortality rate is 100%, if dialysis is not instituted.[14]

Occasionally, an overdistended uterus may cause obstructive uropathy. Ectopic kidney, transplanted kidney, ileal conduit, and ureterosigmoid anastamosis are more likely to be obstructed by the gravid uterus.

A rare but serious cause of ARF in pregnant women is the postpartum hemolytic uremic syndrome. The presence of fibrinoid necrosis in the renal vessels is suggestive of an immune mechanism. The prodrome consists of an influenza-like syndrome leading to a sudden ARF. Hemodialysis and correction of hemolytic anemia are the only hopes for survival.

PRINCIPLES OF MANAGEMENT OF RENAL FAILURE

In the oliguric phase, fluid intake must be limited to the output volume plus 400 ml/day

Table 22–3.   Causes of Acute Renal Failure in Pregnancy

Condition	Probable causes
Antepartum hemorrhage	Abortion, placenta previa, abruption.
Postpartum hemorrhage	Uterine atony, retained placenta.
Preeclampsia	
Disseminated intravascular coagulation	Amniotic fluid embolus, prolonged fetal death, abruption.
Septic shock	Pyelonephritis, chorioamnionitis, septic abortion.
Transfusion reactions	
Nephrotoxins	X-ray contrast media, antibiotics (aminoglycosides, cephalosporin, and amphotericin B). Nonsteroidal antiinflammatory drugs* (acetaminophen, phenbutazone, salicylates, indomethacin).

*–prevent prostaglandin synthesis in the kidney, thereby leading to renal vasoconstriction and renal failure.

Table 22–4. Differences Between Prerenal Azotemia and Acute Tubular Necrosis

Test	Prerenal	ATN
Urine osmolarity (mosm/kg H_2O)	>500	<350
Urine sodium (mEq/L)	<20	>40
Urine/plasma urea nitrogen	>8	<3
Urine/plasma creatinine	>40	<20
Renal failure index	<1	>1
Fractional excretion of filtered sodium	<1	>1
Urine sediment	Not remarkable	Brown granular casts

ATN–Acute tubular necrosis

$$\text{Renal failure index} = \frac{\text{Urinary sodium concentration}}{\text{Urine/plasma creatinine ratio}}$$

for insensible loss. A diet consisting of 40 g of protein, and 100 g of carbohydrates per day must be prescribed. Parenteral hyperalimentation may be needed if the patient is in a catabolic state. Infection must be controlled. Electrolyte and acid-base derangements must be corrected. Hyperkalemia may cause life-threatening cardiac arrhythmias. Management of severe hyperkalemia is summarized in Table 22–5. The following are indications for instituting dialysis: (1) serum K^+ level >6.5 mEq/L; (2) severe volume overload; (3) the presence of uremic encephalopathy; (4) pericardial effusion with circulatory compromise; (5) A BUN level >120 mg/dL; (6) severe metabolic acidosis, and (7) the presence of a dialyzable nephrotoxin. If the patient is pregnant, the current trend is to dialyze early, and frequently, in order to prevent premature labor.

CLINICAL EVALUATION OF PATIENTS WITH RENAL DISEASE

Severe renal disease affects almost every organ in the body and it also causes several important metabolic abnormalities. The following list gives a summary of important clinical features.

Cardiovascular
  Hypertension.
  Pericarditis.
  Cardiac tamponade.
  Cardiomyopathy.
Respiratory
  Batwing infiltrates (uremic lung).
  Mild restrictive lung disease.
  Reduced CO-diffusion.
  Infection.
  Pulmonary calcification.
  Pleural effusion.
Nervous system
  Autonomic neuropathy (Decreased baroceptor action).
  Uremic encephalopathy.
  Peripheral neuropathy (affects lower limbs).
Hemopoietic
  Anemia
  Thrombocytopenia.
  Bleeding tendency.

Table 22–5. Treatment of Hyperkalemia

Treatment	Mechanism	Onset	Duration
Calcium gluconate i.v. 10–30 ml (1–3 ampules).	direct antagonism	immediate	brief
$NaHCO_3$ (45–135 mEq) i.v.	redistribution	minutes	hours
Glucose 10% (500 ml) + Regular insulin 10 U.	redistribution	minutes	hours
Potassium-exchange resin + sorbitol 70% (20 ml oral, 50 ml rectal).	elimination	hours	hours
Hemodialysis.	elimination	hours	hours

Note: If serum K^+ increases above 6.5 mEq/L, and if EKG signs are present, institute therapy immediately. Redistribution causes K^+ to enter the intracellular medium.

Hypoproteinemia.
Hemolysis.
Musculoskeletal
   Renal osteodystrophy.
   Low back pain.
   Compression fracture.
   Soft tissue calcification.
Endocrine
   Secondary hyperparathyroidism.
   Adrenal insufficiency.
   Glucose intolerance (Decreased tissue sensi-
     tivity to insulin).
   Spontaneous hypoglycemia.
Gastrointestinal
   Hepatic dysfunction.
   Mouth ulcers.
   Delayed gastric emptying.
   Hiccough.
   Nausea, vomiting.
Metabolic
   Acid-base disorders.
   Electrolyte disorders.
Immune system
   Hepatitis.
   Immunosuppression.
(For dialysis-related problems, See Table 22–2.)

LABORATORY EVALUATION

In patients with only mild impairment, only routine tests are required. But when impairment is severe, multiple tests may be required for proper evaluation.

1. Complete blood count.
2. Platelet count.
3. Bleeding time, clotting time, prothrombin and partial thromboplastin times.
4. BUN, uric acid, serum cholesterol.
5. Serum creatinine.
6. Creatinine clearance.
7. Serum electrolytes: Na^+, K^+, Ca^{++}, PO_4^{--}, Mg^{++}, HCO_3^-.
8. Complete liver function tests (SMA-12) (Glucose, albumin).
9. EKG (Hypertensive cardiovascular disease, Hyperkalemia).
10. Urinalysis (casts, osmolarity, proteinuria, hematuria, specific gravity, 24-hour proteins).
11. Arterial blood pH and gas tensions.
12. Chest x-ray.

See also Table 22–1 for additional information on renal function tests. The complete blood count (including the platelet count), urinalysis, and measurement of serum creatinine, BUN, serum electrolytes, arterial blood pH, and gas tension are some of the commonly needed tests. In addition, the coagulation system must be evaluated using the partial thromboplastin time and the prothrombin time, also an EKG must be obtained preoperatively.

EFFECTS OF ANESTHESIA ON THE KIDNEY

The effects of anesthesia on the kidney may be immediate or delayed.[15] The immediate effects can either be direct or indirect. The indirect effects are produced by the action of anesthetics on hemodynamics, the sympathetic system, and endocrine function. The anesthetics can directly inhibit certain tubular function. Finally, some anesthetics produce nephrotoxic metabolic byproducts.

IMMEDIATE EFFECTS

In surgical patients with normal kidneys, anesthetics depress GFR, (RBF), and Na^+ excretion. Renal vasoconstriction may occur as a result of systemic hypotension.[15] The reduction in RBF and GFR may be substantial (25 to 35%). Agents that cause sympathetic stimulation (diethyl ether or cyclopropane) may cause a greater degree of renal vasoconstriction than agents such as halothane that do not cause sympathetic activation. The importance of the interaction between the sympathetic system and the anesthetic agent was demonstrated by Berne.[15] He showed that RBF and GFR decreased after induction of anesthesia only in the nondenervated kidney. In the denervated kidney, the RBF and GFR remained unchanged following induction of anesthesia. Thus, anesthetics seem to increase renal vascular resistance by increasing sympathetic activity. Spinal and epidural anesthesia extending to the T5 level interfere only minimally with RPF and GFR provided that the circulating blood volume is maintained. This may be caused by their ability to produce afferent denervation of the kidney.

The effects of anesthetics on the renal autoregulation is controversial. In isolated preparation, anesthesia with 1 MAC (minimum alveolar concentration) halothane has been shown to have no effect on renal autoregulation. But in intact animals, there appears to be some interference with the autoregulation.[15] Autoregulation enables the kidney to maintain a constant GFR over a wide range of mean arterial pressure (MAP) of 80 to 150 mm Hg. When the MAP is higher than normal, the afferent arteriole of the glomerulus acts as a step-down transformer and reduces the hydrostatic pressure in the glomerular capillary, thus maintaining a constant GFR (Fig. 22-6). The lower limit of MAP at which autoregulation fails is 80 mm Hg. (In comparison, cerebral autoregulation has a corresponding value of 50 mm Hg.) Consequently, the protection offered by autoregulation below 80 mm Hg is negliglible. Therefore, every attempt must be made to maintain a normal perfusion pressure and a normal renal vascular resistance in the perioperative period.

The effects of anesthetics on RBF and GFR appear to be dose-related.[16,17] The reduction in RBF is greater than the reduction in GFR, with the result that the filtration fraction increases. The effects are exaggerated in the presence of extracellular volume contraction. Fluid infusion may reverse some of the depressant effects of anesthetics on the renal function. Even balanced anesthesia with N_2O and curare may reduce GFR.[18] The use of spinal anesthesia is associated with only minimal changes in renal function so long as perfusion pressure remains normal.[19]

Anesthesia and surgery may alter renal function indirectly through neuroendocrine mechanisms. Surgical stress may release ADH and catecholamines. ADH causes water retention and both epinephrine and norepinephrine produce marked renal vasoconstriction, causing a reduction in GFR and RBF.[15]

The anesthesia may directly inhibit tubular transport of sodium and organic acids. Anesthetics also interfere with the ability of the kidney slices to uptake para-aminohippuric acid, and with the intrinsic renal clearance of marker drugs.[15]

DELAYED EFFECTS

Many volatile anesthetic agents undergo biotransformation in the body. One of the byproducts of their metabolism is the inorganic fluoride ion (F^-). Fluoride ion is released when methoxyflurane and enflurane are metabolized. With enflurane, serum levels of F^- attain peaks earlier than they do with methoxyflurane. The peaks are smaller and they return to preanesthesia values faster than they do with methoxyflurane (Fig. 22-7). The use of halothane or isoflurane is not associated with any significant F^- release. Nephrotoxicity may occur when the F^- levels exceed 35 μm, and when serum concentrations are sustained at 20 μm, or greater, for 18 hours

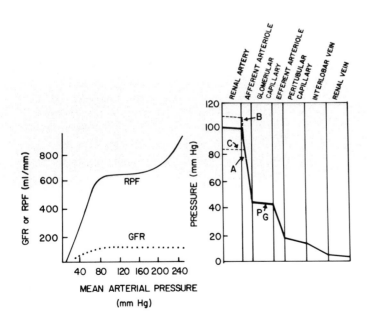

FIG. 22-6. Autoregulation by the kidney. At mean blood pressure, 80–180 mm Hg, the renal plasma flow (RPF) and glomerular filtration rate (GFR) change only minimally. A change in perfusion pressure, however, is expected to affect GFR (left panel). This is prevented by a change in the caliber of the afferent arteriole of the glomerulus (right panel). A = normal mean pressure, B = hypertension, and C = less than normal mean pressure; P_G = glomerular capillary hydrostatic pressure. (From Laiken N, and Fanestil DD: Body fluids and renal function. *In* Best and Taylors Physiologic Basis of Medical Practice. (Edited by West JB.) Baltimore, William and Wilkins, 1985.)

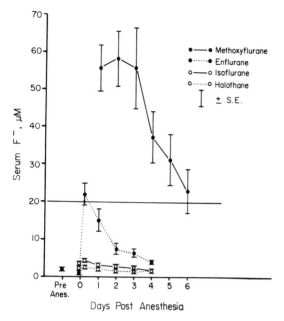

FIG. 22–7. Serum inorganic fluoride concentration before and following anesthesia with different volatile agents. Data are averaged (plus or minus 1 standard error). The F⁻ concentration is much higher with methoxyflurane. With enflurane the F⁻ rises and falls quickly. (From Cousins MJ, Skowronski G, and Plummer JL: Anaesthesia and the Kidney. Anaesth Intens Care *11*:292, 1983.)

or longer.[20] Although oxalic acid is also released during metabolism of methoxyflurane, this is not believed to play a major role in the nephrotoxicity.[15]

Overt nephrotoxicity occurs when anesthesia with methoxyflurane lasts longer than 7 MAC hours. When the exposure is shorter, the toxicity may be mild or subclinical. When renal toxicity develops, it is characterized by vasopressin resistant polyuria; increased serum osmolarity; increased uric acid levels and a diluting-concentration defect in the renal tubules. The toxicity is more likely to occur in obese patients, or in patients who have received either enzyme-inducing drugs (phenobarbital) or other nephrotoxic drugs (aminoglycoside antibiotics). Because of its analgesic properties, methoxyflurane was once a popular agent for obstetric use. It was administered for inhalation analgesia during labor and also for anesthesia for vaginal and abdominal patients.[21] Although no alarmingly high levels of F⁻ have been reported, they may reach the nephrotoxic level in an occasional patient. Methoxyflurane use is best avoided in

patients with renal disease because there are no studies available in obstetric patients with renal disease on this particular issue and other safe techniques and anesthetic agents are available for obstetric anesthesia.

There are case reports of acute renal failure following the use of enflurane. Mazze, et al.[22] has reported that the use of enflurane in patients with preexisting renal disease does not cause further deterioration of renal function.[22] However, there are no studies on obstetric patients. Pregnancy may cause deterioration of renal function. Postpartum renal dysfunction is a leading cause of ARF in young women. For these reasons, enflurane must be used with great caution in pregnant patients with renal disease. Isoflurane or halothane is a safe alternative when a potent volatile agent is needed (blood pressure control in a preeclamptic, asthmatic patient).

ANESTHESIA GUIDELINES

MONITORING

Patients with only mild impairment will not require any extensive monitoring (other than the routine). Patients with severe renal compromise may need CVP monitoring. Patients with cardiovascular compromise may also need a pulmonary artery (PA) catheter. Monitoring of CVP or PA pressures is also helpful not only in detecting preexisting hypovolemia in patients who are on chronic hemodialysis but in avoiding overhydration. Patients with severe hypertension also need an indwelling arterial line. Forearm veins are best avoided for insertion or peripheral lines because they may be needed for the future creation of arteriovenous (A-V) fistula for hemodialysis. A modified V-5 lead may be used to discover possible myocardial ischemia in those with hypertensive cardiovascular disease or lupus coronary artery disease. An indwelling Foley catheter may be required to monitor urinary output, which should be maintained at least at 0.5 ml/kg/hour. Patency of the A-V fistula can be verified using a Doppler flow probe. Extra precautions must be taken to protect the fistula from accidental injury during labor and surgery.

TRANSFUSIONS

Until recently, transfusions were deliberately avoided in a patient with renal failure for fear that the patient might develop antileukocyte antibodies, which could interfere with the survival of a subsequent kidney graft. However, Opelz and Teraski[23] have reported a higher degree of graft survival in patients who received routinely cross-matched packed RBC. The use of frozen RBC is, however, not associated with any increased graft survival. Severe maternal anemia must be corrected before major intervention. Maternal anemia may also hamper fetal oxygenation. Cryoprecipitate transfusion is said to improve renal function in patients with severe renal impairment because of its increased opsonin content.[24] This may be particularly suitable in those with coagulation abnormality.

INTRAVENOUS FLUIDS

In anephric patients, insensible water loss must be replaced with 5% dextrose in water, 500 ml/day. The urine volume must be replaced with 0.45% saline. Blood loss must be adequately restored with packed cells. Any major abdominal surgery results in third-space loss, for which 0.9% saline or salt-poor albumin solutions must be administered at 2 to 5 ml/kg/hour. When available, CVP or PA pressure measurements must be used as guidelines for adequate intravenous fluid therapy.[12]

LABOR ANALGESIA

Meperidine is a popular analgesic for labor pains. It is 60% protein-bound. In some patients with severe renal impairment, normeperidine, a metabolite of meperidine, may accumulate, leading to excitation or CNS irritability.[12] Normeperidine has a half-life of 15 to 20 hours. Morphine sulfate undergoes hepatic metabolism. Its duration of action, however, is prolonged in those with reduced urinary output. The doses of meperidine and morphine should be suitably reduced. Fentanyl in small incremental doses is also safe for analgesia (vide infra).

Amide local anesthestics are metabolized by the liver. 2-chloroprocaine is hydrolyzed by plasma cholinesterase. Lumbar epidural analgesia (LEA) with an amide or an ester derivative is suitable for these patients. There are reports of chronic neurologic damage with the use of 2-chloroprocaine. This is attributed to the antioxidant (sodium bisulphite) contained in the local anesthetic solution. A preparation containing the least amount of the antioxidant is preferable. For more details on neurotoxicity produced by local anesthetics, see Chapter 5. Although epidural anesthesia is not known to worsen neuropathy, this must be carefully discussed with patients presenting with evidence of uremic polyneuritis. An epidural block extending to the T10 level will not affect the renal function, as long as the supine position and systemic hypotension are avoided. In fact, it may cause an increase in renal blood flow by diminishing catecholamine response to labor pains.

Because of the possible coexisting fetal compromise, a paracervical block is not recommended. The use of segmental epidural anesthesia for treating renal colic has been discussed before. Lumbar epidural analgesia may also be useful for relaxing the perineum in patients with urinary diversion, thus avoiding a precipitate labor that may cause injury to the anal sphincter. Patients with ureterosigmoid anastomosis require an intact anal sphincter to be continent of their urine. In the absence of coagulopathy, a spinal block is useful for anesthesia for forceps. If systemic hypotension develops, ephedrine may be administered in 5 mg increments. Although dopamine appears to be a logical choice in patients with renal disease (because of its beneficial effects on renal function), it may reduce uterine blood flow when administered in quantities sufficient to maintain perfusion pressure. Therefore, its routine use for treating maternal hypotension due to regional anesthesia is not recommended.[25]

CESAREAN SECTION

Cesarean section may be needed for obstetric indications or for acute or chronic fetal distress. Regional anesthesia is preferable to general anesthesia. Optimization of circulating fluid volume is essential. Decreased circulating volume is a potent stimulus for renal vasoconstriction. In the absence of severe hypertension or coagulopathy, spinal anesthesia may be considered. If, however, there is superimposed preeclampsia, spinal anesthesia (because of its rapid onset) may cause severe hypotension. When systemic hypotension is avoided and the circulating fluid volume is adequate, spinal anesthesia is associated with only minimal alterations in kidney function[19,26] (Table 22–6). Renal blood flow, renal clearance, and elimination of indicators are not significantly altered even during high spinal anesthesia. A general anesthetic markedly interferes with these parameters. It must be pointed out, however, that a high spinal anesthesia in a patient who is not properly hydrated may affect the RBF and GFR to an equal degree, as does general anesthesia. Chronic renal disease modifies spinal anesthesia in the following ways: it causes a more rapid spread of the anesthetic; it is associated with a slightly higher sensory level; and the duration of action may be shortened. Uremic demyelination of the neurons is believed to be responsible circulation for the faster spread of spinal anesthesia. The hyperdynamic circulation may increase clearance of the drug from the subarachnoid space, thus shortening the duration of anesthesia.[27]

When there is coexisting preeclampsia or severe hypertension, spinal anesthesia may cause a rapid reduction in systemic pressure. When a lumbar epidural analgesia is used for cesarean section, lidocaine or bupivacaine may be used. Acidosis decreases the threshold for local anesthetic induced seizure.[12] Following a regional block, blood levels of local anesthesia increase more rapidly than they would in healthy patients, probably because of the hyperdynamic circulation.[28] Therefore, the total dose of the local anesthetic must be kept to a minimum. The use of epinephrine to prolong the duration of local anesthetics may cause cardiac arrhythmias and/or pulmonary edema in patients who are acidotic and hyperkalemic.[12]

When general anesthesia is needed, patients should be given an antacid preparation preferably sodium citrate to raise the intragastric fluid pH. In patients with severe heartburn, cimetidine may be used. Cimetidine metabolism is not affected in patients with renal impairment. Patients with renal disease and those on chronic hemodialysis often abuse Mg^{++} containing antacids. In addition, hypermagnesemia may occur in renal disease. It is therefore not advisable to use Mg^{++} containing antacids in those patients.[12]

Induction of anesthesia may be done with thiopental. The dose must be reduced because of decreased protein binding and the modification of blood-brain barrier for barbiturates in uremic patients.[29] Although the use of succinylcholine is not associated with any dangers in normokalemic patients with chronic renal disease, serious hyperkalemia may develop in those with a raised serum K^+ prior to anesthesia.[30] Succinylcholine must be avoided when the serum K^+ exceeds 5.5 mMol. An exaggerated hyperkalemic response can also occur in patients with severe uremic polyneuritis.[12] Of the nondepolarizing relaxants, atracurium and vecuronium are not affected by renal failure and are therefore the relaxants of choice. Pancuronium undergoes significant renal excretion, thus its duration of action can be prolonged. Figures 22–8 and 22–9, respectively, show the elimination half-life and clearance rates of commonly used muscle relaxants and the drugs used to reverse the action of muscle relaxants. All reversal agents also undergo renal elimination, and therefore their action is prolonged. Thus recurarization is unlikely when adequate reversal is ensured at the end of the case. When the patient is receiving Mg^{++} therapy for preeclampsia, the dose of neuromuscular blocking agents must be

Table 22–6. Renal Function with General and Spinal Anesthesia

Parameter	Control	GA	Control	Spinal
Cardiac output	4.5 (0.3)	3.4 (0.1)	5.0 (0.5)	6.3 (1.0)
Renal blood flow	0.59 (0.02)	0.37 (0.02)	0.69 (0.06)	0.61 (0.08)
IOH extraction ratio	0.6 (0.01)	0.4 (0.03)	0.76 (0.01)	0.75 (0.03)
IOH clearance	355 (9)	146 (5)	525 (40)	457 (47)
CEF extraction ratio	0.58 (0.05)	0.3 (0.05)	0.77 (0.02)	0.78 (0.05)
CEF clearance	344 (29)	110 (27)	528 (42)	478 (74)

Cardiac output and renal blood flow are in L/min; clearance is in ml/min. IOH–iodohippurate; CEF–cefoxitin. GA–general anesthesia. Data are obtained from Mather LE, et al.[19] and Runciman WB, et al.[26] Values are mean (1SD). Control measurements were done in basal awake state.

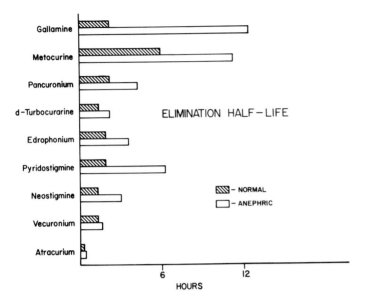

FIG. 22–8. Elimination half-life of different muscle relaxants and reversal agents in patients with normal renal function and in anephric subjects. Vecuronium and atracurium are not affected significantly in anephric subjects. The elimination half-lives of reversal agents are affected, minimizing the chances for recurarization.

carefully adjusted (see Chapter 10 on Hypertensive Disorders).

For maintenance of anesthesia, the balanced technique with fentanyl is preferable because of the rapid nonrenal elimination of fentanyl. Only 10% of fentanyl appears in the urine.[30] Inhalation agents cause a dose-dependent depression of renal function, and are therefore best avoided. However, if systemic hypertension develops during anesthesia, halothane or isoflurane may be used in small concentrations. Droperidol 2.5 to 5 mg is also recommended.[30] Intraoperative supplementation can also be provided with diazepam or midazolam. Excessive doses of both agents have prolonged action in patients with

renal failure;[30] therefore only small doses are recommended. Caution is advised in using enflurane in patients with renal impairment and methoxyflurane must be avoided. It is absolutely essential to maintain intraoperative circulating blood volume to prevent further deterioration in renal function. Any blood loss must be quickly and adequately replaced with packed RBC. Arterial blood pH and gas tensions must be measured and the F_{IO_2} suitably adjusted because of the possibility of arterial hypoxemia.

Hypertension must be adequately controlled with sodium nitroprusside [SNP] or hydralazine before induction of anesthesia and also in the postoperative period. The hydralazine dose

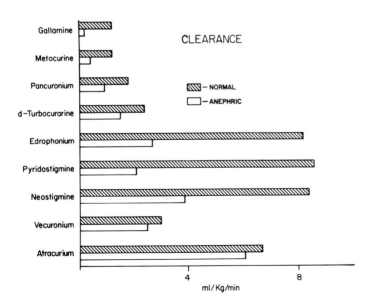

FIG. 22–9. Clearance rates of muscle relaxants and the reversal agents. The clearance rates of vecuronium and atracurium are not significantly affected in anephric subjects. The significant decrease in the clearance rates of reversal agents, makes recurarization unlikely.

must be modified because it depends on renal elimination. In the postoperative period, patients must be kept in the high-risk unit (if available) or in the ICU. Postoperative hypertension may be treated with sodium nitroprusside infusion. Oliguria in the postoperative period must be assessed and treated at the earliest opportunity. Nephrotoxins (aminoglycoside antibiotics, cephalosporins, nonsteroidal anti-inflammatory drugs) must be avoided. Postoperative analgesia with epidural narcotic obviates the need for repeated parenteral narcotic administration.

REFERENCES

1. Brenner BM, and Hofstetter TH: Disturbances of renal function. *In* Harrison's Principles of Internal Medicine. (Edited by Petersdorf RG, et al.) New York, McGraw-Hill, 1983.

2. Laiken N, and Fanestil DD: Body fluids and renal function. *In* Best and Taylors Physiologic Basis of Medical Practice. (Edited by West JB.) Baltimore, Williams and Wilkins, 1985.

3. Davison JM, Katz JI, and Lindheimer MD: Kidney disease and pregnancy. Clin Perinatol 12:497, 1985.

4. Surian M, Imbasciuti E, and Cosci P: Glomerular disease and pregnancy: A study of 123 pregnancies in patients with primary and secondary glomerular diseases. Nephron 36:101, 1984.

5. Gabert HA, and Miller JM Jr.: Renal disease in pregnancy. Obstet Gynecol Sur 40:449, 1985.

6. Burkett G: Lupus nephropathy and pregnancy. Clin Obstet Gynecol 28:311, 1985.

7. Anticardiolipin antibodies: A risk factor for venous and arterial thrombosis. Lancet 1:912, 1985.

8. Ready BL, and Johnson ES: Epidural block for the treatment of renal colic. Can Anaesth Soc J 28:77, 1981.

9. Rudolph JE, Schweizer RT, and Bartus SA: Pregnancy in renal transplant patients. Transplantation 27:26, 1979.

10. Dretchen KL, Morgenroth VH III, Standaert FG, and Walts LF: Azathioprine: Effects on neuromuscular transmission. Anesthesiology 45:604, 1976.

11. Lindsay RM, and Clark WF: Platelet destruction in renal disease. Semin Thromb Hemos 8:138, 1982.

12. Weir PHC, and Chung FF: Anaesthesia for patients with chronic renal disease. Can Anaesth Soc J 31:468, 1984.

13. Knuppel RA, Montenegro R, and O'Brien WF: Acute renal failure in pregnancy. Clin Obstet Gynecol 28: 288, 1985.

14. Pritchard JA, MacDonald PC, and Gant NF: Williams Obstetrics. Norwalk, Appleton-Century-Crofts, 1985.

15. Cousins MJ, Skowronski G, and Plummer JL: Anaesthesia and the kidney. Anaesth Intens Care 11:292, 1983.

16. Halperin BD, and Feeley TW: The effect of anesthesia and surgery on renal function. Int Anesthesiol Clin 22:157, 1984.

17. Mazze RI, et al.: Renal function during anesthesia and surgery: 1. The effects of halothane anesthesia. Anesthesiology 24:279, 1963.

18. Deutch S, et al.: The effects of anesthesia with thiopentone, nitrous oxide, narcotics and neuromuscular blocking drugs on renal function in normal man. Br J Anaesth 41:807, 1969.

19. Mather LE, Runciman WB, and Ilsley AH: Anesthesia induced changes in regional blood flow. Implications for drug disposition. Regional Anesthesia 7:Suppl 45:S23, 1982.

20. Mazze RI, Calverley RK, and Smith NT: Inorganic fluoride toxicity: Prolonged enflurane and halothane anesthesia in volunteers. Anesthesiology 46:265, 1977.

21. Palahniuk RJ, and Cumming M: Plasma fluoride levels following obstetrical use of methoxyflurane. Can Anaesth Soc J 22:291, 1975.

22. Mazze RI, Sievenpiper TS, and Stevenson J: Renal effects of enflurane and halothane in patients with abnormal renal function. Anesthesiology 60:161, 1984.

23. Opelz G, and Terasaki PI: Dominant effects of transfusions on kidney graft survival. Transplantation 29:153, 1980.

24. Annest SJ, et al.: Increased creatinine clearance following cryoprecipitate infusion in trauma and surgical patients with decreased renal function. J Trauma 20:726, 1980.

25. Rolbin SH, et al.: Dopamine treatment of spinal hypotension decreases uterine blood flow in the pregnant ewe. Anesthesiology 51:36, 1979.

26. Runciman WB, et al.: A sheep preparation for studying interactions between blood and drug disposition. IV: The effects of general and spinal anaesthesia on blood flow and cefoxin disposition. Br J Anaesth 57:1239, 1985.

27. Orko R, Pitkanen M, and Rosenberg PH: Subarachnoid anaesthesia with 0.75% bupivacaine in patients with chronic renal failure. Br J Anaesth 58:605, 1986.

28. Strasser K, et al.: Plasma level of etidocaine within the first two hours after axillary plexus block in healthy adults and patients with renal insufficiency. Anaesthetist 30:14, 1981.

29. Hilgenberg JC: Renal Disease, Anesthesia and Coexisting Disease. (Edited by Stoelting RK, Dierdorf SF.) New York, Churchill Livingstone, 1983.

30. Maddern PJ: Anesthesia for patient with impaired renal function. Anaesth Intens Care 11:321, 1983.

CHAPTER 23

DRUG ABUSE

The problem of drug abuse during pregnancy is associated with serious maternal and fetal complications. Unfortunately, the number of young women who abuse drugs is increasing.

Both narcotic and non-narcotic agents may be abused by pregnant women. Table 23–1 gives a list of drugs that may be potentially abused by the pregnant patient. A vast majority of addicts do not seek antenatal medical care and usually go to a hospital only after labor starts.

ALCOHOL

GENERAL ASPECTS

This is the most commonly abused substance by pregnant patients. Regardless of the gestational period, alcohol causes adverse fetal effects.[1] Serious fetal effects are seen only when the mother drinks heavily (5 or more drinks on a single occasion or 45 drinks per month; 1 drink = 15 ml of alcohol). A small risk, however, does exist in moderate drinkers (less than 45 drinks per month but never five or more on a single occasion). Occasional alcohol consumption (less than 15 ml/day) may not be associated with any serious fetal sequelae.[1–3] Increased blood alcohol levels may not only impair metabolism of vital nutrients but may interfere with nucleic acid turnover in the fetal brain. Voluntary reduction of heavy drinking in the third trimester has been shown to improve fetal outcome.

Problem drinkers may also abuse a variety of other substances, including narcotics. Chronic use of alcohol increases cross tolerance to other depressant drugs either because of pharamcodynamic tolerance of the CNS or because of increased metabolism as a result of enzyme induction.[4] The withdrawal syndrome is comprised of tremulousness, hyperreflexia, hallucinations, tremulous delirium, and tonic-clonic seizures. Respiratory alkalosis (with or without reduced serum Mg^{++} levels) is implicated in the genesis of tremulous delirium. Disulfiram and sedatives, which are used for detoxification of alcoholics, are not usually recommended in pregnant subjects because of their teratogenic potential.

Chronic use of alcohol also causes multiple organ damage and nutritional insufficiencies. Fatty necrosis of the liver, cerebral atrophy, polyneuropathy, Wernick's encephalopathy, skeletal myopathy, and cardiomyopathy.[5] The skeletal myopathy may be associated with increased serum creatine phosphokinase. Cardiomyopathy may be associated with decreased cardiac output and increased vasoconstriction. In addition, alcoholics may suffer from dehydration and hypokalemia resulting from vomiting caused by gastritis and/or poor fluid intake.[5]

Heavy drinking is associated with fetal alcohol syndrome.[2] The syndrome consists of pre- or postnatal growth retardation, development delay, impaired intellectual function, characteristic cranial anomalies (maxillofacial anomalies, microcephaly, and/or microphthalmia).[5] The incidence ranges from 3 to 12%. In addition, the

Table 23–1. Commonly Abused Drugs in Pregnancy

Drug	Abstinence syndrome		Teratogenicity	
	Maternal	Fetal	Morphologic	Behavioral
Ethyl alcohol;	Yes	Yes	IUGR; facial anomal-ies; FAS.	Learning disability; delayed mile-stones.
Narcotics	Yes	Yes	IUGR; reduced brain weight (animals).	Learning disability.
Barbiturates	Yes	Yes	None.	—
Benzodiazepines	Yes	Yes	Cleft palate.	—
Stimulants:				
Cocaine	Yes	—	Genitourinary.	?
Amphetamines	Possible	—	—	—
Marijuana	Yes	?	Like fetal alcohol syn-drome.	?
Psychadelics:				
LSD	Yes	No data	No data.	No data.
Phencyclidine	Yes	—	?	No data.

FAS–fetal alcohol syndrome; IUGR–Intrauterine Growth Retardation; LSD–lysergic acid diethylamide; "—" signifies "none reported." "?" signifies that a possibility is suspected.

neonates may develop withdrawal syndrome, which may be delayed 24 hours. The symptoms of neonatal withdrawal include excessive crying, irritability, and seizures. The condition may be treated with phenobarbital 3 to 5 mg/kg.[6]

ANESTHETIC CONSIDERATIONS

If the patient is in tremulous delirium because of alcohol withdrawal, prompt treatment is necessary to prevent circulatory collapse. Hyperthermia may occur if the delirium is not treated promptly. Cooling blankets may be useful in cases of hyperthermia. Dehydration, hypokalemia, hypomagnesemia, and hypoglycemia must be corrected. Caution must be exercised in administering large amounts of glucose because of the possible development of encephalopathy caused by thiamine depletion.[5] Lidocaine is used for treating cardiac arrhythmias. Diazepam in small amounts is used to control the delirium.

All patients who have abused alcohol must have their liver functions properly evaluated. Severe liver disease is associated with resistance to the action of d-tubocurarine caused by increased binding of the drug by gamma-globulin.[7] In patients with hepatic cirrhosis, the onset of action of pancuronium may be delayed but its total duration of action is usually prolonged because of increased volume distribution of the drug.[8] Similarly vecuronium action may be prolonged in patients with liver disease. Whenever a nondepolarizing relaxant is used, a nerve stimulator must be used. Unless the liver disease is so advanced as to decrease the concentration of pseudocholinesterase, the action of succinlycholine is not significantly affected.

Patients with history of alcohol abuse generaly demonstrate resistance to the action of CNS depressant drugs such as pentathal and inhalation agents.[9] The dose of pentothal must be individualized and the drug must be titrated to obtain the desired response. Routine use of excessive doses of pentothal (in view of the possible CNS resistence to the agent) may be hazardous because of diminished protein binding and the possible presence of cardiomyopathy.[10] Similarly, the use of excessive concentrations of volatile agents can lead to cardiovascular depression. Small amounts of narcotics may be used for supplementation when higher then usual concentrations of volatile agents are needed to produce adequate anesthesia. Patients who are acutely intoxicated require less anesthetics and depressant medications. They are also at increased risk for aspiration pneumonia not only because of the increased gastric fluid acidity but also because of impaired laryngeal reflex.

The use of regional anesthesia for labor and for cesarean section obviates some of the problems associated with general anesthesia. However, circulating fluid volume must be optimized to avoid the consequences of sympathetic denervation resulting from regional anesthesia. The presence of polyneuropathy is not a contraindication to regional anesthesia but the anesthesiologist must document the existing neurologic impairment before administering regional anesthesia to avoid future litigation.[10] Regional anesthesia may be hazardous in the presence of coagulopathy caused by advanced liver disease. Two additional factors that may predispose to local anesthetic toxicity are the decreased protein binding (hypoalbuminemia) and the delayed metabolism of amide local anesthetic agents. Thus, even using moderate doses of local anesthetic agents, toxic side effects may be seen.[11] Lidocaine is preferable to bupivacaine because it is less cardiotoxic. 2-chloroprocaine, which is an ester, is ideal under these circumstances. The ester hydrolysis is usually so efficient that in all but those with liver advanced disease, a normal rate of metabolism may be expected.

Whereas only small quantities of local anesthetics are required for labor analgesia, large volumes are required for producing anesthesia for cesarean section. The use of spinal anesthesia may circumvent this problem. Because spinal anesthesia can produce rapid hypotension, meticulous attention must be paid to prophylactic intravenous hydration and proper patient positioning to avoid aortocaval compression. Spinal or epidural opiates may be used for postoperative pain relief. Caution is advised in inserting nasogastric tubes because of the possible occurrence of esophageal varices. Fresh blood is recommended for transfusion to minimize any rise in serum ammonia levels. Ammonia levels are high in stored blood.

NARCOTICS

GENERAL ASPECTS

The use of narcotics such as heroin is on the increase. The abuse of opioids is disturbingly high among the health care professionals. Maternal narcotic addiction affects both the mother and her fetus. The street heroin also contains quinine, talc and/or starch. Frequently, the heroin addict abuses both legal and illegal drugs.

Maternal problems in a drug addict include possible abstinence syndrome and multiple organ dysfunction. When the drug in question is a μ-receptor agonist, withdrawal symptoms appear within 8 to 12 hours after the last dose.[4] Typically the symptoms include (1) anxiety, (2) restlessness, (3) lacrimation, (4) tremors, (5) hot and cold flushes, (6) tachycardia, (7) tachypnea, (8) muscle spasms, and (9) cardiovascular collapse. The cardiovascular collapse may be the result of dehydration, starvation, and disorders of acid-base balance. The withdrawal of methadone takes 24 to 48 hours to produce symptoms, but they are usually less intense. Meperidine abstinence syndrome appears within 2 to 4 hours and reaches a peak within 24 hours.[4]

Patients who have received a high dose of methadone for maintenance may experience withdrawal even when the dose is reduced gradually. Withdrawal also follows discontinuation of semisynthetic opioid drugs such as pentazocine, nalbuphine, butorphanol, and buprenorphine.[12] As a rule, the withdrawal symptoms associated with the semisynthetic drugs are less severe than that seen with heroin withdrawal. The semisynthetic opioids have a differing action on the several opioid receptors. Generally speaking, those which have an antagonistic action on the μ-receptor will precipitate withdrawal in opioid dependent individuals.[12] For instance, when given to a drug addict, pentazocine and nalbuphine, which are partial antagonists of this receptor, may produce withdrawal symptoms. When given in small doses, buprenorphine, which has a partial agonistic action on the μ-receptor, may suppress symptoms caused by morphine withdrawal, but in high doses, it may precipitate withdrawal. A complete description of opioid receptors can be found in Chapter 6 Spinal Opiates. Naloxone and naltrexone are potent antagonists of the μ-receptor and therefore must not be used in opioid dependent patients.[12]

Perinatal problems associated with narcotic use is summarized in Table 23–2. Maternal health complications that may be caused by opioid addiction are presented in Table 23–3. A thorough preanesthetic evaluation of all the systems must be made. Persons who have been previously detoxified may be receiving methadone or 1-α-acetylmethadol (LAAM), which has a longer duration of action than does methadone.[5] Clonidine (α-2 agonist) has been used to

Table 23–2.   Maternal and Neonatal Outcome in Drug Abusers

Problem type	Conditions	Percent of abusers	Percent of controls
Maternal problems.	Meconium stained amniotic fluid	21.2	13.8
	Maternal anemia	13.2	8.2
	Premature membrane rupture	12.2	7.8
	Antenatal hemorrhage	3.0	1.2
	Multiple birth	3.4	1.2
Neonatal condition at birth.	Birth weight (2–2.5 kg)	21	7
	Birth weight (2.5 kg or heavier)	69	89
	Prematurity (<38 weeks)	18.5	9.8
	Apgar <6 (5 min)	7	3.2
Postnatal problems	Jaundice	12.7	8.2
	Aspiration pneumonia	9.2	1.8
	Transient tachypnea	6.6	2.5
	Hyaline membrane disease	3.6	1.5
	Congenital malformations	2.4	0.5

(From Ostrea EM and Chavez CJ: Perinatal problems (excluding neonatal withdrawal) in maternal addiction: A study of 830 cases. J Pediatr *94*:292, 1979.)

Table 23–3.   Complications of Opioid Drug Abuse

Area of condition affected	Complication
Cardiovascular	Endocarditis; EKG abnormalities; Myocardial infarction.
Respiratory	Respiratory infection; Pneumonia (aspiration, infection); Pulmonary foreign body granulomas; Decreased P_{O_2}.
Liver disease	Abnormal SGOT, SGPT, alkaline phosphatase; Hepatitis Cirrhosis.
Renal disease	Nephrotic syndrome; Renal failure.
Musculoskeletal	Osteomyelitis of the vertebra; Rhabdomyolysis (myoglobinuria); Compartment syndrome;* Myopathy.
Nervous system	Necrotizing myelitis; Paraplegia; Isolated neuropathy.
Infective	AIDS; Brain, liver abscesses; Tetanus; Spinal, epidural abscess; Severe thrombophlebitis.

AIDS = Acquired immune deficiency syndrome.
*–Compartment syndrome results from massive swelling of an extremity into which heroin has been injected.

control withdrawal symptoms associated with sympathetic nervous system hyperactivity. Abrupt discontinuation of clonidine may cause symptoms such as anxiety, hypertension, and tachycardia. Therapy with β-blockers and/or sodium nitroprusside may be necessary to control symptoms produced by clonidine withdrawal.[5] Clonidine overdose may cause sedation and hypotension.

Infants born of heroin users have a decreased birth weight compared to those who are on a supervised methadone program.[13] The incidence of fetal distress is the highest in polydrug users. Meconium aspiration and premature delivery are other causes of fetal morbidity. Maternal withdrawal may lead to fetal withdrawal in utero leading to increased fetal oxygen consumption. Maternal withdrawal may also be responsible for initiating uterine contractions, which may further interfere with fetal oxygenation.[14] Human studies have not shown any increased congenital malformations in methadone users. However, animal studies have implicated this drug in causing impaired intellectual function.[15] (see Chapter 18 Teratology). Heroin has been shown to produce congenital cranial anomalies in fetuses exposed to the drug in utero.[15] Methadone administration may also interfere with the ability of the fetus to increase its breathing motion when the mother is given a 5% concentration of CO_2 to inhale, thus demonstrating its profound effect on the fetal central nervous system.[16]

Heroin, methadone, and other opioids cause neonatal withdrawal syndrome characterized by irritability, fever, vomiting, shrill cry, and diarrhea.[13] The symptoms must be recognized and treated promptly to avoid neonatal death. The treatment usually consists of administration of paregoric (camphorated tincture of opium).[6] Phenobarbital may be given if multiple drug exposure is suspected. Diazepam is the least efficacious for the treatment of neonatal abstinence syndrome. Because of accelerated surfactant maturation caused by heroin, the incidence of respiratory distress syndrome is less in these neonates than in those of comparable gestational age.

ANESTHETIC CONSIDERATIONS

Because venipuncture may be a problem in intravenous drug abusers, internal jugular or a subclavian vein cannulation may be needed. Patients must be given their maintenance methadone dose. Regional anesthesia may be used for producing pain relief during labor because it obviates the use of narcotics. If narcotics are required during labor meperidine and/or methadone may be used for producing analgesia. Narcotics, which antagonize μ-receptor activity must not be used lest they should precipitate withdrawal. The withdrawal syndrome may be precipitated by the epidural administration of semisynthetic narcotics such as butophanol.[17]

If general anesthesia is required, pentothal may be used for induction. Maintenance of anesthesia is preferentially done with a powerful inhalation agent. The use of narcotics is not recommended intraoperatively. Isoflurane may be preferable to halothane since it undergoes very little hepatic metabolism. Postoperative pain relief may be provided by epidural injection of local anesthetic injection or morphine, both of which diminish the total narcotic requirement in the postoperative period. Meperidine and/or methadone may be used for parenteral analgesia. The oral route is preferable to the parenteral route for narcotic administration since the intravenous administration is likely to produce euphoria thereby creating a favorable condition for the development of readdiction. Because administration of opioid antagonists such as naloxone precipitates severe withdrawal symptoms, on no account should they be administered to the mother or to the neonate. Patients who are acutely intoxicated must have their airway protected with an endotracheal tube. Hypotension must be treated with vasopressors and intravenous fluid administration. Incremental doses of naloxone are necessary to counteract the respiratory depression.

BARBITURATES

The Domestic Council Drug Abuse Task Force (1975) estimated that 300,000 persons are at risk for suicide, accidental overdose, and other medical complications caused by unsupervised barbiturate use. Tolerance develops more slowly to barbiturates than it does to the use of opioids. An addict may ingest up to 2 g of barbiturate without showing signs of intoxication.[4] Even in those who frequently abuse the drug, the lethal dose does not increase at the same rate at which tolerance develops.[4] With the result that a barbiturate abuser has little room for error. Barbiturates are abused solely for their effects on the CNS, for suppressing withdrawal from alcohol, or to supplement the effects of impure street heroin. A barbiturate abuser may concomitantly abuse benzodiazepines and other sedative drugs.

The manifestations of chronic barbiturism include (1) slow thinking, (2) untidy personal habits, (3) emotional instability, and (4) neurologic signs (cerebellar incoordination, nystagmus, and dysarthria). The electroencephalographic findings during chronic barbiturate use are fast activity of moderate voltage interspersed with some 6 to 8 MHz activity mainly in the frontal and perietal regions.[5] Barbiturate withdrawal is more life-threatening than is narcotic withdrawal. The withdrawal symptoms start within 24 to 72 hours after the last dose of barbiturate.[5] The symptoms include tremors, nervousness, grand mal seizures, and psychosis. When an adult develops sudden seizure or psychosis, the possibility of barbiturate withdrawal must be considered. In many, the EEG shows spike-dome activity, which may or may not be associated with seizure activity.[5] The patient is remarkably sensitive to photic stimulation. Severe hallucinations may also occur. Detoxification is usually done by administering a stabilizing dose of barbiturate. A short acting barbiturate such as pentobarbital (0.2 g orally every 6 hours) or the long acting phenobarbital is used. Phenobarbital produces less fluctuant blood levels than does pentobarbital. Barbiturates are ingested orally, and therefore problems such as endocarditis or hepatitis associated with the use of contaminated hypodermic needles are not usually seen in barbiturate abusers. However, there are other concerns: (1) barbiturates are potent enzyme inducers. They modify the action of several drugs such as anticoagulants. Anesthetic metabolism may also be accelerated, (2) cross-tolerance to other CNS depressants may develop, (3) the neonate usually shows signs of withdrawal, which respond to phenobarbital administration. The chronic use of barbiturates (except when used for treating epilepsy) is not associated with any morphologic teratogenicity. (See Chapter 18 Teratology).

In pregnancy, withdrawal symptoms should be prevented by judicious use of stabilizing doses of pentobarbital. The abuse of other sedatives and/or narcotics must be carefully ruled out. Regional anesthesia or parenteral narcotics may be administered for labor pains. Regional anesthesia or general anesthesia is suitable for cesarean section.

Acute intoxication must be managed with tracheal intubation and positive pressure ventilation. Measurements of blood levels of barbiturate may be helpful. A blood level of 2 mg/dL in a comatose patient is usually the result of secobarbital or pentobarbital poisoning. A blood level of 11 to 12 mg/dL is suggestive of barbital or phenobarbital intake.[5] Barbiturates also cause diminished cardiac output, peripheral vasodilatation and systemic hypotension. To correct hypotension (systolic pressure of less than 90 mm Hg) the patient should be nursed on her side to avoid aortocaval compression, circulating fluid volume should be optimized, and ephedrine should be intermittently injected or continuously infused. The use of pure α-agonists may cause severe reduction in utero-placental perfusion. The fetal heart rate must also be continuously monitored. Forced diuresis and alkali administration are recommended for acclerating the rate of elimination of barbiturates.[5] Occasionally hemodialysis or peritoneal dialysis may be required when the above-mentioned measures fail.

BENZODIAZEPINES

Benzodiazepines including diazepam (or Valium) may be abused by pregnant women. Large doses of the drug may be ingested since tolerance develops. The accumulation of active metabolites of the drug may obscure the development of adaptive changes in the brain. The abstinence syndrome resembles that produced by barbiturate withdrawal. The neonates are also prone to develop withdrawal, which responds to benzodiazepine administration. The use of diazepam in the first trimester is associated with cleft palate in the neonate (see Chapter 18 Teratology). Excessive maternal administration of diazepam also leads to decreased muscle tone in the baby. Diazepam interferes with temperatue regulation in the neonate. (See Chapter 4 on Perinatal Pharmacology and Systemic Medication.)

COCAINE

Five million Americans regularly use cocaine.[18] Some women use cocaine while pregnant. Cocaine is inhaled or self-administered parenterally. The use of cocaine rapidly leads to physical dependence. Unlike the narcotic user, the cocaine user seems to be full of energy immediately after self-administration.[5] They are prone to persecutory delusions. Sudden discontinuation of the drug does not cause any observable changes in behavior, although patients do complain of a craving for the drug, hyperphagia, and depression.[19] Occasionally, a withdrawal syndrome develops consisting of delirium and sleeplessness. There is no need for a slow withdrawal of the drug. The mood changes may be treated with tricyclic antidepressants.

Cocaine prevents the reuptake of catecholamines at the sympathetic synaptic clefts. It produces placental vasoconstriction, hypertension, and tachycardia. It also causes premature uterine contractions, which may result in the onset of premature labor or in spontaneous abortion. The infant's neurobehavior is also affected at birth.[18] The hypertension is said to be responsible for the increased incidence of abruptio placentae in these women.[18] In addition, problems caused by intravenous use of impure cocaine may also develop. Lung damage is known to occur in those who smoke the coca paste.[5] The nasal septum may become ulcerated in those who use the cocaine snuff. Cocaine crosses the placenta and stimulates the fetus with the result that the fetal body movement increases in the third trimester.[18]

General anesthesia may be hazardous in a cocaine abuser because of the possible elevations in circulating catecholamine levels. Hypertension, tachycardia, and cardiac arrhythmias, especially in the presence of sensitizing agents such as halothane or cyclopropane, may occur. In addition, the acute use of cocaine is associated with increased anesthetic requirement.[20] The increased occurrence of abruption immediately after smoking or snorting makes it likely that these patients will require emergency cesarean section. A regional anesthetic technique is suitable both for labor analgesia and cesarean section. General anesthesia for cesarean section usually requires a rapid sequence induction, which may be associated with liberation of catecholamine. The use of epidural anesthesia for this purpose avoids this problem. Regional anesthesia is, however, contraindicated if the placental abruption had caused a coagulopathy.

Acute cocaine intoxication causes excitement, convulsions, tachyarrhythmias, hypermetabolic state, acidosis, and circulatory collapse. Convulsions must be controlled with diazepam and tachyarrhythmias should be controlled with beta-blockers.[21]

CENTRAL NERVOUS SYSTEM STIMULANTS

AMPHETAMINES

The abuse of amphetamines has increased because of the proliferation of drugs marketed for weight reduction. Amphetamine and its d-isomer dextroamphetamine are powerful stimulants. An intravenous dose causes an immediate ecstacy called "flash".[5] The toxic syndrome caused by amphetamine is usually indistinguishable from that caused by cocaine.[4] Amphetamines, like cocaine, block the reuptake of norepinephrine and their effects are believed to be mediated through the dopaminergic sites in the CNS.[4] Tolerance is rapidly developed for the euphorigenic effects of amphetamines but not for the toxic effects; thus increasing the possibility of toxic psychosis.[4] Prolonged use of amphetamines may lead to microvascular damage and depletion of dopamine from the caudate nucleus.[22] Withdrawal symptoms resemble those produced by cocaine withdrawal.[4]

Thus, administration of amphetamine has been shown to increase MAC in animals in a dose-dependent manner. Chronic administration may, however, reduce MAC because of catecholamine depletion in the brain.[23] The use of general anesthetic agents that sensitize the myocardium to circulating catecholamines may be hazardous because of the increased likelihood of cardiac arrhythmias. Cardiac arrest has been reported with the induction of general anesthesia with pentothal in an amphetamine abuser.[24] Sympathetic stimulants, such as ketamine, are thus better avoided. Pulmonary edema occurred in one patient during general anesthesia with halothane.[25] It is interesting to note that pulmonary edema is a frequent complication of tocolytic therapy with a sympathomimetic agent ritodrine (see Chapter 20 Preterm Labor). Because epidural anesthesia diminishes the intensity of sympathetic activity, it is the preferred technique for both labor analgesia and cesarean section. Chronic amphetamine use suppresses appetite and causes ketosis and dehydration.[4] Therefore, circulating fluid volume must be expanded adequately before induction of epidural anesthesia. Ketonuria must be corrected by judicious administration of glucose (see Chapter 2). Chronic amphetamine use may cause depletion of catecholamines by preventing their reuptake into sympathetic nerve endings.[4] To treat systemic hypotension caused by regional anesthesia a direct acting vasopressor such as phenylephrine may be needed, especially when ephedrine fails to restore blood pressure.

Acute toxicity caused by amphetamines, include hypertension, tachycardia, irritability, sweating, hyperpyrexia, and convulsions.[4] Diazepam or chlorpromazine are recommended to control symptoms. Acidification of the urine enhances excretion of the drug.[4] Methylphenidate is another CNS stimulant with a potential for abuse.

CANNABINOIDS (MARIJUANA)

The effects of marijuana are attributed to the 1-Δ-9-tetrahydrocannabinol (THC). A moderate dose of marijuana produces euphoria followed by sleepiness. Higher doses produce hallucinations and delusions.[4] Tachycardia and postural hypotension may occur. THC increases the circulating blood volume by a mechanism that is not understood and it also decreases sweating.[4] Smoking marijuana causes bronchitis and asthma-like syndrome.[4] Tolerance usually develops and sudden withdrawal may result in nervousness, irritability, and insomnia.

Marijuana use is not uncommon among pregnant women.[26,27] Chronic use is associated with premature or precipitate labor and increased incidence of fetal distress. There seems to be increased incidence of intrauterine growth retardation. The babies may have altered response to photic stimulation; altered neurobehavior, as judged by the Brazelton scale; and a peculiar high-pitched cry (cri de chat).[27] A teratogenic effect resembling fetal alcohol syndrome is also described.[27]

PSYCHEDELICS

Lysergic Acid Diethylamide (LSD)

Lysergic acid diethylamide (LSD) produces hallucinations, which may last for hours. The central effects are believed to be mediated by the effects of LSD on the tryptaminergic raphe neurons of the midbrain.[4] Occasionally, the individual may experience a terrifying hallucination, (often referred to as "bad trip"). These experiences may subsequently occur spontaneously, without being provoked by the drug.[28] This is referred to as "flash back" syndrome, which may be exacerbated by the phenothiazine exposure, psychic trauma or the use of alcohol. The syndrome has been reported to occur in the postoperative period also.[29] LSD and related compounds possess in vitro anticholinesterase activity. Thus, there exists a theoretical possibility that the duration of ester drugs may be prolonged in chronic LSD users.[29]

Phencyclidines

Phencyclidines (angel dust) are also abused by pregnant patients. The drugs may be smoked, ingested, or administered intravenously.[5] Users may exhibit catatonic muscular rigidity, sweating, and a neurodissociative state. Phencyclidine prevents the reuptake of dopamine, 5-OH-tryptamine and norepinephrine by synaptosomes.[4] The presence of a PCP receptor has been postulated and this receptor is believed to resemble the σ-opioid receptor.[4] Abrupt withdrawal leads to fear and facial twitching. The infants of mothers who use the drug often manifest neurobehavior changes.[4] Phencyclidine overdose may result in coma, convulsions, respiratory depression, hyperthermia, hypertension, and possible intracranial hemorrhage.[5] Acidification of urine hastens renal excretion of the drug. For the treatment of acute psychosis associated with phencyclidine use, phenothiazines must not be used, because they may potentiate the anticholinergic effect of the agent.[5] Haloperidol is a better choice.[5]

REFERENCES

1. Rosett HL, and Weiner L: Alcohol and pregnancy: A clinical perspective. Ann Rev Med 36:73, 1985.

2. Kruse J: Alcohol use during pregnancy. AFP 29:199, 1984.

3. Mills JL, et al.: Maternal alcohol consumption and birth weight. JAMA 252:1875, 1984.

4. Jaffe JH: Drug addiction and drug abuse. *In* The Pharmacologic Basis of Therapeutics. (Edited by Gilman AG, Goodman LS, Rall TW, and Murad F). New York, Macmillan Publishing, 1985.

5. Petersdorf RG, et al.: Harrison's Principles of Internal Medicine. New York, McGraw-Hill, 1983. pp 1278–1301.

6. Finnegan LP, Michael H, Leifer B, and Desai S: An evaluation of neonatal abstinence modalities. National Institute of Drug Abuse Research Monograph 49:282, 1983.

7. Dundee JW, and Gray TC: Resistance to d-tubocurarine chloride in the presence of liver damage. Lancet 2:16, 1957.

8. Duvaldestein P, et al.: Pancuronium pharmacokinetics in patients with liver cirrhosis. Br J Anaesth 50:1131, 1978.

9. Johnston RE, Kulp RA, and Smith TC: Effects of acute and chronic ethanol administration on isoflurane requirement in mice. Anesth Anal 54:277, 1975.

10. Bruce DL: Alcoholism and anesthesia. Anesth Analg 62:84, 1983.

11. Covino BG, and Vassallo HG: Local Anesthetics. Mechanism of Action and Clinical Use. New York, Grune and Stratton, 1976.

12. Jaffe JH, and Martin WR: Opioid analgesics and antagonists. *In* The Pharmacologic Basis of Therapeutics. (Edited by Gilman AG, Goodman LS, Rall TW, and Murad F.) New York, Macmillan Publishing, 1985.

13. Stimmel B, et al.: Fetal outcome in narcotic dependent women. Am J Drug Alcohol Abuse 9:383, 1982.

14. Ostrea EM, and Chavez CJ: Perinatal problems (excluding neonatal withdrawal) in maternal addiction: A study of 830 cases. J Pediatr 94:292, 1979.

15. Hutchings DE: Behavioral teratology: A new frontier in neurobehavioral research. *In* Teratogenesis and reproductive toxicology. Hand book of Experimental Pharmocology. (Edited by Johnson EM and Kochlar FM) New York, Springer Verlag, 1983.

16. Richardson BS, O'Grady JP, and Olsen GD: Fetal breathing movements and the response to carbon dioxide in patients on methadone maintenance. Am J Obstet Gynecol 150:400, 1984.

17. Weintraub SJ, and Naulty S: Acute abstinence syndrome after epidural injection of butorphanol. Anesth Analg 64:452, 1985.

18. Chasnoff IJ, Burns WJ, Schnoll SH, and Burns KA: Cocaine use in pregnancy. N Eng J Med 336:666, 1985.

19. Kleber HD, and Gawin FH: Cocaine abuse: A review of current and experimental treatments. *In* Cocaine: Pharmacology, Effects and Treatments of Abuse. National Institute of Drug Abuse Monograph Series, 1984.

20. Stoelting RK, Creasser CW, and Martz RC: Effects of cocaine administration on halothane MAC in dogs. Anesthesiology 54:422, 1975.

21. Johnsson S, O'Meara M, and Young JB: Acute cocaine poisoining. Importance of treating seizures and acidosis. Am J Med 75:1061, 1983.

22. Ellinwood EH, Jr: Amphetamines/anorectics. *In* Handbook on Drug Abuse. National Institute on Drug Abuse. U.S. Government Printing Office, Washington DC, 1979.

23. Johnston RR, Way WL, and Miller RD: Alteration of anesthetic requirement by amphetamine. Anesthesiology 36:357, 1972.

24. Samuels SI, Maze A, and Albright G: Cardiac arrest during section in a chronic amphetamine abuser. Anesth Analg 58:528, 1979.

25. Smith DS, and Gutsche BB: Amphetamine abuse and obstetrical anesthesia (letter). Anesth Analg 59:710, 1980.

26. Alpert J, et al.: Maternal alcohol consumption and newborn assessment. Neurobehav Toxicol Teratol 3:195, 1981.

27. Fried P: Marihuana use by pregnant women and effects on offspring: an update. Neurobehav Toxicol Teratol 3:195, 1983.

28. Abraham HD: Visual phenomenology of the LSD flash. Arch Gen Psychiatry 40:884, 1983.

29. Jenkins LC: Anesthetic problems due to drug abuse and dependence. Canad Anaesth Soc J 19:461, 1972.

III

THE NEONATE

CHAPTER 24

ASSESSMENT OF FETAL WELL-BEING

The last two decades have seen great advances in electronic monitoring, which have enabled obstetricians to assess the intrapartum and antepartum fetal well-being. Both biophysical and biochemical methods are used to assess fetal well-being. The anesthesiologist must be familiar not only with fetal responses to hypoxia but also with the different antepartum tests so that he may perform competently during the perinatal period.

INTRAPARTUM ASSESSMENT

The antepartum well-being of the fetus is mainly assessed by recording its heart rate during a uterine contraction and by measuring indices of anaerobic metabolism in the fetal scalp blood. It is necessary to monitor uterine contractions because they reduce uterine blood flow by decreasing uteroplacental perfusion pressure (mean arterial pressure–intra-amniotic pressure). The fetal heart rate may be monitored either noninvasively or invasively.[1] A Doppler transducer is used to record the fetal heart rate noninvasively. A metal spiral, or a clip electrode attached to the fetal scalp is used to monitor the fetal EKG invasively. Uterine activity is monitored externally by placing a tocotransducer on the maternal abdomen. A fluid-filled tube connected to a strain-gauge is used to monitor intraamniotic pressure invasively. Invasive monitoring can be instituted only when the cervix is at least 1 to 2 cm dilated and the presenting part is no higher than −2 station.[1]

THE DOPPLER TRANSDUCER

Johann Christian Doppler first described the Doppler effect in 1842. There was little practical application of the Doppler effect until sonar was developed during World War I. The Doppler effect simply states that the frequency of emitted or reflected sound is affected by the motion of the object that is emitting or reflecting the sound waves.[2] When the object moves toward the observer, the sound is high pitched because the frequency increases. When the object moves away, the sound becomes low-pitched. Similarly, in the case of reflected frequency, the frequency will increase when the reflector moves toward the observer and will decrease when the reflector moves away (Fig. 24–1). The Doppler transducer, when placed on the maternal abdomen, emits an ultrasound wave with a frequency of 2 MHz. The moving myocardium, the valve leaflets, and blood flow in the ventricular outflow tracts reflect the frequency back to the transducer (which is now in the receiving mode). There will be an apparent increase in the frequency of the reflected ultrasound because of the Doppler effect. The difference between the reflected and emitted frequency is the Doppler signal.[2] The Doppler signal can be detected us-

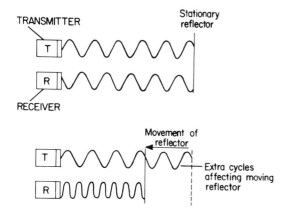

FIG. 24–1.   The Doppler effect: When the reflector is stationary the reflected frequency is similar to the frequency emitted by the transmitter. When the reflector moves towards the transmitter, however, the reflected frequency seems to increase (Doppler effect). (From Sykes MK, Vickers MD, Hull GJ, and Winterburn PJ: Principles of Clinical Measurement. London, Blackwell Scientific Publications, 1981.)

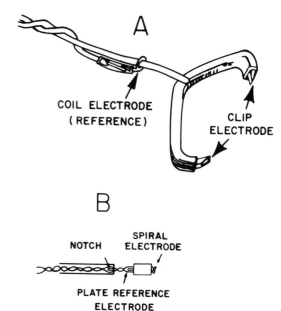

FIG. 24–2.   Scalp electrodes for monitoring fetal EKG. (From Hon EH: An Introduction to Fetal Monitoring. 2nd Edition. Los Angeles, UCLA, Monograph, 1975 [Personal communication]).

ing the heterodyne principle utilizing simple demodulation. The Doppler signal is usually in the audible range (20 to 20,000 Hz) and may therefore be used to drive a loud speaker. The unit demodulates only the spectrum reflected by the valve surfaces. The signal also triggers the cardiotachometer.

Theoretically speaking, motion during systole and diastole may produce two triggering signals that may falsely double the heart rate.[3] To avoid this, the unit automatically goes into a refractory period after each trigger signal is received.[3] Transducers with single crystals are in emission mode only briefly, following which they go into a receiving mode. In the clover-leaf design the receiving crystal is in the center of the transducer and the transmitting crystals are situated on the three sections of the clover-leaf. Such a design is said to minimize loss of signal when the fetus moves.

The major advantage of the Doppler cardiotachometry is that it is noninvasive. However, it is associated with certain disadvantages. The tracing is unsatisifactory in obese patients. The signal may be lost when the mother or the fetus moves. Because the reflected frequency activates the cardiotachometer the triggering may not occur at the same point at each systole, thus it may artificially increase variability.[3] Some units use logic circuits to average the intervals

of the three immediately preceding beats to calculate the rate.[3] Thus, the variability is not really a beat-to-beat variability. Invasive fetal EKG monitoring is required to confirm changes in baseline variability. Two Doppler transducers should not be used simultaneously to record the fetal heart rates of twin fetuses. The frequency reflected by one fetus may be received by the other transducer, leading to erroneous rate calculation. An internal EKG electrode and an external monitor must be used under these circumstances.[3]

INVASIVE MONITORING OF THE FETAL HEART RATE

The fetal heart rate is monitored invasively using a spiral or a clip electrode attached to the fetal scalp (Fig. 24–2). The voltage generated by the fetal myocardium is amplified severalfold by the unit. The intervals between the two consecutive R waves is used to compute the rate. The circuitry uses an automatic gain control to assure near constant voltages of the trigger pulses, regardless of the voltage of the fetal signal.[3] Occasionally the automatic gain control will increase the amplifier gain, especially when the fetal signal is not detectable. Under these circumstances, there is a possibility that any noise artefact may be amplified to a trigger signal, thus resulting in an erroneous reading. To ensure proper function, the connecting plate must be grounded to the maternal thigh (Fig. 24–3).

TOCODYNAMOMETRY

The tocotransducer, a type of force-displacement transducer is used to obtain a noninvasive record of uterine contractions. The hardening uterus displaces a pressure-sensitive projection inward, thus generating a signal. The tocotransducer tracing is at best only qualitative and is not suitable for quantitating uterine activity.

INTERNAL UTERINE PRESSURE MONITORING

This is done by introducing a fluid-filled catheter into the amniotic sac (Fig. 24–3). The free end of the catheter is attached to a previously calibrated transducer. In order to obtain accurate measurements, the transducer must be placed at the level of the patient's xiphoid process. All air bubbles must be excluded from the system. In the early latent phase, the baseline intraamniotic pressure is <5mm Hg but increases to 10 to 12 mm Hg in the active phase. The peak pressure may increase 20 to 30 mm Hg above the baseline pressure at the onset of

first stage, 40 to 50 mm Hg above baseline, in the active phase, and 100 mm Hg above baseline in the second stage, especially during bearing-down efforts.[4]

FETAL HEART RATE RESPONSES TO HYPOXIA

The fetal heart rate is 175 beats per minute in very early pregnancy and decreases as gestation progresses.[5] The normal heart rate for a term fetus is usually between 120 and 160 beats per minute. The fetal heart receives both sympathetic and parasympathetic innervation starting at the 10th week of gestation. The fetal heart rate is also influenced by baroceptor and chemoreceptor mechanisms.[5] The chemoreceptors are of two types: peripheral (carotid and aortic bodies) and central (medulla oblongata) receptors. The medullary chemoreceptors cause tachycardia and hypertension in response to hypoxia, whereas the aortic chemoreceptors cause bradycardia in response to hypoxia.[5] The medulla oblongata exercises the final control not only over the heart rate but also over the fetal heart rate variability. When fetal oxygen supply is severely curtailed, the final response in the fetal heart rate is bradycardia. Subtle differences may be seen, however, in the manner with which bradycardia develops with different conditions. For instance, when hypoxia is caused by re-

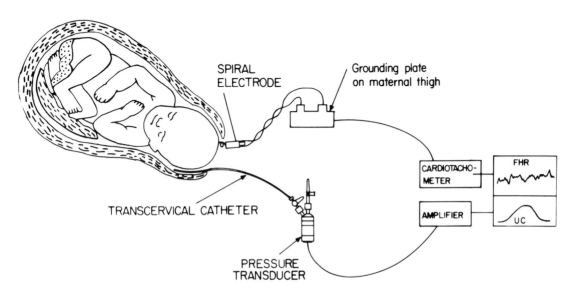

FIG. 24–3. Invasive monitoring of fetal EKG and intraamniotic pressure during labor. FHR-fetal heart rate. UC-uterine contraction.

duced placental oxygen transfer, late decelerations develop because of vagal responses mediated by peripheral chemoreceptors.[5] However, because the fetus is able to maintain myocardial oxygen supply by preferentially redistributing its blood supply (see Chapter 3), the short-term variability of the fetal heart rate will be maintained.[5] When hypoxia is prolonged, however, the short-term variability (see the following section) will usually be lost because of hypoxic myocardial depression.[5,6]

If, however, fetal hypoxia is caused by umbilical cord compression, the heart rate will increase transiently because the compression of the umbilical vein (UV) will decrease the cardiac preload, resulting in tachycardia.[5] As the process of cord compression becomes more complete during the course of a contraction, hypertension develops, which causes bradycardia through the baroceptor mechanism. When the compression is relieved, the heart rate returns to baseline after a brief overshoot. Should hypoxia also ensue during cord compression, the bradycardia will be much more severe because of the chemoreceptor mediated vagal inhibition of the heart.[5] For a discussion of oxygen reserve in the fetus see Chapter 3.

THE NORMAL FETAL HEART RATE

The normal fetal heart rate is usually between 120 and 160 beats per minute. When recorded on chart paper, it has an irregular saw-tooth pattern resulting from constantly changing R-R intervals (Fig. 24–4). This is called the baseline variability. The problem associated with using a Doppler signal to detect baseline variability has already been discussed. The presence of spontaneous accelerations is not unusual and is indeed a sign of fetal well-being (Fig. 24–4).

The baseline variability is of two types: 1) short-term variability and 2) long-term variability. The short-term variability consists of fluctuations (± 10 beats per minute) in heart rate from beat to beat. Long-term variability consists of changes in heart rate occurring in cycles 2 to 6 times a minute.[8] The variability is caused by vagal impulses reaching the heart from the medulla. The presence of good variability signifies fetal well-being.

ABNORMAL FETAL HEART RATE TRACING

Early Deceleration. The decrease in heart rate is cause by increased vagal activity from the compression of the fetal head against the maternal pelvis.[7] The fetal heart rate decreases 10 to 30 beats per minute starting during a contraction. The tracing is U-shaped and reaches nadir at the peak of the concentration but recovers at or before the end of contraction (Fig. 24–5A).[7]

Baseline Bradycardia. The heart rate remains consistently below 120 beats per minute. Idiopathic sinus bradycardia may be seen in postterm healthy fetuses. No undue concern is necessary if the tracing shows good variability.[9] Other causes of consistent bradycardia are maternal β-adrenergic blocker therapy, severe maternal hypothermia and reduced uterine blood flow (variability may be reduced). If the slow heart rate is caused by a cardiac pacemaker that affects other than the sinoatrial node, the variability is usually diminished.[9] Persistent bradycardia caused by atrio-ventricular conduction block may be associated with maternal systemic lupus erythematosus (see Chapter 22) and heart block produced by cytomegalovirus infection and congenital conduction defects (50 to 70 beats per minute).[9]

Baseline Tachycardia. The fetal heart rate decreases with advancing gestational age. The common causes of fetal tachycardia include maternal sepsis (chorioamnionitis) or fetal infection, as well as the maternal use of atropine and sympathomimetic substances (ritodrine, terbutaline) and maternal thyrotoxicosis.[9] Worrisome tachycardia is also caused by severe fetal hypoxia and acidosis. The triad of tachycardia, diminished variability, and subtle late decelerations signifies advanced fetal acidosis and calls for immediate action. Occasionally, rapid supraventricular tachycardia may be seen with fetal congestive heart failure, hydrops fetalis, and atrial fibrillation with a rapid ventricular response.[10]

Variable Decelerations. These are the most common form of fetal heart decelerations (Fig. 24–5C,D). The decelerations are produced by umbilical cord compression. The effect of umbilical cord compression on the fetal chemo- and baroceptor responses have been discussed in this chapter under the section on fetal heart rate

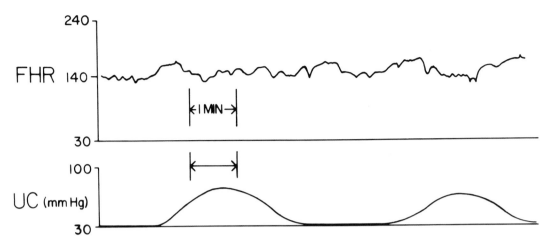

FIG. 24–4.   Normal fetal heart rate (FHR) tracing. Note the saw tooth pattern of the variable baseline. UC-uterine contraction. (From Polin JI, and Frangipane L: Current concepts in the management of obstetric problems for pediatricians: 1. Monitoring the high risk fetus. Ped Clin N 33:621, 1986.)

responses to hypoxia. The variable decelerations start abruptly and recover quickly. Unlike early and late decelerations, variable decelerations do not bear a constant temporal relationship to uterine contractions from one complex to the next. Obviously, the umbilical cord is subject to increased compression in patients with oligo-hydramnios because of diminished fluid buffer.[11] If the deceleration lasts longer than 60 seconds and the heart rate decreases below 70 beats per minute, the deceleration is considered to be severe.[12] Under these circumstances the fetal scalp blood pH is likely to be less than 7.15. When the decelerations last less than 60 sec and/or

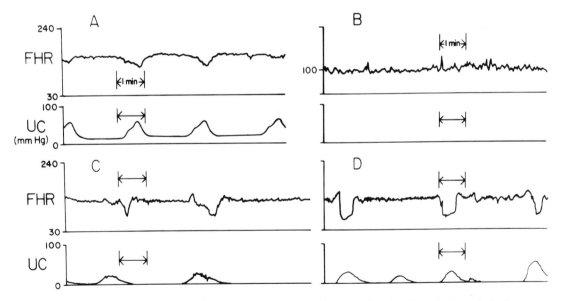

FIG. 24–5.   Periodic decelerations. (A) Early deceleration. Note the deceleration starts early in the course of the contraction and recovers before the end of contraction. (B) Idiopathic sinus bradycardia with good baseline variability. Reproduced with kind permission from Cohen WR and Clin Obstet Gynecol.[9] (C) Variable deceleration with a late component. (D) Variable deceleration with an early component. ((A and D): from Gross TL, Sokol RJ, and Rosen MG: Clinical use of intrapartum monitoring record. Clin Obstet Gynecol, 22:634, 1979. (B): from Cohen WR and Yeh S: The abnormal fetal heart rate baseline. Clin Obstet Gynecol 29:73, 1986. (C): Schneider E, and Tropper PJ: The variable deceleration, prolonged deceleration, and sinusoidial fetal heart rate. Clin Obstet Gynecol 29:64, 1986.)

when the heart beat dose not decrease below 70 beats per minute, the scalp blood pH is usually greater than 7.25.[12] Variable decelerations are likely to start during second stage because the umbilical cord is more likely to be more compressed by the descending fetal part.[11] When there is delayed recovery of the fetal heart rate, when loss of baseline variability is lost and/or when the severity of decelerations increase progressively, fetal scalp blood pH must be measured.

Loss of Baseline Variability (Fig. 24–6A). An internal monitor must be used when doubt exists to the presence or absence of baseline variability. Although baseline variability decreases during fetal sleep, it is never completely lost. Preterm fetuses have a less variable baseline than do term fetuses.[9] Loss of baseline variability may be caused by hypoxic and nonhypoxic factors. The fetuses with diminished variability have a lower scalp blood pH than do those with normal variability.[13] In hypoxic fetuses, late decelerations are particularly ominous when they occur in combination with loss of baseline variability (Fig. 24–6B). Nonhypoxic causes for loss of baseline variability include maternal administration of central nervous system depressants (meperidine, barbiturates, diazepam, alphaprodine, and general anesthestics). Drug induced loss of baseline variability is transient and is not accompanied by periodic decelerations.

Late Decelerations. Late decelerations are perhaps the most serious of all decelerations because they are caused by uteroplacental insufficiency. The decelerations commence typically following a delay of 15 seconds or greater after the contraction has reached its peak (Fig. 24–6B).[7] Because maximum reduction in uteroplacental blood flow occurs only at the height of the contraction, the onset of deceleration is delayed until the intraamniotic pressure has reached the peak. Any factor that reduces uteroplacental blood flow can cause late deceleration. Maternal hypotension caused by regional anesthesia, excessive stimulation by oxytocin and maternal supine position can cause late deceleration.[7] Certain simple corrective measures may be effective in treating late decelerations: (1) turning the patient on her side; (2) discontinuing oxytocin administration; (3) increasing the rate of intravenous fluid administration in order to improve circulating blood volume; and (4) administration of oxygen to the mother (Fig. 24–7).[1] When late decelerations occur repeatedly, further management must be based on fetal scalp blood pH determination.

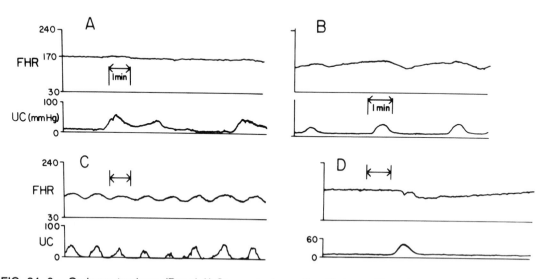

FIG. 24–6.   Ominous tracings. (Panel A) Severe tachycardia with loss of baseline variability. Reproduced with kind permission from Cohen WR and Clin Obstet Gynecol.[9] (Panel B) Loss of baseline variability with late deceleration. (From Gross TL, Sokol RJ, and Rosen MG: Clinical use of intrapartum monitoring record. Clin Obstet Gynecol 22:634, 1979. (Panel C) Sinusoidal heart rate pattern. (From Gimovsky ML, and Bruce SL: Aspects of FHR tracings as warning signals. Clin Obstet Gynecol 29:51, 1986.) (Panel D) Impending fetal death. Note flat tracing with smooth late deceleration. (From Tushuizen PBT, Stoot JEGM, and Ubachs JMH: Fetal heart monitoring of the dying fetus. AM J Obstet Gynecol 120:922, 1974.)

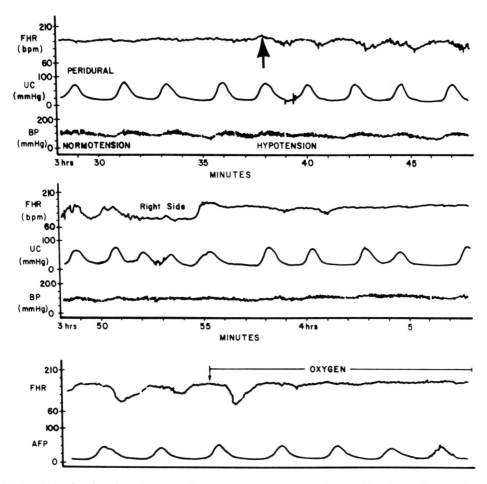

FIG. 24–7.   Late deceleration due to maternal hypotension caused by epidural anesthesia. Turning the patient on her side seems to improve FHR (middle panel). Termination of late deceleration by oxygen (bottom panel). (From Hon EH: An introduction to Fetal Monitoring. 2nd Edition. Monograph, 1975.)

Prolonged Decelerations. A prolonged deceleration is defined as a decrease of 30 beats per minute or more lasting 2 minutes or longer.[8] Severe fetal hypoxia, local anesthetic toxicity (paracervical block), oxytocin-induced tetanic uterine contraction, umbilical cord prolapse, and (rarely) vasa previa that cause sudden fetal hemorrhage may result in prolonged decelerations.[11]

Sinusoidal Pattern (Fig. 24–6C). The tracing assumes an undulant pattern. The characteristic pattern is believed to be caused by the loss of short-term variability with preservation of uniform long-term variability.[14] Severe Rh-isoimmunization, fetal anemia, vasa previa, and fetal acidosis may produce this pattern. Administration of alphaprodine may also cause this pattern to occur but is not usually associated with fetal morbidity. Tissue hypoxia of the medullary car-

diac center is believed to play a role in the genesis of this pattern.[14]

Terminal Pattern. Many fetuses develop prolonged bradycardia before death. The period of bradycardia may be preceded by a period of severe tachycardia loss of baseline variability, or severe variable or late decelerations (Fig. 24–6D).[15] If fetal hypoxia is not corrected quickly, the decelerations become more frequent and severe and deteriorate to the terminal pattern. The best method of diagnosing fetal death is verification of absent fetal heart motion with real-time ultrasonography.

ASSESSMENT OF BIOCHEMICAL FETAL WELL-BEING

During severe hypoxia the fetus has to depend on anaerobic metabolism to fulfill its energy

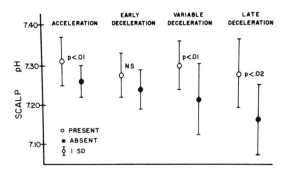

FIG. 24–8. Fetal scalp pH with different periodic heart rate pattern in the presence and absence of variability. (From Zanini B, Paul RH, and Huey JR: Intrapartum fetal heart rate: correlation with scalp pH in the preterm fetus. Am J Obstet Gynecol, 136:43, 1980.)

needs. Since the end product of anaerobic metabolism is lactic acid, the fetal blood pH decreases. To collect fetal blood, the presenting part is exposed with an amnioscope, a small incision is made on the fetal scalp with a special scalpel, and the blood is collected into a preheparinized capillary tube. Special equipment, capable of measuring pH on microsamples are now available. Even a portable device with a disposable cartridge for measuring pH is now used in many centers. The scalp blood pH reflects fetal tissue pH.

The normal scalp blood pH is between 7.25 and 7.35. Values between 7.25 and 7.20 are considered preacidotic and values <7.20 are definitely acidotic. A value of 7.20 calls for a repeat measurement within 15 minutes. If the repeat measurement remains the same or shows further deterioration, immediate action is necessary.[7] Although it is tempting to postulate that a combination of blood pH and lactate may be more predictive of fetal outcome, well-controlled studies have shown that the discriminating powers of the two parameters were not significantly different from one another and that the combination of the two parameters was not more predictive of fetal outcome than was either one of the parameters alone.[16] Late deceleration occurring in combination with lost variability is perhaps associated with worst fetal acidosis (Fig. 24–8).[17] A scalp blood pH of 7.22 signifies that the one-minute Apgar score may be 6 or less. Judged by the clinical condition of the baby at one minute, the fetal blood pH will be falsely

abnormal only in 8% of cases, and falsely normal only in 10% of cases.[18]

RELIABILITY OF FETAL MONITORING

One may be able to predict normal Apgar scores in up to 95% of fetuses when their intrapartum tracings are within normal limits.[3] The diagnostic accuracy depends on the interpreter and the addition of fetal scalp blood pH improves accuracy. In order to obtain reliable information, several complexes must be reviewed. The accuracy dramatically decreases to 50% with abnormal intrapartum tracings associated with evidence of loss baseline variability and other periodic decelerations. Maternal acidosis may cause a falsely low fetal pH.[3] Some of the falsely abnormal cases may be eliminated by a concomitant measurement of maternal arterial blood pH. The cesarean section rate approaches a disturbingly high 25% in some institutions. Some argue that the increased cesarean section rate is a direct result of easy availability of fetal monitoring; it must be pointed out, however, that the diagnosis of fetal distress is the main indicator for cesarean section in only 1% of all the cesarean sections performed in this country.[3,19] The majority of cesarean sections are performed for breech, cephalopelvic disproportions, and for previous cesarean sections. It must, however, be pointed out that in many instances of abnormal fetal heart tracing, measurement of fetal blood pH will help avoid an unnecessary cesarean section.

Continuous electronic fetal monitoring is a sensitive implement for detecting fetal distress. Although the technique may not appreciably reduce the perinatal mortality, it may decrease perinatal morbidity. It was recently reported that the incidence of convulsions was higher in neonates who were monitored with intermittent auscultation during labor than in those who were continuously monitored electronically, signifying undetected intrapartum hypoxia in those who were not continuously monitored.[20]

One must exercise caution in interpreting tracings from postterm neonates because the responses of a postterm neonate to hypoxia differs considerably from those of a term neonate. Perinatal mortality rate increases when gestation is prolonged beyond 42 weeks. Oligohydramnios is common, which puts the fetus at increased

Table 24–1.   Antepartum Fetal Assessment

Test types	Specific tests
Biophysical	Nonstress test. Contraction stress test.* Fetal breathing movement. Fetal body movement. Fetal tone. Amniotic fluid volume.
Biochemical	Lecithin-Sphingomyelin ratio. Urinary estriols. Human placental lactogen.

*–Is not included in the fetal biophysical profile

risk for cord compression. Placental aging further jeopardizes fetal well-being. The heart rate tends to decrease as the gestational age advances, therefore a heart rate of 150 may be considered abnormal in the postterm neonate.[21] An acidotic postterm fetus may pass meconium but may not exhibit the typical late deceleration or the tachycardia. Therefore, a fetal heart tracing even with the slightest abnormality must be persued vigorously and intrapartum hypoxia must be ruled out by measuring scalp blood pH. On the contrary, the preterm fetus responds to hypoxia much in the same way as a term fetus does. However, it has diminished baseline variability.[9] Because the preterm fetus has diminished reserve, it is more likely to benefit from electronic monitoring than the full-term fetus.[3] Continuous fetal scalp pH and P_{O_2} monitoring are new methods that are currently being investigated. Fetal heart rate may also be recorded using phonocardiography and abdominal EKG, but none of the newer methods offers any proven advantage over the methods already established.

ANTEPARTUM FETAL SURVEILLANCE

The fetal well-being may be assessed in the antepartum period by using a battery of tests (Table 24–1). There is no consensus as to which test is the most reliable. However, many feel that combining many tests (Table 24–1) increases accuracy. Both biophysical and biochemical methods are used to assess fetal well-being. A biophysical profile that uses several tests has been claimed to be useful.[7]

BIOPHYSICAL TESTS

Nonstress Test (NST). The fetus is monitored with a Doppler sensor. The fetal heart rate should accelerate with fetal body motion, which is felt by the mother (Fig. 24–9A). If the heart rate accelerates by 15 beats per minute lasting 15 to 20 seconds for at least four times following fetal movement, the test is considered reactive. The test is nonreactive if the accelerations are fewer than four and accelerations are smaller than 15 beats and last <15 seconds (Fig. 24–9B). The total period of observation lasts 20 minutes.[7] Although used extensively, the predictive value of NST is suspect. In diabetic and postdate pregnancies, one should not rely solely on NST for assessing fetal well-being.[7] At best it can be considered a screening test for further assessment. A nonreactive test must be further investigated by contraction stress test (CST) or by fetal biophysical profile. The NST is of limited usefulness in fetuses less than 32 weeks gestation because their central nervous system is too immature to respond with accelerations.[7]

Contraction Stress Testing. Contraction stress testing (CST) is more accurate in identifying fetuses at risk for uteroplacental insufficiency than is NST.[22] When the NST is nonreactive and the contraction stress test is positive, poorest fetal outcome may be expected. To perform the test, uterine contractions are stimulated either by using oxytocin or by asking the patient to massage her nipples. A set of at least 3 contractions in a 10 minute period is necessary to stress the fetus adequately.[7] If late decelerations appear with most contractions, the CST is considered positive (Fig. 24–9C, D). If only occasional late deceleration appears, the test is considered suspicious.[7] Because the CST yields a low false-negative result, the clinician may be fairly certain that the fetus is in good health if the CST is negative.[7] If the test is positive and the fetal heart rate does not show variability at all, the baby must be delivered at the earliest opportunity. If the test is positive but the heart rate shows good variability, other diagnostic tests must be undertaken (biophysical profile).

Fetal Breathing Movement. Fetal breathing movements (FBM) are considered a reliable sign of fetal well-being. The fetal respiratory activity is controlled by the low-voltage cerebral activity.

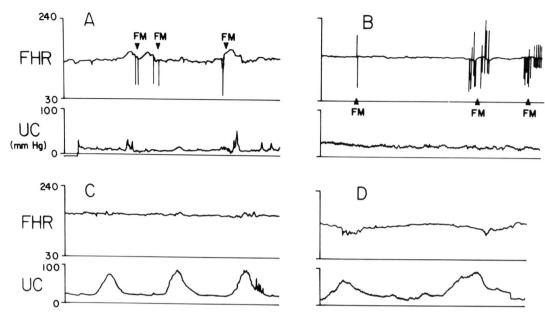

FIG. 24–9. Antepartum fetal surveillance. (A): reactive nonstress test (NST). Note the acceleration with each fetal movement (FM). (B): nonreactive NST. No fetal heart acceleration is noticed with each FM. (C): negative oxytocin challenge test (OCT). No late decelerations are seen with each uterine contraction. (D): positive OCT. Note the development of late decelerations with each uterine contraction. (From Jarrell SE, and Sokol RJ: Clinical use of stressed and nonstressed monitoring techniques. Clin Obstet Gynecol, 22:617, 1979.)

(For the relationship between maternal glucose level and fetal breathing activity see Fig. 3–14. The fetal breathing activity is detected using real-time ultrasonography. It is present from the 20th week of gestation. Human FBM are episodic. Over a 24-hour period they are present 30% of the time. When respiratory activity is present the interbreath interval is 1 to 1.5 seconds in a term fetus and < 1 second in a preterm fetus (faster rate).[23] The apneic intervals may last as long as 122 minutes in term fetuses. Increased activity may be noticed 2 to 3 hours following a maternal meal. The FBM decreases between 9 P.M. and 1 A.M. and increases between 4 A.M. and 7 A.M. signifying a circadian rhythm.[23] In the three days preceding the onset of spontaneous labor and during active labor, the FBM decreases. Maternal alcohol consumption, cigarette smoking, and drug intake may diminish the FBM.[23]

The predictive value of FBM increases when it is used in combination with other tests. The 5 minute Apgar scores may be expected to be less than 7 in 50% of fetuses without FBM, but would be low in only 4% of fetuses with FBM.[24]

The incidence of fetal distress also increases in those fetuses who do not have FBM.[24]

Fetal Body Movement. Mothers notice fetal body movement at 20 weeks of gestation. The test is simple to perform. A sudden decrease in the number of movements, compared to the previous day, requires further active evaluation.[25] When no movements are felt in a 12 hour period, immediate delivery is indicated.[7] Fetal movement rates are influenced by the time of the day, the gestational age (strong rolling body motion are noted at 36 to 38 weeks), and maternal drug intake.[26]

Other Components of the Biophysical Profile. Two other components of a biophysical profile are fetal tone and the volume of amniotic fluid.

When the fetus has normal muscle tone, both his limbs, his head, and trunk are held in flexion. The fetus periodically extends the body and limbs, but he returns them to flexion. The tone is said to be diminished when only trunk flexion is present.

The volume of amniotic fluid is considered to be adequate when the amniotic fluid is detected all through the amniotic cavity and the largest fluid pocket is at least 1 cm in its widest plane.[7,27]

COMPLETE FETAL BIOPHYSICAL PROFILE

All the biophysical variables described above may be used to construct a fetal biophysical profile (Table 24–2).[7,27] When the total biophysical score is 10, the perinatal mortality rate will be 0.3 deaths per 1000 livebirths (a false negative rate). When the score is less than 4, the perinatal mortality may reach 292 deaths per 1000 live births.[27] The accuracy of the test is comparable to contraction stress testing.[7]

BIOCHEMICAL TESTING

Estriol Measurement. The production of estriol from the fetal precursor 16-α-OH-dihydroepiandrosterone has been discussed in Chapter 3. Although both placenta and the fetus contribute to the estriol found in the mother, the measurement of estriol is more predictive of fetal compromise than it is of placental function. Estriol may be measured in maternal plasma or in a 24-hour maternal urine sample. The plasma values are easier to measure and are not dependent on maternal renal function. Because estriol levels fluctuate widely, no norms have been established. A single measurement is therefore not reliable. A sudden decrease from the previous day's value either in urine or plasma value is more diagnostic than a single value.

Measurement of estriol is not useful in all high-risk situations. For instance, the measurement cannot identify a distressed twin-fetus when the other twin is normal. It also is not useful in cases of RH-isoimmunization because the estriol levels are usually within normal limits.[7] Similarly, it is not useful in managing growth-retarded fetuses. Estriols are, however, helpful in managing postterm and diabetic pregnancies. In postterm pregnancies, a plasma value of <12 μg/ml predicts poor outcome. A 40% decrease in the level of unconjugated plasma estriol level signifies poor fetal outcome in patients with diabetes mellitus.[7]

Human Placental Lactogen (HPL). The placental production of this hormone has been discussed in Chapter 3. In general, the measurement of HPL does not aid in predicting outcome or in deciding when to intervene. The test has been abandoned as a diagnostic tool.[7]

Lecithin-sphingomyelin Concentration Ratio (L/S Ratio). The measurement of L/S concentration ratio is the amniotic fluid is widely used in predicting fetal lung maturity. The ratio, which is a measure of the activity of the surfactant function of the fetal lung, may be measured using thin-layer chromatography. The use of the test in diabetic pregnancies is discussed in Chapter 14. Between the 32nd and 34th weeks of a normal pregnancy, the concentration of lecithin increases abruptly in comparison to that of sphingomyelin. This results in an L/S ration that may reach 8:1 in normal pregnancies. If the ratio is at least 2, the chances of the neonate developing RDS is less than 2.2%. If the ratio is less than 1.5, the chances of RDS increases to 73%, and at a ratio 1.5 to 1.9, the risk reaches 50% (transitional zone).[28] The biosynthesis and function of the surfactant is discussed in greater detail in Chapter 25.

REFERENCES

1. Hon EH: An Introduction to Fetal Heart Rate Monitoring. 2nd Edition. Los Angles, UCLA, Monograph, 1975, (Personal communication).

Table 24–2. Fetal Biophysical Profile

Test	Score 2	Score 0
Fetal breathing movements	At least 1 episode lasting 30 sec in 30 min.	Absent or none in 30 sec.
Body movement	At least 3 movements/30 min.	<2.
Fetal tone	At least 1 extension of limbs and trunk returning to flexion.	Slow extension. Partial flexion. Absent movement.
NST	At least 2 episodes of FHR acceleration.	<2.
Amniotic fluid volume	Sufficient.	Inadequate.

Source: Manning FA.[27]

2. Sykes MK, Vickers MD, Hull CJ, and Winterburn PJ: Principles of Clinical Measurement. London, Blackwell Scientific, 1981.

3. Hutson JM, and Petrie RH: Possible limitations of fetal monitoring. Clin Obstet Gynecol 29:104, 1986.

4. Silverman F, and Hutson JM: The clinical and biological significance of the bottom line. Clin Obstet Gynecol 29:43, 1986.

5. Campbell WA, Vintzileos AM, and Nochimson DJ: Intrauterine versus extrauterine management/resuscitation of the fetus/neonate. Clin Obstet Gynecol 29:33, 1986.

6. Harris JL, Krueger TR, and Parer JT: Mechansisms of late decelerations of the fetal heart rate during hypoxia. Am J Obstet Gynecol 144:491, 1982.

7. Polin JI, and Frangipane L: Current concepts in the management of obstetric problems for pediatricians: 1. Monitoring the high risk fetus. Ped Clin North Am 33:621, 1986.

8. Quirk JG, Jr. and Miller FC: FHR tracing characteristics that jeopardize the diagnosis of fetal well-being. Clin Obstet Gynecol 29:12, 1986.

9. Cohen WR, and Yeh S: The abnormal fetal heart rate baseline. Clin Obstet Gynecol 29:73, 1986.

10. Beall MH, and Paul RH: Artifacts, blocks, and arrhythmias: Confusing nonclassical heart rate tracings. Clin Obstet Gynecol 29:83, 1986.

11. Schneider E, and Tropper PJ: The variable deceleration, prolonged deceleration, and sinusoidal fetal heart rate. Clin Obstet Gynecol 29:64, 1986.

12. Kubli FW, Hon EH, Khazin AF, and Takemura H: Observations on heart rate and pH in the human fetus during labor. Am J Obstet Gynecol 104:1190, 1969.

13. Paul RH, et al.: Clinical fetal monitoring III: The evaluation and significance of intrapartum baseline FHR variability. Am J Obstet Gynecol 123:206, 1975.

14. Modanlou HD, and Freeman RK: Sinusoidal fetal heart rate pattern: Its definition and clinical significance. Am J Obstet Gynecol 142:1033, 1982.

15. LaSala AP, and Strassner H: Fetal death. Clin Obstet Gynecol 29:95, 1986.

16. Suidan JS, and Young BK: Outcome of fetuses with lactic acidemia. Am J Obstet Gynecol 150:33, 1984.

17. Zanini B, Paul RH, and Huey JR: Intrapartum fetal heart rate: Correlation with scalp pH in the preterm fetus. Am J Obstet Gynecol 136:43, 1980.

18. Bowe ET, et al.: Reliability of fetal blood sampling. Am J Obstet Gynecol 107:279, 1970.

19. Zalar RW, and Quilligan EJ: The influence of scalp sampling on the cesarean section rate for fetal distress. Am J Obstet Gynecol 135:239, 1979.

20. Boylan P, et al.: The Dublin fetal monitoring trial (Abstract). Society of Perinatal Obstetricians, 1984.

21. Gimovsky ML, and Bruce SL: Aspects of FHR tracings as warning signals. Clin Obstet Gynecol 29:51, 1986.

22. Freeman RK, Anderson G, and Dorchester W: A prospective multi-institutional study of antepartum fetal heart rate monitoring: II Contraction stress test versus nonstress test for primary surveillance. Am J Obstet Gynecol 143:778, 1982.

23. Patrick J, and Challis J: Measurements of fetal breathing movements in healthy pregnancies using real-time scanner. Seminar Perinatol 4:275, 1980.

24. Platt LD, Manning FA, Lemay M, and Sipos L: Human fetal breathing: relationship to fetal condition. Am J Obstet Gynecol 132:514, 1978.

25. Pearson JF, and Weaver JB: Fetal activity and fetal wellbeing: An evaluation. Br Med J 1:1305, 1976.

26. Reece EA, Antoine C, and Montgomery J: The fetus as the final arbiter stress/distress. Clin Obstet Gynecol 29:23, 1986.

27. Manning FA: Assessment of fetal condition and risk: Analysis of single and combined biophysical variable monitoring. Seminar Perinatol 9:168, 1985.

28. Harvey D, Parkinson CE, and Campbell S: Risk of respiratory distress syndrome. Lancet 1:42, 1975.

25

NORMAL AND DEPRESSED NEONATE

Although most neonates require only the use of a bulb syringe for the clearing of secretions from the upper airway, some neonates require extensive resuscitation. The resuscitation of a depressed neonate must be performed by a team of at least two physicians skilled in this field. Under ideal circumstances, the physicians in charge of the neonate should not have any other clinical responsibility. When these conditions cannot be met, the most experienced person must perform the resuscitation. The neonate's ability to adopt to extrauterine life depends on the uninterrupted occurrence of a series of changes in its cardiovascular and respiratory system.

NEONATAL ADAPTATION TO EXTRAUTERINE LIFE

CHANGES IN THE CARDIOVASCULAR SYSTEM

The fetus does not use its lungs for the purposes of oxygenation; therefore up to 90% of the right ventricular output of blood bypasses the lungs via the ductus arteriosus (DA) (Fig. 25–1). The pulmonary vascular resistance (PVR) is increased because of muscular hypertrophy of the precapillary blood vessels.[1] (The caliber of which may be influenced by hypoxia and acidosis.) The umbilical vein (UV) carries the oxygenated blood from the placenta to the fetus. Upon entering the liver, the UV divides into two branches: the ductus venous (DV), which enters the inferior vena cava (IVC), and the portal sinus, which supplies mainly the left lobe of the liver. At midterm, more than 50% of the oxygenated blood reaches the IVC through the DV.[1,2] Thus, the DV is only a partial shunt and allows a significant portion of the oxygenated blood to perfuse the liver. This arrangement places the liver in a strategic position in the fetal circulation, enabling the fetus to metabolize drugs that are transferred across the placenta from the mother.

As the blood enters the right atrium from the IVC, it is divided into two streams by the crista dividens, a projection of the anterior edge of the foramen ovale. The major stream enters the left atrium via the foramen ovale, thereafter to be distributed to the head and the heart. The smaller stream mixes with the blood being carried into the right atrium by the superior vena cava (SVC) and finds its way into the right ventricle. Usually little or no blood from the SVC crosses the foramen ovale. The DA delivers the desaturated blood from the right ventricle to the aorta, which transports blood at a higher oxygen saturation. The mixed stream supplies the lower part of the body and enters the two umbilical arteries. The increased heart rate and decreased systemic vascular resistance (SVR) of the placenta enable the fetus to maintain a high cardiac output (164 ml/kg) relative to its total body sur-

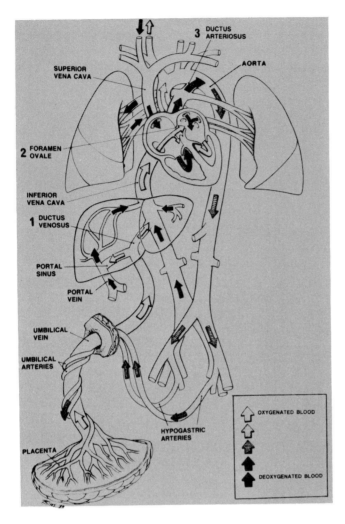

FIG. 25–1. The fetal circulation. Note the position of the ductus venosus, ductus arteriosus, and foramen ovale. Also note that the degree of oxygenation is greater in the umbilical veins than in the ductus arteriosus because of admixture with the aortic blood. Different shades of arrows represent different states of oxygenation. (From Pritchard JA and McDonald PC: Williams Obstetrics. 17th Edition. Norwalk, Appleton-Century-Crofts, 1985. p 150.)

face.[1] Fifty percent of the total cardiac output is pumped to the placenta.

TRANSITION TO ADULT CIRCULATION

Compared to adult circulation, the fetal circulation has increased pulmonary vascular resistance, and decreased systemic vascular resistance because of the presence of the placental low-resistance circuit. In addition, the two ventricles function as two independent units in a series. The onset of respiration and sudden increase in PO_2 decreases the PVR. Clamping the umbilical cord excludes the placenta from the systemic circulation with the result that the SVR increases. This increases the left-side pressure leading to the functional closure of the foramen ovale. The anatomic closure may not occur for a few days and thus the neonate may develop arterial desaturation because of the right-to-left shunt during crying.

Next, the DA closes in response to the increase in arterial PO_2. Striking changes are seen in the ductal lumen when the PO_2 exceeds 50 mm Hg. The size of the ductal lumen is regulated by PO_2 (which constricts it) and prostaglandins (which dilate it). As gestational age increases, the ductus constricts more in response to oxygen and dilates less in response to prostaglandins.[3] In early gestation, the maternal use of prostaglandin inhibitors, particularly indomethacin, has led to the premature closure of the DA in fetal life (see Chapter 22 on Preterm Labor). Because the DA receives mostly deoxygenated blood from the right ventricle, the PO_2 in the ductal blood is lower than in the UA. Even when the mother breathes 100% oxygen, the ductal PO_2 will never rise above 50 mm Hg, thus avoiding premature closure.[4] Anatomic closure

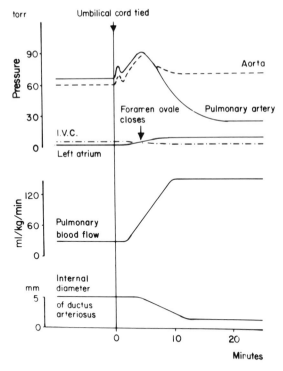

torr

Umbilical cord tied

Pressure

90

60

30

0

Aorta

Foramen ovale closes

Pulmonary artery

I.V.C.

Left atrium

ml/kg/min

120

60

0

Pulmonary blood flow

mm

5

0

Internal diameter

of ductus arteriosus

0   10   20

Minutes

FIG. 25–2. Circulatory adaptation at birth. Note the sudden reduction in the pulmonary artery (PA) pressure and increase in the pulmonary blood flow. (From Dawes GS: Foetal and Neonatal Physiology Chicago, Year Book Medical Publishers, 1968.)

of the ductus may take up to 10 days after birth.[5] In summary, the most important changes in the fetal circulation occurring at birth are closure of the DA, closure of the foramen ovale, decreased PVR, and increased SVR (Fig. 25–2).

CHANGES IN THE RESPIRATORY SYSTEM

In fetal life, the tracheobronchial tree is filled with fluid. The lungs must transform from fluid-filled sacs into airfilled sacs. The surfactant function will begin only when the air-liquid interface is established. Fluid is eliminated from the lungs by the following mechanisms: (1) the fetal chest is compressed by the maternal passages during delivery; (2) the baby's upper airway is suctioned by the delivery room staff; (3) the baby clears some fluid by spitting and coughing; and (4) the lymphatics mobilize fluid from the lung parenchyma.

The sudden decompression of the chest after the baby is born causes passive air movement that is soon followed by the first active breath,

which is unusually large. The first breath mobilizes approximately 50 ml of air, and the intrapleural negative pressure during the first breathing attempt may reach -80 cm H_2O (Fig. 25–3). The expired air volume will be less than the inspired volume during the first few breaths. The retained air volume is used to build its functional residual capacity. As more and more air accumulates in the lungs, the surfactant function becomes well-established. Each breath requires less effort than the previous one, thereby diminishing the intrapleural pressure swings (Fig. 25–4). Immediately after vaginal birth, the neonate has low pH, low Po_2 and high Pco_2. The Pco_2 reaches the adult values within 2 to 3 hours, followed by pH (Fig. 25–5). The Po_2 increases slowly and might take up to 6 weeks to reach adult values. The slow normalization of Po_2 is attributed to increased intrapulmonary shunting (Qs/Qt), which may be as high as 20% in the first few days of life. The causes for increased Qs/Qt are believed to be (1) increased closing volume; (2) increased lung water content; (3) slow clearance of pulmonary fluid by the lymphatics; and (4) elevated PVR. In addition, the hypertrophic pulmonary vascular smooth muscle may take up to six weeks to undergo spontaneous resolution. Some clinically useful measurements relating to neonatal respiratory physiology are listed in Table 25–1.

CHANGES IN BLOOD VOLUME

At birth the negative intrapleural pressure together with the force of uterine contractions facilitate blood flow from the placenta to the fetus via the UA. The blood volume may increase 15 to 20 ml/kg in 3 minutes, if the infant is held below the introitus. The two UA usually constrict vigorously in respose to increased oxygenation; this consequently limits entry of blood into the neonate. The UV is slow to constrict because of the lack of muscular wall. The optimum time for cord clamping is 1 to 2 minutes after the delivery of the baby. Delayed clamping may result in a plethoric infant. Early clamping of the cord may result in neonatal hypovolemia.

THERMOREGULATION

The neonate does not shiver when its body temperature decreases. It produces heat energy

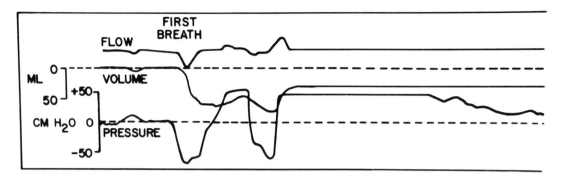

FIG. 25–3.   The first breath. Note the large tidal volume and exaggerated negative pleural pressure. (From Karlberg P: J Pediatr *56*:585, 1980.) (From Karlberg P.: Adaptive changes in the immediate post-natal period with particular reference to respiration. J. Pediatr. *56*:585, 1960.)

by mobilizing energy substrates stored in the brown fat. This process is called the nonshivering thermogenesis (NST). The brown fat tissue is located in the neck, in the interscapular region, the back, and in the perirenal tissues. The brown fat is more cellular and more vascular than the adult adipose tissue and accounts for only 7% of the total body weight. It receives approximately 10% of the total cardiac output under normothermic conditions and up to 25% under hypothermic conditions. During cold exposure, temperature of the brown fat rises, while the rest of the body cools.[1] The veins of the interscapular brown fat drain into the vertebral plexus.

The NST is mediated by the liberation of noradrenaline, which is known to mobilize both glycerol and free fatty acids (FFA) from the adipose tissue. Prolonged exposure to cold will deplete brown fat and seriously impair thermoregulation in the neonate.[6] The neutral thermal environment for the neonate is a narrow range of body temperature at which the neonate's calorific and oxygen demands are at a minimum. When the temperature decreases below the critical range, the oxygen consumption ($\dot{V}O_2$) will increase. In an infant with a normal core temperature, the $\dot{V}O_2$ is at a minimum when the difference between the body temperature and

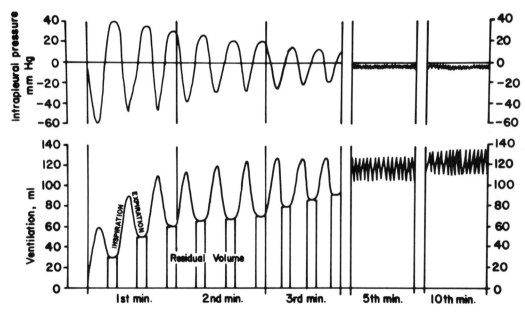

FIG. 25–4.   The development of functional residual capacity. Note that the inspiratory tidal volume is greater than the expiratory tidal volume in the first few minutes of life. The difference is utilized to build the FRC. Also evident is the gradual normalization of intrapleural pressure. (From Karlberg P: Adaptive changes in the immediate post-natal period with particular reference to respiration. J. Pediatr. *56*:585, 1960.)

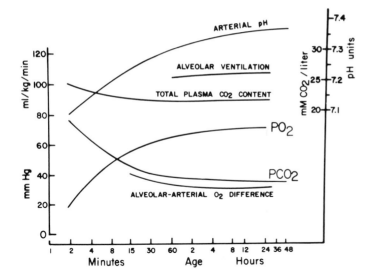

FIG. 25–5. Changes in pulmonary gas exchange in the first few hours of life. Note the increased $AaDo_2$ gradient and the decreased Pao_2 even at 24 hours after birth. See text for explanation. (From Avery GB: Neonatology: Pathophysiology and management of the newborn. 2nd Edition. Philadelphia, J.B. Lippincott, 1981.)

the ambient air is 1.5° or less (Fig. 25–6). In hypoxic animals, the NST is abolished.[7] Hypothermia is associated with the following serious sequelae in the neonate: (1) increased PVR probably caused by norepinephrine; (2) reduced Po_2; (3) acidosis; (4) hypoglycemia caused by exhaustion of hepatic glycogen; and (5) disseminated intravascular coagulation possibly caused by stagnant peripheral circulation.[8]

Wet infants left exposed to room air may experience a decrease in body temperature of up to 2°C in 30 minutes time. Dry infants left under the radiant heater lose only a minimal amount of heat. The baby must be dried and wrapped in a blanket before it is removed from the heater unit.[9] Lowered body temperature is more harmful to the preterm neonate than it is to a term neonate. In spite of the increased number of sweat glands (compared to the adult), the newborn is less capable of losing heat by way of

sweating. Consequently, the risk of hyperthermia is great in an overheated environment. Premature babies almost completely lack the ability to sweat.[6]

The radiant heaters are especially useful during resuscitation because they provide good access to the baby. Several types of heating devices are used to keep the babies warm. The servo-control radiant heaters are probably the most practical ones. A sensor placed on the baby's abdomen is used to regulate the heat output of the overhead radiant heater. The abdominal skin

Table 25–1. Neonatal Pulmonary Physiology

Measurement	Infant	Adult
Rate (min)	35.00	15.00
V_T (ml/kg)	7.00	7.00
Vo_2 (ml/kg/min)	7.00	3.00
V_A (ml/kg/min)	120.00	60.00
V_A (L/M²/min)	2.30	2.30
$\dot{V}/\dot{Q}$ ratio	0.6	0.80
Qs/Qt percentage	15.00	5.00
$AaDo_2$ (mm Hg)	24.00	10.00
CC/FRC	1.17	0.77

Abbreviations: CC = closing capacity; FRC = functional residual capacity. (Source: Avery GB[6])

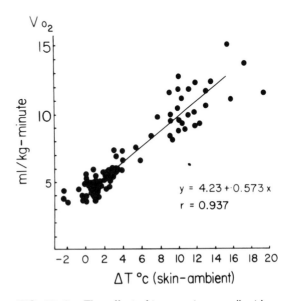

FIG. 25–6. The effect of temperature gradient between skin temperature of the newborn and the ambient temperature (Δ T). The $\dot{V}o_2$ increases markedly when the gradient exceeds 2°C.

temperature maintained at 36.5°C will ensure a neutral thermal environment in most instances. However, the adhesive tape overlying the sensor prevents evaporation from the skin thereby causing localized temperature elevation, causing the servocontrol heater to cycle off. This could result in low core temperature in premature neonates, especially when the relative humidity of the ambient air is low.[10] Therefore, both skin and core temperature must be monitored in small neonates. The other problems associated with radiant heaters include excessive water loss and accidental hyperthermia.[8]

Incubators are used for nursing small preterm neonates. The units with the servocontrols are more practical. Smaller neonates require a higher incubator temperature for the maintenance of thermal neutrality than do term neonates. As in the case of the servo radiant heaters, the skin and core temperature must be monitored frequently. If servocontrol units are used, the heat output of the unit must be adjusted manually several times a day to maintain the baby's thermal neutrality. An infant weighing 1000 g requires an ambient air temperature that is approximately 2°C greater than required by an infant weighing 3000 g.[7]

ASPHYXIA

PATHOPHYSIOLOGY OF ASPHYXIA

Asphyxia may be caused by several factors, which may be generally classified into four types. Labor and delivery predispose to asphyxial insult because of reduction in placental blood flow caused by uterine contractions. Asphyxia may occur as a result of umbilical cord compression; inadequate perfusion of the placental bed (maternal hypotension, supine position); placental factors (infarcts, separation); and neonatal factors (airway obstruction, congenital anomalies of the airway, upper airway obstruction). The fetal circulatory adaptation to intrauterine asphyxia has been described in detail in Chapter 2. Of particular interest is the fact that circulatory adaptations in the unborn fetus are usually in the opposite direction of normally occurring changes vital to extrauterine survival.

Many cases of neonatal asphyxia have their origin in utero. Therefore, the adaptive circu-

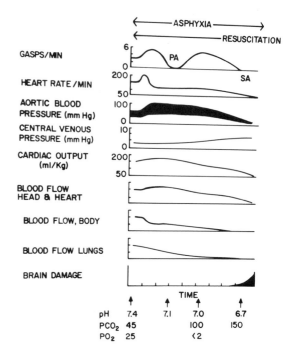

FIG. 25–7. Pathophysiology of the fetal-neonatal asphyxia. Units are not given for the time scale. The interval between divisions depend on the degree of asphyxia. In 100% obstruction, each interval is 1 minute. When asphyxia is less severe, the process takes longer to develop and each division is longer than a minute. With effective resuscitation the entire process is not only reversible (except damage to the brain) but to a degree will retrace its path. Note that the aortic pressure decreases when the peripheral and pulmonary circulations improve. PA–Primary apnea; SA–Secondary apnea. (From Avery GB: Neonatalogy: Pathophysiology and management of the newborn. 2nd Edition. Philadelphia, J.B. Lippincott, 1981.)

latory mechanisms may continue in extrauterine life, especially if the state of oxygenation is not immediately improved. The pathophysiologic changes of fetal asphyxia are described in Figure 25–7. The time scale does not have any units because the rapidity with which the changes develop depends on the severity of the asphyxial insult. In the worst possible case, each interval on the time axis represents a minute.[6]

RESPIRATION

Experiments done in animal fetuses have shown that sudden interruption of oxygen supply causes "gasps" in the fetus, followed by apnea. This apneic period is called the primary

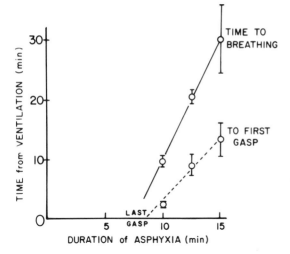

FIG. 25–8.   Response of the asphyxiated neonate to resuscitation. The longer the delay between time of last gasp and the institution of artificial ventilation, the longer it will take the neonate to commence rhythmic spontaneous respiration. (Source: Adamsons K, et al.: Resuscitation by positive pressure ventilation and Tris-hydroxy methylaminomethane of Rhesus monkeys asphyxiated at birth. J. Pediatr 65:807, 1964.)

apnea, to distinguish it from a subsequent terminal or secondary apnea. The majority of babies requiring resuscitation will be in primary apnea and sensory stimuli, such as slapping, will result in onset of breathing. When left to his own devices, the neonate in primary apnea will start gasping again and finally develop secondary or terminal apnea. When resuscitation is instituted at this stage, the baby will start gasping again, and after some time, will start breathing regularly. For every minute delay in instituting manual ventilation, the onset of rhythmic respirations are delayed further by 2 minutes[11] (Fig. 25–8).

Heart rate usually rises immediately after the onset of asphyxia but bradycardia is the rule in later stages. Similarly, blood pressure rises first in response to asphyxial stress but decreased during prolonged asphyxia. Central venous pressure actually rises in prolonged asphyxia because of cardiac failure caused by severe acidosis. The cardiac output may be maintained for 3 to 4 minutes but begins to fall to low levels. Widespread vasoconstriction in skin, lungs and other nonvital organs helps redistribute the available oxygen to the brain and the heart. The

blood pH decreases because of respiratory and lactic acidosis. Blood Po_2 usually reaches values too low to measure within 5 minutes of total asphyxia.

It is often difficult to distinguish between primary and secondary apnea in an asphyxiated infant. Although blood pH measurement is helpful in differentiating the two conditions, it is not available immediately. The differentiation may be made clinically based on the response of the neonate to positive regular ventilation. A neonate in primary apnea usually starts regular respirations soon after institution of positive pressure breathing; whereas a neonate in secondary apnea at the time of birth takes a long time to initiate rhythmic respiratory activity. His circulation will show signs of improvement (increase in heart rate, pink skin) before rhythmic respiratory efforts are established. The differentiation is important because it gives the physician a clue to the duration and severity of the asphyxia. Hypoxic brain damage occurs when hypoxia is prolonged more than 8 to 10 minutes (Fig. 25–6).

Blood Volume. Intrapartum asphyxia usually causes a shift of blood from the placenta to the fetus. Under some exceptional conditions the neonate is likely to be hypovolemic, including (1) selective compression of the UV by the after coming head during breech delivery, which leads to sequestration of the blood in the placenta; (2) hemorrhage from the fetoplacental unit; (3) severe maternal hypotension with the resultant stasis in the placental blood; (4) sudden onset of dystocia that does not allow enough time for placental transfusion to occur; and (5) holding the baby above the level of the introitus before the cord is clamped. Clinical signs of hypovolemia will appear when successful resuscitation reverses the peripheral and pulmonary vasoconstriction.

Effective resuscitation will rapidly reverse most of the pathophysiologic features of asphyxia except brain damage. During recovery from asphyxia, each pathophysiologic feature listed in Fig. 25–7 (except respiratory derangement) will retrace the path it took during the development of asphyxial insult. For instance the CVP and aortic pressure may decrease when the peripheral circulation improves.

Table 25–2.   Loss and Recovery of Apgar Signs

Loss				Recovery
:	1	Color	3	:
:	2	Respirations	2	:
:	3	Tone	5	:
:	4	Reflex response	4	:
:	5	Heart rate	1	:
:				:
:				:

(From Paxon CL: Van Leeuwen's Newborn Medicine, 2nd Edition. Chicago, Year Book Medical Publishers, 1980.)

EVALUATION OF THE ASPHYXIATED NEONATE

The Apgar scoring system remains the simplest and most efficient way of assessing the neonate at birth. The order in which each sign of the Apgar score appears and disappears is given in Table 25–2. During recovery from moderate asphyxia, normalization of heart rate occurs long before the other signs improve.[7] The one-minute Apgar score is indicative of neonatal CNS depression whereas the 5-minute score is predictive of recovery from asphyxia and long-term neurologic abnormality.[7] When the one-minute score is 7 or higher, only gentle clearing of the airway is needed. When the score is 4 to 6, the infant is deemed to be moderately depressed. In this case, the infant is placed under the radiant warmer, the upper airway is cleared of all secretions, and positive pressure breathing is instituted with an Ambu bag and mask. A bulb syringe may be used for clearing secretions from the upper airway. The use of suction catheters in the first five minutes of life may cause bradycardia, arrhythmia, and apneic episodes in 14% of infants.[12] After 5 minutes of extrauterine life the problem seems to be less severe.[12] The heightened vagal activity of the infant who might have suffered mild oxygen deprivation probably accounts for the more frequent occurrence of the problem in the immediate postnatal period. The use of a bulb syringe does not appear to be associated with increased incidence of bradycardia. Similarly, a high flow of oxygen directed at the baby's face may result in bradycardia.[13] When oxygen supplementation is necessary, small flows must be used. The impact of the flow on the baby's face may be lessened by using the finger tip as a baffle, which helps diffuse the flow

somewhat. If the heart rate fails to respond to bag ventilation, endotracheal intubation must be performed.

RESUSCITATION PROCEDURE

The seriously depressed infant (Apgar score of 0 to 3) may be apneic, bradycardic, areflexic, and limp. Meconium, if present should be cleared (vide infra). Meticulous attention must be paid to the maintenance of body temperatue. The EKG and blood pressure must be monitored. A pulse oximeter may be helpful if the infant has fairly reasonable peripheral circulation. The baby must be given a positive pressure breathing with 100% oxygen. Large volume pediatric Ambu bags are preferable to small volume bags because the latter do not deliver a large enough tidal breath.[14] Inflation pressure of 25 to 30 cm H_2O is needed to inflate the lungs during the first breath. Once it can be ascertained by auscultation that the lungs are expanded, inflation pressures may be reduced. If the infant's heart rate does not respond to positive pressure ventilation, endotracheal intubation must be performed.

External cardiac massage is indicated if the heart rate remains below 50 per minute after the onset of assisted ventilation, if no electrical activity is detected in the EKG, or if there is no audible heart beat. The "wrap-around" technique is used for external cardiac massage; both hands are placed behind the infant's chest with the thumbs overlapping in the front (Fig. 25–9) over the midsternum. Downward pressure is exerted 80 to 100 times per minute with a compression to ventilation ratio of 3:1. External cardiac massage must be continued until the baby is able to maintain a spontaneous heart rate of at least 100 beats per minute. It must be kept in mind that many presumed cardiac arrests are actually severe bradycardias that will respond to ventilation. If heart rate fails to increase above 100 despite adequate ventilation and external cardiac massage, an UV catheter must be inserted to establish venous access. The UA may also be cannulated to measure aortic blood pressure and to obtain arterial blood samples.

Drugs. Perhaps in no other situation is the dictum that *airway and breathing* precede *cardiac output and drugs* so appropriate as during newborn resuscitation.[15] A number of drugs

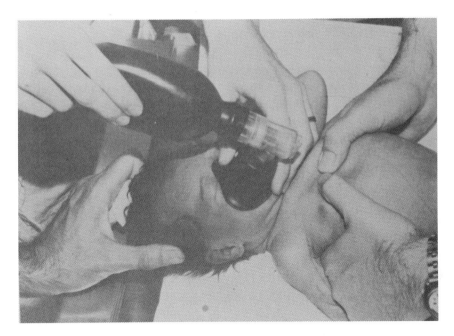

FIG. 25–9. Wrap-around technique for external cardiac massage. A compression to ventilation ratio of 3:1 is used. (From Paxson CL: Van Leuwen's Newborn Medicine. 2nd Edition. Chicago, Medical Yearbook Publishers, 1980.)

have been used for the correction of acidosis and for improving myocardial contractility. However, the use of any drug for these purposes is irrelevant unless effective means of oxygenation can be assured. In addition, some of these agents are implicated in producing severe complications. One must resort to the use of drugs only when the basic life support maneuvers have failed to increase the infant's heart rate above 100 beats per minute.

The drugs in question are sodium bicarbonate (NaHCO₃) and glucose. A rational approach is to ascertain that there is a need for each one of these drugs before administering it. For instance, the use of NaHCO₃ is deferred until the arterial blood pH and gas tensions are actually measured. If a blood sample cannot be obtained from a peripheral artery or from the UA, capillary blood samples may be used (scalp). Blood glucose can be determined easily with glucose oxidase-impregnated test strips. NaHCO₃ is administereed only when the base excess (BE) is less than 10 to 12 mmol/L. For all practical purposes, the extracellular fluid behaves as if it contained 3 g/100 ml of hemoglobin. Base excess value at the 3 g/100 ml of hemoglobin level (BE_3) is particularly suitable for infants. The BE_3 value may be read from a nomogram developed by

Severnghaus[16] or calculated with a hand-held calculator. The dose of NaHCO₃ is 2 to 4 mEq/kg and may be diluted in an equal volume of 50% dextrose solution.[15] The most distressing complication of NaHCO₃ administration is the occasional development of cerebral hemorrhage. The etiology is not clear and has been attributed to osmotically increased circulating blood volume. The following list gives the other complications of NaHCO₃ therapy:

1. Hyperosmolarity.
2. Cerebral hemorrhage.
3. Hypernatremia.
4. Hyperosmolarity.
5. Hypokalemia, hypocalemia.
6. Thrombosis of major blood vessels.

The use of glucose during resuscitation is also shrouded in controversy. Although earlier studies recommended routine use of glucose during newborn resuscitation, recent work has cast doubt on the safety of this practice.[17] During severe asphyxia, hyperglycemia (produced from glucose administration) may lead to increased lactic acidosis and cerebral edema, thus shortening survival.[15,17] Consequently, the only accepted routine during newborn resuscitation in the practice of oxygenation. Drugs are administered only after ascertaining that there does exist a need for them.

When arterial oxygenation has been optimized, metabolic acidosis and hypoglycemia must be immediately corrected. Prolonged intrauterine hypoxia leads to depletion of glycogen stores in the neonate. The possibility of hypoglycemia (<30 mg/dL) must be considered in a neonate whose general condition fails to improve despite good ventilation. Similarly uncorrected metabolic acidosis (BE <15 mmol/L) will seriously hamper myocardial contractility and interfere with drug action. When $NaHCO_3$ and glucose fail to reverse bradycardia, administration of epinephrine (0.5 ml of 1:10,000 solution), atropine (0.01 mg/kg increments) and/or calcium gluconate (1 to 2 mEq/kg) may be tried.

CONTINUED CARE

When tissue oxygenation is being adequately restored, electrolyte abnormalities may be seen. Correction of acidosis may cause hypocalcemia (<7 mg dL) and hypokalemia (<3.0 mEq/L), which may require correction. The reason for these electrolyte disturbances are not known. They are probably related to rapid reversal of acidosis. The reversal of peripheral and pulmonary vasoconstriction may lead to functional hypovolemia. Fluid administration will usually improve the systemic blood pressure. Gross deficits in blood volume caused by conditions decribed under pathophysiology of asphyxia require vigorous treatment. The classical sign of hypovolemic shock namely tachycardia is usually not seen in newborns. A low systolic blood pressure, reduced central hematocrit, persistent metabolic acidosis, low central venous PO_2, and delayed capillary filling (>3 seconds) are some of the clinical features of hypovolemia.

A term neonate with the birth weight of 3.0 kg should have a systolic blood pressure of 65 mm Hg. Approximate normal systolic blood pressure values for preterm and low-birth-weight babies may be obtained by subtracting 0.5 mm Hg of pressure each week the baby is premature and/or 1 mm Hg of pressure for every 100 g the birth weight of the baby is below 3000 g. Thus, a baby weighing 2 kg, born at 34 weeks, will be expected to have an approximate systolic pressure of 50 mm Hg.[7] A 20% reduction is considered hypotension. Fresh, heparinized whole

blood and fresh, partially-packed whole blood must be used to correct hypotension. Packed cells are preferable to whole blood because the newborn has a higher hematocrit than the adult. A packed cell transfusion is indeed a whole blood transfusion for a neonate. If blood is not available, fresh frozen plasma or Ringer's lactate solution may be used to provide volume expansion. The disadvantage of using asanguinous solutions is that they produce significant hemodilution. If banked blood is not available, fetal blood may be used. The blood is collected from the fetal side of the placenta and heparin is added to the blood immediately after collection. A heparin dose of 2 U/ml of blood is necessary to prevent blood coagulation.[18] Heparin doses exceeding 4.5 U/ml may cause prolongation of the baby's partial thromboplastin time. The volume requirement for all sanguinous and asanguinous fluids is approximately 20 ml/kg.[7] The use of albumin is controversial because it may leave the intravascular compartment and accumulate in the interstitial tissue compartment, leading to pulmonary congestion.[7]

When the baby's condition is stabilized, its stomach can be aspirated by gently introducing a suction catheter. It is not unusual for the stomach to be distended after prolonged mask ventilation. Development of a pneumothorax is always a possibility in infants who were subjected to positive pressure ventilation. The only sure way of diagnosing a pneumothorax is with the aid of a chest x-ray. A worsening hypoxia or hypercarbia, in spite of proper ventilation, must arouse suspicion of this condition. Severe tension pneumothorax will cause a severe reduction in cardiac output; therefore this situation does require emergency decompression of the chest with a No. 22-gauge butterfly needle attached to a three-way stop-cock and a syringe. Following this procedure, chest-tube drainage must be instituted as soon as possible. Table 25–3 lists drugs commonly used in neonatal resuscitation and their dosages.

MECONIUM ASPIRATION

During conditions of stress, the babies pass meconium in utero; this is probably caused by hyperperistalsis and the accompanying relaxation of the anal sphincter. Because hypoxia often

Table 25–3. Drugs and Fluids Used in Resuscitation

Drug or fluid	Amount
Atropine	0.01 mg/kg (repeat if needed).
Sodium bicarbonate	2–3 mEq/kg.
Calcium gluconate (9%)	1.0 ml/kg.
Glucose	200 mg/kg.
Epinephrine	0.1 ml/kg, 1:10,000 solution.
Naloxone	10 μg/kg.
Fresh heparinized whole blood	20 ml/kg.
Freshly packed RBC	20 ml/kg.
Fresh frozen plasma	20 ml/kg.
Ringer's lactate	20 ml/kg.
Autologous blood (heparin 2 U/ml)	20 ml/kg.

initiates gasping efforts, meconium often enters the trachea. Meconium is present in 10% of all deliveries. When the amniotic fluid is only lightly stained with meconium, only pharyngeal suctioning with a bulb syringe is indicated. If, however, thick pea-soup meconium is detected, additional measures are necessary. The obstetrician must suction the airway of the baby with a De Lee trap before the shoulders are born. This will prevent aspiration of the meconium when the baby takes the large first breath. The cord is immediately clamped and cut and the baby is handed over to a member of the resuscitation team. The operator must quickly clear meconium from the pharynx, intubate the trachea, and apply oral suction to the endotracheal tube. The operating room mask worn by the operator can be used to trap the meconium. One effective way of clearing the meconium is to withdraw the tube out of the trachea while oral suction is being maintained. Any meconium present in the lumen of the tube is blown off and the baby is reintubated. This procedure may be repeated two or three times. The use of suction catheters for clearing thick meconium is not recommended because they are difficult to introduce into the endotracheal tube and they are too small to mobilize viscid meconium. Endotracheal suctioning must be accomplished swiftly because most babies born with meconium are asphyxiated. Undue delay in ventilation will further worsen their condition. If endotracheal suctioning cannot be performed quickly, the supraglottic airways must be cleared of any meconium and mask ventilation performed forthwith.

The reason for having to clear the meconium from the trachea before positive pressure ventilation is instituted is two-fold; meconium causes mechanical obstruction of the airway and it may cause severe meconium aspiration syndrome. The syndrome is characterized by the development of patchy infiltrates and severe respiratory failure. The mortality may reach 25% in unsuctioned babies.[19] Even with suctioning the babies may develop respiratory symptoms but their chances of survival are markedly improved.[20] Other complications of meconium aspiration include pneumomediastinum, pneumothorax, persistence of fetal circulation, secondary pulmonary infection, and sequelae of intrauterine asphyxia that originally resulted in the passage of meconium by the baby.[7]

UMBILICAL VESSEL CATHETERIZATION

The umbilical artery (UA) and the umbilical vein respectively allow ready access to the aorta and inferior vena cava (IVC) of the neonate. The UV catheter is used for monitoring CVP and to administer medications; the UA catheter may be used to monitor aortic pressure and to obtain arterial blood samples. Umbilical vessel catheterization is associated with serious complications, therefore the risk-benefit ratio must be considered before performing the procedure.[21,22]

The cord and the surrounding abdomen are cleared with an antiseptic solution.[21] The cord is cut with scalpel blade at 1 cm from the umbilicus and the lumen of the vessel is laid open with a pair of forceps. A No. 5 F catheter is used for babies weighing ≥1500 g. The tip of the UV catheter must be advanced into the thoracic portion of the IVC and not left near the portal radicals (Fig. 25–10). Infusion of hypertonic solu-

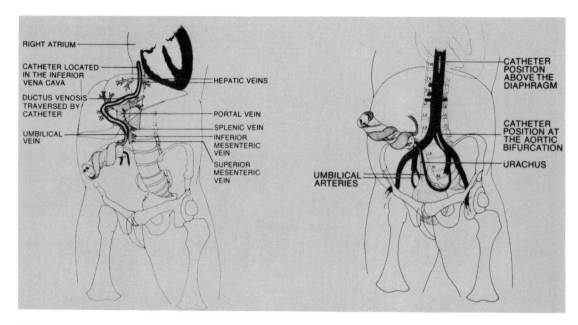

FIG. 25–10. Umbilical venous (UV) catheter (left) and umbilical arterial (UA) catheter (right). Note that the tip of the UV catheter is well above the portal system. The tip of the UA catheter must be positioned either above the diaphragm (high position) or at the aortic bifurcation (low position). (From Hughes WT and Buescher ES: Umbilical vein catheterization, exchange transfusions, and phototherapy. *In* Pediatric Procedures. 2nd Edition. Philadelphia, WB Saunders, 1980.)

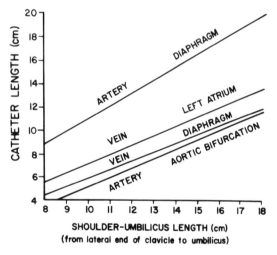

FIG. 25–11. Nomogram for determining the correct length of the umbilical venous and arterial catheters based upon the distance between the lateral end of the clavicle and the umbilicus. The UV catheter may be inserted through the foramen ovale into the left atrium. (From Hughes WT and Buescher ES: Umbilical vein, catheterization, exchange transfusions, and phototherapy. *In* Pediatric Procedures. 2nd Edition. Philadelphia, WB Saunders, 1980.)

tions with osmolarity >300 mosms may result in hepatic necrosis. The length from shoulder to umbilicus of the neonate may be used as a rough index of the length required to reach the desired point in the IVC (Fig. 25–11). Two positions are recommended for the UA catheter, the upper position (above the diaphragm), and the lower position (at the aortic bifurcation) (Fig. 25–10). Leaving the tip of the UA near the renal artery may cause renal artery thrombosis and hypertension.[21] The shoulder to umbilicus length may be used as a guide for proper length. Before hypertonic solutions are injected into the IVC, the position of the tip must be verified radiographically. A simpler way to verify the position of the UV catheter is to seek the typical a, c, and v wave patterns recorded with the aid of a transducer.[22] The complications of the umbilical vessel catheterization are summarized in the following list:

1. Buzzing belly button (A-V fistula).
2. Hepatic necrosis, portal vein thrombosis.
3. Renal artery thrombosis, hypertension.
4. Thrombosis of the aorta, paraplegia.
5. Infection.
6. Organ and vessel trauma.

REFERENCES

1. Stave U: Physiology of the Perinatal Period: Functional and Biochemical Development in Mammals. (Edited by Stave U). New York, Appleton-Century-Croft, 1978.
2. Rudolf AM: Oxygenation in the fetus and the neonate. Semin Perinatol 8:158, 1984.
3. Clayman RI, Heymann EH, and Rudolph AM: Ductus arteriosus responses to prostaglandin E_1 at high and low oxygen concentrations. Prostaglandins 13:219, 1977.
4. Ramanathan S, et al.: Oxygen transfer from mother to fetus during cesarean section under epidural anesthesia. Anesth Anal 61:576, 1982.
5. Hornblad PY: Ductus arteriosus and the mechanism of closure. N Engl J Med 282:566, 1970.
6. Avery GB: Neonatology: Pathophysiology and management of the newborn. 2nd Edition. Philadelphia, J.B. Lippincott, 1981.
7. Paxson CL: Van Leeuwen's Newborn Medicine. Chicago, Year Book Medical Publishers, 1979. pp 43–63, 240–250, 508–523.
8. Chessekks JM, and Wigglesworth JS: Secondary haemorrhagic disease of the newborn. Arch Dis Child 45:539, 1970.
9. Dahm LS, and James LS: Newborn temperature and calculated heat loss in the delivery room. Pediatrics 49:504, 1972.
10. Belgaumar TK, and Scott K: Effects of low humidity on small premature infants in servocontrol incubators. Biol Neonate 26:348, 1975.
11. Adamsons K, et al.: Resuscitation by positive-pressure ventilation and tris-hydroxymethyl-aminomethane of rhesus monkeys asphyxiated at birth. J Pediatr 65:807, 1964.
12. Cordero L, and Hon EH: Neonatal bradycardia following nasopharyngeal stimulation. J Pediatr 78:441, 1971.
13. Brown WU, Ostheimer GW, Gell GC, and Datta SS: Newborn response to oxygen blown over the face. Anesthesiology 44:535, 1976.
14. Field D, Milner AD, and Hopkin IE: Efficiency of manual resucitators at birth. Arch Dis Child 61:300, 1986.
15. Avery M, and Taeusch HW: Epstein's diseases of the Newborn. Philadelphia, WB Saunders, 1984.
16. Severinghaus JW: Acid-base nonogram: a Boston-Copenhagen detente. Anesthesiology 45:539, 1976.
17. Epstein ME, Hartig-Beecken I, and Loo SW: Effect of maternal diabetes on response to hypoxia in the newborn rabbit. Biol Neonate 40:56, 1981.
18. Golden SM, O'Brien WF, and Metz SA: Anticoagulation of autologous cord blood for neonatal resuscitation. Am J Obstet Gynecol 144:103, 1982.
19. Ting P, Brandy JP: Tracheal suction in meconium aspiration. Am J Obstet Gynecol 122:767, 1975.
20. Gregory GA, Goodling CA, Phibbs RH, and Tooley WH: Meconium aspiration in infants: A prospective study. J Pediatr 85:848, 1974.
21. Hughes WT, and Buescher ES: Umbilical vein catheterization, exchange transfusions, and phototherapy. In Pediatric Procedures. 2nd Edition. Philadelphia, WB Saunders, 1980.
22. Fanaroff AA, and Martin RJ: Neonatal-Perinatal Medicine: Diseases of the Fetus and Infant. St. Louis, C.V. Mosby Co, 1983. pp. 179–195.

26

PREMATURITY

The cost of caring for a premature neonate in a neonatal intensive care unit is astronomical.

Any newborn weighing less than 2500 g at birth is considered premature. Serious prematurity related problems usually occur when the birth weight is under 1250 g. Approximately 7% of all babies delivered will weigh under 2500 g and 1% will weigh under 1250 g.[1] Survival is unlikely before 24 weeks gestation because the lungs are mainly canalicular organs incapable of sustaining gas exchange, and the brain is too immature to maintain regular respiration. The smallest surviving infant reported was born at 27 weeks with a weight of 450 g. In many instances however, birth weight below 600 g is not compatible with survival.[1] Because of great advances made in neonatal ventilation in the last 20 years, the chances of survival are steadily improving.

Prolonging gestation, even by a week, may dramatically improve the neonate's survival chances. It is with this hope that many tocolytic agents are used to retard premature labor. Anesthetic considerations in a patient on tocolytic therapy is discussed in Chapter 20. The major determinant of neonatal complication and survival rates is the birth weight.[1,2] In Fig. 26–1, the neonatal mortality is shown at different birth weights. Figure 26–2 gives a list of the most common complications associated with prematurity at different birth weights. These complications include hyaline membrane disease, patent ductus arteriosus, necrotizing enterocolitis, retrolental fibroplasia, bronchopulmonary dys-

plasia, and intraventricular hemorrhage. The prognosis for long-term outcome depends on whether the prematue baby develops one or more of these complications in the postnatal period. For instance, Ruiz, et al. noted that those neonates who required ventilatory support in the neonatal period (when compared to those who did not) were at increased risk for developing neurologic handicaps, retrolental fibroplasia, and bronchopulmonary dysplasia in early childhood.[3]

Many of the complications mentioned above are linked to perinatal asphyxia. Many premature neonates may require some form of assisted ventilation at and/or immediately after birth. In order for the anesthesiologist to be an efficient member of the perinatal team, he should have working knowledge of the problems likely to be encounterd by the premature neonate.

HYALINE MEMBRANE DISEASE (HMD)

Hyaline membrane disease (HMD) affects approximately 1% of all infants born in the United States and is identified as a contributing cause in 20% of all neonatal deaths. The conditions that predispose to HMD include prematurity, cesarean section in a woman who has not previously been in labor, perinatal asphyxia, maternal diabetes mellitus, maternal hemorrhage, and a family history of HMD. The disease affects males more frequently than it does females. The second-born twin is also at increased risk.[4]

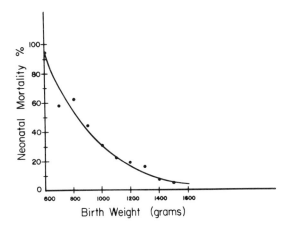

FIG. 26–1. Neonatal death rate and birth weight. (From Avery ME and Taeusch HW: Prematurity. *In* Schaffer's Disease of the Newborn. 5th Edition. Philadelphia, WB Saunders, 1984.)

Avery and Mead were the first to point out the possible relationship between lack of surfactant and the development of HMD.[5] The surfactant is a complex lipoprotein consisting of phosphatidylcholine (78%) and small fractions of phosphatidylglycerol, phosphatidylethanolamine (sphingomyelin) and phosphatidylinositol (Fig. 26–3). Dipalmitoyl phosphatidylcholine (DPCC) accounts for almost 50% of phosphatidylcholine.[5] Another important fraction of the surfactant complex is the phosphatidylglycerol (PG), which appears to enhance the surface activity of DPCC. Thus, determination of PG levels in the amniotic fluid is also predictive of fetal lung maturity. In fact, measurement of PG level together with lecithin/sphingomyelin ration (L/S ratio) is more predictive of fetal lung maturity than is the L/S ratio alone.[5]

The surfactant complex is synthesized by the type II pneumocytes found in the alveolar walls. They are readily identified by the presence of lamellar bodies contained in the cytoplasm (Fig. 26–4). The pneumocytes synthesize phosphatidic acid from dihydroxyacetone phosphate and glycerol-3-phosphate. The surfactant, which is synthesized in the pneumocyte, is extruded into the alveoli. The enzyme phosphatidate phosphohydrolase (PAP-ase) is responsible for the conversion of phosphatidic acid to DPCC and PG. There is evidence to suggest that PG may accelerate the synthesis of phosphatidylcholine by enhancing the activity of the enzyme responsible for biosynthesis.

Fetal lung maturation begins at 28 weeks of gestation. The concentration of lecithin in the amniotic fluid increases several-fold but the sphingomyelin concentration increases only slightly, resulting in an increased L/S ratio. When the gestation reaches 35 weeks, the concentration of PG increases and that of PI decreases (Fig. 26–5). The reaction leading to the formation of PI is reversible, and at late gestation, more PG is formed at the expense of PI, thus explaining the decrease in PI concentration in late pregnancy.[5]

The use of the L/S ratio in the amniotic fluid has been used for many years to assess fetal lung maturity (Fig. 26–6). A sample of amniotic fluid is obtained by amniocentesis. The fluid must not be contaminated by vernix caseosa, meconium, or blood. The L/S ratio is measured using starch-gel electrophoresis. A ratio of 2 to 1 or greater signifies that the fetal lung is mature (see Chapter 24). A ratio of 1.5 to 1 is considered transitional, and a ratio of 1 to 1 signifies a lack of

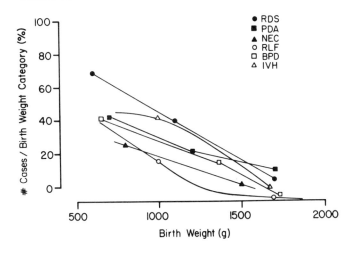

FIG. 26–2. Complications of prematurity and gestational age. RDS = respiratory distress syndrome (Hyaline membrane disease); PDA = patent ductus arteriosus; NEC = necrotizing enterocolitis; RLF = retrolental fibroplasia; BPD = bronchopulmonary dysplasia; IVH = intraventricular hemorrhage. (From Avery ME and Taeusch HW: Prematurity. *In* Shaffer's Diseases of the Newborn. 5th Edition. Philadelphia, WB Saunders, 1984.)

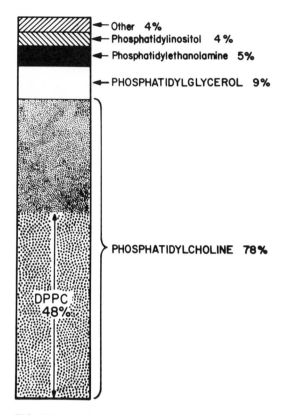

FIG. 26–3. Composition of surfactant. DPPC = dipolmitoyl phosphatidyl choline. (From Pritchard JA, et al.: The morphologic and functional development of the fetus. *In* Williams Obstetrics. 17th Edition. Norwalk, Appleton-Century-Crofts, 1985.)

maturity. In diabetic pregnancies, despite a ratio of 2 to 1, many neonates may develop HMD. A combination of measurements may be used to improve accuracy, including amniotic fluid DPPC (>1000 mg/dL), L/S ratio (>3.5 to 1), and PG concentrations.[5,6] Meconium and blood do not contain DPPC and are therefore not likely to affect the measurement of amniotic fluid DPPC. Similar considerations apply to PG measurement.[5]

The main function of the surfactant is to decrease the intraluminal pressure in the alveoli when lungs deflate during expiration. According to Laplace's law, the intraluminal gas pressure (P), and the wall tension (T) in a sphere with a radius of curvature (R) are related to each other as follows:

$$P = 2\ T/R$$

Therefore when two adjacent communicating al-

veoli have dissimilar sizes but have equal surface tensions on their walls, the small alveolus will empty into the big alveolus because the intraluminal pressure in the smaller alveolus will be greater than that in the larger alveolus (Fig. 26–7, Top). Under normal circumstances all alveoli are not of equal size and do not deflate at similar rates. Thus, the small alveoli may inflate the big alveolus. This will no doubt interfere with lung function. If, however, the wall tension decreases with decreasing alveolar size, then intraluminal pressure will also decrease, leading to uniform inflation of all alveoli (Fig. 26–7 Bottom).[7]

Because the surface activity of the lung will continuously change with the changing size, the pulmonary compliance will also continuously change during the course of a given respiratory cycle. The changing compliance is partially responsible for producing the typical hysteresis loop in the compliance curve of the lung (Fig. 26–8). The lack of surfactant will not only decrease the compliance, but will also diminish the size of the hysteresis loop (Fig. 26–8). Work required to maintain breathing will increase because of diminished compliance. Surfactant deficiency will also lead to alveolar collapse because the end-expiratory intraluminal pressure will be too high to allow reexpansion during the next inspiration. Once total alveolar collapse has occurred, the capillary hydrostatic pressure will cause fluid exudation into the alveolar lumen. In infants with severe HMD, as much as 80% of the cardiac output may be shunted past the airless lungs because of pulmonary vasoconstriction. In addition, uneven distribution of the inspired gas adds to ventilation/perfusion inequalities.

PATHOLOGY OF HMD

On gross examination, the lungs are noted to be unexpanded and often resemble liver tissue in texture.[4] On microscopic examination, the lung appears solid, interspersed with dilated air spaces and expanded respiratory bronchioles. Some respiratory bronchioles, alveolar ducts may be lined with pink staining hyaline-membrane (Fig. 26–9). Capillary damage, capillary congestion, alveolar epithelial damage, and proliferation of type II pneumocytes is also evident.

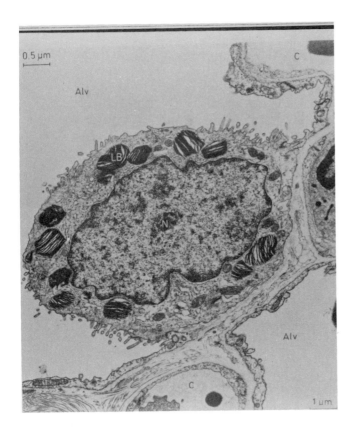

FIG. 26–4. Electron micrograph of alveolar cell type II (Dog). Note the lamellar bodies (LB), which are believed to release surfactant. (From Nunn JF: Applied Respiratory Physiology. 2nd Edition. Boston, Butterworths, 1977.)

A unique necropsy finding is that it is extremely difficult to inflate the lungs.

CLINICAL FEATURES OF HMD

Typically, the infant with HMD is a preterm baby with tachypnea, grunting, and chest retractions. The symptoms may start within minutes after birth, but may occasionally be delayed for several hours.[4] Chest auscultation may reveal fine inspiratory rales and a precardial murmur produced by the patent ductus arteriosus. The infant is prone to hypothermia easily. Some infants also develop pulmonary edema in the early phase of the disease. In addition, the severe hypoxia and diminished cardiac output cause wide-spread organ dysfunction and lactic acidosis. The HMD syndrome produces a typical radiographic appearance of reticulogranular appearance (Fig. 26–10).

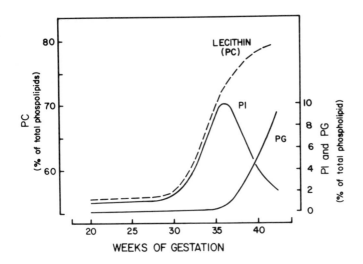

FIG. 26–5. Rate of rise of lecithin (PC), phosphatidyl inositol (PI), and phosphatidyl glycerol (PG) in the amniotic fluid with increasing gestational age. (From Pritchard JA, et al.: The morphologic and functional development of the fetus. In Williams Obstetrics. 17th Edition. Norwalk, Appleton-Century-Crofts, 1985.)

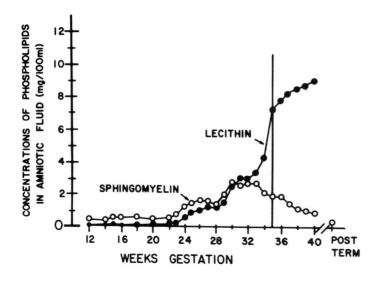

FIG. 26–6. Lecithin and sphingomyelin concentrations in the amniotic fluid with increasing gestational age. Note the upsurge in lecithin concentrations at 32 weeks. (From Gluck L, et al.: Diagnosis of the respiratory distress syndrome by amniocentesis. Am J Obstet Gynecol, *109*:440, 1971.)

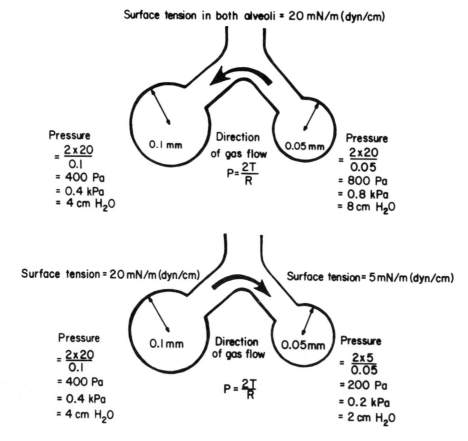

FIG. 26–7. The relationship between surface tension and intraluminal pressure in two spheres communicating with each other. Top: two spheres of dissimilar sizes but with similar surface tension are shown. The intraluminal pressure in the smaller sphere will be higher than that in the bigger one (because of LaPlace relationship), thus the small sphere will empty into the big one. Bottom: The surface tension of the smaller sphere has decreased from 20 to 5 mN/m resulting in the intraluminal pressure becoming greater in the bigger sphere than in the smaller one. The big alveolus will inflate the small alveolus to its size. (From Nunn JF: Applied Respiratory Physiology. 2nd Edition. Boston, Butterworths, 1977.)

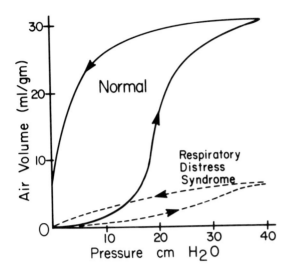

FIG. 26–8. Compliance curve during inspiration (up arrow) and during expiration (down arrow). Note that inspiratory compliance is different from expiratory compliance, which produces the typical hysteresis loop enclosed between the two compliance curves. The loop is much smaller in cases of respiratory distress syndrome probably due to lack of surfactant. (From Lough MD, Doershuk CF, and Stern RC: Pediatric Respiratory Therapy. 2nd Edition. Chicago, Year Book Medical Publishers, 1985.)

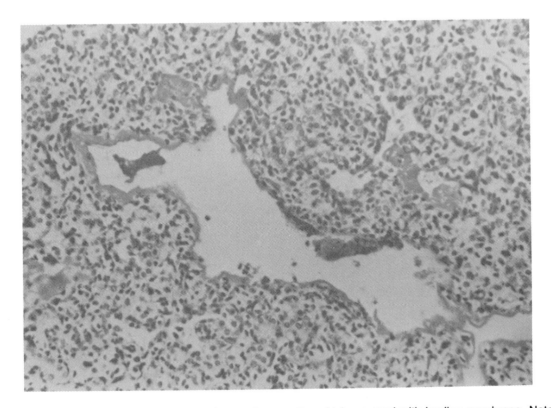

FIG. 26–9. Pathology of hyaline membrane disease. Bronchiole covered with hyaline membrane. Note the extensive collapse of the adjoining capsules. Tissue specimen obtained from the lung of an infant who died of HMD. (From Singer DB: Morphology of hyaline membrane and its pulmonary sequelae. *In* Hyaline Membrane Disease: Pathogenesis and Pathophysiology. (Edited by Stern L) New York, Grune and Stratton, 1984.)

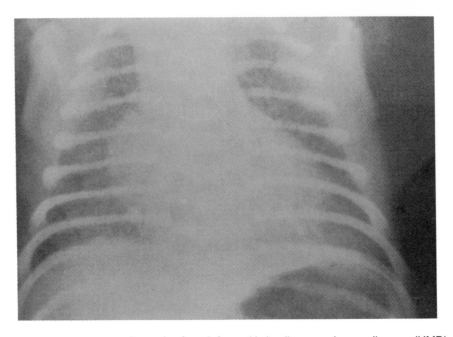

FIG. 26–10. Anteroposterior radiograph of an infant with hyaline membrane disease (HMD). Note the extensive reticulogranular opacities in both lung fields. (From Avery ME and Taeusch HW: Hyaline Membrane Disease. *In* Schaffer's Diseases of the Newborn. 5th Edition. Philadelphia, WB Saunders, 1984.)

The important conditions from which HMD must be differentiated are pneumonia caused by group B streptococcus, transient tachypnea of the newborn, congenital cyanotic heart disease, respiratory tract abnormalities (hypoplastic lungs), and neurologic problems, such as intracranial hemorrhage. Pneumonia caused by streptococcus B is clinically and radiographically indistinguishable from HMD. Maternal sepsis, however, is usually evident in this case. Other conditions mentioned previously may be distinguished by careful clinical examination or by appropriate laboratory tests.[4]

In typical cases, the neonatal condition will deteriorate in the next 48 to 72 hours, following which, there will either be dramatic improvement or a rapid deterioration culminating in death.[6] In many infants, a spontaneous diuresis begins on the second or third day (urine volume greater than 80% of fluid intake) and continues for 64 to 72 hours.[8] The onset of diuresis coincides with an improvement in FRC, pulmonary compliance, and A-A-aDo$_2$ gradient.[6,9] The lack of diuresis or the delayed onset of diuresis may be associated with increased incidence of bronchopulmonary dysplasia.[10]

Furosemide therapy has been used to induce diuresis in patients with HMD. Furosemide therapy has been shown to be associated with a lower mean airway pressure, and improved survival rate.[11] A disadvantage of furosemide therapy is the possible increased incidence of patent ductus arteriosus. This is attributed to furosemide induced renal excretion of prostaglandin E.[12] More randomized clinical trials are needed before diuretic therapy may be routinely prescribed for infants with HMD.

MECHANICAL VENTILATION IN HMD

Mechanical ventilation has been the mainstay of treatment for HMD. Over the last two decades, the outlook for survial has improved, mainly because of the availability of better respiratory therapy equipment. Two indications for ventilator therapy are respiratory acidosis with a pH <7.2, and a Pao$_2$ <50 mm Hg despite a high Fio$_2$ (0.7) and apneic episodes. The goal of therapy is to maintain Pao$_2$ between 50 and 80 mm Hg and Paco$_2$ between 40 to 50 mm Hg and to have a pH of 7.25 to 7.45.[13,14] A milder degree of hypoxia may respond to application of nasal CPAP (constant airway positive pressure) applied with a nasal breathing device (Fig. 26–11). Application of nasal CPAP is possible in neonates because they are obligatory nose

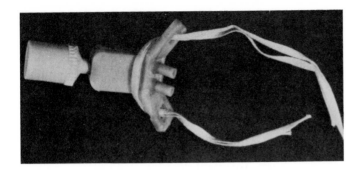

FIG. 26–11. Silastic nasal CPAP mask. (From Lough MD, Doershuk CF, and Stern RC: Pediatric Respiratory Therapy. 2nd Edition. Chicago, Year Book Medical Publishers, 1985.)

breathers. Whatever mode of respiratory assistance used, meticulous attention must be paid to humidification.

Pancuronium has been used for producing muscle paralysis in small infants who seem to fight the respirator.[13] Use of pancuronium has been reported to improve gas exchange,[6,15] to decrease the incidence of barotrauma and bronchopulmonary dysplasia, and to prevent rapid swings in intracranial pressure that accompany "bucking" on the tube.[16] Bucking may also cause fluctuations in cerebral blood flow. The elimination of bucking with pancuronium may therefore reduce the incidence of intracranial hemorrhage.[17] A potential disadvantage of prolonged muscle paralysis is atrophy of skeletal muscles.[18] Pancuronium bromide may also cause tachycardia and hyperbilirubinemia.[17]

Principles of Mechanical Ventilation

Compliance (C, L/cm H_2O) and resistance (R, cm H_2O/L/sec) may be used to calculate the time necessary for a given airway pressure to equilibrate with all alveoli. The product of C and R usually equals one time constant in seconds. For a healthy infant with a Compliance (C) of 0.004 and a Resistance (R) of 30, one time constant equals 0.12 seconds. It takes 0.6 seconds (five time constants) for the airway pressure to completely equilibrate with given instantaneous change in the airway pressure. Similarly, it will take five time constants for exhalation to be completed.

The ventilators that are currently available for neonatal use are of two types: pressure limited and volume limited. The term "limited" implies that the pressure or the volume (as the case may be) rises to a preset value and is held at that level until the cycling variable (inspiratory time) brings it to an end.[14] (Figs. 26–12 and 26–13).

In volume limited ventilation, the ventilator will deliver the tidal volume at a constant flow rate (Fig. 26–12). Airway pressure depends on tidal volume, inspiratory flow rate, airway resistance, and the pulmonary compliance. Any sudden decrease in compliance will cause the airway pressure to rise. With volume-limited ventilation, the tidal volume is affected by leaks in the system. Any respirator intended for neonatal use must be capable of delivering very small tidal volumes at a wide inspiratory-expiratory ratio (I:E ratio).[14] Since it is difficult to meet this requirement, only a few volume-limited ventilators are available on the market today. The Bournes LS 104-150, and the Siemens Servo 900

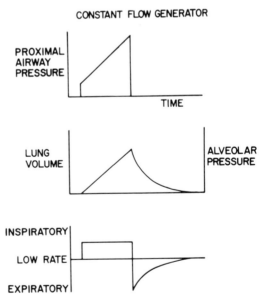

FIG. 26–12. Principle of volume-limited ventilation. Tidal volume is delivered at a constant flow rate which produces the characteristic inspiratory wave forms of pressure-limited ventilation (See Fig. 27–13). (From Lough MD, Doershuk CF, and Stern RC: Pediatric Respiratory Therapy. 2nd Edition. Chicago, Year Book Medical Publishers, 1985.)

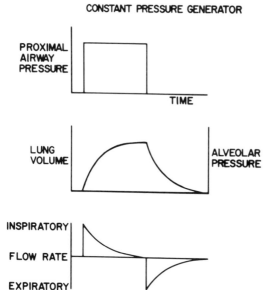

CONSTANT PRESSURE GENERATOR

PROXIMAL AIRWAY PRESSURE

TIME

LUNG VOLUME

ALVEOLAR PRESSURE

INSPIRATORY

FLOW RATE

EXPIRATORY

FIG. 26–13. Principle of pressure-limited ventilation. The proximal airway pressure rises to a preset value and is maintained at that level until the respirator cycles off. Note the changing inspiratory flow rate (compare with Fig. 27–12). Expiratory wave forms are similar in appearance during volume and pressure-limited ventilation because the elastic recoil of the lung produces deflation with both types of ventilation that are illustrated in Figs. 27–12 and 27–13. (From Lough MD, Doershuk CF, and Stern RC: Pediatric Respiratory Therapy. 2nd Edition. Chicago, Year Book Medical Publishers, 1985.)

B are the only volume-limited types. Bournes BP 200, Bear BP 2001, and Sechrist IV-100 are some examples of pressure-limited ventilators.

Pressure-limited ventilators deliver a volume of air until a preset airway pressure is reached. The total delivered tidal volume will not be affected by leaks from the system. The pressure difference between the proximal airway and the alveoli generates the gas flow. During inspiration, the flow rate will decrease as the alveolar pressure approaches the proximal airway pressure. The inspiratory cycle soon gets interrupted and exhalation occurs (Fig. 26–13).[14] The total tidal volume delivered will therefore depend on the difference in the airway pressures at the beginning and the end of the cycle. Assuming that the end inspiratory pressure is atmospheric, the peak inspiratory pressure (PIP) will be a major determinant of delivered tidal volume. When positive end-expiratory pressure (PEEP) is used, the difference between PIP and PEEP will

determine tidal volume (assuming that at least 5 time constants are available for PIP to equilibrate with airway pressure). Lack of adequate inspiratory or expiratory times will decrease tidal volume because of lack of equilibration. Inadequate expiratory time will interfere with alveolar emptying, resulting in higher alveolar pressures. The reduced PIP-PEEP difference will decrease tidal volume delivered during the next inspiration.[14]

Thus, the tidal volume delivered by the respirator is determined by inspiratory and expiratory times (I:E ratio), pulmonary compliance and resistance, PIP and PEEP. Some ventilators do not have a control knob for setting the respiratory rate. The rate is influenced by inspiratory and expiratory times chosen by the operator. For instance, choosing an inspiratory time of 1 second and an expiratory time of 2 seconds will result in a rate of 20 breaths per 60 seconds [$60 \div (1 + 2)$]. Thus two sets of variables (namely pulmonary and respirator-dependent) influence the total minute volume delivered. The interaction between the two sets of variables and the interaction among the individual components of each set is shown in Fig. 26–14.[14]

Many infant respirators also provide a continuous gas flow through the circuit to provide for possible spontaneous breaths by the infant. This flow will not only modify the absolute value of PIP but the wave form as well, thus somewhat influencing the delivered tidal volume.[14] The continuous flow in the circuit also provides for intermittent mandatory ventilation (IMV). During IMV, the infant's spontaneous respiratory activity can trigger a large breath from the respirator 10 times per minute.[4] The use of IMV is particularly useful when the infant is being weaned from mechanical ventilation.

In addition to the parameters discussed above, the *mean airway pressure* is also a determinant of infant oxygenation. The mean airway pressure is determined by inspiratory pressure wave form, I:E ratio, PIP, and PEEP. The rectangular wave form is associated with maximum effect on the mean airway pressure.[13,14] It must, however, be borne in mind that increasing PIP and PEEP to high levels in an attempt to increase the mean pressure will decrease cardiac output. Table 26–1 lists goals of therapy and Table 26–2 lists initial respirator settings that may be used in an infant with HMD. Further

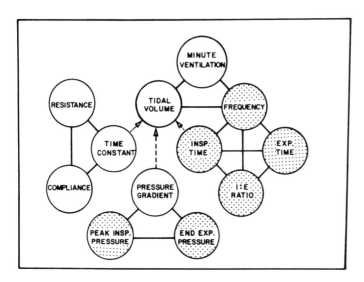

FIG. 26–14. Factors that determine minute ventilation during mechanical ventilation of infants with pressure-limited ventilation. Dots indicate parameters that can be changed using the controls on the respirator. The connections of some circles by solid lines signifies that the relationship between the parameters contained in the two circles may be mathematically derived. For instance, if inspiratory and expiratory time are known, the frequency may be easily calculated. Note that the tidal volume delivered is influenced by (1) time constant (not regulated by the respirator), (2) pressure gradient and (3) inspiratory time. (From Lough MD, Doershuk CF, and Stern RC: Respiratory Therapy. 2nd Edition. Chicago, Year Book Medical Publishers, 1985.)

adjustments of ventilator settings must be made based on repeated measurements of arterial blood pH and gas tensions.[19] For Pa_{O_2} <50 mm Hg at an F_{IO_2} >0.6, an increase in PIP or PEEP may be required. If the upper limit of PIP (25 cm H_2O) has already been reached the I:E ratio may be increased in an attempt to increase the mean airway pressure. When the Pa_{CO_2} is >50 mm Hg, the PIP level may be raised, or if the patient is breathing spontaneously, the IMV rate may be raised. When minute volume needs to be reduced, it is accomplished by reducing the rate rather than by decreasing PIP because the latter will decrease FRC.[14]

The infant may be weaned from the respirator if it has maintained adequate gas exchange at PIP ≤18 cm H_2O, rate ≤10/minutes and at F_{IO_2} ≤0.4. The infant may be given endotracheal CPAP equaling the level of PEEP that it was receiving during mechanical ventilation. A small increase in F_{IO_2} may be necessary when mechanical ventilation is being withdrawn. If the infant is able to maintain adequate oxygenation, the CPAP may be reduced step wise to 2 or 3 cm H_2O before extubation can be accomplished. Low-level CPAP must be maintained before extubation because the presence of the endotracheal tube abolishes laryngeal mechanisms that maintain lung volumes by regulating expiratory flow rate.[13,20] Nasal CPAP may be used in place of endotracheal CPAP during weaning. Nasal CPAP may be particularly useful in small infants intubated with a 2.5 mm tube because the use of endotracheal CPAP may add to the already high resistance to exhalation.[20] Infants who are prone to apneic episodes, infants who have developed bronchopulmonary dysplasia, and extremely small infants require a much slower time-table for weaning. The use of IMV may also be considered during weaning. In the beginning of the weaning process, an IMV rate slightly less than the patient's respiratory rate is used. The IMV rate is then tapered to zero when extubation is performed.[14]

Complications of Mechanical Ventilation

Unfortunately, in small infants, the use of mechanical ventilation is too often associated with complications. Major barotrauma, including

Table 26–1. Mechanical Ventilation: Goals of Therapy

Factor	Goal
Pa_{O_2}	50–80 mm Hg
Pa_{CO_2}	40–50 mm Hg
pH	7.25–7.45

Make adjustments based on measurement of pH and gas tensions.

pneumothorax and interstitial emphysema, occurs in 25% of infants.[4] The association between intracranial hemorrhage and prolonged mechanical ventilation is also striking. However, it cannot be ascertained whether the intracranial hemorrhage is caused by mechanical ventilation or if it is a result of prematurity itself. After extubation, atelectasis of the right upper-lobe has also been noticed recently, even when low-level CPAP is used before extubation.[21] Vigorous chest physiotherapy, and placing the infant on the left side, which delivers maximum pleural pressure to the right side, may minimize the incidence of this complication. Another serious complication of mechanical ventilation is bronchopulmonary dysplasia, which is a form of chronic lung disease. Both intracranial hemorrhage and bronchopulmonary dysplasia will be discussed later in the chapter.

High Frequency Ventilation

Because of the high incidence of barotrauma, ventilatory modes, which achieve gas exchange at low airway pressures, are currently being investigated. The ventilatory modes deliver small volumes at high frequency. The following paragraph describes some of the different ventilatory modes that have been used. High frequency positive pressure ventilation uses commonly available equipment that may be modified using low-compliance tubing. The rate is usually 60 to 150 per minute. In high frequency jet ventilation, the rate varies between 150 to 600 beats per minute. A high gas pressure source is used to deliver a gas jet into the trachea. The volume delivered is mostly independent of the compliance. Lower PIP and mean airway pressures are usually achieved with this technique with improvement in gas exchange.[22] A third ventilatory mode is high frequency oscillation, an acoustic loud speaker or a piston pump is used to deliver small puffs of air into the trachea at a rate of 3000 puffs per minute.[13]. Although numerous publications have attested to the efficacy of high frequency ventilation, the procedure is at best experimental at the time of this writing. Larger well-controlled randomized studies are required before the newer methods may replace the conventional mechanical ventilation for neonatal ventilation.

SURFACTANT THERAPY

Recently, it has been reported that tracheal instillation of surfactant preparations obtained from calf lung improves gas exchange and decreases the need for ventilatory support in infants born at 30 weeks of gestation.[23] The use of surfactant prepared from human amniotic fluid had been shown to improve gas exchange in infants with HMD. Other possible beneficial effects include the fact that it enables the clinician to use a lower F_{IO_2} and a lower mean airway pressure to maintain satisfactory oxygenation. Its use is associated with decreased incidence of pulmonary barotrauma and bronchopulmonary dysplasia, and may reduce overall mortality.[24] Thus the use of exogenous surfactant therapy is soon expected to be a part of the general management of infants with HMD.[6]

FLUID THERAPY

Intravenous fluid therapy assumes paramount importance in infants with HMD because of the delicate balance that exists between dehydration and overhydration. Premature neonates develop dehydration rapidly because of increased insensible water loss and inefficient water conservation by the kidneys. The routine use of infant warmers has further compounded this problem. On the other hand, overzealous hydration may lead to bronchopulmonary dysplasia,[25] prolonged patency of the ductus arteriosus,[26] necrotizing enterocolitis[26] and intraventricular hemorrhage.[27] Increased extracellular fluid (ECF) volume resulting from overhydration is suspected in causing these complications.[28] Consequently, the pendulum seems to be swinging in favor of fluid restriction and even using diuretics to maintain a state of relative dehydration in infants with HMD.

When the fetus grows his total body water (TBW) and ECF shrink. In other words the preterm fetus compared to a term fetus is likely to have an expanded ECF compartment. There is an additional expansion of ECF immediately after birth due to outward migration of intracellular contents.[29] The baby must therefore eliminate the increased ECF waterload in the first few days of extrauterine life. This probably explains not only the apparent negative sodium balance seen in preterm neonates but the excretion of dilute urine in the first few days of extrauterine life.[28]

The handling of sodium and water is inefficient in a preterm neonate. In a term neonate, there is sudden decrease in renal vascular resistance at birth, which increases glomerular filtration rate (GFR). In a preterm neonate, however, this increase in GFR is not seen.[30] The lower GFR puts the preterm infant at increased risk for fluid overload. The preterm neonate has poor renal Na^+ conserving capacity because of insufficient aldosterone production[31] together with diminished response of the renal tubules to aldosterone.[32] The renal concentrating ability is reduced in the preterm infant. This is attributed to decreased response of the renal collecting system to arginine vasopressin.[28] The reduced GRF and diminished Na^+ conserving power put the preterm infant at increased risk for fluid overload and rapid development of a negative Na^+ balance.

An additional feature that complicates fluid therapy in the premature neonate is the increased insensible loss from the skin. The skin of a premature neonate lacks sufficient cornification.[33] The cutaneous water loss differs from infant to infant and therefore no strict guidelines can be prescribed for replacing insensible water loss.[28] Cutaneous cornification proceeds rapidly in the first few weeks of extrauterine life, which necessitates frequent revision of fluid requirements.[34] Placing the infant under a warmer will lead to increased cutaneous water loss. An effective way of minimizing evaporative water loss under these circumstances is to shield the infant from the direct radiant heat with a plastic hood or with a transparent plastic sheet. Other precautions that must be taken to minimize water loss include providing suffecient humidification in the incubator, humidifying inspired gases, and early treatment of hyperthermia and tachypnea (increased respiratory water loss).[28]

Fluid therapy for a neonate with HMD is tailored based on the clinical course of HMD. The clinical course may be divided into three phases: the immediate perinatal period, the diuretic phase, and the postdiuretic phase. Immediately following birth, the cardiovascular and respiratory status of the premature infant must be stabilized. It is important to recognize and treat hypovolemic hypotension and hypoglycemia. Hypovolemia is corrected using whole blood or

saline (20 ml/kg–see Chapter 25). The routine use of $NaHCO_3$ is not recommended. The agent is administered only when the infant's arterial blood pH fails to improve despite satisfactory ventilation (see Chapter 25). Routine administration of glucose is not recommended during resuscitation of an asphyxiated infant (see Chapter 25). The administration must be guided by repeated measurements with glucose oxidase test paper. After the infant's oxygenation has been stabilized, 10% dextrose may be infused at 3 to 4 ml/kg/hr.[28]

Because fluid overload is implicated in causing many complications in preterm babies with HMD, the intravenous fluid therapy must be regulated so that the infant is maintained on the "dry" side. Since the premature neonate is born with an expanded ECF volume, maintenance fluid therapy need not be a major consideration in the first few days of life. During the diuretic phase of HMD, only that volume of fluid sufficient for preventing dehydration must be used. For instance an infant weighing 1000 g must be given 65 ml/kg/day of 12.5% dextrose solution during the first day.[28,35] Sodium chloride (2 to 3 mEq/kg) may be administered in the form of 0.2% saline only when there is evidence of hyponatremia and/or after diuresis is well established. Infants placed under a radiant warmer are given additional volume of fluid (70 ml/kg/day). If the infants are provided with a shield, total fluid volume is decreased to 60 ml/kg/day.[35]

The post-diuresis period is marked by improvement in pulmonary function. Only at this time is fluid administration liberalized to between 100 and 120 ml/kg and the neonate's calorific requirements fulfilled. It must be emphasized that fluid and electrolyte administration must be guided by repeated measurements of blood sugar and electrolytes.[28]

HYPEROSMOLAR STATE

Another serious problem associated with prematurity is the possible development of a hyperosmolar state. The syndrome occurs in infants weighing less than 800 g. The exaggerated water loss, which occurs because of the infant's immature skin, combined with diminished renal excretion of Na^+ probably leads to extreme hyperosmolarity. Hypovolemia, hypernatremia, hyperglycemia, hyperkalemia, and prerenal azotemia may develop in these infants. The hyperglycemia may be caused by inadequate insulin levels, insulin resistance[36] and/or iatrogenic glucose administration. The development of the hyperosmolar state may be prevented by careful monitoring of body weight, which is an index of insensible water loss and proper titration of glucose and Na^+ administration.[28]

PATENT DUCTUS ARTERIOSUS (PDA)

In fetal life, the ductus arteriosus connects the pulmonary artery with the aorta and thus helps right ventricular output bypass the lung. Compared to other muscular arteries, it contains increased amounts of mucoid material in the media and less elastic tissue in its entire wall.[37] When exposed to increasing Po_2, the ductus smooth muscle contracts, which makes the mucoid material coalesce. This forces the intimal cushions to project into the lumen of the vessel causing stagnation of blood. The impaired oxygenation of the media results in necrosis of that layer, eventually leading to fibrosis and closure. Although the ductus is functionally closed in the first two days of life, the potential to reopen does exist in the first week of life.[37] In the fetal life, low Po_2, together with locally synthesized prostaglandin E, assures patency of the ductus.

Prolonged patency of the ductus has been implicated in causing bronchopulmonary dysplasia, necrotizing enterocolitis, cerebral hemorrhage, and congestive heart failure. When a large left to right shunt develops because of the patent ductus arteriosus (PDA), left ventricular failure may follow. The increased pulmonary blood flow will lead to decreased pulmonary compliance. When present, the PDA increases the need for ventilatory support. The symptoms and signs of PDA are summarized in Table 26–3. Classical signs of PDA, such as systolic murmur, may be absent in infants receiving mechanical ventilation.[38]

Some severely ill neonates may require surgical ligation of the patent ductus arteriosus. Surgery for PDA is closely associated with morbidity and mortality.[39] Indomethacin, which inhibits synthesis of prostaglandin, has been found to be efficacious in inducing ductal closure. The

Table 26–2. Mechanical Ventilation: Ventilator Settings in HMD

Variable	Without HMD	With HMD
PIP	12–18 cm H_2O	20–25 cm H_2O
PEEP	2–3 cm H_2O	5 cm H_2O
Rate/minute	20	20–40
I:E ratio	1 to 2	1 to 1 or 1 to 3
$F_{I_{O_2}}$	0.5	0.5

Make adjustments based on measurement of pH and gas tensions. HMD–Hyaline membrane disease; PIP–peak inspiratory pressure.

ductal rate has been shown to be double in those premature neonates who received indomethacin as compared to control groups. The risk of pneumothorax and retrolental fibroplasia may be significantly decreased in infants who receive indomethacin.[38] Thus, whenever the PDA has resulted in hemodynamic impairment, indomethacin is indicated. Infants with birth weights of less than 1000 g will probably benefit the most. Indomethacin is usually administered either orally or intravenously (0.2 mg/kg, three doses). If the ductus reopens, a second course of indomethacin may be prescribed.

PRESERVATION OF DUCTAL PATENCY

While in some instances it is necessary to induce closure of the ductus medically, other conditions may call for maintaining the ductal patency. Neonates with poor pulmonary circulation, transposition of great vessels, or poor systemic perfusion are candidates for preservation of ductal patency.[37] The agent used for this purpose is prostaglandin E_1 (PGE_1). Infants born with pulmonary atresia will improve minutes after PGE_1 infusion is begun. The Pa_{O_2} will increase 20 to 30 mm Hg due to dilatation of the ductus. The lower the preinfusion Pa_{O_2}, the greater the improvement in oxygenation following PGE_1 therapy will be.[40]

Neonates with a transposition of the great vessels will rapidly deteriorate if a communication between the arterial and venous sides is not established. This communication is usually accomplished with an atrial septostomy. Septostomy, in some instances, may not create adequate communication between the two sides. A trial of PGE_1 is indicated under these circumstances. It must, however, be remembered that septostomy is the definitive procedure for transposition and PGE_1 infusion is at best only an adjunct. The use of PGE_1 may render the ductal tissue more friable thus making subsequent surgical ligation more difficult.

Severe congenital aortic stenosis and hypoplastic left heart results in poor systemic perfusion, acidosis, and shock. The right ventricle must, under these conditions, maintain systemic flow by pumping blood through patent ductus. The use of PGE_1 may buy valuable time until surgical correction may be undertaken.[37] Since PGE_1 is metabolized rapidly, it must be infused continuously at a rate of 0.05 μg/kg/min. Side effects include vasodilatation, respiratory depression, apnea, muscular tremors, convulsions, pyrexia, and diarrhea.[37]

PERSISTENT FETAL CIRCULATION

Persistent fetal circulation (PFC) is associated with pulmonary hypertension and large right to left shunts. Clinical manifestations include tachypnea, cyanosis, cardiomegaly, and sometimes also include heart failure. Except for the presence of fetal shunts, the heart is anatomically normal and there is no evidence of pulmonary parenchymal disease. Intrapartum hypoxia, severe HMD, polycythemia, and hyperviscosity are suspected to play a role in the pathogenesis.[41] In infants with PFC, the blood PO_2 in the lower limb arteries (postductal sample) will be lower than that in the upper limb arteries (preductal blood).[37] The treatment is mainly supportive. Mechanical ventilation may be required to produce mild hyperventilation and to improve oxygenation,[41] both of which may lead to a reduction in pulmonary vascular resistance.

BRONCHOPULMONARY DYSPLASIA

Bronchopulmonary dysplasia (BPD) is a term describing lung damage that follows prolonged mechanical ventilation. The severe form, first reported in the early sixties, has been replaced with a more mild form. It is seen in infants exposed to even short durations of mechanical ventilation. With the improving survival of infants with HMD, more and more cases of BPD are being reported. The incidence of BPD is 10 to 20% of all infants who receive mechanical ventilation for HMD.[42]

The condition mainly affects premature neonates who have been exposed to mechanical ventilation. The presence of pneumothorax, intracranial hemorrhage, PDA, meconium aspiration, and bacterial or viral infection necessitate the use of higher peak inspiratory pressure and/or high FIO_2, thus predisposing to the development of BPD. Infants who develop BPD may die because of fulminant respiratory failure or they may improve steadily to a point when they can be weaned off the respirator. However, these infants develop chronic sequelae.

Infants with BPD have varying degrees of respiratory failure because of fibrosis, emphysema, and atelectatic areas. Minute ventilation is increased because of respiratory rate. Pulmonary dynamic compliance is decreased and airway resistance is increased, both of which lead to increased work of breathing. Changes in pulmonary function associated with BPD are shown in Table 26–4. Chronic respiratory failure also leads to significant growth retardation.

Pulmonary hypertension, cardiomegaly, and hypatomegaly may be seen.[43] The radiographic findings in a classical case of BPD include hyperlucent areas alternating with strands of radiodensity caused by collapse and/or fibrosis (Fig. 26–15).

Many conditions produce a clinical picture similar to that produced by BPD. They are Wilson-Mikity syndrome, pulmonary interstitial emphysema, congenital heart disease, pneumonia, recurrent aspiration, and cystic fibrosis. Based on radiographic findings alone it is impossible to distinguish Wilson-Mikity syndrome from BPD. On many occasions, the two conditions may be distinguished from each other only based on early clinical course. Wilson-Mikity syndrome is not associated with prior use of mechanical ventilation, whereas BPD is. In pulmonary interstitial emphysema, the gas coalesces into cystic areas, as seen in BPD. Unlike BPD, however, the clinical and radiographic pattern improves in a few days. The other conditions listed in the differential diagnosis may be distinguished from BPD by using appropriate laboratory tests and/or from clinical history.[42]

The factors that have been held responsible for causing lung damage in patients with BPD are high peak pressure and high inspired con-

Table 26–3.   Features of Patent Ductus Arteriosus

Type of feature	Features
Clinical	Systolic murmur Wide pulse pressure (>35 mm Hg). Tachycardia, Tachypnea. Enlarged liver. Edema.
Laboratory diagnosis	Cardiomegaly (Chest x-ray). Enlarged left atrium, left ventricle (echocardiogram). Doppler rate of flow for the murmur or other contrast studies.

centration of oxygen. Other factors that may play a role are the presence of a PDA and the development of pulmonary edema in the neonatal period. Since all these factors are likely to coexist in a patient with HMD, it is impossible to single out one factor as being causative.[42]

PULMONARY OXYGEN TOXICITY

Breathing high F_{IO_2} for prolonged periods of time has been shown to cause damage to the lung parenchyma and vasculature.[44,45]

Alveolar Damage. Exposure to 100% oxygen causes interstitial edema and destruction of type I pneumocytes, initially. During continued exposure to 100% oxygen, there is hyperplasia of type II cells. Invasion by fibroblasts and macrophages is evident at this point. The thickness of the alveolar capillary membrane increases several-fold leading to diffusion defects.

Bronchiolar Damage. Bronchiolar destruction also occurs characterized by mucosal necrosis, peribronchiolar edema, and obstruction.

Damage to the Growing Pulmonary Vasculature. The growth and development of pulmonary vasculature is also influenced by hyperoxia.[45] Immediately following exposure to oxygen, there is diminished branching of the pulmonary vasculature in newborn animals. The number of capillaries per unit area is decreased

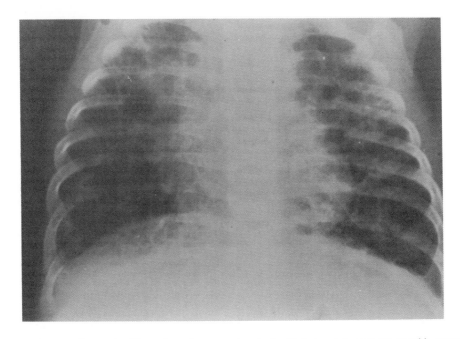

FIG. 26–15.   Chest radiograph of bronchopulmonary dysplasia. Note hyperlucent areas with course streak-like densities. (From Fletcher BD: The radiology of respiratory distress syndrome and its sequelae. *In* Hyaline Membrane Disease: Pathogenesis and Pathophysiology. (Edited by Stern L). New York, Grune and Stratton, 1984.)

Table 26–4. Pulmonary Function in Bronchopulmonary Dysplasia

Factor	Dysplastic response
Dynamic compliance	Decreased
Airway resistance	Increased
FRC	Increased
VD/VT ratio	Increased
Inspired gas distribution	Uneven
Nitrogen clearance	Delayed
P_{O_2}	Decreased
P_{CO_2}	Increased
V/Q mismatch	Increased
Minute ventilation	Increased

in the first 6 days of exposure. When, however, the animals are allowed to recover in room air, the number of capillaries increases.

The pathologic effect of oxygen is attributed to its cytotoxic effects. Increased concentrations of oxygen lead to the formation of highly cytotoxic free radicals listed in Table 26–5. Many of these free radicals can be rendered inactive by naturally occurring substances (Table 26–5). For instance, the superoxide radical can be effectively neutralized by superoxide dismutase enzyme. Although it is tempting to postulate that deficiency of one of the endogenous defense factors may lead to oxygen toxicity, no clear-cut evidence is still available to support such a contention.

PATHOLOGY OF BPD

Histologic examination of the lungs of an infant who died of BPD shows areas of emphysema surrounded by areas of atelectasis (Fig. 26–16). Bronchial and bronchiolar lumen may be obstructed with mucosal hypertrophy and/or with excessive mucus.[42] In addition, there may be peribronchial smooth muscle hypertrophy. The alveolar-capillary membrane may be thickened as a result of interstitial edema and increased fibrosis. The lymphatics may be dilated and tortuous. Thus, histopathologic changes of BPD closely resemble those produced by oxygen toxicity.

PREVENTION OF BPD

During mechanical ventilation of premature infants the lowest possible airway pressures must be used. With intelligent use of PEEP, the FI_{O_2} may be kept at the minimum possible level. Fluid administration must be based on guidelines discussed previously. Medical or surgical closure of PDA (if present) must be attempted.[42] There is no known treatment for BPD. However, progression of the disease may be arrested by attempting to wean the neonate off mechanical ventilation (vide supra). Survivors of BPD may require prolonged oxygen therapy at home. Water and salt intake may be restricted, and diuretic therapy may be tried in those who develop cor pulmonale.[42] The overall prognosis for long-term outcome has improved in recent years because of early detection and treatment of hypoxia, which decreases the likelihood of the development of cor pulmonale. The pulmonary pathology may take many years to resolve and in many instances does not resolve completely.[42]

RETINOPATHY OF PREMATURITY

Hyperoxia damages not only the lung tissue but the retina as well.

Prematurity increases the vulnerability of the neonate to oxygen induced retinopathy. Annually, 250 to 500 infants lose their vision as a result of retinopathy.[46] Other risk factors include duration of exposure to hyperoxic environment, the level of FI_{O_2} and the use of mechanical ventilation.[47] No safe level of arterial oxygen saturation of Pa_{O_2} has been established.[47] The Pa_{O_2} must be maintained at a minimum possible value compatible with neonatal well-being (50 to 80 mm Hg).

The normal developing human retina does not contain blood vessels until the fourth month of gestation. Vascular tissue starts growing from the region of the optic disk towards the periphery. Although the nasal quadrant of the retina is fully vascularized at 8 months of gestation, the temporal quadrant does not become fully vascularized until after term birth.[46] Thus, the temporal retina is more suceptible to oxygen damage than is any other portion. The earliest sign of oxygen toxicity is vasoconstriction followed by permanent vascular closure. Depending on the severity and the duration of oxygen exposure, the retinopathy may deteriorate from just vascular proliferation (Stage I) to total retinal detachment (Stage V, Table 26–6). Spontaneous

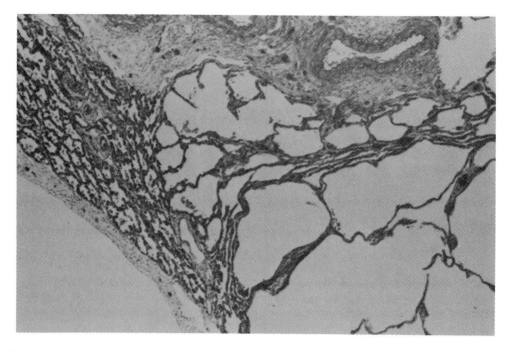

FIG. 26–16. Histopathology of bronchopulmonary dysplasia. Note the areas of emphysema surrounded by areas of atelectasis. (From Bancalari E, Gerhart T: Bronchopulmonary dysplasia. Pediatr Clin N Am, *33*(1):1, 1986.)

regression can occur if the disease has not progressed beyond Stage II. In more severe cases, residual cicatricial changes are usually the rule.[46] Cicatricial sequelae may vary from minor peripheral scarring of the retina forms to total fibrosis with phthisis in more advanced cases (Table 26–6).

Any infant who has been exposed to oxygen in the perinatal period must be followed closely by the ophthalmologist familiar with retinopathy of prematurity. The opthalmoscopic examination must be made at discharge from the nursery and at 3 to 6 months. Infants who develop BPD may

Table 26–5. Oxygen Toxicity

Toxic molecular species	Protective systems
Superoxide radical	Superoxide dismutase
Hydrogen peroxide	Catalase
Hydroxyl radical	Glutathione peroxidase
Singlet oxygen	Glutathione reductase
Peroxy radical	Vitamin E
Alkoxy radical	Dioxygenases
	Vitamin A (antioxidant)

Roberts RJ: Pulmonary oxygen toxicity in the premature and full-term infant—Its relationship to the development and pathogenesis of respiratory distress syndrome and its complications. *In* Hyaline Membrane Disease. (Edited by Stern L), New York, Grune and Stratton, 1984.

be prescribed nasal oxygen therapy at home. These infants are also at risk and must therefore be followed closely. Stage III retinopathy may require laser or cryotherapy. Vitamin E therapy administered early in the course of the disease may favorably alter the course of the condition.[46]

PERIVENTRICULAR-INTRAVENTRICULAR HEMORRHAGE

Another serious complication associated with prematurity is the increased incidence of periventricular-intraventricular hemorrhage (PV-IVH).[48] The availability of computed tomography and cranial ultrasonography has made the detection of PV-IVH easy and accurate. The PV-IVH usually occurs in the germinal matrix, which are the portions of the brain in the ventricular and subventricular areas. Neuronal and glial cells develop in these areas in the subependymal strata and slowly migrate to various layers of the cortex. The germinal matrix is quite extensive in early gestation but eventually disappears when the fetus is near term.

Intracranial hemorrhage occurs readily in the germinal matrix because it contains immature blood vessels that are poorly supported by the surrounding tissue. These blood vessels carry a major portion of the cerebral blood flow. The germinal tissue is also rich in fibrinolytic activity, especially in early gestation.[49] Some evidence suggests that blood may be hypocoagulable in premature neonates,[48] which further increases the likelihood of intracranial hemorrhage.

Conditions that increase the fetal cerebral blood flow (CBF) predispose to subependymal hemorrhage (SEH) or PV-IVH. These conditions include perinatal asphyxia, fetal hypertension, hypercapnia, and hemorrhagic hypovolemia. Fetal hypertension results in increased CBF because the fetal brain lacks autoregulation. During hemorrhagic hypovolemia, blood is shunted to the brain because of peripheral vasoconstriction and cerebral vasodilation. The CBF increases further when the neonate is given intravenous fluids (after birth) to treat hypovolemia probably because the circulatory adaptions set in motion during hypovolemia are somewhat irreversible.[50]

Several factors predispose to the development of PV-IVH in infants with HMD. The wide fluctuations seen in cerebral blood flow in infants with HMD can result in PV-IVH. The efficacy of muscle paralysis in smoothing these fluctuations in CBF in mechanically ventilated infants has already been described.[17] The other important risk factors are hypernatremia and hyperosmolarity produced by $NaHCO_3$ infusion, PDA, mechanical ventilation, fluid resuscitation, the use of vasoconstrictors to maintain blood pressure, and the development of major chest barotrauma.[48]

In severe cases, the PV-IVH may start with seizures, coma, apnea, and a rapidly developing decerebrate state. When the hemorrhage is small, the clinical picture may be less conclusive. Abnormal eye signs, lack of visual tracking, and a tight popliteal angle may be indicative of the lesion.[51] However, in many instances PV-IVH may occur without any neurologic sign. With the advent of refined techniques in ultrasonography, many centers routinely obtain cranial scans in all infants below 35 weeks of gestation.[48] The ultrasonography scan is used to grade the severity of PV-IVH. When a scan is performed, information must be obtained as to the presence or absence of intraparenchymal hemorrhage (IPH), which are large areas of hemorrhagic infarcts in the white matter. Whereas the size of the IVH predicts the possibility of developing post-IVH hydrocephalus, the presence of IPH indicates poor neurologic outcome.[48]

Post hemorrhagic ventricular dilatation is the most common long-term complication of PV-IVH. Hydrocephalus may develop without apparent evidence of increased cephalic size.[52] In all infants with IVH, with or without IPH, weekly cranial scans must be done. In addition, the occipital-frontal circumference of their head must be measured. If the circumference increases at a rate greater than 2 cm/week and signs of increased intracranial pressure appear, the diagnosis of posthemorrhagic hydrocephalus may be made. Repeated lumbar punctures and/or external ventricular drainage may be used repeatedly until the infant reaches a body weight of 2000 g when a ventriculo-peritoneal shunt may be placed. Following suitable ventricular drainage procedures reexpansion of the compressed brain parenchyma is likely to occur. If the ventricular scan shows only ventriculomegaly without evidence of hydrocephalus, no specific therapy is needed except for periodic evaluation of head circumference.[48] Although infants with small IVH or subependymal hemorrhage may be expected to have a normal neurologic outcome, those with large IVH or IPH will suffer long-term developmental problems.

ANEMIA OF PREMATURITY

In preterm neonates (with normal body weight for gestational age), the cord blood hemoglobin concentration is 17 G/dL.[53] This is close to the values found in term neonates. Hemoglobin concentration steadily declines in the first few weeks of life. The level may decrease to 7 G/dL in some neonates by the 8th week of extrauterine life. At birth, there is a significant amount of fetal hemoglobin in neonatal blood. The fetal hemoglobin will be gradually replaced by adult hemoglobin. This transition will depend on the actual post-conceptual age rather than on the postnatal age.[54] However, the actual change in the P_{50} (the Po_2 at which hemoglobin is 50% saturated) of the neonatal hemoglobin is influenced by the birth process, regardless of the gestational age at which birth occurs.

The affinity of neonatal blood for oxygen cannot be predicted relying only on the concentration of fetal hemoglobin[53] because of 2 to 3 diphosphoglyceraldehyde (2-3 DPG) assumes a greater role in regulating oxygen affinity at birth. During fetal life, the red cell concentration of 2-3 DPG increases with gestational age and at term its concentration in the neonatal RBC is close to that found in adult cells. During the first weeks of extrauterine life, the ability of fetal hemoglobin to interact with 2-3 DPG steadily increases. The P_{50} increases and tissue oxygen delivery improves. A 2 mm Hg increase in P_{50} may actually double oxygen delivery to tissues.[53]

Because of increased ability of adult hemoglobin to interact more avidly with 2-3 DPG, replacing fetal cells with adult cells improves oxygen delivery to fetal tissues. Consequently, blood reticulocyte counts and erythropoietin levels (which are the classical hallmarks of functionally significant anemia) are lower in infants who receive exchange transfusion with adult red cells. Since a right shifted curve lowers the mixed venous PO_2 ($P\bar{v}O_2$) oxygen uptake at the lungs will improve. This is particularly useful in infants who develop hypoxemia as a result of severe right to left shunting.[55] Decreasing levels of $P\bar{v}O_2$ are associated with increasing blood erythropoietin concentrations.[56]

In addition to the physiologic anemia described above, blood samples taken for routine laboratory measurements may cause anemia in the neonate. Feeding difficulties, dyspnea, tachypnea, tachycardia, and pallor are the classical signs of anemia in neonates. However, clinical signs alone do not predict the need for transfusion therapy. Many centers use the actual hemoglobin concentration as an index of the need for transfusion therapy. However, for a given hemoglobin level, the degree of functional impairment is widely variable from infant to infant. For instance, some premature infants may develop symptoms even at a hemoglobin concentration of 10.5 g/dL.[53,57]

Indices of oxygen delivery to tissues are advocated by some authorities.[53,57] The decreases in $P\bar{v}O_2$ seem to be a reliable predictor of the need for transfusion. The normal $P\bar{v}O_2$ is greater than 38 mm Hg. At a $P\bar{v}O_2$ of less than 30 mm Hg, most neonates will have abnormally high erythropoietin levels, signifying a clinically significant anemia. A hemoglobin concentration of 9G/dL is usually associated with a $P\bar{v}O_2$ of 30 mm Hg. Another useful index of oxygen delivery is to calculate the volume of available oxygen.[57] Available oxygen represents volume of oxygen released per 100 ml of blood. For deriving available oxygen, the hemoglobin concentration and P_{50} must be known. If P_{50} cannot be measured available oxygen is calculated from the Wardrop's equation.[57] The equation is based on the predictable decline in fetal hemoglobin concentration with increasing post-conceptual age (gestational age + postnatal age).[57]

$$\text{Available oxygen (ml/dL blood)} = [0.54 + (0.005 \times \text{postconceptual age in weeks})] \times \text{Hb (g/dL)}$$

The measured or calculated available oxygen may be used to predict the need for oxygen therapy especially in infants of a gestational age of less than 32 weeks. An available oxygen value of less than 7 ml/dL is usually associated with clinically significant anemia.[53]

NEONATAL POLYCYTHEMIA AND HYPERVISCOSITY

Neonatal polycythemia must be suspected whenever the venous hematocrit exceeds 65%. The capillary hematocrit may be 15% higher than the venous hematocrit, therefore they are not reliable.[58] Conditions that predispose to neonatal hyperviscosity include maternal diabetes, intrauterine growth retardation, perinatal asphyxia, intrauterine twin-twin transfusion, delayed cord clamping and Beckwith's syndrome (macrosomia, hypoglycemia, umbilical hernia, and macroglossia). Maternal diabetes causes polycythemia probably by elevating erythropoietin levels. Perinatal hypoxia may cause hyperviscosity by shifting blood from the placenta to the fetus and also by causing increased erythropoietin production. The clinical signs and symptoms are listed in Table 26–7. They mainly include cardiorespiratory distress, congestive heart failure, and central nervous system symptoms. The treatment is to perform exchange transfusion with crystalloid or commercially

Table 26–6.   Retinopathy of Prematurity

Change	Development	Description
Acute	Stage 1	Early peripheral vascularization.
Acute	Stage 2	Advanced peripheral vascularization. Dilated and tortuous blood vessels.
Acute	Stage 3	Vascularization of the vitreous humor. Traction on the vitreous.
Acute	Stage 4	Localized retinal detachment.
Acute	Stage 5	Total retinal detachment.
Cicatricial	Grade I	Peripheral scarring, Myopia.
Cicatricial	Grade II	Disc distortion, vision 20/40–20/200.
Cicatricial	Grade III	Temporal retinal fold traction; vision 20/200–5/200.
Cicatricial	Grade IV	Incomplete retinal fibrotic mass. Only finger counting possible.
Cicatricial	Grade V	Complete retinal mass: cataracts, glaucoma, phthisis. Only light perception possible.

available albumin solutions. Only symptomatic patients must be treated. The prognosis depends on the primary cause of hyperviscosity.

NECROTIZING ENTEROCOLITIS

Necrotizing enterocolitis (NEC) is one of the most serious complications of prematurity. The syndrome of NEC may start within 24 hours of birth or may be delayed for several days. In the majority of cases, risk factors such as perinatal asphyxia, hyaline membrane disease, umbilical vessel catheterization, polycythemia, and patent ductus arteriosus are present.[60] NEC occurs in relation to oral feedings in up to 95% of infants. Perinatal asphyxia is associated with NEC possibly because the blood is shunted away from the intestines during asphyxial insult. In a given institution, NEC usually occurs sporadically, but occasionally, it may reach a disturbingly high rate. The most commonly isolated bacterial pathogens are Escherichia coli, Klebsiella, Enterobacter, Pseudomonas, Salmonella, and Clostridia species. Coronavirus, rotavirus, and other enteroviruses have also been implicated.[60]

Abdominal distention and bloody stools are the common presenting symptoms. Sepsis, metabolic acidosis, and shock rapidly develop. Episodes of apnea and bradycardia often occur. In advanced cases, disseminated intravascular coagulation, intestinal perforation, and gangrene may develop. Radiographic examination of the abdomen shows distention, paralytic ileus, and

Table 26–7.   Clinical Picture of Polycythemia-Hyperviscosity Syndrome

Disorder	Symptoms
Plethora	
CNS symptoms	Jitteriness, irritability, lethargy, seizures, apnea.
Cardiorespiratory	Tachypnea, respiratory distress, congestive heart failure.
Gastrointestinal	Necrotizing enterocolitis, bloody diarrhea.
Renal	Acute renal failure.
Metabolic	Hypoglycemia, jaundice (increased cell destruction).

ascites. The specific radiographic signs of NEC include demonstration of linear streaks of gas in the intestinal wall (pneumatosis intestinalis) and gas in the intrahepatic portal vasculature.[60] Hydrogen gas is one of the major constituents of the intestinal gas.[61]

The treatment mainly consists of discontinuing oral feeding, supportive measures, broad-spectrum and antibiotic therapy, and maintaining fluid and electrolyte balance. Laparotomy is reserved for intestinal perforation or for removal of gangrenous bowel. Late sequelae include intestinal strictures, persistent melena and malabsorption syndrome, and septicemia.

INFANT APNEA

The possible relationship between infant apnea and sudden infant death syndrome (SIDS) has aroused a great deal of interest in this subject. Premature infants are prone to apneic episodes probably because of immaturity of the central nervous system. In addition the upper airway musculature of the premature neonates may have poor tone.[12] The tone in the genioglossus muscle is believed to be necessary for maintaining upper airway patency.[63] In addition, the chest wall of an infant is extremely compliant, making it difficult for him to maintain lung volume.

Apnea in an infant is defined as absence of respiratory activity lasting more than 15 seconds. When accompanied by a heart rate of less than 100 beats per minute, even shorter duration of apnea will place the infant in the apnea prone category. Apnea is not always related to sleep. In many instances, apnea is noted to occur within an hour before or after feeding.[62] When apnea occurs during sleep, it is more frequent during REM (deep) sleep than during quiet sleep.[64] Birth asphyxia, central nervous system anomalies, sepsis, and hypoglycemia may also increase the risk of infant apnea. A family history of sudden death of a sibling or history of sudden infant death syndrome in a twin are other risk factors.[62]

Infants who are at risk for apnea may be studied using a thermistor pneumocardiogram (TPC).[62] A thermistor probe is used to detect exhalation from the nares, while an impedance device records thoracic cage activity during respiration. Nasal exhalation can also be detected using a capnograph. Heart rate must also be recorded simultaneously. Based on the TPC findings the infant apnea may be classified into four types.

Obstructive Apnea. The apnea is caused by upper airway obstruction; the TPC will show an absent exhalation when the chest wall continues to move. Patients with obstructive apnea may also show a sudden decrease in the esophageal pH (measured by an indwelling pH electrode) due to a concomitant gastroesophageal reflux. The poor tone in the upper airway muscles probably leads to airway obstruction.

In Central Apnea. Both exhalation and thoracic cage motion cease, signifying lack of CNS activity.

With Mixed Apnea. Both central and obstructive apnea may occur in combination.

Periodic breathing is described as lasting less than 10 seconds, alternating with normal respiratory activity. At least three such cycles must be present for the diagnosis to be made. Although periodic breathing does not definitely predispose to SIDS, the risk may increase if apneic spells also coexist.

The use of home cardiorespiratory monitoring may be valuable in identifying infants at risk. In infants with central apnea, theophylline has been used to stimulate respiration.[62] Theophylline increases ventilatory response to inhaled CO_2 and improves efficiency of diaphragmatic contraction.[65] Caffeine citrate (10 to 20 mg/kg/dose, tid) has been used for this purpose.

REFERENCES

1. Avery ME, and Taeusch HW: Prematurity. *In* Schaffer's Diseases of the Newborn. 5th Edition. Philadelphia, WB Saunders, 1984.
2. Bowes WA: Delivery of the very low birth weight infant. Symposium on Difficult Labor and Delivery. Clin Perinatol 8:182, 1981.
3. Ruiz M, et al.: Early development of infants of birth weight less than 1000 g with reference to mechanical ventilation in the newborn period. Pediatrics 68:330, 1981.
4. Farrell P, and Avery ME: Hyaline membrane disease: State of the art. Am Rev Resp Dis 111:657, 1975.
5. Pritchard JA, et al.: The morphologic and functional development of the fetus. *In* Williams Obstetrics. 17th Edition. Norwalk, Appleton-Century-Crofts, 1985.
6. Stark AR, and Frantz ID: Respiratory Distress Syndrome. Pediatr Clin North Am 33:533, 1986.
7. Nunn JF: Applied Respiratory Physiology. 2nd Edition. Boston, Butterworths, 1977.
8. Langman CB, et al.: The diuretic phase of respiratory distress syndrome and its relationship to oxygenation. J Pediatr 98:462, 1981.
9. Heaf DP, et al.: Changes in pulmonary function during the diuretic phase of respiratory distress syndrome. J Pediatr 101:103, 1982.
10. Spitzer AR, Fox WW, and Delivoria-Papadopoulos M: Maximum diuresis–a factor in predicting recovery from respiratory distress syndrome and the development of bronchopulmonary dysplasia. J Pediatr 98:476, 1981.
11. Green TP, et al.: Diuresis and pulmonary function in premature infants with respiratory distress syndrome. J Pediatr 103:618, 1983.
12. Green TP, et al.: Furosemide promotes patent ductus arteriosus in premature infants with respiratory-distress syndrome. N Engl J Med 308:743, 1983.
13. Carlo WA, and Martin RJ: Principles of neonatal assisted ventilation. Pediatr Clin North Am 33:221, 1986.
14. Lough MD, Doershuk CF, and Stern RC: Pediatric Respiratory Therapy. 2nd Edition. Chicago, Year Book Medical Publishers, 1985.
15. Pollitzer MJ, et al.: Pancuronium during mechanical

ventilation speed recovery of lungs of infants with hyaline membrane disease. Lancet 1:346, 1981.

16. Finer NM, and Tomney PM: Controlled evaluation of muscle relaxation in the ventilated neonate. Pediatrics 67:641, 1981.

17. Perlman JM, et al.: Reduction in intraventricular hemorrhage by elimination of fluctuating cerebral blood-flow velocity in preterm infants with respiratory distress syndrome. N Engl J Med 312:1353, 1985.

18. Rutledge M, Hawkins E, and Langston C: Skeletal muscle atrophy induced in newborns by chronic pancuronium treatment. Pediatr Res 19:361A, 1985.

19. Spitzer AR, and Fox WW: The use and abuse of mechanical ventilation. In Hyaline Membrane Disease: (Pathogenesis and Pathophysiology.) (Edited by Stern L) New York, Grune & Stratton, 1984.

20. Fox WW, et al.: Tracheal extubation of the neonate at 2-3 cm H$_2$O continuous positive airway pressure. Pediatrics, 59:257, 1977.

21. Finer NN, et al.: Postextubation atelectasis: A retrospective study and a prospective controlled study. J Pediatr 94:110, 1979.

22. Carlo WA, et al.: Decrease in airway pressure during high-frequency jet ventilation in infants with respiratory distress syndrome. J Pediatr 104:101, 1984.

23. Enhorning G, et al.: Prevention of neonatal respiratory distress syndrome by tracheal instillation of surfactant: A randomized clinical trial. Pediatrics, 76:145, 1985.

24. Hallman M, et al.: Exogenous human surfactant for treatment of severe respiratory distress syndrome: A randomized prospective clinical trial. J Pediatr, 106:963, 1985.

25. Brown R, et al.: Bronchopulmonary dysplasia: Possible relationships to pulmonary edema. J Pediatr, 92:982, 1978.

26. Bell EF, et al.: Effect of fluid administration on the development of symptomatic patent ductus arteriosus and congestive heart failure in premature infants. N Engl J Med, 302:598, 1980.

27. Papile L, et al.: Relationship of intravenous sodium bicarbonate infusions and cerebral intraventricular hemorrhage. J Pediatr, 93:834, 1978.

28. Coastrino A, and Baumgart S: Modern fluid and electrolyte management of the critically ill premature infant. Ped Clin North Am 33:153, 1986.

29. Cassady G: Effect of caesarian section on neonatal body water spaces. N Engl J Med 285:887, 1971.

30. Aperia A, et al.: Postnatal development of renal function in pre-term and full-term infants. Acta Pediatr Scand, 70:183, 1981.

31. Sulyok E, et al.: Relationship between maturity, electrolyte balance, and the function of renin-angiotensin-aldersterone system in newborn infants. Biol Neonate, 36:60, 1979.

32. Sulyok F, et al.: Postnatal development of sodium handling in premature infants. J Pediatr, 95:787, 1979.

33. Baumgart, et al.: Radiant warmer power and body size as determinants of insensible water loss in the critically ill neonate. Pediatr Res, 15:1495, 1981.

34. Hammarlund K, et al.: Transepidermal water loss in newborn infants: VIII. Relation to gestational age and

postnatal age in appropriate and small for gestational age infants. Acta Paediatr. Scand, 72:721, 1983.

35. Baumgart S: Fluid and electrolyte therapy in the premature infant. In Workbook Exercises in Neonatology. (Edited by Burg F and Polin RA). Philadelphia, WB Saunders, 1983.

36. Fisher DA: Endocrine physiology. In The Physiology of the Newborn Infant. 4th Edition. (Edited by Smith CA and Nelson NM). Springfield, Illinois, Charles C. Thomas, 1976.

37. Gersony WM: Patient ductus arteriosus in the neonate. Pediatr Clin North Am 33(3):545, 1986.

38. Dudell GG, and Gersony WM: Patient ductus arteriosus in neonates with severe respiratory disease. J Pedatr 104(6):915, 1984.

39. Peckham GJ, et al.: Clinical course to 1 year of age in premature infants with patent ductus arteriosus: Results of a multicenter randomized trial of indomethacin. J Pediatr, 105(2):285, 1984.

40. Freed MD, et al.: Prostaglandin E$_1$ in infants with ductus arteriosus dependent congenital heart disease. Circulation, 64:899, 1981.

41. Avery MA, and Taeusch HW: Persistent fetal circulation. In Schaffer's Diseases of the Newborn. 5th Edition. Philadelphia, WB Saunders, 1984.

42. Bancalari E, and Gerhardt T: Bronchopulmonary dysplasia. Pediatr Clin North Am 33(1):1, 1986.

43. Melnick G, et al.: Normal pulmonary vascular resistance and left ventricular hypertrophy in young infants with bronchopulmonary dysplasia: An echocardiographic and pathologic study. Pediatrics, 66:589, 1980.

44. Winter PM, and Smith G: The toxicity of oxygen. Anesthesiology 37:210, 1975.

45. Roberts RJ: Pulmonary oxygen toxicity in the premature and full-term infant–Its relationship to the development and pathogenesis of respiratory distress syndrome and its complications. In Hyaline Membrane Disease. (Edited by Stern L) New York, Grune and Stratton, 1984.

46. Payne JW: Retinopathy of prematurity. In Schaffer's Diseases of the Newborn. (5th Edition). (Edited by Avery ME and Taeush HW). Philadelphia, WB Saunders, 1984.

47. Kinsey VE, et al.: Pa$_{O_2}$ levels and retrolental fibroplasia: A report of the cooperative study. Pediatrics 60:655, 1977.

48. Allan WC, and Volpe JJ: Periventricular-intraventricular hemorrhage. Pediatr Clin North Am 33:47, 1986.

49. Gilles FH, et al.: Fibrinolytic activity in the ganglionic eminence of the premature human brain. Biol Neonate, 18:426, 1971.

50. Goddard-Feingold J, and Michael LH: Cerebral blood flow and experimental intraventricular hemorrhage. Pediatr Res, 18:7, 1984.

51. Dubowitz LMS, et al.: Neurologic signs in neonatal intraventricular hemorrhage: A correlation with real-time ultrasound. J Pediatr 99:127, 1981.

52. Larroche JC: Post-hemorrhagic hydrocephalus in infancy: Anatomical study. Biol Neonate, 20:287, 1972.

53. Stockman JA: Anemia of prematurity: current concepts in the issue of when to transfuse. Pediatr Clin North Am 33(1):111, 1986.

54. Bard H: The postnatal decline of hemoglobin F synthesis

in normal full term infants. J Lab Clin Invest, 55:395, 1975.

55. Rossoff L, et al.: Changes in blood P$_{50}$. Effects on oxygen delivery when arterial hypoxemia is due to shunting. Chest, 77:142, 1980.

56. Stockman JA, et al.: Anemia of prematurity: Determinants of the erythropoietin response. J Pediatr, 105:786, 1984.

57. Wardrop CA, et al.: Nonphysiological anemia of prematurity. Arch Dis Child, 53:855, 1978.

58. Oh W, and Lind J: Venous and capillary hematocrit in newborn infants and placental transfusion. Acta Pediatr Scand, 55:38, 1966.

59. Oh W: Neonatal polycythemia and hyperviscosity. Pediatr Clin North Am, 33(3):523, 1986.

60. Walsh MC and Kliegman RM: Necrotizing Enterocolitis: Treatment Based on Staging Criteria. Pediatric Clin North Am 33:179, 1986.

61. Engel RR, et al.: Origin of mural gas in necrotizing enterocolitis. Pediatr Res, 7: 292, 1973.

62. Spitzer AR, and Fox WW: Infant apnea. Pediatr Clin North Am 33:561, 1986.

63. Brouillette RT, and Thach BT: Control of genioglossus inspiratory activity. J Appl Physiol 49:801, 1980.

64. Schulte FJ: Developmental aspects of neuronal control of breathing. *In* Human Growth: A Comprehensive Treatise: Developmental Biology; Prenatal Growth, Vol. 1. 2nd Edition. New York, Plenum Publishing, 1979.

65. Aubier M, et al.: Aminophylline improves diaphragmatic contractility. New Engl J Med 305:249, 1981.

27

NEONATAL EMERGENCIES

LIFE-THREATENING CONGENITAL ANOMALIES

The neonate who requires resuscitation for perinatal asphyxia may often have congenital anomalies that are either coincidental to or directly responsible for the asphyxia. Routine endotracheal ventilation alone will not guarantee a satisfactory outcome unless the coexisting anomaly is recognized and special precautions are instituted. A basic knowledge of these anomalies will enable the anesthesiologist to anticipate the problem and act accordingly. For instance, in an infant with tracheal agenesis, endotracheal intubation is almost impossible. One may take advantage of the possible coincidental occurrence of tracheoesophageal fistula, and intubate the esophagus with the hope of providing some pulmonary ventilation through the fistula.

The obstetric anesthesiologist is often needed to help in the management of deformed infants because not only is he skilled in airway management, but often he may be the only person available to attend to the baby. Some anomalies are readily noticeable and others are not. Some produce profound physiologic effects at birth, whereas others produce delayed manifestations. Table 27–1 gives a list of some congenital malformations that may be encountered in the neonate.

RESPIRATORY EMERGENCIES

DIAPHRAGMATIC HERNIA

The delivery room care of an infant born with congenital diaphragmatic hernia (CDH) is perhaps one of the most challenging clinical situations. Delay in recognition of the condition leads to considerable morbidity and mortality. The presence of maternal hydramnios may serve as a clue to the possibility of the neonate being born with CDH. The diaphragm develops from four components: the ventral, dorsal, lateral, and pleuroperitoneal components (Fig. 27–1).[1] The ventral component is formed from the septum transversum form the 3rd to the 5th week of gestation. Gradually extending dorsally, it envelopes the esophagus, inferior vena cava, and the aorta, and finally fuses by the 8th week with the foregut mesentery (the dorsal component). The lateral components of the diaphragm then develop from the muscles of the body wall. The pleuroperitoneal membranes finally fuse with the central membranous portion to complete the framework (Fig. 27–1). The diaphragmatic closure is complete by the 9th week of gestation.

During this period the esophagus develops and the midgut herniates into the umbilical coelom. The midgut then partially returns into the

Table 27–1.   Neonatal Emergencies

Category	Disorder	Incidence ratio
Respiratory emergencies	Diaphragmatic hernia.	1:5000
	Esophageal atresia (TE fistula).	1:3000
External tracheal compression	Cystic hygroma.	
	Vascular rings.	
	Lung cysts.	
	Lobar emphysema.	
Intrinsic anomaly of the airway lumen	Choanal atresia.	1:8,000
	Laryngeal web.	1:10,000
	Laryngo and tracheomalacia.	
	Congenital subglottic stenosis and subglottic hemangioma.	
	Laryngotracheoesophageal cleft.	
	Branchial arch syndromes.	
Cardiovascular emergencies	Transposition of the great arteries.	1:500
	Tetralogy of Fallot	1:5000
	Pulmonary stenosis.	1:14,000
	Pulmonary atresia.	1:14,000
	Tricuspid atresia.	1:18,000
	Ebstein's anomaly.	1:80,000
Gastrointestinal emergencies	Omphalocele.	1:5800
	Gastroschisis.	1:15,000

The incidence (when known) is indicated on the right.

abdominal cavity. If the return of the midgut occurs before the pleuroperitoneal membranes fuse with the central membranous portion of the developing diaphragm, the abdominal contents may enter the pleural cavity resulting in a diaphragmatic hernia. The lungs develop as a ventral bud from the foregut. The buds repeatedly divide to form the conducting airways and this process is complete by the 17th week of gestation. By the 24th week, the airways are completely differentiated with a well-established lumen. The alveolar development begins at 24 weeks and proceeds at a steady pace even postnatally. The presence of abdominal contents in

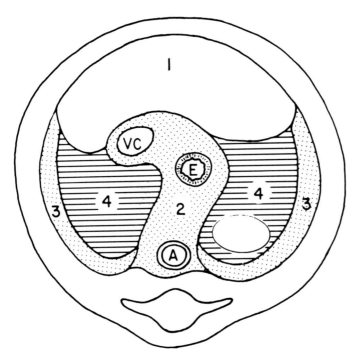

FIG. 27–1. Developmental components of the diaphragm. Components: (1) ventral component, derivative of septum transversum; (2) dorsal component, derivative of posterior mesentery; (3) lateral component, derivative of body wall; and (4) pleuroperitoneal canals. The encircled area to the right shows the approximate defect through which diaphragmatic hernia occurs. (From Cullen ML, Klein MD, and Philippart AI: Congenital diaphragmatic hernia. Surg Clin North Am., *65*:1115, 1985.)

the pleural cavity will hinder proper development of the airways and the alveoli. It is therefore not surprising that babies born with CHD also have hypoplastic lungs. The number and size of the alveoli and bronchi, together with the size of the pulmonary vascular bed are reduced.[2] The earlier the hernia occurs in gestation, the more severe the pulmonary hypoplasia is.

Almost all neonatal CDH occur through the left posterolateral surface of the diaphragm, which lies over part of the pleuroperitoneal membrane (Bochdalek hernia) (Fig. 27–1). Right-sided hernias are more common in older children. When herniation occurs early in gestation, the contents may not be enclosed in a sac (eventration). Bilateral hernias are usually fatal.

The advent of ultrasonography has made it possible to diagnose CDH before birth. The sonogram will reveal the presence of intestine in the chest of the neonate. In the majority of patients, hydramnios will also be detected. If CDH is diagnosed prenatally, the infant must be delivered in an institution with facilities for neonatal surgery.[3] The classical findings in CDH include cyanosis, dyspnea, rightward displacement of the apical impulse, scaphoid abdomen and diminished or absent breath sounds in the left hemithorax. Bowel sounds may also be heard in the side of the chest. Chest x-ray shows loops of bowel in the abdomen (Fig. 27–2). Infants born with CDH are particularly susceptible to group B streptococcal pneumonia. On occasions, the pneumonia may make its appearance before clinical or radiologic signs of CDH appear.[4]

Immediately after the diagnosis is made a No. 10 nasogastric tube must be placed in the stomach to avoid further distention of the intestines, which causes further herniation and respiratory embarrassment. The baby must be intubated and ventilated with small tidal volumes (60% of the expected normal) at a rapid rate. Large tidal volumes may increase the airway pressure leading to barotrauma of the lung. A pulse oximeter must be used for monitoring oxygen saturation in the delivery room. In addition, the umbilical artery may be cannulated for obtaining arterial blood samples. A Pa_{O_2} of less than 80 mm Hg, a Pa_{CO_2} of greater than 50 mm Hg, and a pH of 7 or less, predict poor outcome[1], as does hypercarbia that is unresponsive to rigorous ventila-

tion.[5] Babies who develop symptoms within the first 6 hours of life have increased mortality rate.[6]

The surgical correction of CDH is done through an abdominal incision. The hernia is reduced, the sac (if present) is excised, and the defect in the diaphram is closed. Prosthetic material may be used to close large defects the edges of which cannot be easily approximated. Too tight a closure of the abdominal wall may cause obstruction to the vena cava. To avoid this, blood pressure must be measured continuously when the surgeon tightens the abdominal stitches. A reduction in blood pressure or an increase in airway pressure usually signifies a tight closure.[1] A prosthetic membrane may also be used to bridge the gap in the abdominal wall.

Immediately following surgical repair, babies seem to improve (this period is nicknamed the honeymoon period) only to deteriorate rapidly. The neonatal circulation reverts back to fetal circulation because of intense pulmonary vasoconstriction. This leads to increased right-to-left shunting through the ductus arteriosus.[7] Tolazoline has been used to decrease pulmonary vasoconstriction.[8] The indications for using tolazoline are a postductal P_{O_2} less than 80 mm Hg at an F_{IO_2} of 1 and/or the difference between the pre and postductal P_{O_2} exceeds 25 mm Hg. The response to tolazoline therapy (1 to 2 mg/kg iv followed by an infusion at 1 to 4 mg/kg/hour) occurs within an hour. Lack of response usually indicates very poor outcome.[9] The mechanism of action of tolazoline is believed to be caused by its vasodilating property and to its ability to decrease the synthesis of thromboxane by the platelets.[10] Patients who do not respond to tolazoline therapy may require oxygenation with extracorporeal membrane oxygenator (ECMO). The experience with this method has been limited, but to date a 50% salvage rate has been achieved.[1] Disadvantages of ECMO include the need for total heparinization, the need to ligate the carotid artery, and an exorbitant cost.[1] High frequency ventilation has also been used.[11]

Another serious complication of CDH is the occurrence of major pulmonary barotrauma. Development of serious tension pneumothorax often results in the death of the neonate.[12] In the perioperative period, pneumothorax may develop on the ipsilateral or on the contralateral side. The development of pneumothorax on the normal side causes severe cardiorespiratory dis-

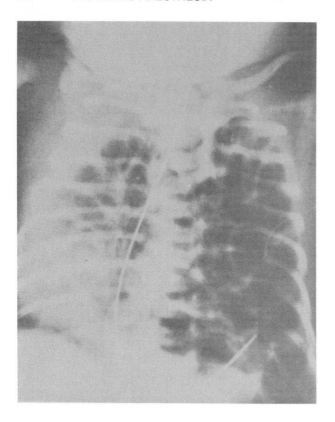

FIG. 27–2. Roentgenograph of CDH. Note the gas-filled loops of intestine in the left hemothorax. (From Todres ID, and Firestone S: Neonatal emergencies. *In* A Practice of Anesthesia for Infants and Children. (Edited by Ryan JF, et al.) New York, Grune and Stratton, 1986.)

tress.[12] The possibility of barotrauma must always be considered in a neonate when the infant's condition suddenly deteriorates. A needle thoracentesis may be performed to relieve tension and this often results in dramatic improvement (albeit temporary) in the patient's condition. Limiting airway pressure to less than 34 cm H_2O is likely to minimize this complication.[12]

ESOPHAGEAL ATRESIA (TRACHEOESOPHAGEAL FISTULA)

The trachea develops with the rest of the respiratory system as a diverticulum from the ventral wall of the foregut. The tracheoesophageal septum separates the developing trachea from the esophagus. The laryngotracheal tube grows much faster than the esophagus. If the esophageal growth is delayed, the rapidly elongating laryngotracheal tube will separate the esophagus into proximal and distal segments resulting in esophageal atresia (EA) and tracheoesophageal fistula (TEF).

In 90% of cases, esophageal atresia occurs in association with tracheoesophageal fistula (TEF); in other instances, it may also occur alone. In up to 85% of the cases, the upper

esophagus ends in a blind pouch with the fistula connecting the lower esophageal segment with the trachea.[13] The fistulous connection enters the trachea just above the carina (Fig. 27–3). Twenty percent of infants born with TEF will weigh under 2000 g at birth,[14] and one-third will also have an additional congenital malformation, the most common one being congenital heart disease. Musculoskeletal and anorectal malformations may also occur. Occasionally, TE fistula may occur in combination with VATER association (Vertebral anomalies, imperforate anus, tracheosophageal fistula, radial and renal dysplasia).[15]

Maternal polyhydramnios is often associated with EA because of the inability of the fetus to swallow the amniotic fluid. The presence of EA must be suspected in newborn infants who salivate excessively or develop frequent cyanotic spells. Simple suction usually causes a dramatic improvement in the patient's condition. Cyanotic spells, coughing, and choking during feeding are other classical symptoms of TE fistula. Occasionally, increased gastric distention following bag-ventilation during resuscitation may give a clue as to the presence of the condition. The presence of EA may be excluded by

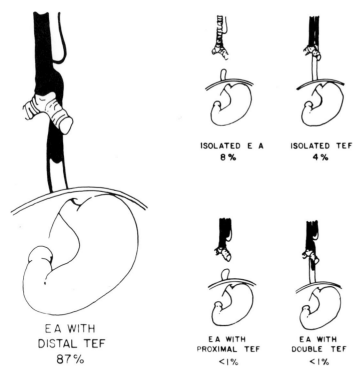

ISOLATED E A
8%

ISOLATED TEF
4%

E A WITH
DISTAL TEF
87%

E A WITH
PROXIMAL TEF
<1%

E A WITH
DOUBLE TEF
<1%

FIG. 27–3. The different types of tracheoesophageal fistula (TEF) with frequency of occurrence shown as percentage of the total number. EA = Esophageal atresia. (From Holder TM, and Ashcraft KW: Developments in the care of patients with esophageal atresia and tracheoesophageal fistula. Surg Clin North Am. 61:1051, 1981.)

passing a sufficiently rigid catheter into the stomach. If the catheter does not readily pass into the stomach, EA must be suspected. The diagnosis may be confirmed with a lateral radiograph of the neck, which will show the tip of the catheter present in the proximal esophageal pouch. A soft suction catheter should not be used for confirming esophageal patency because it may coil in the upper esophagus and thus give a false negative result.[16] Rarely, the catheter may pass into the trachea from where it may reach the stomach via the fistula. When this happens, the tonal quality of the infant's cry will change because of the presence of a foreign body between the vocal cords.

Injecting 0.5 ml of lipiodol through the catheter will provide a definitive diagnosis during radiographic examination[16] (Fig. 27–4A). One must avoid excessive volume of the contrast medium for fear that it may overflow into the larynx and cause respiratory distress (Fig. 27–4B). The contrast medium must be emptied as soon as the examination is finished.[16] When the radiograph reveals the presence of air in the abdomen, it indicates a fistula between the trachea and the lower esophagus (Fig. 27–4A). Total absence of abdominal air shadow in the radiograph is highly suggestive of a lack of communication between the trachea and esophagus (Fig. 27–4C).[13]

Immediate corrective surgery is necessary to prevent aspiration pneumonitis, which is associated with a 70% mortality rate. When the infant cries, the glottis is closed, thus forcing air into the stomach through the fistula. Gastric distention will not only interfere with diaphragmatic excursions but will lead to aspiration of gastric contents through the fistula. If the diagnosis is made in the delivery room, the infant must be intubated and the tip of the endotracheal tube placed distal to the opening of the fistula into the trachea. A similar placement of the endotracheal tube is recommended for administering anesthesia for the repair. In many centers, gastrostomy is routinely performed under local anesthesia to prevent the potential hazard of gaseous gastric distention. If a gastrostomy tube is available, it can be used to verify proper positioning of the endotracheal tube in the trachea. The outer end of the gastric tube is immersed in water and the endotracheal tube is positioned so that no air leak occurs during ventilation[17] (Fig 27–5). During anesthesia the anesthesiologist must repeatedly ascertain that the endotracheal tube has not inadvertently slipped into one of the bronchi. Alternately, the endotracheal tube may be passed into the bronchus and withdrawn slowly into the carina until breath sounds become equal.[18]

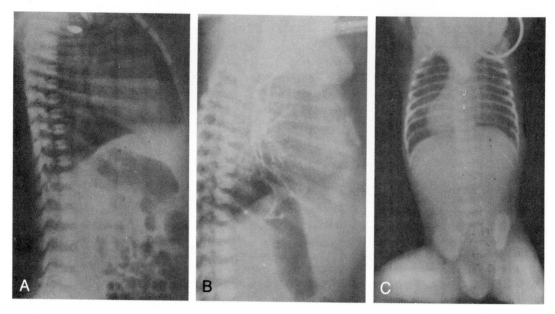

FIG. 27–4. Radiographic confirmation of TE fistula. (A) small amount of X-ray contrast medium has been placed in the upper segment of the esophagus. Also note the presence of gas in the abdomen. (B) The use of excessive amount of contrast medium has resulted in the overflow of the medium into the tracheo-bronchial tree. (C) Roentgenograph of a patient with esophageal atresia. Note the lack of gas in the abdomen signifying absence of communication between the trachea and the esophagus. (A and C From Martin LW, and Alexander F: Esophageal Atresia. Surg Clin North Am, *65*:1099, 1985.) (B From Ein SH, and Friedberg J: Esophageal atresia and tracheoesophageal fistula: Review and update. Otolaryngol Clin North Am, *14*:219, 1981.)

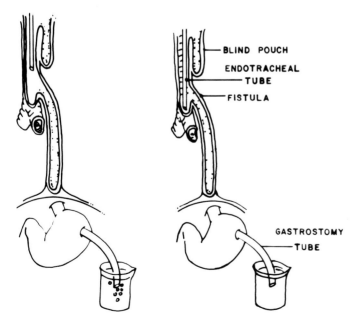

FIG. 27–5. Verifying proper placement of the endotracheal tube during anesthesia for tracheoesophageal (TE) fistula repair. The tip of the endotracheal tube must be distal to the opening of the fistula into the carina. If air bubbles are seen escaping from the tip of the gastrostomy tube, the endotracheal tube tip is probably located proximal to the fistulous opening. The tube must be advanced until leakage stops. Advancing the endotracheal tube into the bronchus must be avoided. (From Dierdorf SF, and Krishna G: Anesthetic management of neonatal surgical emergencies. Anesth Analg, *60*:204, 1981.)

Surgical correction of the anomaly as soon as possible is the only hope for survival of the infant. Aspiration pneumonia must be treated preoperatively with antibiotics. The stomach and the blind esophageal pouch must be free of secretions before surgery to prevent further aspiration. The surgical goal is to divide the fistula from the trachea and anastomose the two ends of the esophagus. If the two ends of the esophagus cannot be brought together for a primary anastomosis, a colon conduit may be performed when the baby is a year old. In premature babies (weight below 2000 g) some prefer to complete the definitive procedure in stages because of the complications associated with primary anastomosis (anastomosis leakage, massive atelectasis, recurrence of the fistula, esophageal stricture). The surgical correction is performed in the following three stages: Stage 1–a gastrostomy is performed soon after birth; Stage 2–the fistula is divided at one week of life; and Stage 3–esophageal anastomosis is performed when the baby's body weight reaches 3000 g. Gastrostomy feeding and/or parenteral nutrition is usually necessary before anastomosis can be successfully performed.[13]

Occasionally, tracheal agenesis may occur in combination with several components of VATER association. Polyhydramnios is usually present in the mothers. The babies will be cyanotic at birth without an audible cry. Tracheal intubation is usually not possible. However, the bag-mask ventilation may be possible because of the TE fistula. Ventilation through an esophageal tube or bag ventilation may be tried, if tracheal intubation fails.

EXTRINSIC TRACHEAL COMPRESSION

CYSTIC HYGROMA

A congenital cystic hygroma originates from the tracheal epithelial rests that are entrapped when the first and second branchial arches unite in the midline. Some cysts may be formed from the tuberculum impar of His, which contributes to the formation of the tongue and the floor of the mouth. Congenital cystic hygromas may attain large size and may produce dystocia or airway obstruction at birth (Fig. 27–6).[19] Endotracheal intubation may be difficult to perform. If orotracheal intubation cannot be accomplished, a blind nasal intubation or a tracheostomy may be needed.

In dire emergencies a 3.5 mm flexible bronchofiberscope may be passed into the trachea through the nose. A 3.5 mm bronchoscope has been used in infants weighing as little as 700 g.[20] The suction channel of the bronchoscope may be used to deliver manual jet ventilation (see Chapter 9). Since exhaled gases escape through the space between the bronchoscope and the tracheal wall, any obstruction to exhalation will rapidly result in barotrauma. Consequently, the following precautions must be taken during manual jet ventilation: (1) minimum possible driving pressure and tidal breaths must be used, (2) sufficient exhalation time must be allowed and (3) one must watch for signs of chest hyperinflation. The cystic hygroma may be diagnosed prenatally with the aid of ultrasound examination. If the hygroma is large enough to preclude vaginal delivery, a cesarean section may be performed. The anesthesiologist must be fully prepared to manage any possible neonatal airway obstruction.

VASCULAR RINGS

Six pairs of branchial arches develop between the third and fourth week of gestation.[21] Only the third, fourth, and sixth arches contribute to normally present vascular structures. There are several abnormalities associated with arch development. Only a few, however, produce respiratory obstruction; these include the following: a double aortic arch, a right arch with ligamentum arteriosum, an anomalous innominate or left common carotid artery, an aberrant subclavian artery, a pulmonary artery sling, and aneurysmal dilatation of the pulmonary artery. Stridor, starting a few days to a few weeks after birth, is the most common symptom of tracheal obstruction by a vascular ring. Occasionally, respiratory obstruction may be noticeable at birth. Hyperextension of the head usually lessens the degree of obstruction. A flexible fiberoptic bronchoscope may be used to locate the site of the obstruction. An attempt must be made to pass the tip of the endotracheal tube beyond the obstruction site.

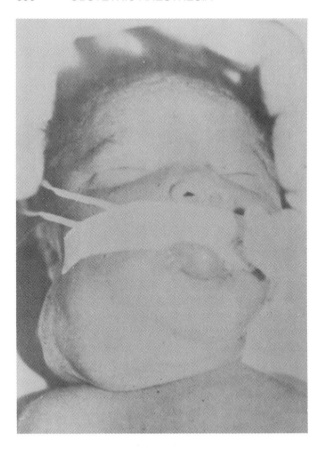

FIG. 27–6.   Cystic hygroma. (From Tepas JJ, Deen HG, McArtor R, and Southern TE: Giant cystic choristoma of the head and neck in a neonate: successful management of a life-threatening respiratory emergency. J Pediatr Surg, *17*:184, 1982.)

LARYNGEAL AND BRONCHIAL CYSTS

Occasionally, the trachea or the larynx may be compressed extramurally by cysts arising from the isolated rests of the respiratory epithelium.[21,22] The classic example is a bronchial cyst that may cause respiratory obstruction in the neonate. In many the onset of symptoms may be delayed for a few weeks. The laryngeal cyst is an atavistic remnant of the lateral air sacs found in apes. It may cause severe respiratory obstruction and stridor at birth. The airway must be quickly established with an endotracheal tube. If the size of the cyst precludes endotracheal intubation, needle aspiration of the cyst or a tracheostomy may be needed to establish the airway.

Bronchogenic cysts are cysts containing nonfunctioning pulmonary tissue. The cysts may attain enormous sizes and may cause respiratory obstruction at birth. The cyst may obstruct the trachea or the bronchus and is most commonly located in the superior mediastinum at the level of the carina. Immediate surgery is needed to relieve respiratory distress. Endotracheal intu-bation or the passing of a rigid bronchoscope through the trachea may be required to relieve tracheal compression in the neonatal period.

Congenital adenomatoid cystic malformation of the lung is associated with multiple cysts throughout the lung.[21] Some of these cysts grow rapidly and may cause rapid respiratory distress in the neonate.

CONGENITAL LOBAR EMPHYSEMA (FIG. 27–7)

This condition occurs more frequently in males than in females, and most commonly affects the left upper lobe. The cyst often enlarges because of air trapping, which leads to compression of functional lung tissue in both the normal and the affected sides.[21] Tachypnea, cyanosis, and acute respiratory distress may develop in the first few days of life or may be delayed for a few weeks. Severe cardiovascular compromise may occur because of obstruction of venous return to the heart.[18] Chest roentgenograph is usually diagnostic of the condition. The etiology of congenital lobar emphysema is not fully under-

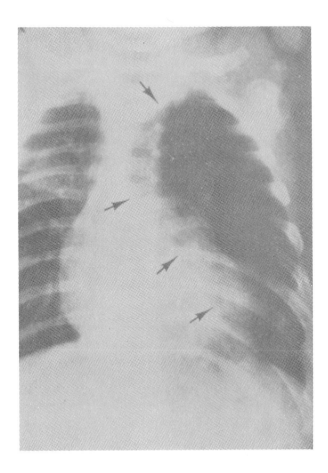

FIG. 27–7. Congenital lobar emphysema. Note the hyperlucent lung field. (From Todres ID, and Firestone S: Neonatal emergencies. *In* A Practice of Anesthesia for Infants and Children. (Edited by Ryan JF, et al.) New York, Grune and Stratton, 1986.)

stood and is believed to be caused by bronchial obstruction or failure of the static lung recoil during expiration. Respiratory distress in a newborn associated with hyperresonant lung fields should arouse suspicion as to the presence of this condition. Should endotracheal ventilation be necessary, low inflating pressures must be used. Aspiration of air with a needle must be avoided because it may lead to the rapid development of pneumothorax. Emergency surgical removal of the emphysematous lobe is the treatment of choice in infants who become symptomatic in the neonatal period. Bronchoscopy is usually performed before thoracotomy to detect a ball-valve type of mucus plugs. Aspiration of the mucus plug will occasionally lead to spontaneous regression of the air-filled cyst.[18,23]

INTRINSIC ANOMALY OF THE AIRWAY LUMEN

CHOANAL ATRESIA

Atresia of the airway between the nasal passage and the nasopharynx is called the choanal atresia. The obstruction is usually caused by a bony plate and rarely by a thin membrane.[24] It occurs in association with Treacher Collins syndrome, palatal anomalies, congenital heart disease, TE fistulas, and mental retardation.[24] Newborns are obligatory nose-breathers, thus nasal obstruction will usually lead to respiratory distress. The diagnosis must be suspected when the infant has marked chest retractions and attempts to breath through the mouth. The inability to pass a suction catheter through the nose or actual visualization of the obstruction with an otoscope introduced into the nose will confirm the diagnosis.[24] To relieve respiratory distress, an oral airway must be promptly inserted. Carbon dioxide laser has been used to remove choanal obstruction caused by a thin bony plate or by a membrane.[25] Thick bony obstruction must be excised with a rongeur.

LARYNGEAL WEB

Laryngeal webs obstruct the airway level of the true vocal cords. The web may cover a part or whole of the glottic chink. Incomplete recanalization of the developing laryngeal airway results in the web formation. Complete webs cause life-threatening emergency. Incomplete webs cause stridor. Direct laryngoscopy will immediately reveal the problem. An attempt must be made to rupture the web forcibly with an endotracheal tube bearing a stylet.[18] If this is not possible an emergency tracheostomy must be performed. A rigid bronchoscope may be used to maintain an airway temporarily until a treacheostomy can be performed.[22] Partial webs may be treated with excision through a rigid bronchoscope, or with repeated dilatation.[26]

LARYNGOMALACIA

This condition, which is also called simple congenital laryngeal stridor, is associated often with pes escavatum. The stridor, which is usually inspiratory, is only occasionally noticed at birth. The laryngeal framework is less rigid and the epiglottic folds are shorter than usual, which leads to collapse of the larynx during inspiration. In severe cases, suprasternal retractions may be noticeable.

TRACHEOMALACIA

The tracheal framework is less rigid than normal and the trachea collapses during inspiration. If respiratory distress is noticed at birth, the infant must be intubated with an endotracheal tube. The condition is self-limiting.

CONGENITAL SUBGLOTTIC STENOSIS–SUBGLOTTIC HEMANGIOMA

The stenosis is located 2 mm below the glottic chink. Cricoid cartilage may be deformed. The stridor is usually noticeable at birth. Treatment is tracheostomy in severe cases.[22] Occasionally, a subglottic hemangioma may produce the same picture as subglottic stenosis. The presence of stridor in an infant with other facial cutaneous hemangioma will point to the diagnosis.[27] Diagnosis may be made using a flexible fiberoptic bronchoscope. The lesion is usually soft and compressible.[22] An atraumatic endotracheal intubation may be performed to relieve the stridor. A tracheostomy may be needed in severe cases.[27] The lesions usually shrink as the child grows older.

LARYNGOTRACHEOESOPHAGEAL CLEFT

The malformation occurs as a result of failure of rostral development of the tracheoesophageal septum. A communicating cleft is thus established between the trachea and the esophagus. Choking, coughing, and cyanotic spells are frequent because of entry of saliva into the trachea, a problem that is likely to be exaggerated during feeding. Treatment consists of passing an endotracheal tube into the trachea. The endotracheal tube separates the two edges of the cleft (which are usually in contact with each other) and thus aids in detection of the condition during endoscopy.[22] A gastrostomy is performed for feeding and all oral feeds are discontinued. When the infant's condition is stabilized, reconstructive surgery must be performed.[22]

CONGENITAL CYANOTIC HEART DISEASE

Congenital cardiac anomalies constitute 10% of all malformations. Ventricular septal defect is probably the most common type of congenital heart disease. Whereas respiratory distress caused by pulmonary pathology is associated with flaring of the ala nasi, chest retractions and grunting, these signs are conspicuous by their absence when respiratory distress is caused by congenital heart disease. The only consistent respiratory sign in such infants is tachypnea (50 to 60 beats per minute). Tachycardia (150 to 200 beats per minute) and cyanosis are other signs of congenital heart disease. Although in many cases of congenital heart disease the symptoms may be delayed for a few days, some infants may become symptomatic soon after birth. In addition, certain conditions may cause intrauterine congestive heart failure. Consequently, the baby may need additional supportive measures at birth.[28]

Persistent cyanosis that does not respond to the usual measures should arouse a high degree of suspicion of cyanotic heart disease. The absence of murmur does not eliminate the diagnosis of heart disease because in many severe anomalies a murmur is not heard. A forceful murmur, if present may, however, alert the clinician as to the possibility of a cardiac anomaly. Measurements of arterial P_{O_2}, pH, and oxygen saturation (pulse oximetry) and a chest x-ray are useful in the diagnosis and management of serious cardiac anomalies.[28]

TRANSPOSITION OF THE GREAT ARTERIES

The aorta arises from the right ventricle and the pulmonary artery from the left ventricle. The pulmonary and the systemic circuits are arranged in parallel rather than in series with little or no admixture between the two circuits.[28] The fetus with this condition grows normally in utero because the hemodynamics of transposition is only slightly different from that of normal fetal circulation. However, soon after birth, the ductus arteriosus closes with the result that the admixture between the two circuits decreases leading to rapid deterioration of the neonate. Survival is possible only when bidirectional shunting occurs through the foramen ovale, which permits oxygenated blood to reach the aorta from the right ventricle and deoxygenated blood from the aorta to reach the lungs for oxygenation. The diagnosis is established by echocardiography.[29] The posterior vessel is identified at its origin from the left ventricle and is traced to its bifurcation into left and right branches. Cardiac catheterization will also confirm the diagnosis. Immediate therapeutic measures include correction of acidosis, improving oxygenation with endotracheal ventilation, and using prostaglandin E1 to open the ductus arteriosus. The use of PGE_1 for maintaining of ductal patency is discussed in Chapter 26. Atrail balloon septostomy may be attempted when the baby's condition is stabilized. Corrective surgery is performed at 6 months of age.

TETRALOGY OF FALLOT

Ventricular septal defect, pulmonary stenosis, right ventricular hypertrophy and the dextroposition of the aorta, which appears to override the interventricular septum causing the aorta to receive venous and arterial blood, are the four individual abnormalities that constitute the tetralogy of Fallot. The neonate born with this condition appears to be normally grown because there is little hemodynamic impairment while in utero. The severity of the clinical picture depends on the extent of the pulmonic stenosis. The important clinical findings include cyanosis, which may become evident as the ductus arter-

iosus begins to close. Because of shunt reversal, cyanosis may develop during crying. The infant is prone to tetralogy spells, which are characterized by attacks of dyspnea and severe cyanosis. The chest x-ray usually reveals a bloodless field and the echo cardiogram may show aortic overriding. Cardiac catheterization is needed to assess the degree of pulmonary stenosis.

The aorta is markedly dilated because it receives the output from both ventricles. In infants with severe pulmonic stenosis, collateral circulation through the bronchial vessels may maintain arterial oxyhemoglobin saturation at 75%. Prostaglandin E_1 infusion may be tried to maintain ductal patency (see Chapter 26). Creation of Blalock-Taussig shunt between the subclavian and pulmonary arteries may be considered once the infant is stabilized.

PULMONARY STENOSIS

The pulmonic orifice is narrowed and the right ventricle may be either normal sized or slightly hypoplastic. If the pulmonic stenosis occurs later in gestation, the right ventricle may be of normal size.[30] The left ventricle may be hypertrophic, because in fetal life, the stiffened right ventricle causes diversion of the right atrial flow to the left heart through the foramen ovale. Correction of hypoxia with endotracheal ventilation and correction of acidosis with bicarbonate may reduce pulmonary vascular resistance. Severe cases of hypoxia may require PGE_1 therapy to maintain ductal patency. In severe cases, emergency pulmonary valvotomy may be needed.

PULMONARY ATRESIA

In pulmonary atresia, the pulmonic valve is represented by a membrane and the right ventricle is hypoplastic. The tortuous ductus arteriosus maintains pulmonary blood flow for a few hours after birth after which it closes. The condition of the neonate markedly deteriorates, leading to hypoxia and acidosis. The right atrium and left ventricle are hypertrophic and these changes are noticeable both in the EKG and echocardiogram. In the initial phases of stabilization, endotracheal ventilation must be instituted. Acidosis must be corrected. Infusion of PGE_1 may be necessary to improve ductal blood flow (see Chapter 26 for details). If arterial saturation remains below 60% despite these maneuvers, a vascular shunt must be placed between the systemic and pulmonary circulation.

TRICUSPID ATRESIA

The tricuspid valve fails to develop with the result that the left ventricle maintains pulmonary blood flow through a large ventricle septal defect. The deoxygenated blood from the right side reaches the left side through the foramen ovale. Other anomalies, such as pulmonic stenosis or atresia may coexist.[31] The great arteries may be normally situated or may be transposed. In infants with marked pulmonic stenosis, cyanosis appears soon after birth. As long as the fetal shunts remain open, the arterial oxygenation is fair. Once they start closing, the condition of the neonate rapidly deteriorates. The echocardiogram may reveal the absence of the tricuspid valve and the presence of a hypertrophic left ventricle and a dilated aorta. Appropriate oxygen therapy, treatment of acidosis, and PGE_1 infusion may be needed during the stabilization period. Palliative Blalock shunting between pulmonary and systemic arteries may be considered in severe cases.

EBSTEIN'S ANOMALY

A part of the tricuspid valve is attached to the right ventricular wall instead of to the septum resulting in an enlarged right atrium. (See Chapter 12 for more details). The atrioventricular orifice is stenotic and often regurgitant. The remainder of the right ventricle may be small. The condition is associated with multiple cardiac defects. The pulmonary blood flow is usually reduced. The condition may cause cardiac failure in the unborn neonate. Cardiac failure may also develop soon after birth.

A pansystolic murmur of tricuspid regurgitation may be heard. The EKG may show Wolff-Parkinson-White syndrome and evidence of right atrial hypertrophy (see Chapter 16). Right atrial enlargement and diminished pulmonary vascularity may be noticeable in the chest x-ray. Of all congenital cardiac defects, Ebstein's anomaly is perhaps associated with the largest heart size in chest roentgenograms. Since the pulmonary vascular resistance decreases during the first few weeks of life, infants may often show a marked improvement. Infants with severe hypoxia may respond to PGE_1 therapy. Only palliative surgical shunting procedures are available for treating this condition.

TRUNCUS ARTERIOSUS

The single arterial trunk, which arises from the base of the heart, supplies the pulmonary, systemic, and coronary blood vessels. There is only minimal cyanosis at birth but the left ventricle, which is overworked from birth, soon begins to fail. Consequently, the cardiac failure often develops in the first week of life. The treatment consists of digitalis preparations and diuretics, and pulmonary artery bonding to reduce pulmonary blood flow.[28]

TOTAL ANOMALOUS PULMONARY VENOUS RETURN

The pulmonary veins do not open into the left atrium; instead, they open into the right atrium, innominate vein, portal vein, ductus venosus, azygos, or superior vena cava. The right ventricle is enlarged.[28] Pulmonary blood flow increases leading to pulmonary edema. Cyanosis is often present. Echocardiography is useful in detecting the presence of anomalous communication of the pulmonary veins. The recommended treatment is surgery.

GASTROINTESTINAL ANOMALIES

OMPHALOCELE

During early development, the midgut usually herniates into the umbilical cord, but soon returns to the abdominal cavity leaving a defect. By the 10th week of gestation, both rectus muscles close the defect. If the closure does not happen, omphalocele develops (Fig. 27–8). Occasionally, the sac covering the intestine ruptures, which results in eventeration of the intestine. The omphalocele may contain one or many of the abdominal organs including liver, spleen, stomach, uterus, and ovaries. Infants born with omphalocele have other coexisting anomalies, such as congenital heart disease, trisomy syndromes, and diaphragmatic hernia. Oc-

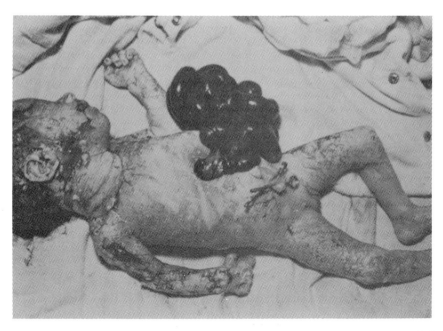

FIG. 27–8. Omphalocele. (From Martin LW, and Torres AM: Omphalocele and gastroschisis. Surg Clin North Am, 65:1235, 1985.)

casionally, omphalocele may be a manifestation of Beckwith syndrome (macroglossia, omphalocele, and hypoglycemia) or pentalogy of Cantrell (omphalocele, diaphragmatic hernia, intracardiac defects, and in exteme cases, bifid sternum and ectopia cardis).[32] The absence of the xiphoid process is usually suggestive of the presence of the pentalogy. Duodenal obstruction or midgut volvulus may necessitate further surgery in the neonatal period.

Immediate care of the neonate born with omphalocele includes the treating of hypoglycemia (in cases of Beckwith syndrome), and the establishing of adequate ventilation when a coexisting diaphragmatic hernia, macroglossia, or congenital heart disease causes respiratory distress. The intestines must be covered with wet towels to minimize evaporative water loss. The definitive treatment of omphalocele is surgical repair. Reducing a large omphalocele into the tight abdominal cavity may cause respiratory and cardiovascular embarrassment. Large omphaloceles are reduced gradually over a period of a week, thus allowing the abdominal wall to stretch. During this time, the omphalocele is protected by sewing a silastic silo around it.

GASTROSCHISIS

Gastroschisis is the name given to the defect in the abdominal wall that is remote from the umbilicus and is separated from it by a stretch of skin (Fig. 27–9). The contents of the hernial sac are variable, as they are in the case of omphalocele. Unlike omphalocele, however, gastroschisis occurs more frequently in premature infants and is not associated with many congenital malformations, particularly cardiac defects.[33] The lack of congenital malformations probably accounts for the lower mortality rate in patients with gastroschisis compared to those born with omphalocele. However, the incidence of bowel atresia is more common with gastroschisis.[33] The recommended form of treatment is surgery. Larger defects may require a staged correction.

MALFORMATIONS OF THE UPPER AIRWAY

Occasionally, airway obstruction may develop in neonates born with distorted upper airway because of branchial arch defects. These conditions include mandibulofacial dysostosis (Treacher Collins syndrome) and Pierre Robin syndrome. The Treacher Collins syndrome includes the following abnormalities: micrognathia, receding chin, and glossoptosis). The condition rarely produces cyanotic spells. The Pierre Robin triad, which includes microgna-

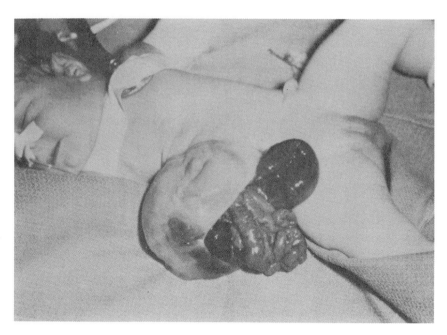

FIG. 27–9.   Gastroschisis. Note that a segment of normal skin intervenes between the umbilicus and the herniated bowel. (From Martin LW, and Torres AM: Omphalocele and gastroschisis. Surg Clin North Am, 65:1235, 1985.)

thia, glossoptosis, and cleft palate often results in cyanotic spells and sternal retractions. Intubation of the trachea is difficult in patients with micrognathia. Blind nasal intubation has been successfully performed by placing the infant in the prone position with the head hyperextended.[34]

REFERENCES

1. Cullen ML, Klein MD, and Philippart AI: Congenital diaphragmatic hernia. Surg Clin North Am, 65:1115, 1985.
2. Levin DL: Morphologic analysis of the pulmonary vasculature in congenital left-sided diaphragmatic hernia. J Pediatr Surg, 92:805, 1978.
3. Adzick NS, Harrison MR, and Glick PL: Diaphragmatic hernia in the fetus: Prenatal diagnosis and outcome in 94 cases. J Pediatr Surg, (In press).
4. Banagale RC, and Watters JH: Delayed right-sided diaphragmatic hernia. Surg Clin N Am, 61:1023, 1981.
5. Bohn DJ, et al.: The relationship between Pa_{CO_2} and ventilation parameters in predicting survival in congenital diaphragmatic hernia. J Pediatr Surg, 19:666, 1984.
6. Harrison MR, and De Lorimier AA: Congenital diaphragmatic hernia. Surg Clin North Am, 61:1023, 1981.
7. Dibbons AW, and Weiner ES: Mortality from neonatal diaphragmatic hernia. J Pediatr Surg, 9:653, 1976.
8. Ein SH, et al.: The pharmacological treatment of newborn diaphragmatic hernia: A two year evaluation. J Pediatr Surg, 15:384, 1980.
9. Bloss RS, Aranda JV, and Beardmore HE: Vasodilator response and prediction of survival in congenital diaphragmatic hernia. J Pediatr Surg, 16:118, 1981.
10. Ford WDA, James MJ, and Walsh JA: Congenital diaphragmatic hernia: association between pulmonary vascular resistance and plasma thromboxane concentrations. Arch Dis Child, 59:143, 1984.
11. Karl SR, Ballantine TVN, and Snider MT: High frequency ventilation at rates of 375-1800 cycles per minute in four neonates with congenital diaphragmatic hernia. J Pediatr Surg 18:822, 1983.
12. Gibson C, and Fonkalsrud EW: Iatrogenic pneumothorax and mortality in congenital diaphragmatic hernia. J Pediatr Surg,18:555, 1983.
13. Martin LW, and Alexander F: Esophageal atresia. Surg Clin North Am, 65:1099, 1985.
14. Hicks LM, and Mansfield PB: Esophageal atresia and tracheoesophageal fistula. J Thorac Cardiovasc Surg, 81:358, 1981.
15. Milstein JM, Lau M, and Bickers RG: Tracheal agenesis in infants with VATER association. Am J Dis Child 139:77, 1985.
16. Ein SH, and Friedberg J: Esophageal atresia and tracheoesophageal fistula: Review and update. Otolaryngol Clin North Am, 14:219, 1981.
17. Dierdorf SF, and Krishna G: Anesthetic Management of neonatal surgical emergencies. Anesth Analg, 60:204, 1981.
18. Todres ID, and Firestone S: Neonatal emergencies. In A Practice of Anesthesia for Infants and Children. (Edited by Ryan JF, et al.) New York, Grune and Stratton, 1986.
19. Tepas JJ, Deen HG, McArtor R, and Southern TE:

Giant cystic choristoma of the head and neck in a neonate: Successful management of a life-threatening respiratory emergency. J Pediatr Surg, *17*:184, 1982.

20. Wood RE: Spelunking in the pediatric airways: Explorations with the flexible fiberoptic bronchoscope. Pediatr Clin North Am, *31*:785, 1984.

21. Deluca FG, and Wesselhoeft CW: Surgically treatable causes of neonatal respiratory distress. *In* Diagnosis and Management of Respiratory Disorders in the Newborn. (Edited by Stern L.) California, Addison-Wesley Publishing, 1983.

22. Richardson MA, and Cotton RT: Anatomic abnormalities of the pediatric airway. Pediatr Clin North Am., *31*:821, 1984.

23. Avery ME, and Taeusch HW: Air leak and air trapping. *In* Schaffer's Diseases of the Newborn (Fifth Edition). Philadelphia, W.B. Saunders, 1984.

24. Avery ME, and Taeusch HW: Nasal obstructions. *In* Schaffer's Diseases of the Newborn (Fifth Edition). Philadelphia, W.B. Saunders, 1984.

25. Healy G, et al.: Management of choanal atresia with the carbon dioxide laser. Ann Otol Rhinol Laryngol, *87*:658, 1978.

26. Avery ME, and Taeusch HW: Stridors in the newborn.

In Schaffer's Diseases of the Newborn (Fifth Edition). Philadelphia, W.B. Saunders, 1984.

27. Lee MH, Ramanathan S, Chalon J, and Turndorf H: Subglottic hemangioma. Anesthesiology *45*:459, 1976.

28. Freed MD: Congenital cardiac malformations. *In* Schaffer's Diseases of the Newborn (Fifth Edition). (Edited by Avery ME, and Taeusch HW). Philadelphia, W.B. Saunders, 1984.

29. Aziz KU, et al.: M-mode echocardiographic assessment of D-transposition of the great arteries and associated defects. Pediatr Cardiol, *2*:11, 1982.

30. Rudolph AM: Congenital diseases of the Heart. Chicago, Year Book Medical Publishers, 1974.

31. Dick M, Fyler DC, and Nadas AS: Tricuspid atresia: Clinical course in 101 patients. Am J Cardiol, *36*:327, 1975.

32. Martin LW, and Torres AM: Omphalocele and Gastroschisis. Surg Clin North Am, *65*:1235, 1985.

33. Mayer T, Black R, Matlak ME, and Johnson DG: Gastroschisis and Omphalocele: An eight-year review. Ann Surg, *192*:783, 1980.

34. Populaire C, Lundi JN, and Souron R: Elective tracheal intubation in the prone position for a neonate with Pierre Robin syndrome. Anesthesiology, *62*:214, 1985.

INDEX

Page numbers set in *italics* indicate figures; numbers followed by "t" indicate tables.